D0706910

Paramedic Care: Principles & Practice

Fifth Edition

Volume 5

Special Considerations and Operations

BRYAN E. BLEDSOE, DO, FACEP, FAAEM, EMT-P
Professor of Emergency Medicine
University of Nevada, Las Vegas School of Medicine
University of Nevada, Reno School of Medicine
Attending Emergency Physician
University Medical Center of Southern Nevada
Medical Director, MedicWest Ambulance
Las Vegas, Nevada

RICHARD A. CHERRY, MS, EMT-P
Director of Training
Northern Onondaga Volunteer Ambulance
Liverpool, New York

LEGACY AUTHOR

ROBERT S. PORTER

Pearson

330 Hudson Street, NY, NY 10013

Publisher: Julie Levin Alexander
Publisher's Assistant: Sarah Henrich
Editor: Sladjana Repic Bruno
Editorial Assistant: Lisa Narine
Development Editor: Sandra Breuer
Copyeditor: Deborah Wenger
Director, Publishing Operations: Paul DeLuca
Team Lead, Program Management: Melissa Bashe
Team Lead, Project Management: Cynthia Zonneveld
Manufacturing Buyer: Maura Zaldivar-Garcia
Art Director: Mary Siener
Cover and Interior Designer: Mary Siener
Managing Photography Editor: Michal Heron
Vice President of Sales & Marketing: David Gesell
Vice President, Director of Marketing: Margaret Waples
Senior Field Marketing Manager: Brian Hoehl
Marketing Assistant: Amy Pfund
Senior Producer: Amy Peltier
Media Producer and Project Manager: Lisa Rinaldi
Full-Service Project Manager: iEnergizer Aptara®, Ltd.
Composition: iEnergizer Aptara®, Ltd.
Printer/Binder: LSC Communications
Cover Printer: LSC Communications
Cover Image: ollo/Getty Images, Rudi Von Briel/Getty Images

Notice

The author and the publisher of this book have taken care to make certain that the information given is correct and compatible with the standards generally accepted at the time of publication. Nevertheless, as new information becomes available, changes in treatment and in the use of equipment and procedures become necessary. The reader is advised to carefully consult the instruction and information material included in each piece of equipment or device before administration. Students are warned that the use of any techniques must be authorized by their medical advisor, where appropriate, in accordance with local laws and regulations. The publisher disclaims any liability, loss, injury, or damage incurred as a consequence, directly or indirectly, of the use and application of any of the contents of this book.

Copyright © 2017, 2013, 2009, 2006 by Pearson Education, Inc. All rights reserved. Manufactured in the United States of America. This publication is protected by Copyright, and permission should be obtained from the publisher prior to any prohibited reproduction, storage in a retrieval system, or transmission in any form by any means, electronic, mechanical, photocopying, recording, or likewise. To obtain permission(s) to use material from this work, please submit a written request to Pearson Education, Inc., Permission Department, 221 River Street, Hoboken, New Jersey 07030, or you may fax your request to 201-236-3290.

Library of Congress Cataloging-in-Publication Data

Names: Bledsoe, Bryan E., author. | Cherry, Richard A., author. | Porter, Robert S., author.
Title: Paramedic care : principles & practice | Bryan E. Bledsoe, Richard A. Cherry, Robert S. Porter.
Description: Fifth edition. | Boston : Pearson Education, Inc., 2016- | Includes bibliographical references and index.
Identifiers: LCCN 2016009904 | ISBN 9780134449753 (pbk. : alk. paper) | ISBN 0134449754 (pbk. : alk. paper)
Subjects: | MESH: Emergencies | Emergency Medical Services | Emergency Medical Technicians
Classification: LCC RC86.7 | NLM WB 105 | DDC 616.02/5—dc23 LC record available at http://lccn.loc.gov/2016009904

4 17

Pearson

ISBN 10: 0-13-444975-4
ISBN 13: 978-0-13-444975-3

This text is respectfully dedicated to all EMS personnel
who have made the ultimate sacrifice. Their memory
and good deeds will forever be in our thoughts and prayers.

BEB, RAC

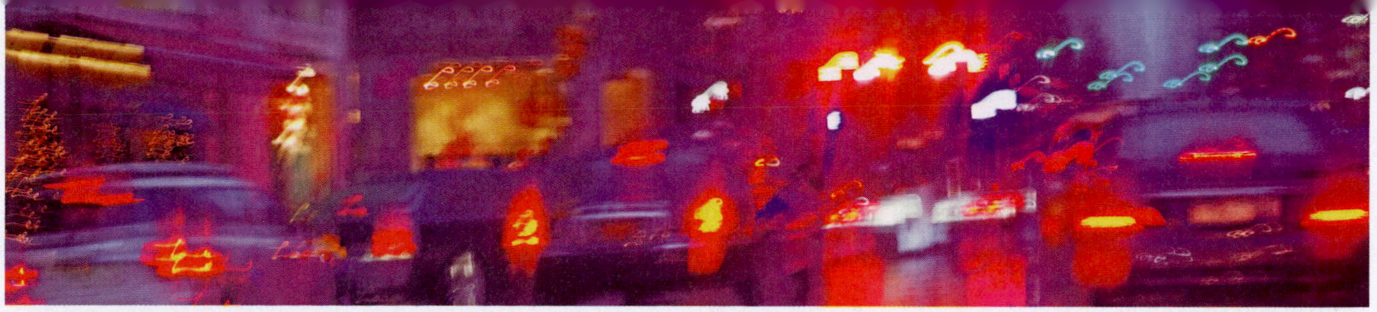

Contents

Preface to Volume 5 xi
Acknowledgments xiv
About the Authors xvi

1 Gynecology 1

Introduction 3
Anatomy and Physiology 3
  Female Reproductive Organs 3
  The Menstrual Cycle 6
Assessment of the Gynecologic Patient 8
  History 8
  Physical Exam 10
Management of Gynecologic Emergencies 10
Specific Gynecologic Emergencies 11
  Medical Gynecologic Emergencies 11
  Traumatic Gynecologic Emergencies 13

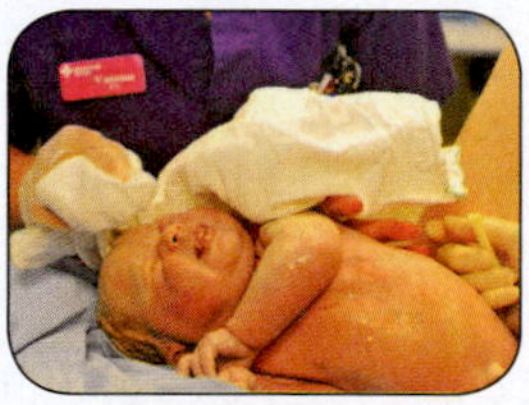

2 Obstetrics 18

Introduction 19
The Prenatal Period 19
  Anatomy and Physiology of the Obstetric Patient 19
General Assessment of the Obstetric Patient 25
  Primary Assessment 25
  History 25
  Physical Examination 27
General Management of the Obstetric Patient 28
Complications of Pregnancy 28
  Trauma 28
  Medical Conditions 29
  Medical Complications of Pregnancy 32
The Puerperium 36
  Labor 36
  Management of a Patient in Labor 37
  Field Delivery 38
  Neonatal Care 40
  Abnormal Delivery Situations 42
  Other Delivery Complications 44
  Maternal Complications of Labor and Delivery 45
  Cardiac Arrest in Pregnancy 47

3 Neonatology 53

Introduction 54
General Pathophysiology, Assessment, and Management 55
  Epidemiology 55
  Pathophysiology 55
  Assessment 59
  Treatment 62
The Distressed Newborn 63
  Resuscitation 64
  Maternal Narcotic Use 69
  Neonatal Transport 70
Specific Neonatal Situations 70
  Meconium-Stained Amniotic Fluid 70
  Apnea 71
  Diaphragmatic Hernia 71
  Bradycardia 71
  Prematurity 72
  Respiratory Distress/Cyanosis 72
  Hypovolemia 73
  Seizures 73
  Fever 73
  Hypothermia 74
  Hypoglycemia 74
  Vomiting 75
  Diarrhea 75
  Common Birth Injuries 75
  Cardiac Resuscitation, Postresuscitation, and Stabilization 76

4 Pediatrics 79

Introduction 81
Role of Paramedics in Pediatric Care 81
  Continuing Education and Training 81
  Improved Health Care and Injury Prevention 81
  Advanced Life Support Skills in Pediatrics 82

General Approach to Pediatric Emergencies 82
Communication and Psychological Support 82
Responding to Patient Needs 82
Responding to Parents or Caregivers 83
Growth and Development 83
Newborns (First Hours after Birth) 83
Neonates (Birth to 1 Month) 83
Infants (Ages 1 to 5 Months) 84
Infants (Ages 6 Months to 1 Year) 84
Toddlers (Ages 1 to 3 Years) 84
Preschoolers (Ages 3 to 5 Years) 85
School-Age Children (Ages 6 to 12 Years) 85
Adolescents (Ages 13 to 18 Years) 86
Anatomy and Physiology 86
Head 86
Airway 86
Chest and Lungs 87
Abdomen 89
Extremities 89
Skin and Body Surface Area 89
Respiratory System 89
Cardiovascular System 89
Nervous System 89
Metabolic Differences 89
General Approach to Pediatric Assessment 90
Basic Considerations 90
Scene Size-Up 90
Primary Assessment 91
Secondary Assessment 95
Reassessment 99
General Management of Pediatric Patients 99
Basic Airway Management 99
Advanced Airway and Ventilatory Management 104
Circulation 109
C-Spine Stabilization 113
Transport Guidelines 113
Specific Medical Emergencies 116
Infections 116
Respiratory Emergencies 116
Specific Respiratory Emergencies 118
Shock (Hypoperfusion) 123
Neurologic Emergencies 129
Gastrointestinal Emergencies 130
Metabolic Emergencies 131
Poisoning and Toxic Exposure 133
Trauma Emergencies 134
Mechanisms of Injury 134
Special Considerations 136
Specific Injuries 138
Sudden Infant Death Syndrome 140
Apparent Life-Threatening Event 141
Child Abuse and Neglect 141
Perpetrators of Abuse or Neglect 141
Types of Abuse 141
Assessment of the Potentially Abused or Neglected Child 142
Management of the Potentially Abused or Neglected Child 143
Resources for Abuse and Neglect 143
Infants and Children with Special Needs 143
Common Home Care Devices 143
General Assessment and Management Practices 145
Multiple-Casualty Incidents Involving Children 146
Using the JumpSTART System 146

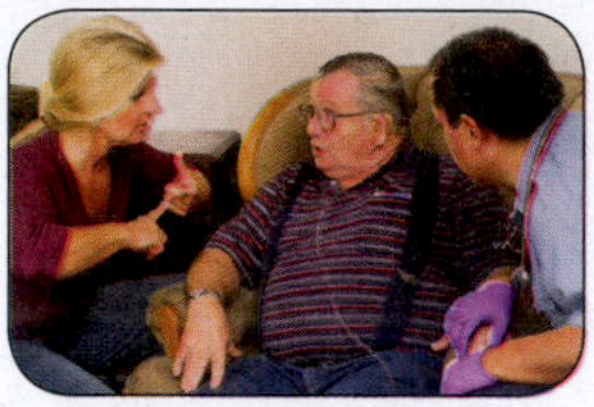

5 Geriatrics 151

Introduction 153
Epidemiology and Demographics 154
Population Characteristics 154
Societal Issues 154
Financing and Resources for Health Care 157
General Pathophysiology, Assessment, and Management 159
Pathophysiology of the Elderly Patient 160
Assessment Considerations 163
Management Considerations 166
System Pathophysiology in the Elderly 167
Respiratory System 168
Cardiovascular System 169
Nervous System 169
Endocrine System 170
Gastrointestinal System 170
Thermoregulatory System 170
Integumentary System 170
Musculoskeletal System 171
Renal System 171
Genitourinary System 171
Immune System 171
Hematologic System 172
Common Medical Problems in the Elderly 172
Pulmonary/Respiratory Disorders 172
Cardiovascular Disorders 175
Neurologic Disorders 178
Metabolic and Endocrine Disorders 181
Gastrointestinal Disorders 182
Skin Disorders 183
Musculoskeletal Disorders 184
Renal Disorders 186
Urinary Disorders 186
Environmental Emergencies 186
Toxicologic Emergencies 187

Substance Abuse 191
Behavioral/Psychological Disorder 192
Trauma in the Elderly Patient 193
Contributing Factors 193
General Assessment 193
General Management 194
Specific Injuries 195

6 Abuse, Neglect, and Assault 199

Introduction 200
Partner Abuse 201
Reasons for Not Reporting Abuse 201
Identification of Partner Abuse 201
Characteristics of Partner Abusers 201
Characteristics of Abused Partners 202
Approaching the Abused Patient 202
Elder Abuse 203
Identification of Elder Abuse 203
Theories about Domestic Elder Abuse 203
Characteristics of Abused Elders 203
Characteristics of Elder Abusers 204
Child Abuse 204
Characteristics of Child Abusers 204
Characteristics of Abused Children 204
Identification of the Abused Child 205
Recording and Reporting Child Abuse 207
Sexual Assault 207
Characteristics of Victims of Sexual Assault/Rape 207
Characteristics of Sexual Assailants 208
Date Rape Drugs 208
EMS Responsibilities 209
Human Trafficking 209
Hate Crimes 211

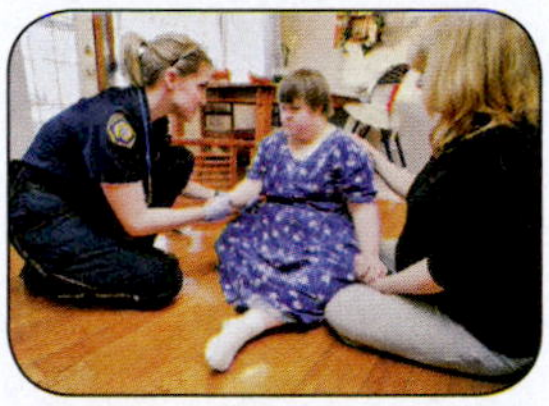

7 The Challenged Patient 214

Introduction 215
Physical Challenges 216
Hearing Impairment 216
Visual Impairments 217
Speech Impairments 218
Obesity 219
Paralysis 221
Mental Challenges and Emotional Impairments 221
Developmental Disabilities 221
Accommodations for Developmental Disabilities 222
Down Syndrome 222
Fetal Alcohol Syndrome 223
Pathological Challenges 223
Arthritis 223
Cancer 223
Cerebral Palsy 224
Cystic Fibrosis (Mucoviscidosis) 225
Multiple Sclerosis 225
Muscular Dystrophy 225
Poliomyelitis 226
Previous Head Injuries 226
Spina Bifida 227
Myasthenia Gravis 227
Other Challenges 227
Culturally Diverse Patients 227
Terminally Ill Patients 228
Patients with Communicable Diseases 228
Patients with Financial Challenges 228

8 Acute Interventions for the Chronic Care Patient 231

Introduction 233
Epidemiology of Home Care 233
Patients Receiving Home Care 233
ALS Response to Home Care Patients 234
General System Pathophysiology, Assessment, and Management 239
Assessment 239
Transport and Management Treatment Plan 242
Specific Acute Home Health Situations 242
Respiratory Disorders 242
Vascular Access Devices 250
Cardiac Conditions 251
GI/GU Crisis 252
Acute Infections 254
Maternal and Newborn Care 255
Hospice and Comfort Care 256

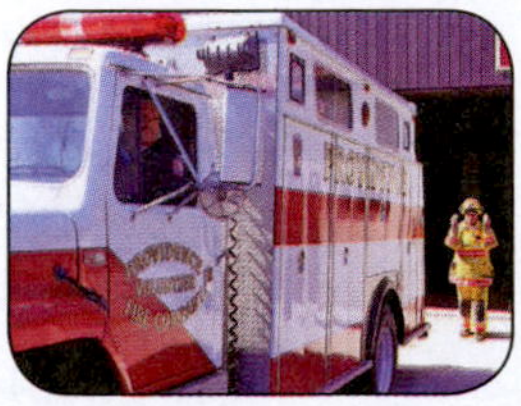

9 Ground Ambulance Operations 260

Introduction 261
Ambulance Standards 261
Ambulance Design 261
Medical Equipment Standards 262
Additional Guidelines 261
Checking Ambulances 263
Ambulance Deployment and Staffing 264
Traffic Congestion 265
Operational Staffing 265

Safe Ambulance Operations 265
Educating Providers 266
Reducing Ambulance Collisions 266
Standard Operating Procedures 267
The Due Regard Standard 267
Lights and Siren: A False Sense of Security 268
Escorts and Multiple-Vehicle Responses 269
Parking and Loading the Ambulance 269
The Deadly Intersection 269

10 Air Medical Operations 274

Introduction 275
History 277
Aircraft 278
Fixed-Wing Aircraft 278
Rotor-Wing Aircraft 279
Role in EMS 281
Uses 281
Limitations 284
Staffing 285
Controversies 285
Scene Operations 286
Initial Information 286
Landing Zone 286
Helicopter Approach 287
Patient Handoff 288
Aircraft Loading 289
Aircraft Departure 289

11 Multiple-Casualty Incidents and Incident Management 293

Introduction 295
Origins of Emergency Incident Management 297
Regulations and Standards 297
A Uniform, Flexible System 298
Command 299
Establishing Command 299
Incident Size-Up 299
Singular versus Unified Command 300
Identifying a Staging Area 301
Incident Communications 301
Resource Utilization 301
Command Procedures 302
Termination of Command 303
Support of Incident Command 303
Command Staff 303
Finance/Administration 304
Logistics 304
Operations 305
Planning/Intelligence 305
Division of Operations Functions 305
Branches 305
Units 305
Sectors 305
Functional Groups within an EMS Branch 305
Triage 306
Morgue 313
Treatment 313
On-Scene Physicians 314
Staging 314
Transport Unit 315
Extrication/Rescue Unit 315
Rehabilitation (Rehab) Unit 315
Communications 316
Disaster Management 316
Mitigation 317
Planning 317
Response 317
Recovery 317
Meeting The Challenge of Multiple-Casualty Incidents 317
Common Problems 317
Preplanning, Drills, and Critiques 318
Disaster Mental Health Services 318

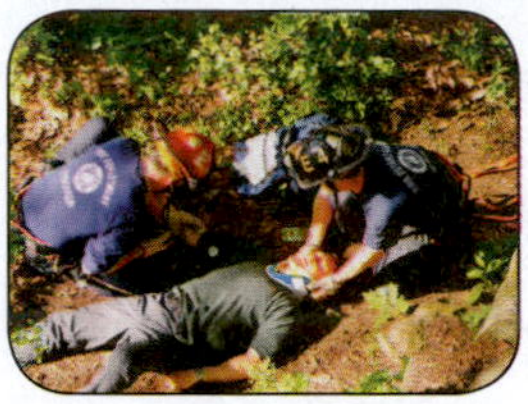

12 Rescue Awareness and Operations 322

Introduction 323
Role of The Paramedic 324
Protective Equipment 325
Rescuer Protection 325
Patient Protection 326
Safety Procedures 327
Rescue SOPs 327
Crew Assignments 327
Preplanning 327
Rescue Operations 328
Phase 1: Arrival and Size-Up 328
Phase 2: Hazard Control 329
Phase 3: Patient Access 329
Phase 4: Medical Treatment 330
Phase 5: Disentanglement 331
Phase 6: Patient Packaging 332
Phase 7: Removal/Transport 332
Surface Water Rescues 333
General Background 333
Moving Water 334
Flat Water 337
Hazardous Atmosphere Rescues 340
Confined-Space Hazards 340
Cave-Ins and Structural Collapses 342

Highway Operations and Vehicle Rescues 342
Hazards in Highway Operations 342
Auto Anatomy 344
Rescue Strategies 345
Hazardous Terrain Rescues 346
Types of Hazardous Terrain 347
Patient Access in Hazardous Terrain 347
Patient Packaging for Rough Terrain 348
Patient Removal from Hazardous Terrain 349
Extended Care Assessment and Environmental Issues 350

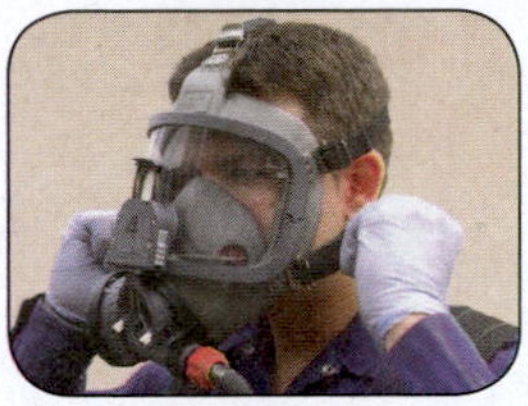

13 Hazardous Materials 354

Introduction 356
Role of the Paramedic 356
Requirements and Standards 357
Levels of Training 357
Incident Size-Up 357
ICS and Hazmat Emergencies 357
Incident Awareness 358
Recognition of Hazards 359
Identification of Substances 361
Hazardous Materials Zones 364
Specialized Terminology 364
Terms for Medical Hazmat Operations 364
Toxicologic Terms 365
Contamination and Toxicology Review 365
Types of Contamination 367
Routes of Exposure 367
Cycles and Actions of Poisons 367
Treatment of Common Exposures 367
Approaches to Decontamination 369
Methods of Decontamination 369
Decontamination Decision Making 370
Field Decontamination 371
Hazmat Protection Equipment 372
Medical Monitoring and Rehabilitation 373
Entry Readiness 373
Post-Exit Rehab 373
Heat Stress Factors 374
Importance of Practice 374

14 Crime Scene Awareness 377

Introduction 378
Approach to the Scene 379
Possible Scenarios 379
Specific Dangerous Scenes 381
Highway Encounters 381
Violent Street Incidents 382
Drug-Related Crimes 383
Clandestine Drug Laboratories 383
Domestic Violence 384
Tactical Considerations 384
Safety Tactics 385
Situational Awareness 386
Tactical Patient Care 387
EMS at Crime Scenes 388
EMS and Police Operations 388
Preserving Evidence 389

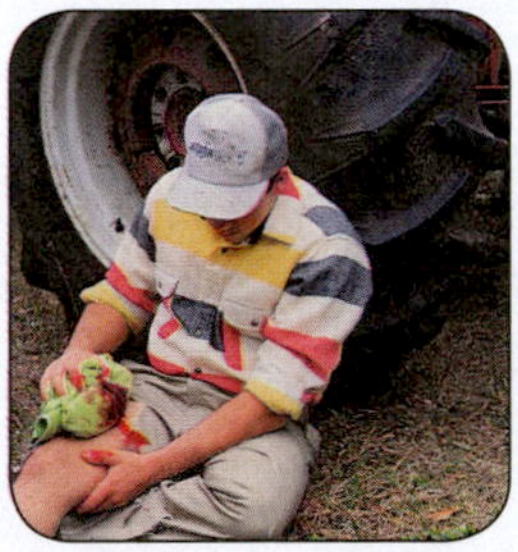

15 Rural EMS 393

Introduction 395
Practicing Rural EMS 395
Special Problems 395
Creative Problem Solving 397
Typical Rural EMS Situations and Decisions 398
The Distance Factor 398
Agricultural Emergencies 399
Recreational Emergencies 405

16 Responding to Terrorist Acts 409

Introduction 410
Explosive Agents 411
Nuclear Detonation 412
Nuclear Incident Response 413
Radioactive Contamination 413
Chemical Agents 413
Nerve Agents 414
Vesicants (Blistering Agents) 415
Pulmonary Agents 415
Biotoxins 415
Incapacitating Agents 416
Other Hazardous Chemicals 416
Recognition of a Chemical Agent Release 416
Management of a Chemical Agent Release 416
Biological Agents 417
Pneumonia-Like Agents 418
Encephalitis-Like Agents 418

Other Biological Agents 419
Protection against Biological Agent Transmission 419
Mass Shootings 420
General Considerations Regarding Terrorist Attacks 420
Scene Safety 420
Recognizing a Terrorist Attack 420
Responding to a Terrorist Attack 421
Precautions on Bloodborne Pathogens and Infectious Diseases 423
Suggested Responses to "You Make the Call" 425
Answers to Review Questions 431
Glossary 433
Index 443

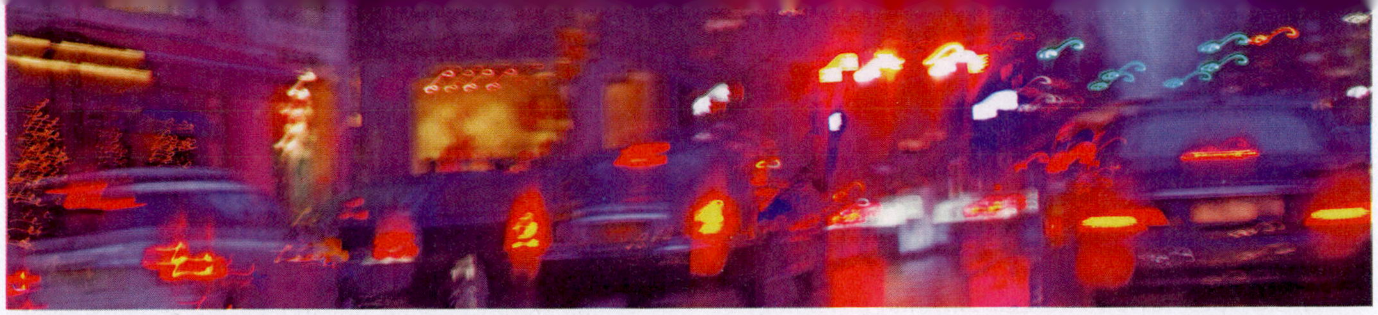

Preface to Volume 5

Today's paramedics are professional health care clinicians and practitioners of emergency field medicine. The present paramedic curriculum provides both a broad-based medical education and a specific intensive training program designed to prepare paramedics to perform their traditional role as providers of emergency field medicine. The curriculum also provides a broad foundation in anatomy and physiology, patient assessment, pathophysiology of disease, and pharmacology that allows paramedics to expand their roles in the health care industry. The five-volume ***Paramedic Care: Principles & Practice*** and, in particular, *Volume 5, Special Considerations and Operations,* reflect these broad and specific purposes.

This volume provides paramedic students with information they need about special populations and paramedic operations.. The first eight chapters discuss medical emergencies involving special patient populations: gynecology, obstetrics, neonatology, pediatrics, geriatrics, abused/neglected/assaulted patients, patients with special challenges, and patients who require chronic care. The next eight chapters examine special circumstances that the paramedic may face at any time, including multiple-casualty incidents, rescue operations, hazardous materials, crime scenes, rural practice, and terrorist incidents.

Overview of the Chapters … and What's New in the 5th Edition?

CHAPTER 1 Gynecology is devoted to the recognition and treatment of emergencies arising from the female reproductive system. The chapter provides an overview of female reproductive anatomy and physiology. This is followed by a discussion of common gynecologic emergencies.

CHAPTER 2 Obstetrics pertains to both normal delivery of a baby in the prehospital setting and various abnormal conditions and emergencies that may occur in association with childbearing. Following a review of the anatomic and physiologic changes that occur with pregnancy, the chapter addresses emergencies that may arise before, during, or after childbirth.

New in the 5th Edition: A detailed section, **cardiac arrest in pregnancy**, which includes information on estimating gestational age, chest compressions, aortocaval compression, defibrillation, airway management, use of emergency drugs, and transport destinations for the pregnant cardiac arrest patient.

CHAPTER 3 Neonatology introduces the paramedic student to the specialized world of neonates. The neonate is a child less than one month of age. These patients have very different problems, and their treatment must be modified to accommodate their size, anatomy, and physiology. This chapter presents a detailed discussion of neonatology with a special emphasis on neonatal resuscitation in the field setting.

New in the 5th Edition: The chapter, particularly the sections on treatment and resuscitation of the newly born baby, has been extensively updated to reflect the 2015 American Heart Association guidelines.

CHAPTER 4 Pediatrics presents a detailed discussion of pediatric emergencies. Children are not "small adults." They have special needs and must be approached and treated differently from adults. This chapter provides an overview of the common and uncommon pediatric emergencies encountered in prehospital care, with special emphasis on recognition and treatment. Specialized pediatric assessment techniques and emergency procedures are presented in detail.

New in the 5th edition: comparative outcomes of pediatric **endotracheal intubation vs. BVM ventilation**; use of **lidocaine** in pediatric advanced life support; updated instructions for pediatric **spinal stabilization**; use of **nebulized epinephrine in management of croup**; **infant nasal suctioning to relieve respiratory arrest**; a **pneumonia vaccine** now available for children; and dehydration and accidental ingestion of diabetic medications as possible **causes of hypoglycemia in nondiabetic children**.

CHAPTER 5 Geriatrics is a detailed presentation of emergencies involving elderly patients. The elderly are the fastest-growing group in our society. A significant number of EMS calls involve elderly patients. This chapter reviews the anatomy and physiology of aging. It then presents a detailed discussion of the assessment and treatment of emergencies commonly seen in the elderly.

New in the 5th edition: discussion of **new anticoagulant medications** (in addition to warfarin) that may be prescribed for the patient: dabigatran (Pradaxa), rivaroxaban (Xarelto), and apixaban (Eliquis).

CHAPTER 6 Abuse, Neglect, and Assault presents a timely discussion of the needs of victims of abuse, neglect, or assault. This chapter provides important information that will aid the paramedic in detecting abusive or otherwise dangerous situations. EMS personnel are often the first, and occasionally the only, health care personnel to encounter the victim of abuse, neglect, or assault. Therefore, it is essential that abusive situations be recognized early and the appropriate personnel and authorities notified.

New in the 5th edition: A major new section on **human trafficking**.

CHAPTER 7 The Challenged Patient addresses patients with special physical, mental, or cultural needs. Paramedics must be familiar with techniques for successful assessment and treatment of these patients. Because a medical emergency can be an extremely frightening event for the challenged patient, the paramedic must be skilled in strategies that reduce stress for these special patients.

CHAPTER 8 Acute Interventions for the Chronic Care Patient offers an important discussion of the role of EMS personnel in treating home care patients and patients with chronic medical conditions. With declining hospital revenues, more and more patients are being cared for at home—either by family members or by home care personnel. Paramedics are often summoned when a home care patient deteriorates or otherwise suffers a medical or trauma emergency. It is essential that prehospital personnel have a fundamental understanding of home health care as well as a basic knowledge of the medical devices and technology routinely used in home care. This chapter details the paramedic's role in assessing, treating, and managing home care patients.

CHAPTER 9 Ground Ambulance Operations discusses the special world of EMS ambulance operations, in which patient care begins long before the call is received. The paramedic is responsible for keeping the ambulance and medical equipment in a constant state of readiness. In addition, the paramedic must understand the various EMS system operations to be able to act appropriately.

CHAPTER 10 Air Medical Operations looks at the use of aircraft for emergency patient transport. Both rotor-wing and fixed-wing aircraft have become vital assets in the emergent transport of seriously ill or injured patients from the scene or between health care facilities, as well as bringing specialty teams to remote locations. Aircraft are also essential for organ transport, search and rescue missions, and disaster assistance. Air medical transport should be considered a medical procedure with benefits and risks that must be weighed against each other. Like any other asset or tool, air medical transport must be used responsibly and EMS providers must be familiar with their capabilities and protocols.

New in the 5th edition: FAA terminology change: **the term "helicopter EMS (HEMS)" replaced with the term "helicopter air ambulance (HAA)."**

CHAPTER 11 Multiple-Casualty Incidents and Incident Management provides an overview of situations that can result in multiple-casualty incidents. The chapter then presents a detailed discussion of the National Incident Management System (NIMS)—a system developed and mandated by the U.S. Department of Homeland Security for managing resources at the scene of a multiple-casualty incident, particularly at scenes involving many ambulances and multiple agencies. Paramedics must intimately understand the workings of the Incident Management System and apply them in daily operations.

CHAPTER 12 Rescue Awareness and Operations presents a comprehensive discussion of rescue operations. The level of EMS involvement with rescue operations varies significantly. In many EMS systems, paramedics are responsible for rescue operations. In others, paramedics are primarily responsible for patient care, whereas rescue operations are carried out by specially trained and equipped rescue teams. Regardless, the modern paramedic must have a thorough understanding of rescue operations, with an emphasis on scene safety.

CHAPTER 13 Hazardous Materials recognizes that more and more emergency scenes involve hazardous materials (hazmat). Although most hazardous materials scenes are handled by specialized hazmat teams, paramedics are often responsible for recognizing a hazmat incident, for activating the proper response and resources, and, of course, for patient care during the incident. Because the hazardous materials scene can be extremely dangerous, the paramedic must have a fundamental understanding of various hazardous materials and of hazmat operations.

CHAPTER 14 Crime Scene Awareness details the importance of protecting the crime scene. EMS personnel are often the first to arrive at a crime scene. Although their principal responsibilities are personal safety and patient care, they should take great effort to avoid disturbing important aspects of the crime scene. This chapter provides an overview of crime scene operations essential for effective paramedic functioning at the scene.

New in the 5th edition: a new section on **situational awareness.**

CHAPTER 15 Rural EMS provides an overview that enhances awareness of the special challenges, such as distance, faced by rural EMS personnel and the creative problem solving necessary to provide high-quality care to those who live or pursue recreation in rural or wilderness areas.

CHAPTER 16 Responding to Terrorist Acts discusses the types of agents likely to be used in terrorist attacks (conventional explosives, nuclear devices, chemical agents, and biological agents) with emphasis on the strategies paramedics need to ensure scene safety and the skills necessary to recognize and respond to a terrorist attack.

New in the 5th edition: A brief discussion of **mass shootings** as terrorist acts.

Acknowledgments

Chapter Contributors

We wish to acknowledge the remarkable talents of the following people who contributed to this five volume series. Individually, they worked with extraordinary commitment. Together, they form a team of highly dedicated professionals who have upheld the highest standards of EMS instruction.

Paul Ganss, MS, NRP (Volume 1, Chapter 2)
Michael F. O'Keefe (Volume 1, Chapter 5)
Wes Ogilvie, MPA, JD, LP (Volume 1, Chapter 7)
Kevin McGinnis, MPS, EMT-P (Volume 1, Chapter 9)
Jeff Brosious, EMT-P (Volume 1, Chapter 10)
W.E. Gandy, JD, NREMT-P (Volume 1, Chapter 15)
Darren Braude, MD, MPH, FACEP (Volume 1, Chapter 15)
Joseph R. Lauro, MD, EMT-P (Volume 2, Chapter 6)
Brad Buck, NRP, CCEMT-P (Volume 3, Chapter 10)
Andrew Schmidt, DO, MPH (Volume 4, Chapter 10)
Justin Sempsrott, MD (Volume 4, Chapter 10)
David Nelson, MD, FAAP, FAAEM (Volume 5, Chapter 4)
Mike Abernethy, MD, FAAEM (Volume 5, Chapter 10)
Ryan J. Wubben, MD, FAAEM (Volume 5, Chapter 10)
Louis Molino, NREMT-I (Volume 5, Chapter 11)
Dale M. Carrison, DO, FACEP, FACOEP (Volume 5, Chapter 14)
Dan Limmer, AS, NRP (Volume 5, Chapter 14)
Deborah J. McCoy-Freeman, BS, RN, NREMTP (Volume 5, Chapter 15)

BEB, RAC

Instructor Reviewers

The reviewers of *Paramedic Care: Principles & Practice, Fourth Edition, Volume 5* have provided many excellent suggestions and ideas for improving the text. The quality of the reviews has been outstanding, and the reviews have been a major aid in the preparation and revision of the manuscript. The assistance provided by these EMS experts is deeply appreciated.

Fifth Edition

Michael Smith, MS, Educator, Kilgore College, Longview, TX

Edward Lee, A.A.S., BS, Ed.S., NRP, CCEMT-P, EMT Paramedic Program Coordinator, Trident Technical College, Summerville, SC

Ryan Batenhorst, BA, NRP, EMS-I, Program Director, Paramedic Program, Southeast Community College, Milford, NE

Brett Peine, BS, NRP, Director, Southern State University, Joplin, MO

Fourth Edition

John L. Beckman, AA, BS
FF/EMT-P I/C
Addison Fire Protection District
Technology Center of DuPage
Addison, IL

Bryon Bellinger, NREMT-P, BA, RN
Lead Instructor Paramedic Specialist Program
Indian Hills Community College
Ottumwa, IA

Brian Bird, AS, EMS
Firefighter/Paramedic
Santa Fe Fire Department
Santa Fe, NM

L. Kelly Kirk, III, AAS, BS, EMT-P
Director of Distance Education, Paramedic
Randolph Co. Community College/Davidson County EMS
Asheboro, NC/Lexington, NC

Gregory M. Reardon, BS, NREMT-P
Paramedic, Adjunct Faculty Cecil College/Maryland Fire and Rescue Institute
Baltimore Washington International Airport Fire and Rescue Department
Baltimore, MD

Billy Respass, NCEMT-P
EMS Programs Instructor
Beaufort County Community College
Washington, NC

Mike Smertka, EMT-P
Assistant EMS Instructor
Graduate Student of Medicine/Medical University of Silesia
Katowice, Poland

Kelly Weller, MA, RN, LP, EMS-C
EMS Program Director
Lone Star College-Montgomery
Conroe, TX

We also wish to express appreciation to the following EMS professionals who reviewed the third edition of Paramedic Care: Principles & Practice. Their suggestions and perspectives helped to make this program a successful teaching tool.

Mike Dymes, NREMT-P
EMS Program Director
Durham Technical Community College
Durham, NC

Ginger K. Floyd, BA, NREMT-P
Assistant Professor
Austin Community College EMS Professions
Austin, TX

Darren P. Lacroix, AAS, EMT-P
Del Mar College
Emergency Medical Service Professions
Corpus Christi, TX

Greg Mullen, MS, NREMT-P
National EMS Academy
Lafayette, LA

Deborah L. Petty, BS, EMT-P I/C
Training Officer
St. Charles County Ambulance District
St. Peters, MO

B. Jeanine Riner, MHSA, BS, RRT, NREMT-P
GA Office of EMS and Trauma
Atlanta, GA

Aaron Weitzman, BS, NREMT-P
Lieutenant (ret.)
Faculty, Emergency Medical Services
Baltimore City Community College
Baltimore, MD

Brian J. Wilson, BA, NREMT-P
Education Director
Texas Tech School of Medicine
El Paso, TX

Photo Acknowledgments

All photographs not credited adjacent to the photograph or in the photo credit section below were photographed on assignment for Brady/Prentice Hall/Pearson Education.

Organizations

We wish to thank the following organizations for their assistance in creating the photo program for this project:

Michael J. Grant, President & CEO
Ambitrans Medical Transport, Inc., Punta Gorda, FL

Alan J. Skavroneck, Vice-President & COO
Ambitrans Medical Transport, Inc.

Debbie Harrington, BS, NREMT, Director
Community Relations, Ambitrans Medical Transport, Inc.

Companies

The following companies assisted in our photo program by donating EMS products to use in our photo shoots:

Persys Medical. NIO and BIG interosseous

Pyng Medical. FAST interosseous

Teleflex Corp. LMAs

Photo Coordinators/ Technical Advisors

Thanks to the following for valuable assistance directing the medical accuracy of the shoots and coordinating models, props, and locations for our photos:

Skippi Farley, EMT-P

Rodney VanOrsdol, FF/EMT-P

Photographers who have contributed to this project

Michael Gallitelli, Michal Heron, Kevin Link and Richard Logan

Photographer for the Fifth edition

Maria Lyle/Maria Lyle Photography
Sarasota, Florida

Models

Thanks to the following people from the Flower Mound Fire Department, Flower Mound, Texas, and from Winter Park Fire-Rescue, Winter Park, Florida, who provided locations and/or portrayed patients and EMS providers in our photographs.

FAO/Paramedic Wade Woody
FF/Paramedic Tim Mackling
FF/Paramedic Matthew Daniel
FF/Paramedic Jon Rea
FF/Paramedic Waylon Palmer
FF/EMT Jesse Palmer
Captain/EMT Billy McWhorter
Linda Kirk, Director, Winter Park Towers, Winter Park, FL
Andrew Isaacs
Richard Rodriguez
Tod Meadors
Jeff Spinelli
Mark Vaughn
Victoria Devereaux
Teresa George

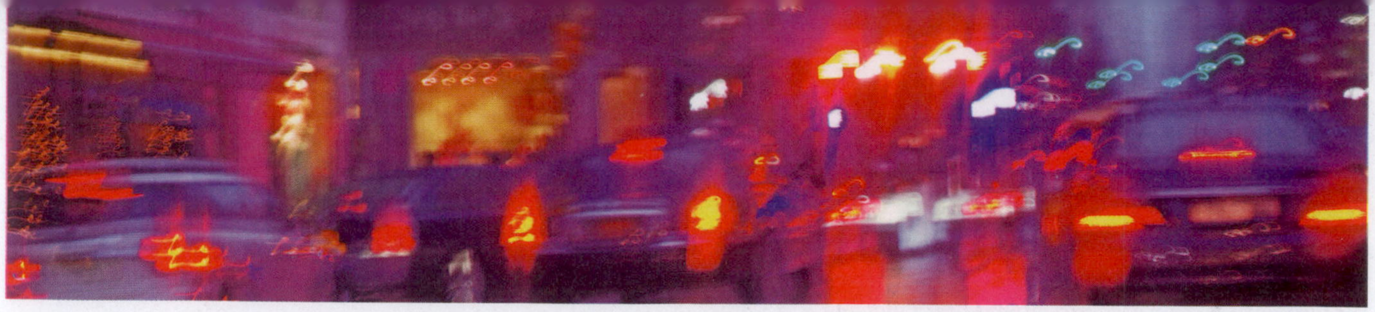

About the Authors

BRYAN E. BLEDSOE, DO, FACEP, FAAEM, EMT-P

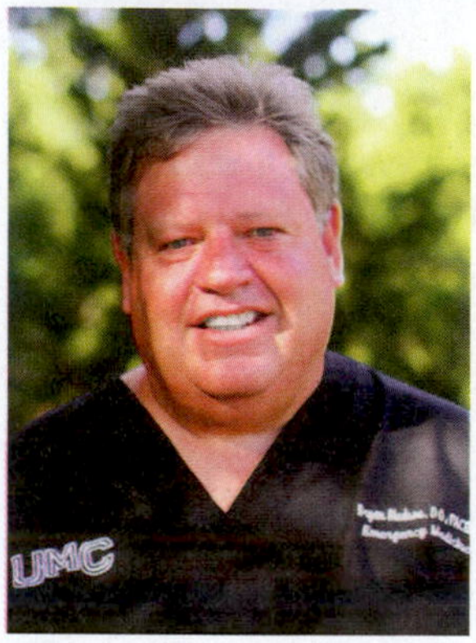

Dr. Bryan Bledsoe is an emergency physician, researcher, and EMS author. Presently he is Professor of Emergency Medicine at the University of Nevada School of Medicine and an Attending Emergency Physician at the University Medical Center of Southern Nevada in Las Vegas. He is board-certified in emergency medicine and emergency medical services. Prior to attending medical school, Dr. Bledsoe worked as an EMT, a paramedic, and a paramedic instructor. He completed EMT training in 1974 and paramedic training in 1976 and worked for six years as a field paramedic in Fort Worth, Texas. In 1979, he joined the faculty of the University of North Texas Health Sciences Center and served as coordinator of EMT and paramedic education programs at the university.

Dr. Bledsoe is active in emergency medicine and EMS research. He is a popular speaker at state, national, and international seminars and writes regularly for numerous EMS journals. He is active in educational endeavors with the United States Special Operations Command (USSOCOM) and the University of Nevada at Las Vegas. Dr. Bledsoe is the author of numerous EMS textbooks and has in excess of 1 million books in print. Dr. Bledsoe was named a "Hero of Emergency Medicine" in 2008 by the American College of Emergency Physicians as a part of their 40th anniversary celebration and was named a "Hero of Health and Fitness" by *Men's Health* magazine as part of their 20th anniversary edition in November of 2008. He is frequently interviewed in the national media. Dr. Bledsoe is married and divides his time between his residences in Midlothian, TX, and Las Vegas, NV.

RICHARD A. CHERRY, MS, EMT-P

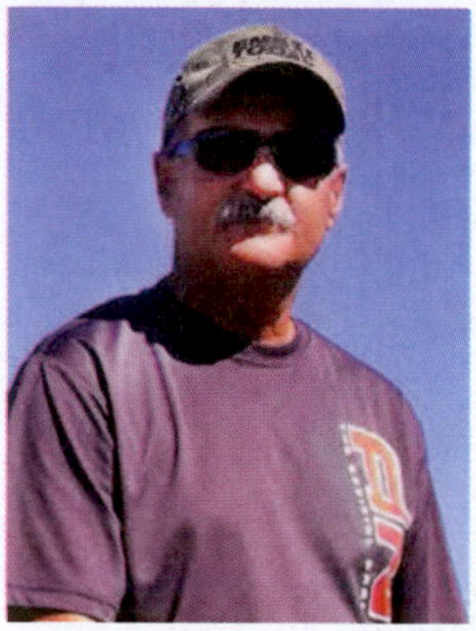

Richard Cherry is the Director of Training for Northern Onondaga Volunteer Ambulance (NOVA) in Liverpool, New York, a suburb of Syracuse. He recently retired from the Department of Emergency Medicine at Upstate Medical University where he held the positions of Director of Paramedic Training, Assistant Emergency Medicine Residency Director, Clinical Assistant Professor of Emergency Medicine, and Technical Director for Medical Simulation. His experience includes years of classroom teaching and emergency fieldwork. A native of Buffalo, Mr. Cherry earned his bachelor's degree at nearby St. Bonaventure University in 1972. He taught high school for the next ten years while he earned his master's degree in education from Oswego State University in 1977. He holds a permanent teaching license in New York State.

Mr. Cherry entered the emergency medical services field in 1974 with the DeWitt Volunteer Fire Department, where he served his community as a firefighter and EMS provider for more than 15 years. He took his first EMT course in 1977 and became an ALS provider two years later. He earned his paramedic certificate in 1985 as a member of the area's first paramedic class.

Mr. Cherry has authored several books for Brady. Most notable are *Paramedic Care: Principles & Practice, Essentials of Paramedic Care, Intermediate Emergency Care: Principles & Practice,* and *EMT Teaching: A Common Sense Approach.* He has made presentations at many state, national, and international EMS conferences on a variety of teaching topics. He and his wife, Sue, run a summer horse-riding camp for children with special needs on their property in West Monroe, New York. He also plays guitar in a Christian band.

A GUIDE TO KEY FEATURES

Emphasizing Principles

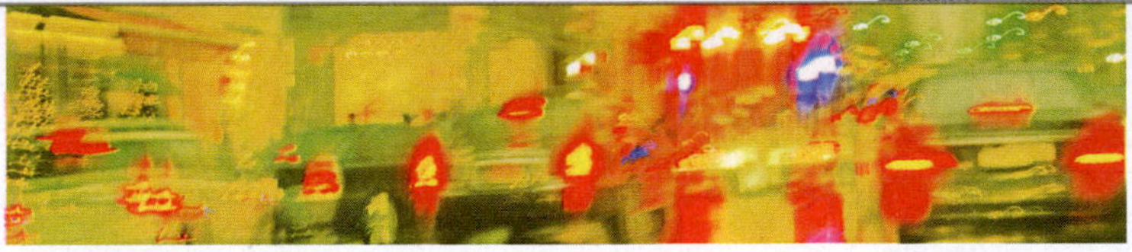

Chapter 1

Introduction to Paramedicine

Bryan Bledsoe, DO, FACEP, FAAEM

STANDARD
Preparatory (EMS Systems)

COMPETENCY
Integrates comprehensive knowledge of EMS systems, the safety and well-being of the paramedic, and medical–legal and ethical issues, which is intended to improve the health of EMS personnel, patients, and the community.

Learning Objectives

Terminal Performance Objective: After reading this chapter your should be able to discuss the characteristics of the profession of paramedicine.

Enabling Objectives: To accomplish the terminal performance objective, you should be able to:

1. Define key terms introduced in this chapter.
2. Compare and contrast the four nationally recognized levels of EMS providers in the United States.
3. Describe the requirements that must be met for EMS professionals to function at the paramedic level.
4. Discuss the traditional and emerging roles of the paramedic in health care, public health, and public safety.
5. List and describe the various health care settings paramedics may practice in with an expanded scope of practice.

KEY TERMS

Advanced Emergency Medical Technician (AEMT), p. 3
community paramedicine, p. 4
critical care transport, p. 7
Emergency Medical Responder (EMR), p. 3
Emergency Medical Services (EMS) system, p. 2
Emergency Medical Technician (EMT), p. 3
mobile integrated health care, p. 4
National Emergency Medical Services Education Standards: Paramedic Instructional Guidelines, p. 5
Paramedic, p. 3
paramedicine, p. 4

1

LEARNING OBJECTIVES

Terminal Performance Objectives and a separate set of Enabling Objectives are provided for each chapter.

KEY TERMS

Page numbers identify where each key term first appears, boldfaced, in the chapter.

more rapid are the pulse and respiratory rates.

3.0 and 3.5 kg. Because of the excretion of extracellular

As newborns make the transition from fetal to pulmonary circulation in the first few days of life, several important

Table 11-1 Normal Vital Signs

	Pulse (Beats per Minute)	Respiration (Breaths per Minute)	Blood Pressure (Average mmHg)	Temperature	
Infancy:					
At birth:	100–180	30–60	60–90 systolic	98–100°F	36.7–37.8°C
At 1 year:	100–160	30–60	87–105 systolic	98–100°F	36.7–37.8°C
Toddler (12 to 36 months)	80–110	24–40	95–105 systolic	96.8–99.6°F	36.0–37.5°C
Preschool age (3 to 5 years)	70–110	22–34	95–110 systolic	96.8–99.6°F	36.0–37.5°C
School-age (6 to 12 years)	65–110	18–30	97–112 systolic	98.6°F	37°C
Adolescence (13 to 18 years)	60–90	12–26	112–128 systolic	98.6°F	37°C
Early adulthood (19 to 40 years)	60–100	12–20	120/80	98.6°F	37°C
Middle adulthood (41 to 60 years)	60–100	12–20	120/80	98.6°F	37°C
Late adulthood (61 years and older)	*	*	*	98.6°F	37°C

*Depends on the individual's physical health status.

TABLES

A wealth of tables offers the opportunity to highlight, summarize, and compare information.

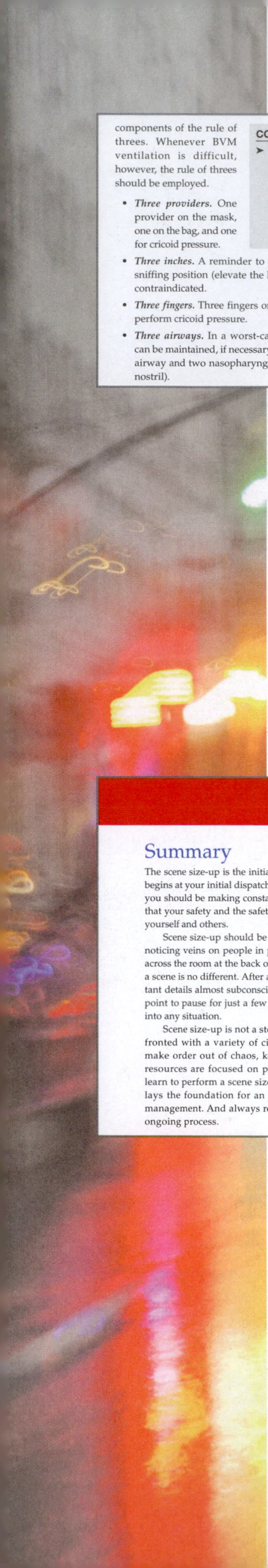

CONTENT REVIEW

Content review boxes set off from the text are interspersed throughout the chapter. They summarize key points and serve as a helpful study guide—in an easy format for quick review.

components of the rule of threes. Whenever BVM ventilation is difficult, however, the rule of threes should be employed.

> **CONTENT REVIEW**
>
> ➤ The Rule of Threes for Optimal BVM Ventilation
> - Three providers
> - Three inches
> - Three fingers
> - Three airways
> - Three PSI
> - Three PEEP

- ***Three providers.*** One provider on the mask, one on the bag, and one for cricoid pressure.
- ***Three inches.*** A reminder to place the patient in the sniffing position (elevate the head three inches) if not contraindicated.
- ***Three fingers.*** Three fingers on the cricoid cartilage to perform cricoid pressure.
- ***Three airways.*** In a worst-case scenario, the airway can be maintained, if necessary, with an orophrayngeal airway and two nasopharyngeal airways (one in each nostril).

PHOTOS AND ILLUSTRATIONS

Carefully selected photos and a unique art program reinforce content coverage and add to text explanations.

index, and middle finger of one hand. If a lesser-trained provider is performing the maneuver, you should confirm that they are in the correct position (Figure 15-47).

Use caution not to apply so much pressure as to deform and possibly obstruct the trachea; this is a particular danger in infants. The necessary pressure has been estimated as the amount of force that will compress a capped 50-mL syringe from 50 mL to the 30 mL marking. In the event that the patient actively vomits, it is imperative to release the pressure to avoid esophageal rupture. Similarly, if cricoid pressure is being performed during intubation, reduce or release the pressure if the intubator is having difficulty visualizing the vocal cords.

Optimal BVM Ventilation Using the Rule of Threes

The *rule of threes* was developed to help providers recall the components of optimal BVM ventilation. Many patients can be easily oxygenated and ventilated without using all

- ***Three PSI.*** A gentle reminder to use the lowest pressure necessary to see the chest rise.
- ***Three seconds.*** A reminder to ventilate slowly and allow time for adequate exhalation.
- ***Three PEEP.*** Or up to 15 cm/H_2O positive-end expiratory pressure (PEEP) as needed to improve oxygen saturations.

Bag-Valve Ventilation of the Pediatric Patient

The differences in the pediatric patient's anatomy require some variation in ventilation technique. First, the child's relatively flat nasal bridge makes achieving a mask seal more difficult. Pressing the mask against the child's face to improve the seal can actually obstruct the airway, which is more compressible than an adult's. You can best achieve the mask seal with the two-person BVM technique, using a jaw-thrust to maintain an open airway.

For BVM ventilation, the bag size depends on the child's age. Full-term neonates and infants will require a pediatric BVM with a capacity of at least 450 mL. For children up to 8 years of age, the pediatric BVM is preferred, although for patients in the upper portion of that age range you can use an adult BVM with a capacity of 1,500 mL if you do not maximally inflate it. Children older than 8 years require an adult BVM to achieve adequate tidal volumes. Additionally, be

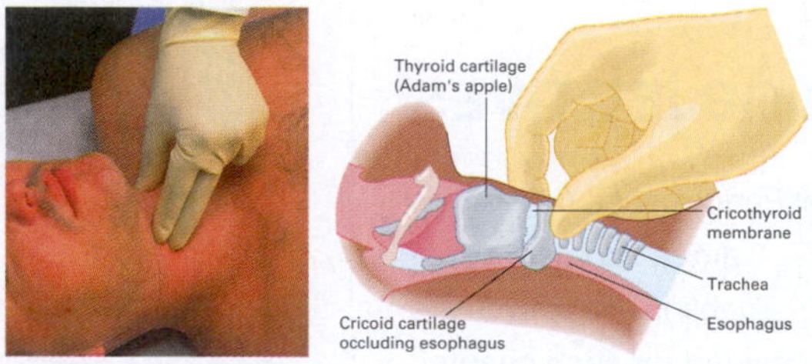

FIGURE 15-47 Cricoid pressure.

Summary

The scene size-up is the initial step in the patient care process. Sizing up the scene and situation begins at your initial dispatch and does not end until you are clear of the call. As the call unfolds, you should be making constant observations and adjustments to your plan of action. Remember that your safety and the safety of your partner are paramount—it is hard to effectively treat both yourself and others.

Scene size-up should be practiced so much that it becomes second nature to you. It is like noticing veins on people in public after you begin starting IVs. (You have all done it—looked across the room at the back of someone's hand and noticed what nice veins they had.) Sizing up a scene is no different. After a while, you begin to notice mechanisms of injury and other important details almost subconsciously. But be careful and do not get complacent! Always make it a point to pause for just a few seconds and consciously look around the scene before proceeding into any situation.

Scene size-up is not a step-by-step process, but a series of decisions you make when confronted with a variety of circumstances that are often beyond your control. It is a way to make order out of chaos, keep yourself and your crew safe, and ensure that all necessary resources are focused on patient care and outcomes. With time and experience, you will learn to perform a scene size-up quickly and focus on important issues. Your careful size-up lays the foundation for an organized and timely approach toward patient care and scene management. And always remember that scene size-up is not a one-time occurrence. It is an ongoing process.

SUMMARY

This end-of-chapter feature provides a concise review of chapter information.

YOU MAKE THE CALL

A scenario at the end of each chapter promotes critical thinking by requiring students to apply principles to actual practice.

airway management in every patient, you should learn and use advanced skills such as intubation, RSI, and cricothyrotomy. You must maintain proficiency in all airway skills, especially the more advanced techniques, through ongoing continuing education, physician medical direction, and testing with each EMS service. If you cannot do this, it is in the patient's best interest to focus on less sophisticated airway skills. If you anticipate that every airway will be complicated, apply basic airway skills before using advanced procedures, and perform frequent reassessments, you will give the patient his best chance for meaningful survival.

You Make the Call

You and your paramedic partner, Preston Connelly, are assigned to District 4, a quiet suburban neighborhood, on a warm Saturday in June. At 2:00 P.M., you are dispatched to care for a choking child at the Happy Hotdog Restaurant on Main Street. On your way to the location, the dispatcher advises you that they are currently giving prearrival choking instructions to the bystanders at the scene. On arrival, you find a frantic mother who tells you that her 6-year-old son was eating a hot dog and drinking a soda when he started coughing and gasping for air. She keeps yelling for you to do something. Bystanders surround the child and are attempting to perform the Heimlich maneuver without success. On your primary assessment, you find a 6-year-old boy lying on the floor, unconscious and apneic, with a pulse rate of 130. There is cyanosis surrounding his lips and fingernail beds, with a moderate amount of secretions coming from his mouth. There are no signs of trauma. You and Preston immediately start management of this child.

1. What is your primary assessment and management of this child?
2. What are your first actions?
3. What are your options for managing the airway after the obstruction is relieved?
4. What are the major anatomic differences between pediatric and adult patients in terms of airway management?

See Suggested Responses at the back of this book.

REVIEW QUESTIONS

These questions ask students to review and recall key information they have just learned.

Review Questions

1. When you couple the physical assessment findings with the patient's medical history, you are able to derive a list of __________
   a. clinical diagnostics.
   b. field prognoses
   c. chief complaints
   d. differential field diagnoses.
2. The pain, discomfort, or dysfunction that caused your patient to request help is known as the __________
   a. primary problem.
   b. nature of the illness.
   c. differential diagnosis.
   d. chief complaint.
3. You are assessing a patient who complains of cardiac-type chest pain that is felt in the jaw and down the left arm. This pattern of pain is known as __________
   a. sympathetic pain.
   b. tenderness.
   c. referred pain.
   d. associated pain.
4. Your patient has smoked 2 packs of cigarettes each day for the past 35 years. He is a __________ pack/year smoker.
   a. 35 c. 730
   b. 70 d. 25,550
5. The CAGE questionnaire is used as an evaluation tool to assess a patient with what type of history?
   a. Alcoholism c. Allergies
   b. Lung disease d. Pregnancy
6. What interviewing mnemonic should be used for each presenting problem a patient has?
   a. SAMPLE
   b. DCAP–BTLS
   c. OPQRST–ASPN
   d. AEIOU–TIPS
7. The mnemonic GPAL is used to evaluate a patient's __________
   a. alcoholism.
   b. allergies.
   c. pregnancy history.
   d. endocrine dysfunction.

Match the following elements of the present illness of the patient with a chief complaint of chest pain with their respective examples:

1. O	**a.** Pain is 6 on a scale of 1–10
2. P	**b.** Patient also complains of shortness of breath and nausea
3. Q	**c.** Pain had a sudden onset
4. R	**d.** Pain began 2 hours ago
5. S	**e.** Pain worsens while lying down
6. T	**f.** Patient denies dizziness
7. AS	**g.** Pain goes through to the back
8. PN	**h.** Pain is heavy and vise-like

See Answers to Review Questions at the back of this book.

6. Which radio frequencies may be used by cities and municipalities for their ability to better transmit through concrete and steel?
   a. UHF c. 800-mHz
   b. VHF d. none of the above
7. Which frequency band is typically used by county and suburban agencies due to its ability to transmit over various terrains and longer distances?
   a. UHF c. 800-mHz
   b. VHF d. none of the above
8. What is the name of the basic communications system that uses the same frequency to both transmit and receive?
   a. Multiplex c. Simplex
   b. Duplex d. Complex
9. A communications system that uses a different transmit and receive frequency allowing for simultaneous communications between two parties is called __________
   a. multiplex.
   b. duplex.
   c. simplex.
   d. complex.
10. __________ communications systems are capable of transmitting both voice and electronic patient data simultaneously.
    a. Multiplex c. Simplex
    b. Duplex d. Complex

See answers to Review Questions at the back of this book.

References

1. Department of Homeland Security. SAFECOM. (Available at http://www.dhs.gov/safecom/)
2. National EMS Information System (NEMSIS). The NEMSIS Technical Assistance Center (TAC). (Available at http://www.nemsis.org//.)
3. American College of Emergency Physicians (ACEP). "Automatic Crash Notification and Intelligent Transportation Systems." *Ann Emerg Med* 55 (2010): 397.
4. National Emergency Number Association (NENA). National Emergency Number Association. (Available at: http://www.nena.org)
5. Association of Public-Safety Communications Officials (APCO). [Available at: http://www.apco911.org/]
6. Department of Transportation, Research and Innovative Technology Administration. Next Generation 911. (Available at: http://www.its.dot.gov/ng911/.)
7. Centers for Disease Control and Prevention. Recommendations from the Expert Panel: Advanced Automatic Collision Notification and Triage of the Injured Patient. (See NHTSA summary at http://www.nhtsa.gov/Research/Biomechanics+&+Trauma/Advanced+Automatic+Collision+Notification+-+AACN)
8. Wilson, S., M. Cooke, R. Morrell et al. "A Systematic Review of the Evidence Supporting the Use of Priority Dispatch of Emergency Ambulances." *Prehosp Emerg Care* 6 (2002): 42–29.
9. Billittier, A. J., 4th, E. B. Lerner, W. Tucker, and J. Lee. "The Lay Public's Expectations of Prearrival Instructions When Dialing 911." *Prehosp Emerg Care* 4 (2000): 234–237.
10. Munk, M. D., S. D. White, M. L. Perry, et al. "Physician Medical Direction and Clinical Performance at an Established Emergency Medical Services System." *Prehosp Emerg Care* 13 (2009): 185–192.
11. Cheung, D. S., J. J. Kelly, C. Beach, et al. "Improving Handoffs in the Emergency Department." *Ann Emerg Med* 55 (2010): 171–180.
12. Chan, T. C., J. Killeen, W. Griswold, and L. Lenert. "Information Technology and Emergency Medical Care during Disasters." *Acad Emerg Med* 11 (2004): 1229–1236.
13. DREAMS Ambulance Project. (See article at: https://www.ems1.com/ems-products/technology/articles/1183110-DREAMS-revolutionizes-communication-between-ER-and-ambulance/.)
14. Haskins, P. A., D. G. Ellis, and J. Mayrose. "Predicted Utilization of Emergency Medical Services Telemedicine in Decreasing Ambulance Transports." *Prehosp Emerg Care* 6 (2002): 445–448.

Further Reading

Bass, R., J. Potter, K. McGinnis, and T. Miyahara. "Surveying Emerging Trends in Emergency-related Information Delivery for the EMS Profession." *Topics in Emergency Medicine* 26 (April–June 2004): 2, 93–102.

Fitch, J. "Benchmarking Your Comm Center." *JEMS* 2006: 98–112.

McGinnis, K. K. "The Future of Emergency Medical Services Communications Systems: Time for a Change." *N C Med J* 68 (2007): 283–285.

McGinnis, K. K. *Future EMS Technologies: Predicting Communications Implications.* National Public Safety Telecommunications Council, National Association of State EMS Officials, National Association of EMS Physicians, June, 2010.

McGinnis, K. K. "The Future Is Now: Emergency Medical Services (EMS) Communications Advances Can Be as Important as Medical Treatment Advances When It Comes to Saving Lives." *Interoperability Today* (SafeCom, U.S. Department of Homeland Security), Volume 3, 2005.

McGinnis, K. K. *Rural and Frontier Emergency Medical Services Agenda for the Future.* National Rural Health Association Press: October 2004.

REFERENCES

This listing is a compilation of source material providing the basis of updated data and research used in the preparation of each chapter.

FURTHER READING

This list features recommendations for books and journal articles that go beyond chapter coverage.

CASE STUDY

This feature at the start of each chapter draws students into the reading and creates a link between text content and real-life situations.

cleaning, p. 70
Code Green Campaign, p. 78
disinfection, p. 70
exposure, p. 70
isotonic exercise, p. 61
pathogens, p. 65
personal protective equipment (PPE), p. 66
sterilization, p. 70
stress, p. 74
stressor, p. 74
Tema Conter Memorial Trust, p. 78

Case Study

Howard is a 15-year veteran of a high-volume, inner-city EMS service. When he first started his career, Howard thought he knew what he was getting into, but the years have taught him differently.

Right now, Howard is in the spotlight for saving the life of a police officer who was shot in a hostage situation. "That call forced me to reflect on a few important things," he says. "Two years ago, I had a minor heart problem, and it was a good wake-up call. Since then I've been lifting weights and running, so I was able to get to the officer with enough strength to carry him to safety.

"Another thing is that I always use personal protective equipment. I never go to work without steel-toed boots and I never leave the ambulance without a pair of disposable gloves. Can you believe there are still paramedics who knock the concept of infection control? If any one of my partners sticks a needle into the squad bench in my ambulance, they know I'll speak up."

Howard, a mild-mannered, nondescript man, doesn't realize that his young colleagues regard him as a role model. They've seen him handle himself at chaotic scenes as well as when a situation demands sensitivity, patience, and gentleness. "Howard is the man I'd want to tell bad news to my mother," one of his partners says. "He can handle people involved in just about any circumstance—death situations, panicked parents, lonely elderly people, and even hostile drunks. I've never seen anyone treat others with such dignity and respect. He's the best partner anyone could want, especially when we have to manage patients who are thrashing around. But that was not always so, was it, Howard?"

"No, it wasn't," Howard replies. "There was a time when no one wanted to work with me. I was a rebel, and I figured there was only one way to do things: my way. But an incident that occurred a few years ago changed all that. It's a long story. But the upshot is that when I recovered from the stress, my outlook had been altered. I realized that though I couldn't save the world, I could save myself. That's when I learned how to deal with the effects of a stressful job. I started eating right, lost a lot of weight, and adopted a new attitude. Anyway, if I can maintain my own well-being, I can do a lot more to help others. Right? Isn't that what we're about?"

Introduction

The safety and well-being of the workforce is a fundamental aspect of top-notch performance in EMS.[1] As a paramedic, it includes your physical well-being as well as your mental and emotional well-being. If your body is fed well and kept fit, if you use the principles of safe lifting, observe safe driving practices, and avoid potentially addictive and and insidious infections. If you let your spirit appreciate the fear and sadness on other faces, you will find ways to combat your prejudices and treat people with dignity and respect. By doing all these things, you will also be able to promote the benefits of well-being to your EMS colleagues.

Death, dying, stress, injury, infection, fear—all these threaten your wellness and conspire to interfere with your good intentions. However, you can do something about

PROCEDURE SCANS

Visual skill summaries provide step-by-step support in skill instruction.

Procedure 7-4 Reassessment

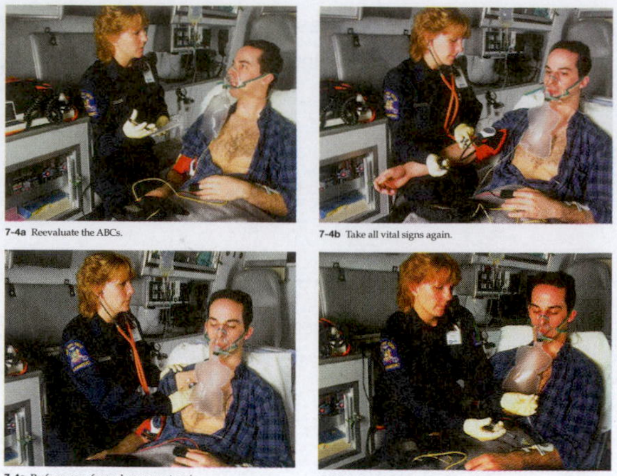

7-4a Reevaluate the ABCs.

7-4b Take all vital signs again.

7-4c Perform your focused assessment again.

7-4d Evaluate your interventions' effects.

laryngospasm may be occurring. Airway and breathing management requires constant reevaluation.

oxygenation. Lip cyanosis indicates central hypoxia (overall oxygen status), whereas peripheral cyanosis indicates decreased oxygen to the tissues. Pallor and coolness sug-

Special Features

PATHO PEARLS

Offer a snapshot of pathological considerations students will encounter in the field.

the present illness. Common sense and clinical experience will determine how much of the following history to use.

Preliminary Data

For documentation, always record the date and time of the physical exam. Determine your patient's age, sex, race, birthplace, and occupation. This provides a starting point for the interview and establishes you as the interviewer. Who is the source of the information you receive about your patient? Is it the competent patient himself, his spouse, a friend, or a bystander? Are you receiving a report from a first responder, the police, or another health care worker? Do you have the medical record from a transferring facility?

After you have gathered the information, you should establish its reliability, which will vary according to the source's knowledge, memory, trust, and motivation. Again, reconfirm the information with the patient, if possible. This is a judgment call based on your experience. For example, if the patient information you received from a particular EMT first responder has been accurate in the past, you probably will trust it again. On the other hand, if the nurse at a physician's office has repeatedly provided you with erroneous information, you probably will doubt its accuracy.

scious patient, the chief complaint becomes what someone else identifies or what you observe as the primary problem. In some trauma situations, for instance, the chief complaint might be the mechanism of injury, such as "a penetrating wound to the chest" or "a fall from 25 feet."

Patho Pearls

The renowned Canadian physician Sir William Osler said, "Listen to the patient, and he will tell you what is wrong." This advice is as true today as it was 100 years ago. A great deal of information can be determined from a skillful history taking. As you listen to a patient's medical history, try to understand the underlying pathophysiologic processes that might cause the symptoms the patient describes. This will help you to fully comprehend the disease process or processes affecting the patient.

For example, consider the following case. Mrs. J. Franklin is a 72-year-old pensioner, twice widowed, who lives in an older section of town. She summons EMS with what initially seem like vague complaints. She reports to the dispatcher, when queried, that she is "just sick." You arrive and begin an assessment, starting with a pertinent history. The patient reports that her symptoms began about two weeks ago after several family members came to her house with dinner, which included a baked ham. Since that time, she has developed some fatigue, progressive dyspnea, and occasional chest pain. She now reports that she often wakes up at 3:00 A.M. with breathing trouble that resolves when she walks around the room or

LEGAL CONSIDERATIONS

Offer a snapshot of pathological considerations students will encounter in the field.

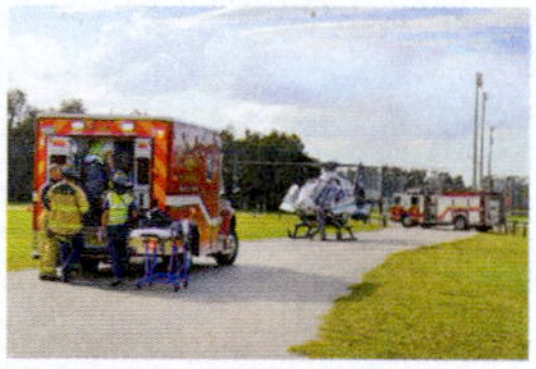

FIGURE 2-11 Patients may be transported by ground or air. Medical helicopter transport was introduced in the 1950s during the Korean War. *(© Ed Effron)*

Vietnam, and success of military evacuation procedures led to their use in civilian ambulance systems. In 1970, the Military Assistance to Safety and Traffic (MAST) program was established. This demonstration project set up 35 helicopter transportation programs nationwide to test the feasibility of using military helicopters and paramedics in

Legal Considerations

Emergency Department Closures. Numerous factors have resulted in emergency department closures and ambulance diversions. This can have a significant impact on the EMS system. All systems must address this situation so that patient care does not suffer.

In 1974, in response to a request from the DOT, the General Services Administration (GSA) developed the "KKK-A-1822 Federal Specifications for Ambulances." This was the first attempt at standardizing ambulance design to permit intensive life support for patients en route to a definitive care facility. The act defined the following basic types of ambulance:

- ***Type I (Figure 2-13).*** This is a conventional cab and chassis on which a module ambulance body is mounted, with no passageway between the driver's and patient's compartments.
- ***Type II (Figure 2-14).*** A standard van, body, and cab form an integral unit. Most have a raised roof.

CULTURAL CONSIDERATIONS

Provide an awareness of beliefs that might affect patient care.

An important part of patient assessment is gathering information that is accurate, complete, and relevant to the present emergency. To begin, you must identify the patient's chief complaint. Although dispatch probably will have given you an idea of what the emergency is about, it is

Cultural Considerations

Eye contact is a major form of nonverbal communication. Short eye contact is often seen as friendly, whereas prolonged eye contact may be interpreted as threatening. Thus, timing is an important factor in how a person interprets eye contact.

One's culture also influences how eye contact is interpreted. Eye contact can mean respect in one culture and disrespect in another. Often, Asians will avoid eye contact even when they have nothing to hide. Eye contact between people of different sexes is problematic in Muslim cultures, in which a prolonged look in the face of a member of the opposite sex might be misinterpreted. Because of this, people in Middle Eastern countries might look a person of the same sex in the eye and not look into the eyes of a person of the opposite sex.

If you work in a culturally diverse community, you should learn the customs of eye contact and other forms of nonverbal communication of those you might encounter during the course of your work.

unexpected but important facts. For example, instead of asking your patient with abdominal pain, "Did you have breakfast today?" which can be answered with either a "yes" or a "no," ask: "What have you eaten today?"

- ***Use direct questions when necessary.*** Direct questions, or **closed questions**, ask for specific information. ("Did you take your pills today?" or "Does the abdominal pain come and go like a cramp, or is it constant?") These questions are good for three reasons: They fill in information generated by open-ended questions. They help to answer crucial questions when time is limited. And they can help to control overly talkative patients, who might want to tell you about their gallbladder surgery in 1969 when their chief complaint is a sprained ankle.
- ***Ask only one question at a time, and allow the patient to complete his answers.*** If you ask more than one question, the patient may not know which one to answer and may leave out portions of information or become confused. Equally important is having one person do the interview. Don't force your patient to discern questions from multiple interviewers.
- ***Listen to the patient's complete response before asking the next question.*** By doing so, you might find that

ASSESSMENT PEARLS

Offer tips, guidance, and information to aid in patient assessment.

Provocation/Palliation

What provokes the symptom (makes it worse)? Does anything palliate the symptom (make it better)? In many

Assessment Pearls

Chest pain is a common reason that people summon EMS. However, the causes of chest pain are numerous. In emergency medicine or EMS, we often look to exclude the most serious causes before determining whether chest pain is of a benign origin. Internal organs do not have as many pain fibers as do such structures as the skin and other areas. Pain arising from an internal organ tends to be dull and vague. This is because nerves from various spinal levels innervate the organ in question. The heart, for example, is innervated by several thoracic spinal nerve segments. Thus, cardiac pain tends to be dull and is sometimes described as pressure. It also tends to cause referred pain (i.e., pain in an area somewhat distant to the organ), such as pain in the left arm and jaw. Dull pain that is hard to localize (or to reproduce with palpation) may be due to cardiac disease. One sign often seen with patients suffering cardiac disease is Levine's sign. With Levine's sign, the patient will subconsciously clench his fist when describing the chest pain. Levine's sign is associated with pain of a cardiac origin (e.g., angina or acute coronary syndrome).

Ask about any activity, medication, or other circumstance that either alleviates or aggravates the chief complaint.

Quality

How does your patient perceive the pain or discomfort? Ask him to explain how the symptom feels, and listen carefully to his answer. Does your patient call his pain crushing, tearing, oppressive, gnawing, crampy, sharp, dull, or otherwise? Quote his exact descriptors in your report.

Region/Radiation

Where is the symptom? Does it move anywhere else? Identify the exact location and area of pain, discomfort, or dysfunction. Does your patient complain of pain "here," while holding a clenched fist over the sternum, or does he grasp the entire abdomen with both hands and moan? If your patient has not done so, ask him to point to the painful area. Identify the specific location, or the boundary of the pain if it is regional.

Determine whether the pain is truly pain (occurring independently) or **tenderness** (pain on palpation). Also determine whether the pain moves or radiates. Localized pain occurs in one specific area, whereas radiating pain

PEDIATRIC PEARLS

Offer tips, guidance, and information on how to deal with pediatric patients encountered in the field.

the result of a head injury, hypothermia, severe hypoxia, or drug overdose. Bradycardia is a common finding in the well-conditioned athlete, but it may be found in almost anyone. Treat bradycardia only if it compromises your patient's cardiac output and general circulatory status.

Tachycardia usually indicates an increase in sympathetic nervous system stimulation as the body compensates for another problem, such as blood loss, fear, pain, fever, drug overdose, or hypoxia. It is an early indicator of shock and may indicate ventricular tachycardia, a life-threatening cardiac dysrhythmia.

The pulse's quality can be weak, strong, or bounding. Weak, thready pulses indicate a decreased circulatory status, such as shock. Strong, bounding pulses may indicate high blood pressure, heat stroke, or increasing intracranial pressure. The pulse location may be another indicator of your patient's clinical status. The presence of a carotid pulse generally means that his systolic blood pressure is at least 60 mmHg. The presence of peripheral pulses indicates a higher blood pressure; their absence suggests circulatory collapse. Practice locating each of the pulse locations (Figure 5-12). As with other vital signs, take your patient's pulse frequently in the emergency setting and note any trends.

To take the pulse of a conscious adult or large child, the most accessible and commonly used location is the radial artery. With the pads of your first two or three

Pediatric Pearls

In infants and small children, use the brachial artery or auscultate for an apical pulse. Remember that auscultating an apical pulse does not provide information about your patient's hemodynamic status. To locate the brachial artery, feel just medial to the biceps tendon. Auscultate the apical pulse just below the left nipple.

fingers, compress the radial artery onto the radius, just below the wrist on the thumb side (Procedure 5-1b). In the unconscious patient, begin by checking his carotid pulse. To locate the carotid pulse, palpate medial to and just below the angle of the jaw. Locate the thyroid cartilage (Adam's apple) and slide your fingers laterally until they are between the thyroid cartilage and the large muscle in the neck (sternocleidomastoid).

First, note your patient's pulse rate by counting the number of beats in 1 minute. If his pulse is regular, you can count the beats in 15 seconds and multiply that number by 4. If his pulse is irregular, you must count it for a full minute to obtain an accurate total. Also note the pulse's rhythm and quality.

Blood Pressure

Blood pressure is the force of blood against the arteries' walls as the heart contracts and relaxes. It is equal to cardiac output times the systemic vascular resistance. Any

CUSTOMER SERVICE MINUTE

Shows how extending extra kindness and compassion can make an important difference to patients and families coping with an emergency.

Customer Service Minute

Following Up. Last week, a man took his dog to the vet for an upper respiratory infection. The dog was pretty sick, but the vet assured the owner that she was not critical, and with antibiotics she would be better in a few days, so he brought her home. The next day, the veterinarian called to find out how the dog was doing. She called every day until the dog was back to normal. Needless to say, the man was delighted in the service he received from that vet.

Physicians' offices, dentists' offices, and veterinary offices often call their patients a few days following a visit to see how things are going. Why don't we? Before you leave your patient and the family, why not ask them for permission to call the next day or in a few days to see how they're doing? If they say no or are hesitant to give permission, drop it. If they give permission, call them and see if there is anything you can do for them.

The follow-up has many benefits. You get to reconnect with the people in your community. It is great for public relations. It is educational because you can see whether your diagnosis was accurate. It's a winner from every angle. When they hang up, they'll be thinking, "Wow!"

Introduction

Patient assessment means conducting a problem-oriented evaluation of your patient and establishing priorities of your patient en route to the hospital to detect changes in patient condition.

Your proficiency in performing a systematic patient assessment will determine your ability to deliver the highest quality of prehospital **advanced life support** (ALS) to sick and injured people. Paramedic patient assessment is a straightforward skill, similar to the assessment you might have performed as an EMT. It differs, however, in depth and in the kind of care you will provide as a result.

Your assessment must be thorough, because many ALS procedures are potentially dangerous. Safely and appropriately performing advanced procedures such as administration of drugs, defibrillation, synchronized cardioversion, needle decompression of the chest, or endotracheal intubation will depend on your assessment and correct field diagnosis. If your assessment does not reveal your patient's true problem, the consequences can be devastating.

As always, common sense dictates how you proceed in the field. When you assess the responsive medical patient, the history reveals the most important diagnostic information and takes priority over the physical exam. For the trauma patient and the unresponsive medical patient, the reverse is true. However, trauma may cause a medical emergency, and, conversely, a medical emergency may cause trauma. Only by performing a thorough patient assessment can you discover the true cause of your patient's problems. This chapter provides problem-oriented patient assessment examples based on the information and techniques presented in the previous six chapters.

IN THE FIELD

Provides extra tips that can help ensure success in real-life emergency situations.

In the Field

The Tools of Your Trade: *The Ophthalmoscope*

An **ophthalmoscope** (Figure 5-27) is a medical instrument used to examine the internal eye structures, especially the retina, located at the back of the eye. Although it is most often used to diagnose eye conditions, you can discover information that may be relevant to other medical and traumatic events.

The ophthalmoscope is basically a light source with lenses and mirrors. It has a handle, which houses the batteries, and a head, which includes a window through which you visualize the internal eye; an aperture dial, which changes the width of the light beam; a lens dial to bring the eye into focus; and a lens indicator, which identifies the lens magnification number (i.e., 0 to +40 or 0 to –20). You examine the eye by looking through a monocular eyepiece into the eye of your patient. You can view different depths of the eye at different magnifications by rotating a disk of varying lenses within the instrument itself.

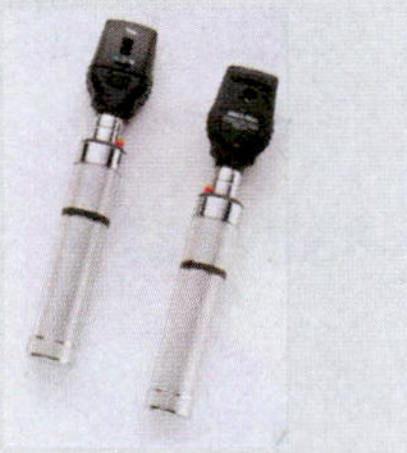

FIGURE 5-27 An ophthalmoscope is used to visualize the interior of your patient's eyes.

eye while the patient continues to fix his gaze on an object in the distance. Adjust the lens disk as needed to focus on the retina. Farsighted patients will require more "plus" diopters (black or green numbers), whereas nearsighted patients will require more "minus" diopters (red numbers) to keep the retina in focus.

Try to keep both your eyes open and relaxed. The optic disk should come into view when you are about 1.5 to 2 inches from the eye while you are still aiming your light 15 to 25 degrees nasally. If you are having difficulty finding the disk, look for a branching (bifurcation) in a retinal blood vessel. Usually the bifurcation will point toward the disk.

Follow the vessel in the direction of the bifurcation and you should arrive at the optic disk. The disk should appear as a yellowish-orange to pink round structure. Within the center of the disk there should be a central physiologic cup, which normally appears as a smaller, paler circle. The cup should be less than half the diameter of the disk. An enlarged cup may indicate chronic open-angle glaucoma. Indistinct borders or elevation of the optic disk may indicate papilledema, which is a marker of increased intracranial pressure.

Next, look at the arteries and veins of the retina. The arteries are usually brighter and smaller than the veins. Spontaneous venous pulsations are normal. Abnormalities of the retina such as hemorrhages, arteriovenous (AV) nicking, and cotton wool spots may indicate local or systemic disease such as retinal vein occlusion, hypertension, or many other conditions.

Finally, look at the fovea and surrounding macula. This area is where vision is most acute. It is located about two disk diameters temporal to the optic disk. You may also find the macula by asking the patient to look directly into the light of your ophthalmoscope. Prepare for a fleeting glimpse as this area is very sensitive to light and may be uncomfortable for your patient to maintain. A "cherry red" macula with surrounding pallor of tissue in the setting of acute painless monocular visual loss indicates a central retinal artery occlusion. Irreversible damage occurs

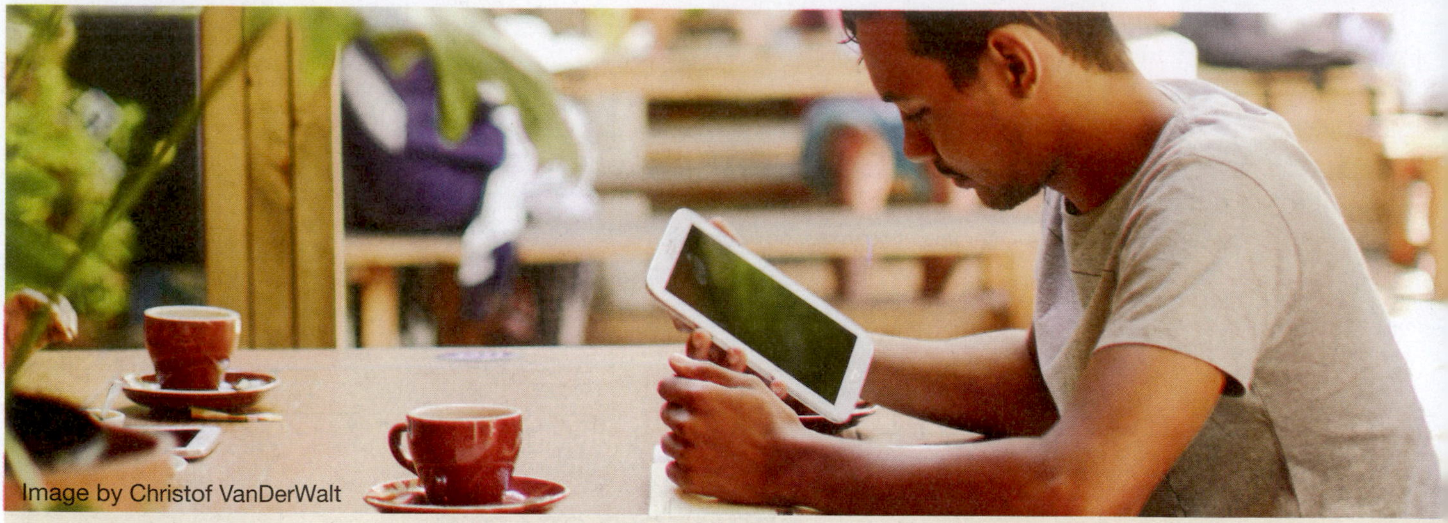

MyBRADYLab®

Our goal is to help every student succeed.
We're working with educators and institutions to improve results for students everywhere.

MyLab & Mastering is the world's leading collection of online homework, tutorial, and assessment products designed with a single purpose in mind: to improve the results of higher education students, one student at a time. Used by more than 11 million students each year, Pearson's MyLab & Mastering programs deliver consistent, measurable gains in student learning outcomes, retention, and subsequent course success.

Highlights of this Fully Integrated Learning Program

- Gradebook: A robust gradebook allows you to see multiple views of your classes' progress. Completely customizable and exportable, the gradebook can be adapted to meet your specific needs.
- Multimedia Library: allows students and instructors to quickly search through resources and find supporting media.
- Pearson eText: Rich media options let students watch lecture and example videos as they read or do their homework. Instructors can share their comments or highlights, and students can add their own, creating a tight community of learners in your class.
- Decision-Making Cases: take Paramedic students through real-life scenarios that they typically face in the field. These cases give students the opportunity to gather patient data and make decisions that would affect their patient's health.

For more information,
please contact your BRADY sales representative at 1-800-638-0220,
or visit us at www.bradybooks.com

ALWAYS LEARNING

PEARSON

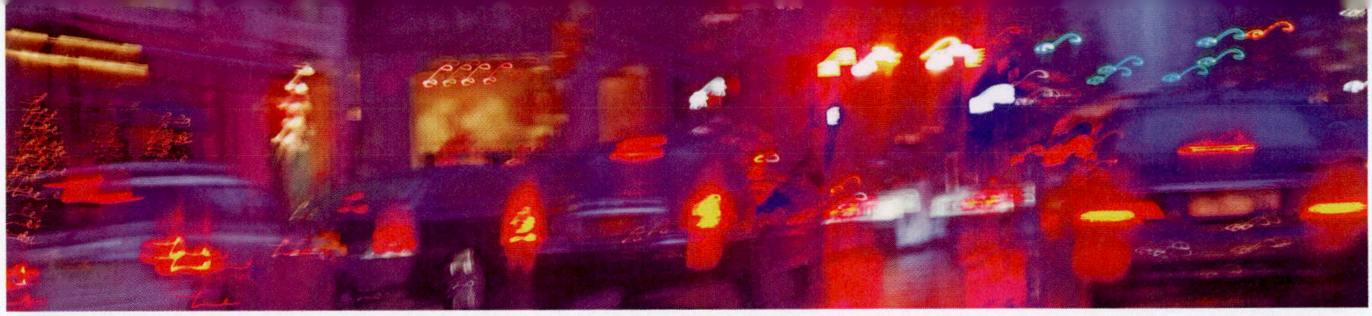

Chapter 1

Gynecology

Bryan Bledsoe, DO, FACEP, FAAEM, EMT-P

STANDARD

Medicine (Gynecology)

COMPETENCY

Integrates assessment findings with principles of epidemiology and pathophysiology to formulate a field impression and implement a comprehensive treatment/disposition plan for a patient with a medical complaint.

Learning Objectives

Terminal Performance Objective: After reading this chapter, you should be able to integrate patient assessment findings, patient history, and knowledge of anatomy, physiology, pathophysiology, and basic and advanced life support interventions to recognize and manage patients with gynecologic emergencies.

Enabling Objectives: To accomplish the terminal performance objective, you should be able to:

1. Define key terms introduced in this chapter.
2. Review and discuss the pertinent anatomy and physiology of the female reproductive system, including organs, structures, hormones, and the menstrual cycle.
3. Use a process of clinical reasoning to guide and interpret the medical history and patient assessment findings for patients with specific gynecologic complaints.
4. Discuss how to adapt the major phases of patient assessment for a female patient with complaints and presentations related to gynecologic emergencies.
5. Discuss how to adapt the major phases of patient assessment for a female patient with complaints and presentations specific to sexual assault.
6. Given a variety of scenarios, discuss the integration of assessment and management guidelines as they relate to gynecologic emergencies.

KEY TERMS

cystitis, p. 12
dysmenorrhea, p. 8
dyspareunia, p. 8
dysuria, p. 12
ectopic pregnancy, p. 12
endometriosis, p. 12
endometritis, p. 12
endometrium, p. 5
gynecology, p. 3
menarche, p. 6
menopause, p. 8
menorrhagia, p. 13
menstruation, p. 7
miscarriage, p. 12
mittelschmerz, p. 12
myometrium, p. 6
obstetrics, p. 3
ovulation, p. 6
pelvic inflammatory disease (PID) , p. 11
perimetrium, p. 6
premenstrual dysphoric disorder (PMDD) , p. 8
premenstrual syndrome (PMS) , p. 8

Case Study

It is near dusk on a warm summer evening when you and your partner, Sam Rusk, are dispatched from quarters to a nearby community park for an "assault." Within 4 minutes, you pull up to the park access gate near the security office, where you meet a police officer and the park security supervisor. The police officer tells you that your 28-year-old female patient was found wandering in the park by a security officer just as the park was closing. He tells you that the Crime Scene Unit is en route. The supervisor reports that the officer who found her is sitting with her in the office.

You enter the security office as Sam gets the stretcher and jump kit from the back of the medic unit. The patient is seated on a cot facing away from the door. The security officer is sitting on a chair next to the cot, talking quietly to her. The patient has a white cotton blanket, provided by the officer, wrapped tightly over her shoulders and around her body. You observe that her hair is tangled and matted, with leaves and small twigs sticking from it. As you approach her, you identify yourself, and introduce Sam, as paramedics who are there to help her. She turns her tear-stained, battered face toward you and nods, saying "I know" so quietly that you can barely hear her. The park officer stands and tells you that your patient's name is Stephanie. He then excuses himself, telling her that she is in good hands and that he will be right outside.

You pull up the chair that had been used by the officer and position it in front of Stephanie to complete your primary assessment. Although your priority is the assessment of her ABCs, you cannot ignore her obvious injuries. She has dried blood on her nose and mouth and her left eye is bruised and nearly swollen shut. You tell her that you need to perform some simple procedures to make sure that she is okay, and you ask her permission to do so. Again she nods, her eyes never leaving your face. In a soft hoarse voice, she says quietly, "He raped me, even though I begged him not to."

Stephanie's airway is open and her breathing is regular in rate and depth. You ask her if you can check her pulse, and she unwraps the blanket just enough to let her right forearm extend toward you. You find that her pulse is strong but rapid and her skin is cool and dry. You notice an abrasion around her wrist that makes you wonder if she had been tied down. You also observe that she has several broken nails on the trembling hand she extends toward you. Again with her permission, you gently unwrap the blanket to reveal a torn, dirty T-shirt that is splattered with blood. She is wearing nothing else. Her inner thighs are covered with dried blood, as well as with dirt and leaves. You limit your rapid trauma assessment to merely a search for life-threatening injuries, as Stephanie will undergo a thorough exam by the sexual assault nurse examiner (SANE). Stephanie's blood pressure is 108/70 mmHg. Her pulse is strong and regular at 110 beats per minute. Her breathing is quiet and nonlabored at a rate of 24 breaths per minute, with a pulse oximeter reading of 99 percent on room air.

Explaining exactly what you're going to do and asking her permission to do so, you and Sam help her stand and then pivot her onto the stretcher, leaving her wrapped in the blanket in which you found her. You move her to the medic unit. As you get her settled, and before beginning the short drive to the hospital, Sam contacts medical direction and requests that the SANE meet you at the hospital.

En route, you complete Stephanie's history. She denies allergies and reports that the only medication she takes is a multivitamin tablet daily. Stephanie denies any significant past medical history. She ate a chef's salad for lunch about mid-afternoon. Stephanie says that she was grabbed from behind while she was jogging and that she was dragged off the path and into the woods. You reassure her that she is safe now and no one will hurt her. Within minutes, you arrive at the hospital.

Emma Cannise, RN, the SANE coordinator, meets you at the emergency entrance to the hospital. You introduce Stephanie to Emma, who then accompanies you to the evaluation unit located behind the main emergency department. You give her a brief report, and she signs off on your patient care report.

Returning to quarters, you and Sam discuss how ironic it was that this month's continuing medical education (CME) program was a presentation by Emma Cannise on caring for victims of sexual assault.

Introduction

The term **gynecology** is derived from the Greek *gynaik*, meaning "woman." Gynecology is the branch of medicine that deals with the health maintenance and the diseases of women, primarily of their reproductive organs. **Obstetrics** is the branch of medicine that deals with the care of women throughout pregnancy. This chapter focuses on the assessment and care of nonpregnant patients with problems of the reproductive system. The assessment and care of the obstetric patient is the subject of the chapter "Obstetrics."

Anatomy and Physiology

It is essential that you have a thorough understanding of the anatomy and physiology of the female reproductive system. This knowledge will allow you to better understand, recognize, and treat gynecologic emergencies when they arise.

Female Reproductive Organs

The most important female reproductive organs are internal and are located within the pelvic cavity. These include the ovaries, fallopian tubes, uterus, and vagina, which are essential to reproduction. The external genitalia have accessory functions, in that they protect body openings and play an important role in sexual functioning.

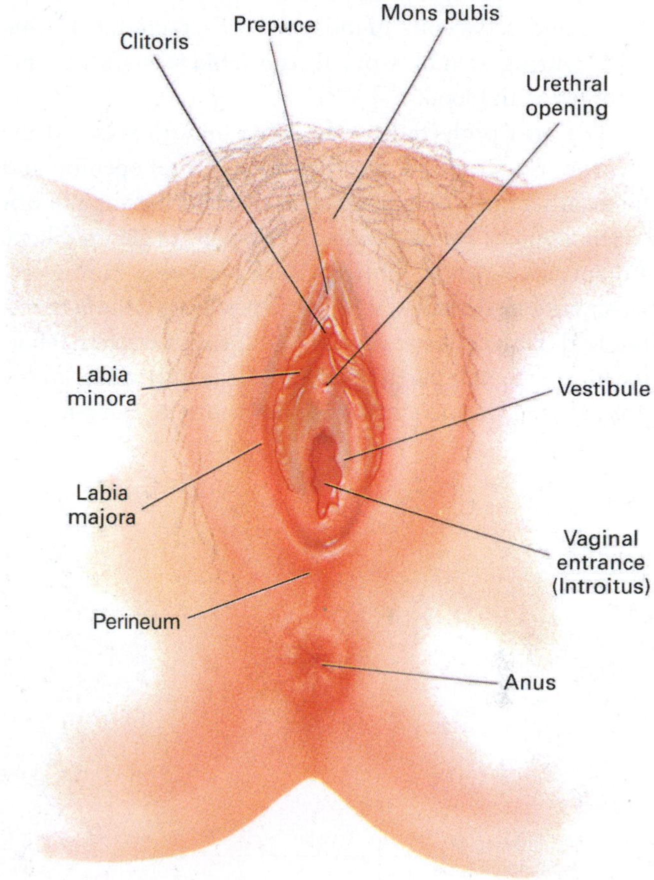

FIGURE 1-1 The vulva.

External Genitalia

The female external genitalia are known collectively as the *vulva*, or *pudendum* (Figure 1-1).

PERINEUM The *perineum* is a roughly diamond-shaped, skin-covered area of muscular tissues separating the vagina and the anus. These tissues form a slinglike structure that supports the internal pelvic organs and that is able to stretch during childbirth. This area is sometimes torn as a result of sexual assault or during childbirth. An *episiotomy*, or incision of the perineum, may be performed to facilitate delivery of the baby and to prevent spontaneous tearing, which could cause significant injury to the perineum and adjacent structures. Sometimes the term *perineum* is used to include the entire vulvar area.

MONS PUBIS The *mons pubis* is a fatty layer of tissue over the *pubic symphysis*, the junction of pubic bones. During puberty, the hormone *estrogen* causes fat to be deposited under the skin, giving it a moundlike shape. This serves as a cushion that protects the pubic symphysis during intercourse. Also during puberty, the mons becomes covered with pubic hair and its sebaceous and sweat glands become more active.

LABIA The *labia* are the structures that protect the vagina and the urethra. There are two distinct sets of labia. The *labia majora* are located laterally, whereas the *labia minora* are more medial. Both sets of labia are subject to injury during trauma to the vulvar area, such as that which occurs with sexual assault.

The labia majora are two folds of fatty tissue that arise from the mons pubis and extend to the perineum, forming a cleft. During puberty, pubic hair grows on the lateral surface, and sebaceous glands on the hairless medial surface begin to secrete lubricants. The labia majora serve to protect the inner structures of the vulva. The labia minora, lying medially within the labia majora, are two smaller, thinner folds of highly vascular tissue, well supplied with nerves and sebaceous glands, which secrete lubricating fluid. During sexual arousal, the labia minora become engorged with blood.

The area protected by the labia minora is called the *vestibule.* The vestibule contains the urethral opening and the external opening of the vagina, called the vaginal orifice, or *introitus.* The secretions of two pairs of glands (Skene and Bartholin glands) lubricate these structures during sexual stimulation. Located within the vestibule is the *hymen,* a thin fold of mucous membrane that forms the external border of the vagina, partly closing it. It is only intact in the virginal state (women who have not had intercourse).

CLITORIS The *clitoris* is highly innervated and richly vascular erectile tissue that lies anterior to the labia minora. This cylindrical structure is a major site of sexual stimulation and orgasm in women. The *prepuce* is a fold of the labia minora that covers the clitoris.

URETHRA Although not truly a part of the female reproductive system, the *urethra,* which drains the urinary bladder, is superior and anterior to the vagina. In the human female, the urethra is only 2 to 3 centimeters in length, which enables bacteria to travel more easily to the bladder than in the male. For this reason, the female is more susceptible to bladder infections than the male. As a rule, bladder infections occur more often in women once they become sexually active. In fact, after periods of prolonged sexual activity, it is not uncommon for a woman to develop a bladder infection. Sometimes this is referred to as "honeymoon cystitis."

Internal Genitalia

The internal female reproductive organs are the vagina, the uterus, the fallopian tubes, and the ovaries (Figures 1-2 and 1-3).

VAGINA The *vagina* is an elastic canal of primarily smooth muscle, 9 to 10 centimeters in length, that connects the external genitalia to the uterus. It lies between

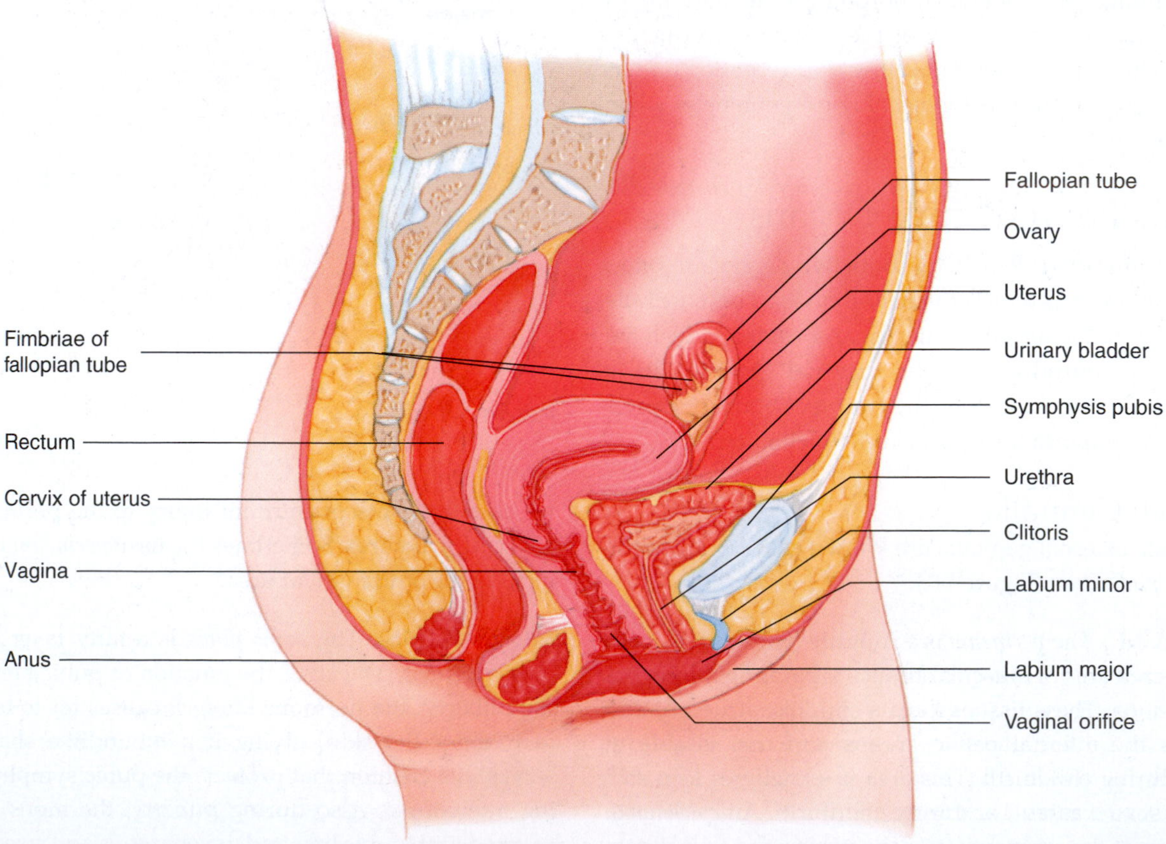

FIGURE 1-2 Cross-sectional anatomy of the female reproductive system.

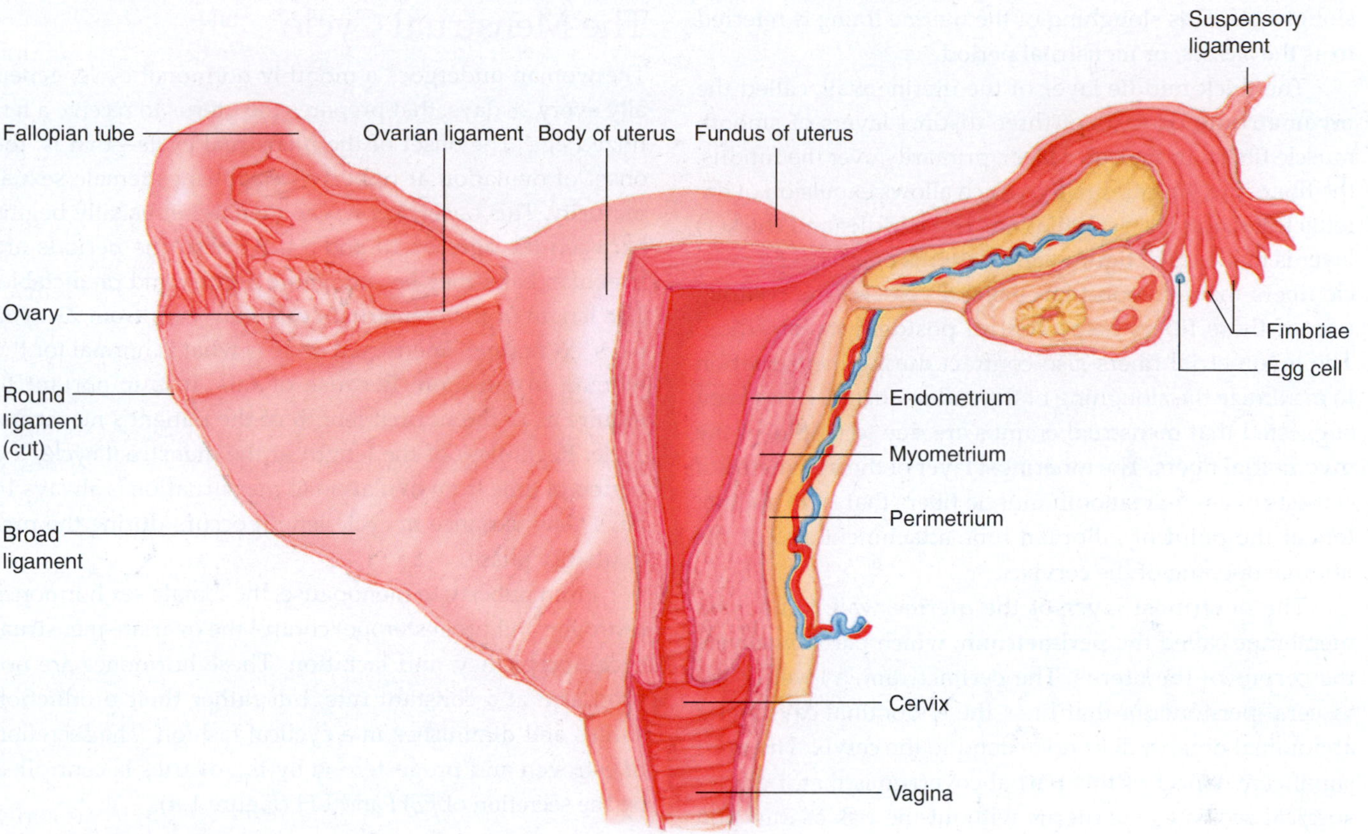

FIGURE 1-3 The uterus, fallopian tubes, and ovaries.

the urethra/bladder and the anus/rectum. Lined with mucous membrane, the vagina extends up and back from the vaginal orifice to the lower end of the uterus (cervix). The vaginal walls are crisscrossed with ridges that allow it to stretch during childbirth, allowing passage of the fetus. The vagina's primary blood supply is the vaginal artery. The pudendal nerve innervates the lower third of the vagina and the external genitalia.

The vagina has three functions:

- It is the female organ of copulation and receives the penis during sexual intercourse.
- Often called the *birth canal*, it forms the final passageway for the infant during childbirth.
- It provides an outlet for menstrual blood and tissue to leave the body.

UTERUS The *uterus* is a hollow, thick-walled, muscular, inverted-pear-shaped organ that connects with the vagina. It lies in the center of the pelvis and is flexed forward between the bladder and rectum above the vagina. Approximately 7.5 centimeters (3 inches) long and 5 centimeters (2 inches) wide, the uterus is held loosely in position by ligaments, peritoneal folds, and the pressure of adjacent abdominal structures. The primary function of the uterus is to provide a site for fetal development. During pregnancy, the uterus stretches to a size capable of containing the fetus, placenta, and the associated membranes and amniotic fluid. At term, the gravid uterus measures approximately 40 centimeters (16 inches) in length. The uterus has an extensive blood supply, primarily from the uterine arteries, which are branches of the internal iliac artery. The autonomic nervous system innervates the uterus. In a nonpregnant state, the uterine cavity is flat and triangular.

The uterus has two major parts: the *body* (or corpus) and the *cervix*, or neck. The upper two-thirds of the uterus forms the body and consists of smooth muscle layers. The lower third is the cervix.

The rounded uppermost portion of the body of the uterus is the *fundus*, which lies above the point at which the fallopian tubes attach. Measurement of fundal height (distance from the pubic symphysis to the fundus) may be used to estimate gestational age during pregnancy. The fundal height, measured in centimeters, is generally comparable to the weeks of gestation. For instance, if the fundal height is 30 centimeters, the gestational age is about 30 weeks. This method of assessing uterine size is most accurate from 22 to 34 weeks.

The body of the uterus has three layers of tissue that make up the uterine wall. The innermost layer or lining is called the **endometrium**. Each month, stimulated by estrogen and progesterone, the endometrium builds up in preparation for the implantation of a fertilized ovum. If fertilization does not occur, the lining degenerates and sloughs off. This sloughing of the uterine lining is referred to as the *menses*, or menstrual period.

The thick middle layer of the uterine wall, called the **myometrium**, consists of three distinct layers of smooth muscle fibers. In the outer layer, primarily over the fundus, the fibers run longitudinally, which allows expulsion of the fetus following cervical dilation. The middle (and thicker) layer is made up of figure-eight patterns of interlaced muscle fibers that surround large blood vessels. The contraction of these fibers helps control postdelivery bleeding. The myometrial fibers also contract during menstruation to maximize the sloughing of the endometrium. It has been suggested that menstrual cramps are due to fatigue of the myometrial fibers. The innermost layer of the myometrium consists of circular smooth muscle fibers that form sphincters at the point of fallopian tube attachment and at the internal opening of the cervix.

The outermost layer of the uterine wall is a serous membrane called the **perimetrium**, which partially covers the corpus of the uterus. The perimetrium, a layer of the visceral peritoneum that lines the abdominal cavity and abdominal organs, does not extend to the cervix. The most significant aspect of this partial coverage is that it allows surgical access to the uterus without the risk of infection that is associated with peritoneal incisions.

The cervix, or neck of the uterus, extends from the narrowest portion of the uterus to connect with the vagina. That distance forms the cervical canal and is only approximately 2.5 centimeters (1 inch) in length. Elasticity characterizes the cervix. During labor, it dilates to a diameter of approximately 10 centimeters to allow delivery of the fetus.

OVARIES The *ovaries* are the primary female gonads, or sex glands. Almond shaped, the ovaries are situated laterally on either side of the uterus in the upper portion of the pelvic cavity. The ovaries have two functions. One function is the secretion of the hormones estrogen and progesterone in response to stimulation from follicle-stimulating hormone (FSH) and luteinizing hormone (LH) secreted from the anterior pituitary gland. The second function of the ovaries is the development and release of eggs (ova) for reproduction.

FALLOPIAN TUBES The two *fallopian tubes*, also called *uterine tubes*, are thin flexible tubes that extend laterally from the uterus and curve up and over each ovary on either side. Each tube is approximately 10 centimeters (4 inches) in length and about 1 centimeter in diameter (about the size of a pencil lead), except at its ovarian end, which is trumpet shaped. Each fallopian tube has two openings, a fimbriated (fringed) end that opens into the abdominal cavity in the area adjacent to the ovaries and a minute opening into the uterus. The function of the tubes is to conduct the egg from the space around the ovaries into the uterine cavity via peristalsis (wavelike muscular contractions). Fertilization usually occurs in the distal third of the fallopian tube.

The Menstrual Cycle

The woman undergoes a monthly hormonal cycle, generally every 28 days, that prepares the uterus to receive a fertilized egg. The onset of the menstrual cycle—that is, the onset of ovulation at puberty—establishes female sexual maturity. This onset, known as **menarche**, usually begins between the ages of 10 and 14. At first, the periods are irregular. Later they become more regular and predictable. The length of the menstrual cycle may vary from 21 to 32 days. A "normal" menstrual cycle is what is normal for the woman in question. Because of this, it is important to inquire as to the normal length of the patient's menstrual cycle. Regardless of the length of the menstrual cycle, the period of time from ovulation to menstruation is always 14 days. Any variance in cycle length occurs during the preovulatory phase.

From puberty to menopause, the female sex hormones (estrogen and progesterone) control the ovarian–menstrual cycle, pregnancy, and lactation. These hormones are not produced at a constant rate, but rather their production surges and diminishes in a cyclical fashion. The secretion of estrogen and progesterone by the ovaries is controlled by the secretion of FSH and LH (Figure 1-4).

Proliferative Phase

The first two weeks of the menstrual cycle, known as the *proliferative phase*, are dominated by estrogen, which causes the uterine lining (endometrium) to thicken and become engorged with blood. In response to a surge of LH at approximately day 14, **ovulation** (release of an egg) takes place.

At birth, each female's ovary contains some 200,000 ova within immature ovarian follicles known as *graafian follicles*. This is the woman's lifetime supply of ova, which are gradually "used up" through ovulation during her lifetime.

In response to FSH and increased estrogen levels, once during every menstrual cycle, a follicle reaches maturation and ruptures, discharging its egg through the ovary's outer covering into the fallopian tube. The ruptured follicle, under the influence of LH, develops the *corpus luteum*, a small yellowish body of cells, which produces progesterone during the second half of the menstrual cycle. If the egg is not fertilized, the corpus luteum will atrophy about three days prior to the onset of the menstrual phase. If the egg is fertilized, the corpus luteum will produce progesterone until the placenta takes over that function.

The cilia (fine, hairlike structures) on the fimbriated ends of the fallopian tubes draw the egg into the tube and sweep it toward the uterus. If the woman has had sexual intercourse within approximately 24 hours of ovulation, fertilization may take place. If the egg is fertilized, it normally implants in the thickened lining of the uterus, where the fetus subsequently develops. If it is not fertilized, it passes into the uterine cavity and is expelled.

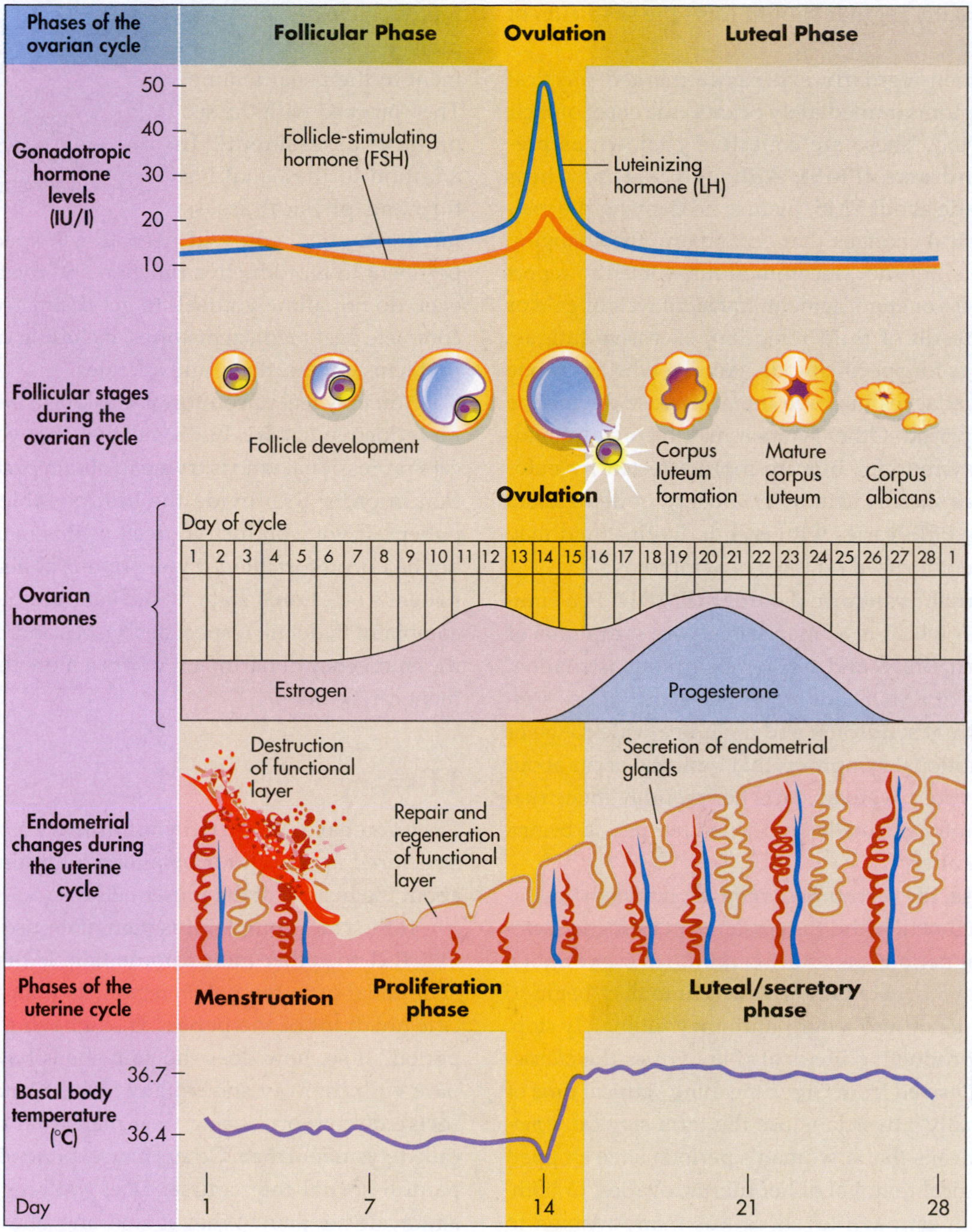

FIGURE 1-4 Phases of the menstrual cycle.

Secretory Phase

The stage of the menstrual cycle immediately surrounding ovulation is referred to as the *secretory phase*. If the egg is not fertilized, the woman's estrogen level drops sharply while the progesterone level dominates. Uterine vascularity increases during this phase in anticipation of implantation of a fertilized egg.

Ischemic Phase

If fertilization does not occur, estrogen and progesterone levels fall. Vascular changes cause the endometrium to become pale and small blood vessels to rupture.

Menstrual Phase

During the menstrual phase, the ischemic endometrium is shed, along with a discharge of blood, mucus, and cellular debris, a process known as **menstruation**. A "normal" menstrual cycle depends on the regular pattern in the individual woman. The first day of the menstrual cycle is the day on which bleeding begins; the menstrual flow usually lasts from three to five days, although this varies from woman to woman. An average blood loss of about 50 mL is common. The absence of a menstrual period in any woman in the childbearing years (generally ages 12 to 55) who is sexually active and whose periods are usually regular should raise the suspicion of pregnancy.

Some women regularly experience marked physical signs and symptoms immediately prior to the onset of their menstrual period. These are collectively known as **premenstrual syndrome (PMS)**. Although you may hear crude jokes made about PMS, there is no denying the reality of the physical changes that accompany the changing hormonal levels. It is not uncommon for women to report breast tenderness or engorgement, transient weight gain or bloating as a result of fluid retention, excessive fatigue, and/or cravings for specific foods. Women who are prone to migraine headaches may see them increase during the premenstrual period. Other women may have only minimal physical symptoms, but are more affected by emotional responses such as irritability, anxiety, or depression. The severity of PMS varies with each individual and may require treatment focused on relief of symptoms.[1]

Premenstrual dysphoric disorder (PMDD) is a similar condition in which a woman has severe symptoms of depression, irritability, and tension before menstruation. The symptoms of PMDD are more severe than those seen with premenstrual syndrome and include a wide range of physical or emotional symptoms that typically occur about 5 to 11 days before a woman starts her monthly menstrual cycle. The symptoms usually stop when her period begins or shortly thereafter.[2]

Menopause, the cessation of menses, marks the cessation of ovarian function and the cessation of estrogen secretion. Menstrual periods generally continue to occur until a woman is 45 to 55 years old, at which time they begin to decline in frequency and length until they ultimately stop. The end of reproductive life is also known as the *climacteric,* which is derived from Greek meaning "critical time of life." Occasionally, physicians use the term *surgical menopause,* which means that a woman's periods have stopped because of surgical removal of her uterus, ovaries, or both. The decrease in estrogen levels causes many women to experience hot flashes, night sweats, and mood swings during menopause. It is not uncommon for hormone replacement therapy (oral estrogen or estrogen and progesterone) to be prescribed to help relieve these complaints and to provide other health benefits associated with continuing adequate levels of these hormones.

Assessment of the Gynecologic Patient

Beyond labor and delivery, the most common emergency complaints of women in the childbearing years are abdominal pain and vaginal bleeding. Abdominal pain in women in the childbearing years is often due to problems of the reproductive organs. Complete the primary assessment in the usual manner. Then proceed with the secondary assessment. In addition to the usual history and physical assessment activities, you will need to ask specific questions pertinent to reproductive function and dysfunction. However, do not allow yourself to get distracted from getting complete past medical histories, including chronic medical problems, medications, and allergies.

CONTENT REVIEW

➤ Most Common Emergency Gynecologic Complaints
- Abdominal pain
- Vaginal bleeding

You may feel uncomfortable asking a patient about her reproductive history, but remember that you are a health care professional who is trying to obtain pertinent information in order to provide the best possible care for your patient. If you conduct yourself in this manner, it should not be uncomfortable for you or your patient. Assess your patient's emotional state. If she is reluctant to discuss her complaint in detail, respect her wishes and transport her to the emergency department, where a more thorough assessment can be done.

History

Once you have completed your primary assessment, use a structured approach for obtaining additional information about the history of the present illness.

If the chief complaint is pain, then use the mnemonic OPQRST to gather more information. Is the patient's pain abdominal or in the pelvic region? Is it localized in a specific quadrant of the pelvis? Is she having her menstrual period? If so, how does the pain she is having now compare with the way she usually feels? Some women have severe discomfort during their menstrual periods. This is called **dysmenorrhea**. Others may experience **dyspareunia**, painful sexual intercourse. Does walking or defecation aggravate her pain? What, if anything, alleviates her pain? Does positioning herself on her back or side with her knees bent relieve her discomfort?

You need to determine whether there are any associated signs or symptoms that will be helpful in determining what is wrong with your patient. For instance, does your patient report a fever or chills? Is she reporting signs of gastrointestinal problems, such as nausea, vomiting, diarrhea, or constipation? Is she complaining of urinary problems, such as frequency, painful urination, or "colicky" urinary cramping? Does she report a vaginal discharge or bleeding? If so, obtain information about the color, amount, frequency, or odors associated with either vaginal bleeding or discharge. If she reports vaginal bleeding, how does the amount compare with the volume of her usual menstrual period? Does she report dizziness with changes in position (orthostatic hypotension), syncope, or diaphoresis?

You will need to obtain specific information about her obstetric history. Has she ever been pregnant? *Gravida (G)* is the term used to describe the number of times a woman has been pregnant, including this one if she is pregnant. How many of those pregnancies ended in the delivery of a viable infant? *Para* or *parity (P)* refers to the number of deliveries. *Abortion (Ab)* refers to any pregnancy that ends before 20 weeks of gestation, regardless of cause. You may see this information recorded in shorthand—for example, G_3 P_2 Ab_1, or gravida 3, para 2, ab 1. This means that the woman has been pregnant three times and had two prior deliveries and one pregnancy that ended before 20 weeks' gestation. These terms refer to the number of pregnancies and deliveries, not the number of infants delivered, so even twins or triplets count only as one pregnancy and one delivery.

You will also need to obtain a gynecologic history. Question the patient about previous ectopic pregnancies, infections, cesarean sections, pelvic surgeries such as tubal ligation, abortions (either elective or therapeutic), and dilation and curettage (D&C) procedures. Also ask the patient about any prior history of trauma to the reproductive tract. It is often helpful to find out whether the patient, if she is sexually active, has had pain or bleeding during or after sexual intercourse.

It is important to document the date of the patient's last menstrual period, commonly abbreviated LMP (or LNMP for "last normal menstrual period"). Ask whether the period was of a normal length and whether the flow was heavier or lighter than usual. An easy way for women to estimate menstrual flow is by the number of pads or tampons used. The patient can easily compare this number to her routine usage. It is also important to inquire how regular the patient's periods tend to be. Ask her what form of birth control she uses, if any. Also, find out whether she uses it regularly. Direct questions such as "Could you be pregnant?" are generally unlikely to get an accurate response. Indirect questioning is often more helpful in determining the likelihood of pregnancy, such as "When did your last menstrual period start?" If you suspect pregnancy, inquire about other signs, including a late or missed period, breast tenderness, bloating, urinary frequency, or nausea and vomiting. Until proven otherwise, you should assume that any missed or late period is due to pregnancy even though your patient may deny it.

Contraception, or the prevention of pregnancy, takes many forms, with variable degrees of effectiveness. You should have some familiarity with the various forms, their method of action, and their reliability (Table 1-1). Remember that many contraceptives are medications, so ask about their use. With the exception of oral contraceptives ("the pill") and intrauterine devices (IUDs), side effects caused by contraceptives are relatively rare. Oral contraceptives have been associated with hypertension, rare incidents of stroke and heart attack, and possibly pulmonary embolism.

Table 1-1 Contraceptives

Type of Contraceptive	Method of Action	Effectiveness
Rhythm method	Abstinence during fertile phase—follows six to eight months of monitoring the menstrual cycle to determine fertile phase	Effective if abstinent during fertile phase; however, this is difficult to judge with precision
Coitus interruptus (withdrawal)	Penis withdrawn prior to ejaculation	Oldest and least reliable form of contraception
Condom	Barrier prevents transport of sperm	Reliable if used consistently and properly; additional benefit is that latex condoms prevent disease transmission
Vaginal ring (NuvaRing)	Transparent, flexible ring that secretes hormones similar to birth control pills; placed deep in the vagina and left for three weeks, then removed for one week (to allow for menses) and another inserted	As effective as birth control pills (99%)
Diaphragm	Barrier covers cervix to prevent entry of sperm	Reliable if fit properly and used consistently
Spermicide	Destroys sperm or neutralizes vaginal secretions to immobilize sperm	Limited effectiveness, but increases when used with a barrier device
Intrauterine device (IUD)	Unclear; either prevents implantation of fertilized egg or affects sperm motility through cervix	Highly effective
Oral contraceptives (birth control pill)	Combination of estrogen and progesterone inhibits release of egg	Highly effective
Norplant	Progestin-containing capsules cause changes in cervical mucus to inhibit sperm penetration*	Highly effective and continuous (up to six years) but requires surgical implantation
Depo-Provera	Suppresses ovulation	Highly effective and continuous (three months)
Tubal ligation	Prevents egg from being fertilized by blocking tube	Highly effective but requires surgery

IUDs can cause perforation of the uterus, uterine infection, or irregular uterine bleeding. This is especially true for IUDs that have remained in place longer than the time recommended by the manufacturer, which rarely exceeds two years.

Physical Exam

Physical examination of the gynecologic patient is limited in the field. More than at any other time, the patient's comfort level should guide your actions. Respect your patient's modesty and maintain her privacy. This may mean that you need to exclude parents from the room when assessing adolescent patients or that you need to exclude spouses of married patients. Recognizing that most people are not comfortable discussing matters related to sexuality or reproductive organs, take your cues from the patient. Maintain a professional demeanor. Explain all procedures thoroughly so your patient can understand them before you initiate any care. Some women may feel more comfortable if they can be cared for by a female paramedic.

As always, the level of consciousness is the best indicator of your patient's status. Assess your patient's general appearance, paying particular attention to the color of her skin and mucous membranes. Cyanosis and pallor may indicate shock or a gas-exchange problem, whereas a flushed appearance is more indicative of fever.

Remember that vital signs are useful clues to the nature of your patient's problem. Pain and fever tend to cause an increase in pulse and respiratory rates along with a slight increase in blood pressure. Significant bleeding will cause increased pulse and respiratory rates, as well as narrowing pulse pressures (the difference between systolic and diastolic pressures). Perform a tilt test to assess for orthostatic changes in her vital signs (a decrease in blood pressure and an increase in pulse rate when the patient rises from a supine or seated position), which again points to significant blood loss.

Assess your patient for evidence of vaginal bleeding or discharge. If possible, estimate blood loss. The use of more than two sanitary pads per hour is considered significant bleeding. If serious bleeding is reported or evident, it may be necessary to inspect the patient's perineum. Document the color and character of the discharge, as well as the amount, and the presence or absence of clots. *Do not perform an internal vaginal exam in the field.*

Pay particular attention to the abdominal examination. Auscultate the abdomen and note whether bowel sounds are absent or hyperactive. Gently palpate the abdomen. Document and report any masses, distention, guarding, localized tenderness, or rebound tenderness. In thin patients, a palpable mass in the lower abdomen may be an intrauterine pregnancy. At 3 months, the uterus is barely palpable above the symphysis pubis. At 4 months, the uterus is palpable midway between the umbilicus and the symphysis pubis. At 5 months (approximately 20 weeks), the uterus is palpable at the level of the umbilicus.

Legal Considerations

The Gynecologic Physical Exam. Fortunately, paramedics seldom have to examine a woman's genitalia. Even when necessary, all that is required is a brief look at the external structures for injury and for any evidence of hemorrhage. Always have a chaperone when examining the genitalia of any person of the opposite sex, or even of the same sex. This will protect you from possible allegations of sexual assault or inappropriate touching. Always explain to the patient what you are planning to do and talk to her throughout the examination.

With the exception of emergent treatment for a breech birth (to maintain the infant's airway) or for a prolapsed cord (to keep the baby's head off the cord), there is no reason to perform an internal vaginal examination in the field. Even significant vaginal bleeding (unless caused by a tear in the labia or introitus) cannot be controlled with packing. These patients require immediate transport, treatment for shock, and rapid gynecologic examination at the hospital.

Management of Gynecologic Emergencies

In general, the management of the patient experiencing a gynecologic emergency is focused on supportive care. Rely on your primary assessment to guide your decision making about the need for oxygen therapy, intravenous access, and analgesia. If your patient is hypoxic by pulse oximetry, administer oxygen or assist ventilation as necessary. As a rule, intravenous access and fluid replacement are usually not indicated. However, if your patient has excessive bleeding or demonstrates signs of shock, then establish at least one large-bore IV and administer normal saline at a rate indicated by the patient's presentation. You may also want to initiate cardiac monitoring if your patient is unstable. Analgesics are often required for pain management.

Continue to monitor and evaluate serious bleeding. *Do not pack dressings in the vagina.* Discourage the use of tampons to absorb blood flow. If your patient is bleeding heavily, count and document the number of sanitary pads used. If shock is not a consideration, then position your patient for comfort in the left lateral recumbent position or supine with her knees bent, as this decreases tension on the peritoneum. Opiate analgesics can help to mitigate or alleviate moderate to severe pain.

Because it is not appropriate to perform an internal vaginal exam in the field, most patients with gynecologic complaints will be transported to be evaluated by a physician. Some problems may require surgical intervention, so you should consider emergency transport to the appropriate facility based on your local protocols.

Psychological support is particularly important when caring for patients with gynecologic complaints. Keep calm. Maintain your patient's modesty and privacy. Remember that this is likely to be a very stressful situation for your patient, and she will appreciate your gentle, considerate care.

Specific Gynecologic Emergencies

Gynecologic emergencies can be generally divided into two categories—medical and traumatic.

Medical Gynecologic Emergencies

Gynecologic emergencies of a medical nature are often hard to diagnose in the field. The most common symptoms of a medical gynecologic emergency are abdominal pain and/or vaginal bleeding.

Gynecologic Abdominal Pain

PELVIC INFLAMMATORY DISEASE Probably the most common cause of nontraumatic abdominal pain is **pelvic inflammatory disease (PID)**, an infection of the female reproductive tract that can be caused by a bacterium, virus, or fungus. The organs most commonly involved are the uterus, fallopian tubes, and ovaries (Figure 1-5). Occasionally the adjoining structures, such as the peritoneum and intestines, become involved. PID is the most common cause of abdominal pain in women in the childbearing years, occurring in 1 percent of that population. The highest rate of infection occurs in sexually active women ages 15 to 24. The most common causes of PID are gonorrhea (*Neisseria gonorrhoeae*) or chlamydia (*Chlamydia trachomatis*), although rarely streptococcus or staphylococcus bacteria may cause it. Commonly, gonorrhea or chlamydia progresses undetected in a woman until frank PID develops.

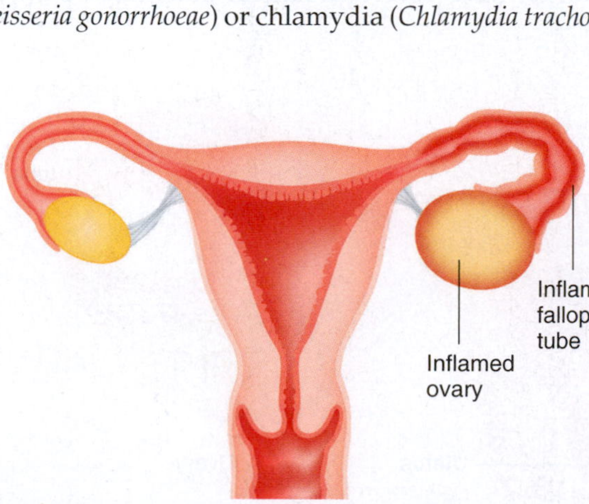

FIGURE 1-5 Pelvic inflammatory disease (PID).
(© Dorling Kindersley)

Predisposing factors include multiple sexual partners, prior history of PID, recent gynecologic procedure, or an IUD. Postinfection damage to the fallopian tubes is a common cause of infertility. PID may be either acute or chronic. If it is allowed to progress untreated, sepsis may develop. Additionally, PID may cause adhesions, in which the pelvic organs "stick together." Adhesions are a common cause of chronic pelvic pain and increase the frequency of infertility and ectopic pregnancies.

Although it is possible for a patient with PID disease to be asymptomatic, most patients with PID complain of abdominal pain, which is often diffuse and located in the lower abdomen. It may be moderate to severe, which occasionally makes it difficult to distinguish it from appendicitis. Pain may intensify either before or after the menstrual period. It may also worsen during sexual intercourse, as movement of the cervix tends to cause increased discomfort. Patients with PID tend to walk with a shuffling gait, as walking often intensifies their pain. In severe cases, fever, chills, nausea, vomiting, or even sepsis may accompany PID. Occasionally, patients have a foul-smelling vaginal discharge, often yellow in color, as well as irregular menses. It is common also to have midcycle bleeding.

Generally, on physical examination, the patient with PID appears acutely ill or toxic. The blood pressure is normal, although the pulse rate may be slightly increased. Fever may or may not be present. Palpation of the lower abdomen generally elicits moderate to severe pain. Occasionally, in severe cases, the abdomen will be tense with obvious rebound tenderness. Such cases may be impossible to distinguish from appendicitis in the prehospital setting.

The primary treatment for PID is antibiotics, often administered intravenously over an extended period. Once the causative organism is determined, the sexual partner may also require treatment. In the field, the primary goal is to make the patient as comfortable as possible. Place the patient on the ambulance stretcher in the position in which she is most comfortable. She may wish to draw her knees up toward her chest, as this decreases tension on the peritoneum. *Do not perform a vaginal examination.* If your patient has signs of sepsis, administer oxygen (if the patient is hypoxic) and establish intravenous access.[3]

RUPTURED OVARIAN CYST *Cysts* are fluid-filled pockets. When they develop in the ovary, they can rupture and be a source of abdominal pain. When an egg is released from the ovary, a cyst, known as a *corpus luteum cyst*, is often left in its place (Figure 1-6). Occasionally, cysts develop independent of ovulation. When the cysts rupture, a small amount of blood is spilled into the abdomen. Because blood irritates the peritoneum, it can cause abdominal pain and

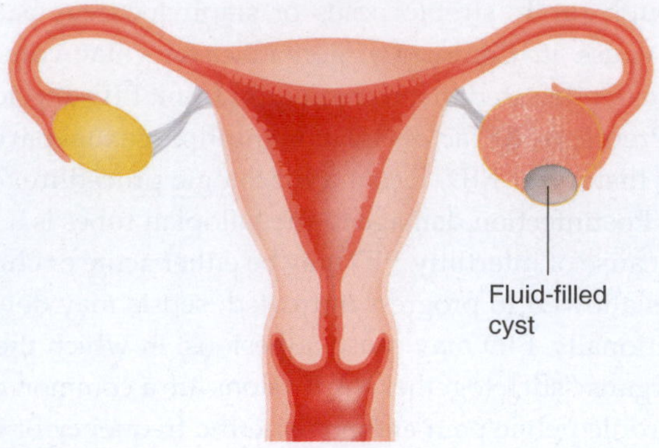

FIGURE 1-6 Large ovarian cyst.
(© Dorling Kindersley)

rebound tenderness. Ovarian cysts may be found during a routine pelvic examination. However, in the field setting, your patient is likely to complain of moderate to severe unilateral abdominal pain, which may radiate to her back. She may also report a history of dyspareunia, irregular bleeding, or a delayed menstrual period. It is not uncommon for patients to rupture ovarian cysts during intercourse or physical activity. This often results in immediate, severe abdominal pain, causing the patient to immediately stop intercourse or other physical activity. Ruptured ovarian cysts may be associated with vaginal bleeding.

CYSTITIS Urinary bladder infection, also called urinary tract infection (UTI) or **cystitis**, is a common cause of abdominal pain. Bacteria usually enter the urinary tract via the urethra, ascending into the bladder and ureters. The bladder lies anterior to the reproductive organs and, when inflamed, causes pain, generally immediately above the pubic symphysis. If untreated, the infection can progress to the kidneys. In addition to abdominal pain, your patient may report urinary frequency, pain or burning with urination (**dysuria**), and a low-grade fever. She may also complain of trouble starting and stopping her urinary stream (hesitancy). Occasionally the urine may be blood tinged.

MITTELSCHMERZ Occasionally, ovulation is accompanied by midcycle abdominal pain known as **mittelschmerz**. It is thought that the pain is related to peritoneal irritation due to follicle rupture or bleeding at the time of ovulation. The unilateral lower quadrant pain is usually self-limited and may be accompanied by midcycle spotting. Although some women may report a low-grade fever, it should be noted that body temperature normally increases at the time of ovulation and remains elevated until the day prior to the onset of the menstrual period. Treatment is symptomatic.

ENDOMETRITIS An infection of the uterine lining called **endometritis** is an occasional complication of **miscarriage**, childbirth, or gynecologic procedures such as D&C. Commonly reported signs and symptoms include mild to severe lower abdominal pain; a bloody, foul-smelling discharge; and fever (101°F to 104°F). The onset of symptoms is usually 48 to 72 hours after the gynecologic procedure or miscarriage. These infections often mimic the presentation of PID and can be quite serious if not quickly treated with the appropriate antibiotics. Complications of endometritis may include sterility, sepsis, or even death.

ENDOMETRIOSIS **Endometriosis** is a condition in which endometrial tissue is found outside the uterus. Most commonly it is found in the abdomen and pelvis, although it has been found virtually everywhere in the body, including the central nervous system and lungs. Regardless of its site, the tissue responds to the hormonal changes associated with the menstrual cycle and thus bleeds in a cyclic manner. This bleeding causes inflammation, scarring of adjacent tissues, and the subsequent development of adhesions, particularly in the pelvic cavity.

Endometriosis is usually seen in women between the ages of 30 to 40 and is rarely seen in postmenopausal women. The exact cause is unknown. The most common symptom is dull, cramping pelvic pain that is usually related to menstruation. Dyspareunia and abnormal uterine bleeding are also commonly reported. Painful bowel movements have also been reported when the endometrial tissue has invaded the gastrointestinal tract. It is not uncommon for endometriosis to be diagnosed when the patient is being evaluated for infertility. Definitive treatment may include medical management with hormones, analgesics, and antiinflammatory drugs, and/or surgery to remove the excessive endometrial tissue or adhesions from other organs.

ECTOPIC PREGNANCY An **ectopic pregnancy** is the implantation of a fetus outside the uterus. The most common site is within the fallopian tubes. This is a surgical emergency, because the tube can rupture, triggering a massive hemorrhage (Figure 1-7). Patients with ectopic pregnancy often have severe unilateral abdominal pain that

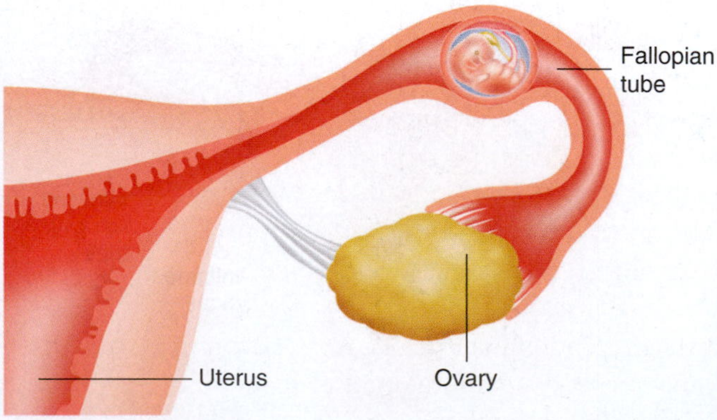

FIGURE 1-7 Ectopic (tubal) pregnancy shown in the fallopian tube.
(© Dorling Kindersley)

CONTENT REVIEW

➤ Treatment for Abdominal Pain
- Make the patient comfortable.
- Transport the patient.

may radiate to the shoulder on the affected side, a late or missed menstrual period, and, occasionally, vaginal bleeding. Additional discussion of ectopic pregnancy is presented in the "Obstetrics" chapter.[4]

Management of Gynecologic Abdominal Pain

Any woman with significant abdominal pain should be treated and transported to the hospital for evaluation. Administer oxygen (if the patient is hypoxic) and establish intravenous access if indicated. Refer to the earlier section on management of gynecologic emergencies for additional information.

Nontraumatic Vaginal Bleeding

Nontraumatic vaginal bleeding, often called *dysfunctional uterine bleeding,* is rarely seen in the field unless it is severe. Refer to the earlier section in this chapter on completing a patient history. You should not presume that vaginal bleeding is due to normal menstruation. Occasionally a woman will experience **menorrhagia**, or excessive menstrual flow, but rarely is it the cause for a 911 call. Hemorrhage, regardless of cause, is always potentially life threatening, so be alert for signs of impending shock.

The most common cause of nontraumatic vaginal bleeding is a spontaneous abortion (miscarriage). If it has been more than 60 days since your patient's LMP, you should assume that this is the cause. Vaginal bleeding due to miscarriage is often associated with cramping abdominal pain and the passage of clots and tissue. The loss of a pregnancy, even at a very early phase, is a significant emotional event for your patient, so your kind and considerate care is important. Spontaneous abortion and other causes of bleeding in the obstetric patient are discussed further in the "Obstetrics" chapter.

Another common cause of vaginal bleeding in the nonpregnant woman is the presence of uterine fibroids. Uterine fibroids—or, more correctly, *leiomyomas*—are noncancerous tumors that develop in the uterus. They are the most common pelvic tumor and can be found in 1 in 5 women of childbearing age. They typically affect women in their 30s (fourth decade of life) and are more common in African Americans than in those of Caucasian descent. The signs and symptoms of uterine fibroids include vaginal bleeding (usually between periods), heavy periods (menorrhagia), abdominal fullness or swelling, and pain during intercourse (dyspareunia). Fibroids often shrink when a woman goes through menopause and the estrogen effect is lost. Other potential causes of vaginal bleeding include cancerous lesions, PID, or the onset of labor.

Management of Nontraumatic Vaginal Bleeding

CONTENT REVIEW

➤ Treatment for Vaginal Bleeding
- Absorb blood flow, but do not pack the vagina.
- Transport the patient.
- Initiate oxygen therapy (if the patient is hypoxic) and IV access based on the patient's condition.

Your field management of patients suffering nontraumatic vaginal bleeding will depend on the severity of the situation and your assessment of the patient's status. Absorb the blood flow. *Do not pack the vagina.* If your patient is passing clots or tissue, save these for evaluation by a physician. Transport your patient in a position of comfort. The initiation of oxygen therapy (if the patient is hypoxic) and intravenous access should be guided by the patient's condition.

Traumatic Gynecologic Emergencies

Most cases of vaginal bleeding result from obstetric problems or are related to the menstrual period. However, trauma to the vagina and perineum can also cause bleeding and abdominal pain.

Causes of Gynecologic Trauma

The incidence of genital trauma is increasing, with vaginal injury occurring far more commonly than male genital injury. Gynecologic trauma may occur at any age. Blunt trauma occurs more frequently than penetrating trauma. Straddle injury (such as that which may occur while riding a bicycle) is the most common form of blunt trauma. Vaginal injuries are most often lacerations due to sexual assault. Other causes of gynecologic trauma include blunt force to the lower abdomen due to assault or seat belt injuries, direct blows to the perineal area, foreign bodies inserted into the vagina, self-attempts at abortion, and lacerations following childbirth.

Management of Gynecologic Trauma

Injuries to the external genitalia should be managed by direct pressure over the laceration or a chemical cold pack applied to a hematoma. In most cases of vaginal bleeding, the source is not readily apparent. If bleeding is severe or your patient demonstrates signs of shock, establish IV access to maintain intravascular volume and monitor vital signs closely. Blunt force may cause organ rupture, leading to the development of peritonitis or sepsis. *Never* pack the vagina with any material or dressing, regardless of the severity of the bleeding. Expedite transport to the emergency department because surgical intervention is often required.

Sexual Assault

Sexual assault continues to represent the most rapidly growing violent crime in America. More than 700,000 women are sexually assaulted annually. Unfortunately, it is estimated that more than 60 percent of all sexual assaults are never reported to authorities. Male victims represent 5 percent of reported sexual assaults. Sexual abuse of children is reported even less frequently. It is estimated that the incidence of sexual abuse in children ranges from 50,000 to 350,000 per year. There is no "typical victim" of sexual assault. No one, from small children to elderly adults, is immune.

Most victims of sexual assault know their assailants. Friends, acquaintances, intimates, and family members commit the vast majority (80 percent) of sexual assaults against women. Acquaintance rape is particularly common among adolescent victims. Sexual assault is a crime of violence, not passion, that is motivated by aggression and a need to control, humiliate, or inflict pain. There are very few predictors of who is capable of committing sexual assault, as age, economic status, and ethnic origins vary widely. Common behavioral characteristics found among rapists include poor impulse control, the need to achieve sexual satisfaction within the context of violence, and immaturity.

The definition of sexual assault varies from state to state. The common element of any definition is sexual contact without consent. Generally, rape is defined as penetration of the vagina or rectum of an unwilling female or the rectum in an unwilling male. In most states, penetration must occur for an act to be classified as rape. Sexual assault also includes oral–genital sex. Regardless of the legal definition, sexual assault is a crime of violence with serious physical and psychological implications.

ASSESSMENT The victim of sexual assault is a unique patient with unique needs. Your patient needs emergency medical treatment and psychological support. Your patient also needs to have legal evidence gathered. *Your* objectivity is essential, as your attitude may affect long-term psychological recovery. As a rule, victims of sexual abuse *should not* be questioned about the incident in the field. Do not ask questions about specific details of the assault. It is not important, from the standpoint of prehospital care, to determine whether penetration took place. Do not inquire about the patient's sexual practices. Confine your questions to the physical injuries the patient received. Even well-intentioned questions may lead to guilt feelings in the patient. Do not ask questions, for instance, such as "Why did you go with him or get in his car?"

The psychological response of sexual assault victims is widely variable. The victim of sexual assault may be withdrawn or hysterical. Some use denial, anger, or fear as defense mechanisms. Approach the patient calmly and professionally. Allay the patient's fear and anxiety. Respond to the patient's feelings, but be aware of your own. If the patient is incompletely dressed, a cover should be offered. Respect the patient's modesty. Explain all procedures and obtain the patient's permission before beginning them. Avoid touching the patient other than to take vital signs or examine other physical injuries. *Do not* examine the genitalia unless there is life-threatening hemorrhage.

In some instances, the patient may have been drugged. Flunitrazepam (Rohypnol) is the classic "date rape" drug, but any medication that alters mental status, including alcohol, can be used.[5] More recently, some of the "designer drugs," including gamma-hydroxybutyric acid (GHB), have been associated with rape. These can be placed in the victim's drink—often without the victim's knowledge.[6] Paramedics should always be concerned about the possibility of medication ingestion in any rape.

MANAGEMENT In most situations, psychological and emotional support is the most important help you can offer. Maintain a nonjudgmental attitude and assure the patient of confidentiality. If the patient is female, allow her to be cared for by a female EMT or paramedic (if available). If the patient desires, have a woman accompany her to the hospital. Provide a safe environment, such as the back of a well-lit ambulance. Respond to the patient's feelings and respect the patient's wishes. Unless your patient is unconscious, do not touch the patient unless given permission. Even when your patient appears to have an altered level of consciousness, explain what is going to be done before initiating any treatment.

Preservation of physical evidence is important. When the patient arrives at the hospital, a physician or sexual assault nurse examiner will complete a sexual assault examination to gather physical evidence. To protect this evidence, it is important that you adhere to the following guidelines:

- Consider the patient a crime scene and protect that scene.
- Handle clothing as little as possible, if at all.
- If you must remove clothing, bag separately each item that must be bagged.
- Do not cut through any tears or holes in the clothing.
- Place bloody articles in brown paper bags.
- Do not examine the perineal area.
- If the assault took place within the hour or the patient is bleeding, put an absorbent underpad (e.g., Chux) under the patient's hips to collect that evidence.
- If you cover the patient with a sheet or blanket, turn that over to the hospital as evidence.
- Do not allow patients to change their clothes, bathe, or douche (if female) before the medical examination.
- Do not allow patients to comb their hair, brush their teeth, or clean their fingernails.
- Do not clean wounds, if at all possible.
- If you must initiate care on scene, avoid disruption of the crime scene.

DOCUMENTATION When completing your patient care report, keep the following documentation guidelines in mind:

- State the patient's remarks accurately.
- Objectively state your observations of the patient's physical condition, environment, or torn clothing.
- Document any evidence (e.g., clothing, sheets) turned over to the hospital staff and the name of the individual to whom you gave it.
- Do *not* include your opinions as to whether rape occurred.

Summary

The vast majority of gynecologic emergency patients will present with abdominal pain, vaginal bleeding, or both. Even though it may be uncomfortable for the patient, it is beneficial to obtain a detailed history, including whether the patient is sexually active. Because of women's short urethras, urinary tract infections are commonplace in women, especially following periods of prolonged sexual activity.

Additional causes of abdominal pain in sexually active women can include pelvic inflammatory disease and ectopic pregnancy. In either case, the treatment for the patient remains predominantly the same, including supportive care and IV therapy as necessary to maintain normotension. If the patient does not want to divulge information, treat her for the worst-case scenario. Keep in mind that many times, especially with young teens, patients will deny having a sexual relationship even though they may have indeed had one.

When dealing with nontraumatic vaginal bleeding, the best historian will be the patient. Menarche occurs as early as the age of 10 and is the beginning of further development into sexual maturity. Initial cycles may have a slight variation to the dates and eventually lead to a regular 28-day cycle. The patient should be able to tell you where she is in her cycle and whether this type of bleeding is normal. Remember that you should *never* pack anything into the vagina, but use 5 × 9 or trauma dressings to absorb the blood flow and keep any tissue or clots that are passed. Keep the patient comfortable and treat hypotension with IV and oxygen therapy (if the patient is hypoxic).

There are few differences between the treatment of traumatic vaginal bleeding and any other traumatic bleeding. Here, again, do not pack the vagina, but apply pressure to the injury site. If the injury is secondary to an assault, keep in mind the importance of preservation of evidence, but remember to make patient care your number-one priority. Here again, treatment with IV and oxygen therapy will be largely symptom based.

Unfortunately, a paramedic can do very few things for gynecologic emergencies. General supportive care and basic IV therapy are the primary weapons for paramedics transporting patients with these types of emergencies. The patient should be placed in a position of comfort, which may include a position in which she is able to draw her knees up.

There are a variety of etiologies for female abdominal pain or vaginal bleeding. It is more important that the patient be treated symptomatically with dignity and respect than it is to have a definitive field diagnosis of endometriosis or ruptured ovarian cysts. Remember that patient care is the paramedic's top priority beyond self-safety.

You Make the Call

Late one evening in early winter, you are dispatched to a dormitory at the local university for a female patient with abdominal pain. When you arrive, the resident assistant escorts you to the room of your 17-year-old patient. There, the resident assistant introduces you to your patient and tells her that she will wait in the other room. Your patient is a slightly built young female who appears to be acutely ill. She is lying on her left side with her knees drawn up to her chest, crying quietly. Her skin is slightly flushed and diaphoretic. The tearful patient complains of excruciating lower abdominal pain that has increased in intensity over the past several hours. She says that she has not eaten today because she was too nauseated, but she denies vomiting or diarrhea.

The patient's blood pressure is 82/64 mmHg. Her pulse is 116 and thready. Respirations are 24 per minute, with a pulse oximetry reading of 95 percent. Her temperature is 104°F. Lung sounds are clear and equal bilaterally. The abdominal exam reveals diffuse tenderness over both lower quadrants. She denies any past medical problems and says that she takes no medications, including birth control pills. She denies any allergies. Her LMP was seven weeks ago, but reports that earlier that evening she noticed a foul-smelling, bloody discharge. After questioning, she admits that she found out she was pregnant a week ago, but when she told her boyfriend, he told her to "get rid of it." She reports that three days ago she had an abortion at a local clinic. Her obstetric history is gravida 1, para 0, ab 1.

1. What is your first priority?
2. What else should you do?
3. What do you suspect is the likely cause of her signs and symptoms?
4. Because your patient is a minor, do you have any legal requirements to notify her parents or obtain their consent before treating her?

See Suggested Responses at the back of this book.

Review Questions

1. The female external genitalia are known collectively as the _____
   a. labia.
   b. vulva.
   c. mons pubis.
   d. perineum.

2. What are the names for the two folds of fatty tissue that arise from the mons pubis and extend to the perineum, forming a cleft?
   a. Pudendum
   b. Labia minora
   c. Labia majora
   d. Sebaceous glands

3. The serous membrane that forms the outermost layer of the uterine wall is called the _____
   a. myometrium.
   b. endometrium.
   c. perimetrium.
   d. ectometrium.

4. Regardless of the length of the menstrual cycle, the period of time from ovulation to menstruation is typically how many days?
   a. 10
   b. 14
   c. 18
   d. 20

5. What term is used to describe the number of times a woman has been pregnant?
   a. Para (Pa)
   b. Parity (P)
   c. Gravida (G)
   d. Abortion (Ab)

6. Abdominal pain associated with ovulation is called _____
   a. dysuria.
   b. endometritis.
   c. mittelschmerz.
   d. endometriosis.

7. The most common cause of nontraumatic vaginal bleeding is _____.
   a. pelvic inflammatory disease.
   b. the onset of labor.
   c. a spontaneous abortion.
   d. a cancerous lesion.

8. In the case of sexual assault, the paramedic should _____
   a. determine whether any life-threatening physical injuries exist.
   b. respect the patient's wishes whenever possible and offer emotional support.
   c. make every effort to preserve physical evidence.
   d. do all of the above.

See Answers to Review Questions at the end of this book.

References

1. Futterman, A. and A. J. Rapkin. "Diagnosis of Premenstrual Disorders." *J Reprod Med* 51 (2006) (2 Suppl): 349–358.
2. DiGiulo, G. and E. D. Reissing. "Premenstrual Dysphoric Disorder: Prevalence, Diagnostic Considerations, and Controversies." *J Psychosom Obstet Gyneacol* 27 (2006): 201–210.
3. Crossman, S. H. "The Challenge of Pelvic Inflammatory Disease." *Am Fam Physician* 73 (2006): 859–864.
4. Kruszka, P. S. and S. J. Kruszka. "Evaluation of Acute Pelvic Pain in Women." *Am Fam Physician* 82 (2010): 141–147.
5. Schwartz, R. H., R. Milteer, and M. A. LeBeau. "Drug-Facilitated Sexual Assault ('Date Rape')." *South Med J* 93 (2000): 558–561.
6. Nemeth, Z., B. Kun, and Z. Demetrovics. "The Involvement of Gamma-Hydroxybutyrate in Reported Sexual Assaults: A Systematic Review of the Literature." *J Psychopharmacol* 24 (2010): 1281–1287.

Further Reading

Greenspan, F. S. and G. J. Strewler. *Basic & Clinical Endocrinology.* 7th ed. Stamford, CT: Appleton & Lange, 2004.

Ladewig, P. W., M. L. London, and S. B. Olds. *Contemporary Maternal-Newborn Maternal Care.* 5th ed. Menlo Park, CA: Addison Wesley Longman, 2001.

McCance, K. L. and S. E. Huether. *Pathophysiology: The Biologic Basis for Disease in Adults and Children.* 4th ed. St. Louis: C.V. Mosby, 2001.

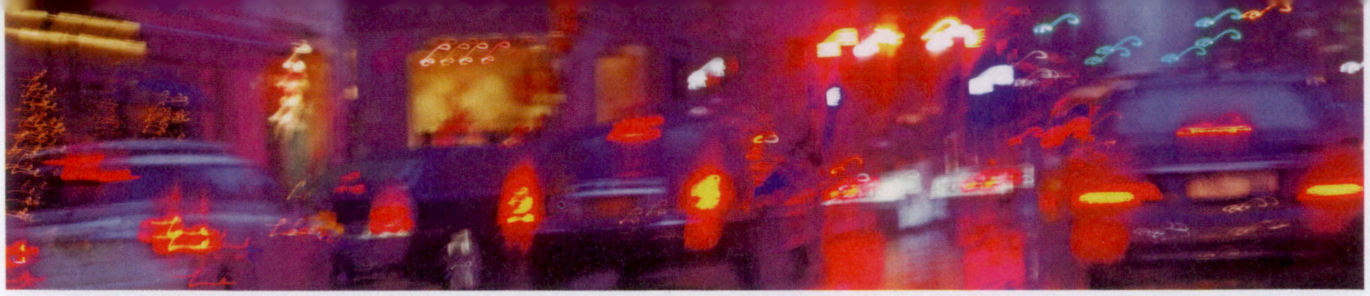

Chapter 2
Obstetrics

Bryan Bledsoe, DO, FACEP, FAAEM, EMT-P

STANDARD
Special Patient Populations (Obstetrics)

COMPETENCY
Integrates assessment findings with principles of epidemiology and pathophysiology and knowledge of psychosocial needs to formulate a field impression and implement a comprehensive treatment/disposition plan for patients with special needs.

Learning Objectives

Terminal Performance Objective: After reading this chapter, you should be able to integrate patient assessment findings, patient history, and knowledge of anatomy, physiology, pathophysiology, and basic and advanced life support interventions to recognize and manage patients with obstetric presentations.

Enabling Objectives: To accomplish the terminal performance objective, you should be able to:

1. Define key terms introduced in this chapter.
2. Relate the anatomy and physiology of pregnancy, stages of fetal development, and their effect on a woman's major body systems.
3. Use a process of clinical reasoning to guide and interpret the medical history and patient assessment findings for patients with specific obstetric presentations.
4. Discuss how to adapt the major phases of patient assessment for a female patient with complaints and presentations of both medical and traumatic etiologies related to obstetric emergencies.
5. Discuss how the paramedic should recognize, assess, and manage the female patient with preterm labor.
6. Identify indications of imminent obstetric delivery, the steps of normal delivery, and the role the paramedic has in facilitating prehospital delivery.
7. Briefly discuss the routine management of the neonate, APGAR scoring, and neonatal resuscitation.
8. Identify the types of abnormal delivery situations and other delivery complications, and the paramedic's approach to the assessment and management of these emergencies.

KEY TERMS

abortion, p. 29
afterbirth, p. 20
amniotic fluid, p. 21
amniotic sac, p. 21
aortocaval compression, p. 49
crowning, p. 28
effacement, p. 35
estimated date of confinement (EDC), p. 23
labor, p. 36
lochia, p. 37
manual lateral uterine displacement (LUD), p. 49
neonate, p. 19
ovulation, p. 20
placenta, p. 20
puerperium, p. 36
tocolysis, p. 35
umbilical cord, p. 20

Case Study

The crew members of Fire Station 32 are relaxing in the television room when, suddenly, they hear an automobile screech to a halt at the station door. The captain rushes to the door and finds an old station wagon parked out front with a man standing beside it yelling, "Help! My wife needs help!"

The whole crew spills out the door. In the back seat of the station wagon, they see a pregnant woman. She keeps saying, "The baby is coming! The baby is coming!" The ambulance normally based at Station 32 has gone out for gas. The captain notifies fire dispatch, which orders the ambulance to return. Meanwhile, the paramedics assigned to the engine learn that the patient is 29 years old and that this is her sixth pregnancy. She exclaims that she feels as if she has to move her bowels.

Now the patient begins to scream. "I've got to push! I've got to push!" she yells. The paramedics take Standard Precautions and the senior paramedic checks for crowning. He easily spots the top of the baby's head during a contraction. One member of the crew retrieves an OB kit and an oxygen bottle from the medic box on the fire engine. Shortly thereafter, the patient gives birth to a baby girl in the back of the station wagon.

At the time of delivery, the ambulance crew arrives. They assist the engine crew in cutting the cord, then dry and wrap the baby in a warming blanket. APGAR scores are 8 at 1 minute and 9 at 5 minutes. The mother receives fundal massage and an IV of normal saline solution. The paramedics then transport both mother and daughter to the hospital without incident. The father follows in the station wagon.

The next morning, as the Station 32 crewmembers are walking to their cars, they see a stork artfully painted on the window of the car belonging to the paramedic who delivered the baby.

Introduction

Pregnancy, childbirth, and the potential complications of each are the focus of this chapter. Pregnancy is a normal, natural process of life that results from ovulation and fertilization. Complications of pregnancy are uncommon, but when they do occur, you must be prepared to recognize them quickly and manage them appropriately. Complications such as hypertension or eclampsia may result from the pregnancy itself. In addition, complications such as diabetes or cardiac diseases may result from the body's responses to the pregnancy. In some cases, complications are a consequence of trauma.

Childbirth occurs daily, usually requiring only the most basic assistance, although childbirth complications do occasionally occur. These include preterm labor, multiple births, abnormal presentations, bleeding, or distressed neonates, to name but a few.

This chapter will prepare you to assess and care for the female patient throughout her pregnancy and delivery of her child.

The Prenatal Period

The *prenatal period* (literally, "prebirth period") is the time from conception until delivery of the fetus. During this period, fetal development takes place. In addition, significant physiologic changes occur in the mother. Health care visits during pregnancy are referred to as "prenatal visits" or "prenatal care."

Anatomy and Physiology of the Obstetric Patient

As you learned in the "Gynecology" chapter, the first two weeks of the menstrual cycle are dominated by the hormone estrogen, which causes the endometrium (the inner lining of the uterus) to thicken and become engorged with blood. In response to a surge of luteinizing hormone (LH) and follicle-stimulating hormone (FSH), **ovulation**, or release of an egg (ovum) from the ovary, takes place. The egg travels down the fallopian tube to the uterus. If the egg has been fertilized, it becomes implanted in the uterus and pregnancy begins. If the egg has not been fertilized, menstruation (discharge of blood, mucus, and cellular debris from the endometrium) takes place 14 days after ovulation. (The time from ovulation to menstruation is always exactly 14 days. However, the time from menstruation to the next ovulation may vary by several days from the average of 14 days, which is why it can be difficult for couples to find the optimal time of the month to conceive, or to avoid conceiving, a baby.)

If the woman has had intercourse within 24 to 48 hours before ovulation, fertilization may occur. The man's seminal fluid, carrying numerous spermatozoa, or male sex cells, enters the vagina and uterus and travels toward the fallopian tubes. Fertilization, which usually takes place in the distal third of the fallopian tube, occurs when a male spermatozoon fuses with the female ovum (Figure 2-1). After fertilization, the ovum begins cellular division immediately, which continues as it moves through the fallopian tube to the uterus. The ovum then becomes a *blastocyst* (a hollow ball of cells). The blastocyst normally implants in the thickened uterine lining, which has been prepared for implantation by the hormone progesterone, where the fetus and placenta subsequently develop.

Approximately three weeks after fertilization, the placenta develops on the uterine wall at the site where the blastocyst attached (Figure 2-2). The **placenta**, known as the "organ of pregnancy," is a temporary, blood-rich structure that serves as the lifeline for the developing fetus. It transfers heat while exchanging oxygen and carbon dioxide; delivering nutrients, such as glucose, potassium, sodium, and chloride; and carrying away wastes, such as urea, uric acid, and creatinine. The placenta also serves as an endocrine gland throughout pregnancy, secreting hormones necessary for fetal survival as well as the estrogen and progesterone required to maintain the pregnancy. Additionally, the placenta serves as a protective barrier against harmful substances. (However, some drugs, such as narcotics, steroids, and some antibiotics, are able to cross the placental membrane from the mother to the fetus.) When expelled from the uterus following birth of the child, the placenta and accompanying membranes are called the **afterbirth**.

The placenta is connected to the fetus by the **umbilical cord**, a flexible, ropelike structure approximately 2 feet (0.6 m) in length and 0.75 inch (1.9 cm) in diameter. Normally, the umbilical cord contains two arteries and one vein. The umbilical vein transports oxygenated blood to the fetus, and the umbilical arteries return relatively deoxygenated blood to the placenta.

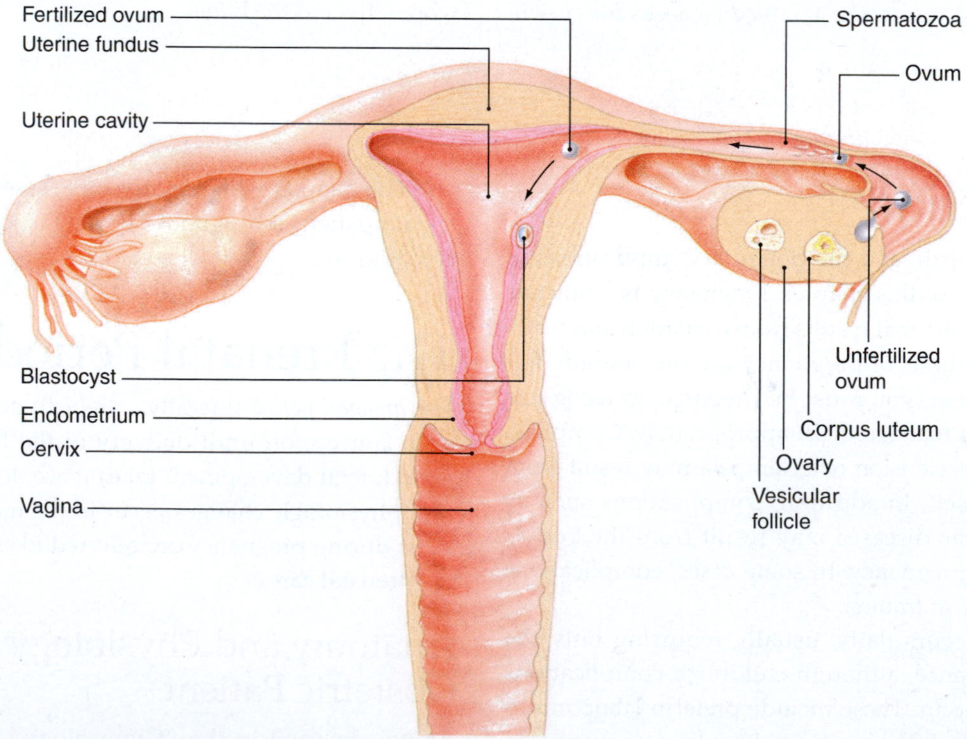

FIGURE 2-1 Fertilization and implantation of the ovum.

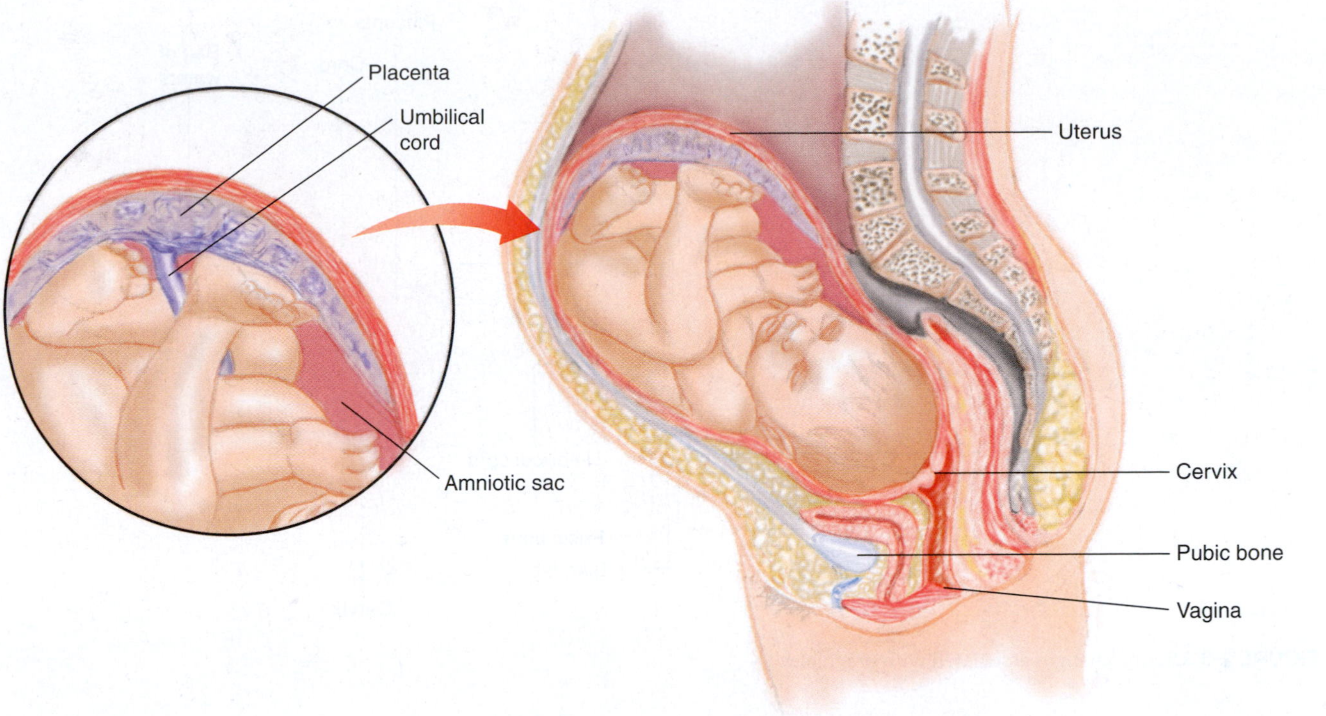

FIGURE 2-2 Anatomy of the placenta.

The fetus develops within the **amniotic sac**, sometimes called the "bag of waters" (BOW). This thin-walled membranous covering holds the **amniotic fluid** that surrounds and protects the fetus during intrauterine development. The amniotic fluid increases in volume throughout the course of the pregnancy. After the 20th week of gestation, the volume varies from 500 to 1,000 mL. The presence of amniotic fluid allows for fetal movement within the uterus and serves to cushion and protect the fetus from trauma. The volume changes constantly as amniotic fluid moves back and forth across the placental membrane. During the latter part of the pregnancy, the fetus contributes to the volume by secretions from the lungs and urination. Although it may rupture earlier, the amniotic sac usually breaks during labor, and the amniotic fluid or "water" flows out of the vagina. This is called *rupture of the membranes* (ROM). This is what has happened when the pregnant woman says, "My water has broken."

Physiologic Changes of Pregnancy

The physiologic changes associated with pregnancy are due to an altered hormonal state, the mechanical effects of the enlarging uterus and its significant vascularity, and the increasing metabolic demands on the maternal system. It is important for you to understand the physiologic changes associated with pregnancy so you can better assess your pregnant patients.

REPRODUCTIVE SYSTEM It is understandable that the most significant pregnancy-related changes occur in the uterus. In its nonpregnant state, the uterus is a small pear-shaped organ weighing about 60 g (2 oz) with a capacity of approximately 10 mL. By the end of pregnancy, its weight has increased to 1,000 g (slightly more than 2 pounds), and its capacity is now approximately 5,000 mL (Figure 2-3). Another notable change is that during pregnancy, the vascular system of the uterus contains about one-sixth (16 percent) of the mother's total blood volume.

Other changes occurring in the reproductive system include the formation of a mucus plug in the cervix that protects the developing fetus and helps to prevent infection. This plug will be expelled when cervical dilation begins prior to delivery. Estrogen causes the vaginal mucosa to thicken, vaginal secretions to increase, and the connective tissue to loosen to allow for delivery. The breasts enlarge and become more nodular as the mammary glands increase in number and size in preparation for lactation.

RESPIRATORY SYSTEM During pregnancy, maternal oxygen demands increase. To meet this need, progesterone causes a decrease in airway resistance. This results in a 20 percent increase in oxygen consumption and a 40 percent increase in tidal volume. There is only a slight increase in respiratory rate. The diaphragm is pushed up by the enlarging uterus, resulting in flaring of the rib margins to maintain intrathoracic volume.

CARDIOVASCULAR SYSTEM Various changes take place in the cardiovascular system during pregnancy

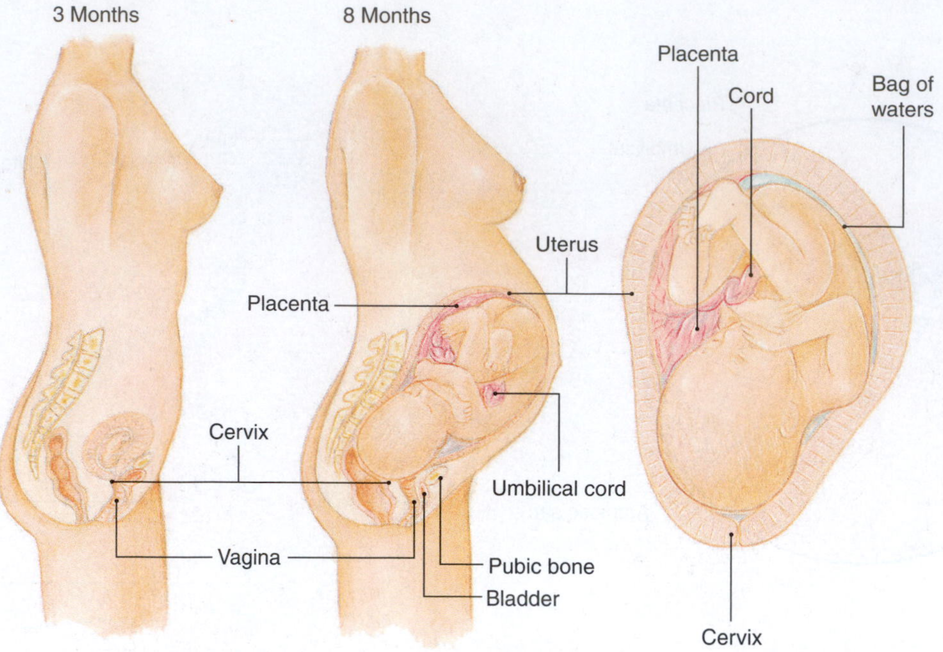

FIGURE 2-3 Uterine changes associated with pregnancy.

(Figure 2-4). Cardiac output increases by 30 to 50 percent throughout pregnancy, peaking at 6 to 7 liters/minute by the time the fetus is fully developed. Systemic vascular resistance decreases. The maternal blood volume increases by 45 percent and, although both red blood cells and plasma increase, there is slightly more plasma, resulting in a relative anemia. To combat this anemia, pregnant women receive supplemental iron to increase the oxygen-carrying capacity of their red blood cells. Because of the increase in blood volume, the pregnant woman may suffer an acute blood loss of 30 to 35 percent without a significant change in vital signs. The maternal heart rate increases by 10 to 15 beats/minute. Blood pressure decreases slightly during the first two trimesters of pregnancy and then rises to near nonpregnant levels during the third trimester.

Supine hypotensive syndrome occurs when the gravid uterus compresses the inferior vena cava when the mother lies in a supine position, causing decreased venous return to the right atrium, which lowers blood pressure. Current research suggests that the abdominal aorta may also be compressed. The enlarging uterus also may press on the pelvic and femoral vessels, causing impaired venous return from the legs and venous stasis. This may lead to the development of varicose veins, dependent edema, and postural hypotension. Some patients are predisposed to this problem because of an overall decrease in circulating blood volume or because of anemia. Assessment and management of supine hypotensive syndrome are discussed later in this chapter.

GASTROINTESTINAL SYSTEM Nausea and vomiting are common in the first trimester as a result of hormone levels and changed carbohydrate needs. Peristalsis is slowed, so delayed gastric emptying is likely and bloating or constipation is common. As the uterus enlarges, abdominal organs are compressed, and the resulting compartmentalization of abdominal organs makes assessment difficult.

URINARY SYSTEM Renal blood flow increases during pregnancy. The glomerular filtration rate increases by nearly 50 percent in the second trimester and remains elevated throughout the remainder of the pregnancy. As a result, the renal tubular absorption also increases. Occasionally, glucosuria (large amounts of sugar in the urine) may result from the kidney's inability to reabsorb all of the glucose being filtered. Glucosuria may be normal or may indicate the development of gestational diabetes. The urinary bladder gets displaced anteriorly and superiorly, increasing the potential for rupture. Urinary frequency is common, particularly in the first and third trimesters, as a result of uterine compression of the bladder.

MUSCULOSKELETAL SYSTEM Loosened pelvic joints caused by hormonal influences account for the waddling gait that is often associated with pregnancy. As the uterus enlarges and the mother's center of gravity changes, postural changes take place to compensate for anterior growth, causing low back pain.

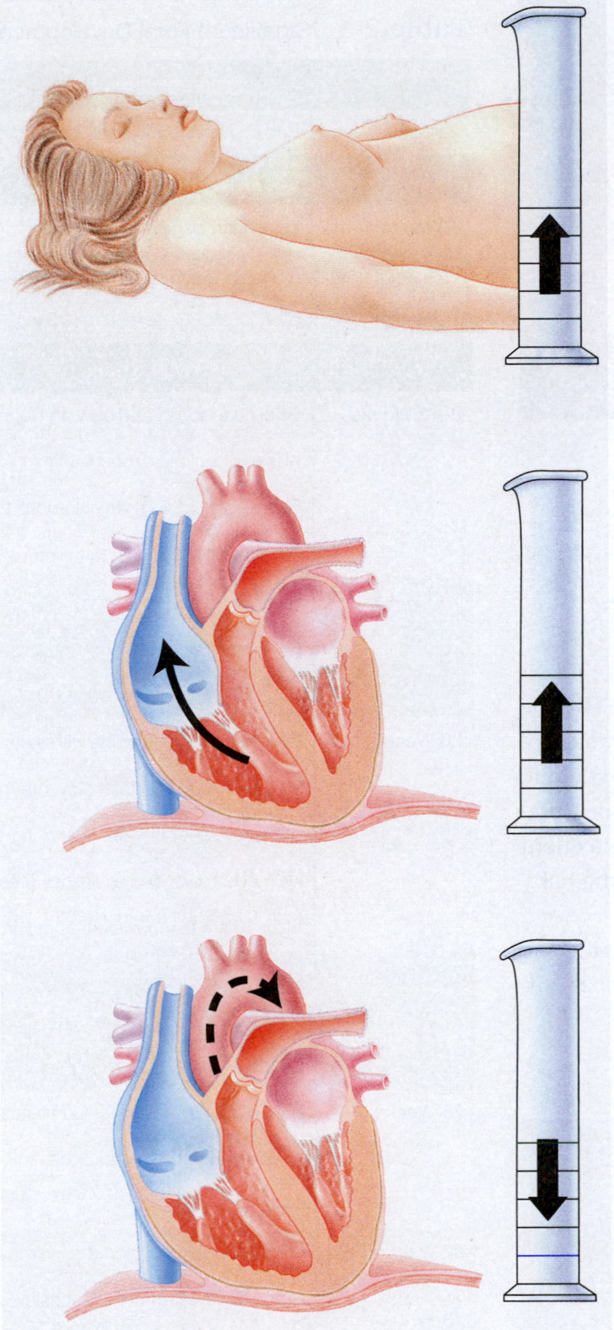

FIGURE 2-4 The hemodynamic changes of pregnancy.

Fetal Development

Fetal development begins immediately after fertilization and is quite complex. The time at which fertilization occurs is called *conception*. Because conception occurs approximately 14 days after the first day of the last menstrual period, it is possible to calculate, with fair accuracy, the approximate date the baby should be born. This estimate is usually made during the mother's first prenatal visit. The normal duration of pregnancy is 40 weeks from the first day of the mother's last menstrual period. This is equal to 280 days, which is 10 lunar months or, roughly, 9 calendar months. This estimated birth date is commonly called the *due date*. Medically, it is known as the **estimated date of confinement (EDC)** or *estimated date of delivery (EDD)*. Generally, pregnancy is divided into *trimesters*. Each trimester is approximately 13 weeks, or 3 calendar months, long.

During the course of pregnancy, several different terms are used to describe the stages of development. The *preembryonic stage* covers the first 14 days following conception. The *embryonic stage* begins at day 15 and ends at approximately 8 weeks (Figures 2-5 and 2-6). The period from 8 weeks until delivery is known as the *fetal stage*. As a paramedic, you should be familiar with some of the significant

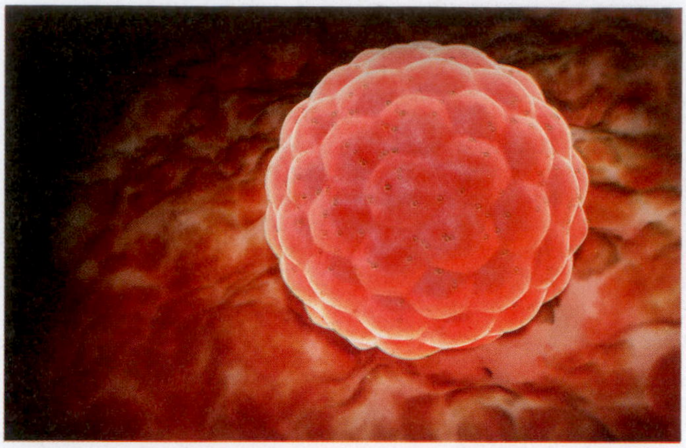

FIGURE 2-5 Human embryo at time of implantation.
(© MedicalRF/Science Source)

developmental milestones that occur during these three periods (Table 2-1).

During normal fetal development, the sex of the infant can usually be determined by 16 weeks' gestation. By the 20th week, *fetal heart tones (FHTs)* can be detected by stethoscope. The mother also has generally felt fetal movement. By 24 weeks, the baby may be able to survive if born prematurely. Fetuses born after 28 weeks have an excellent chance of survival (Figure 2-7). By the 38th week the baby is considered *term*, or fully developed.

Most of the fetus's organ systems develop during the first trimester. Therefore, this is when the fetus is most vulnerable to the development of birth defects.

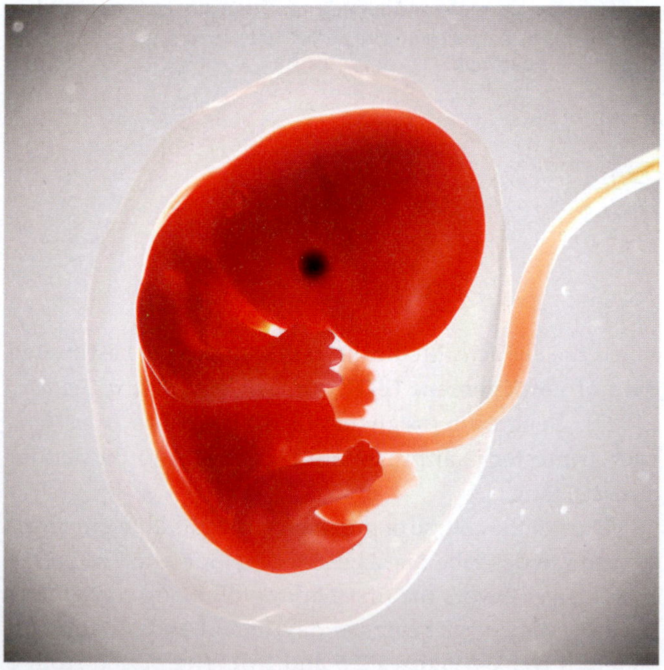

FIGURE 2-6 Human fetus at 7 weeks of development.
(© SciPro/Science Source)

Table 2-1 Significant Fetal Development Milestones

Preembryonic Stage	
2 Weeks	Rapid cellular multiplication and differentiation
Embryonic Stage	
4 Weeks	Fetal heart begins to beat
8 Weeks	All body systems and external structures are formed Size: approximately 3 cm (1.2 in.)
Fetal Stage	
8–12 Weeks	Fetal heart tones audible with Doppler Kidneys begin to produce urine Size: 8 cm (3.2 in.), weight about 1.6 oz Fetus most vulnerable to toxins
16 Weeks	Sex can be determined visually Swallowing amniotic fluid and producing meconium Looks like a baby, although thin
20 Weeks	Fetal heart tones audible with stethoscope Mother able to feel fetal movement Baby develops schedule of sucking, kicking, and sleeping Hair, eyebrows, and eyelashes present Size: 19 cm (8 in.), weight approximately 16 oz
24 Weeks	Increased activity Begins respiratory movement Size: 28 cm (11.2 in.), weight 1 lb 10 oz
28 Weeks	Surfactant necessary for lung function is formed Eyes begin to open and close Weighs 2–3 lb
32 Weeks	Bones are fully developed but soft and flexible Subcutaneous fat being deposited Fingernails and toenails present Weighs 3–4 lb
38–40 Weeks	Considered to be full term Baby fills uterine cavity Baby receives maternal antibodies

Fetal Circulation

The fetus receives its oxygen and nutrients from its mother through the placenta. Thus, while in the uterus, the fetus does not need to use its respiratory system or its gastrointestinal tract. Because of this, the fetal circulation shunts blood around the lungs and gastrointestinal tract.

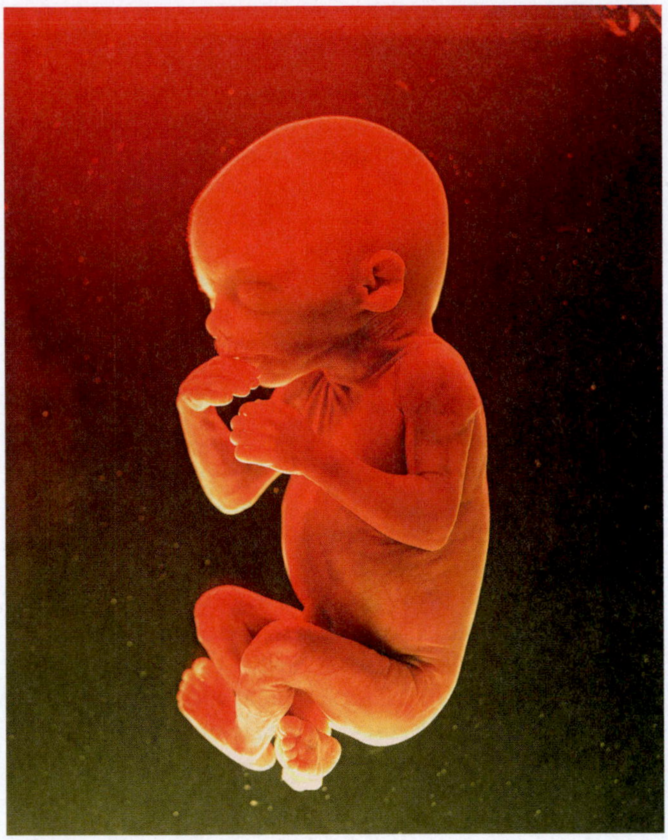

FIGURE 2-7 Mature human fetus.

(© James Stevenson/Science Source)

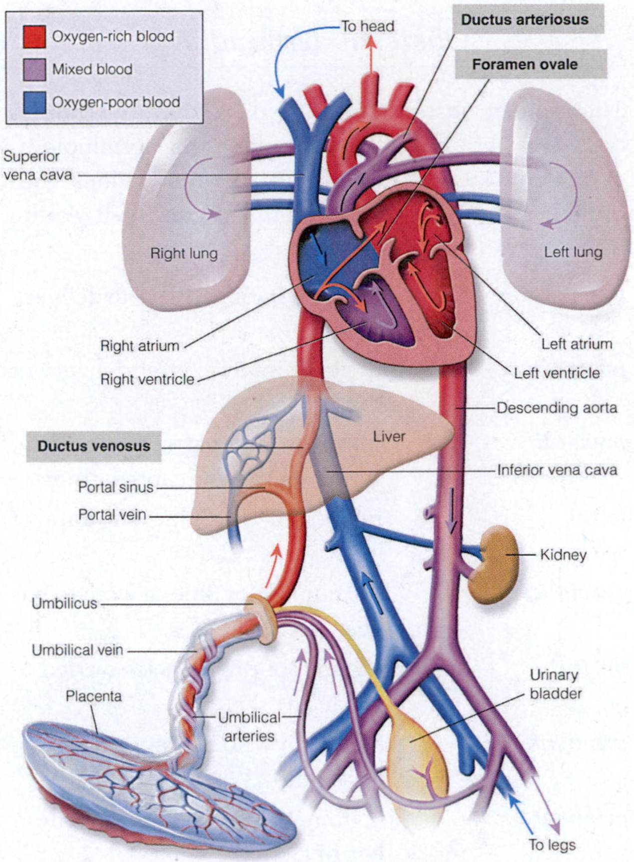

FIGURE 2-8 The maternal-fetal circulation.

The infant receives his blood from the placenta by means of the umbilical vein (Figure 2-8). The umbilical vein connects directly to the inferior vena cava by a specialized structure called the *ductus venosus.* Blood then travels through the inferior vena cava to the heart. The blood enters the right atrium and passes through the tricuspid valve into the right ventricle. It then exits the right ventricle and travels through the pulmonic valve into the pulmonary artery. The fetus's heart has a hole between the right and left atria, termed the *foramen ovale,* which allows mixing of the oxygenated blood in the right atrium with that leaving the left ventricle bound for the aorta. This serves to aid in blood flow bypassing the lungs.

At this time, the blood is still oxygenated. Once in the pulmonary artery, the blood enters the *ductus arteriosus,* which connects the pulmonary artery with the aorta. The ductus arteriosus causes blood to bypass the uninflated lungs. Once in the aorta, blood flow is basically the same as in extrauterine life. Deoxygenated blood containing waste products exits the fetus, after passage through the liver, via the umbilical arteries.

The fetal circulation changes shortly after birth. As soon as the baby takes his first breath, the lungs inflate, greatly decreasing pulmonary vascular resistance to blood flow. The ductus arteriosus closes, diverting blood to the lungs. In addition, the ductus venosus closes, stopping blood flow from the placenta. The foramen ovale also closes as a result of pressure changes in the heart, which stops blood flow from the right to left atrium.

General Assessment of the Obstetric Patient

Primary Assessment

The initial approach to the obstetric patient should be the same as for the nonobstetric patient, with special attention paid to the developing fetus. Complete the primary assessment quickly and then obtain essential obstetric information.

History

The SAMPLE history will allow you to gain specific information about the mother's situation, as well as her pertinent medical history.

General Information

You will want to obtain information about the pregnancy, such as the mother's gravidity and parity, the length of

Obstetric Terminology

The field of obstetrics has its own unique terminology. You should be familiar with this terminology, as patient documentation and communications with other health care workers and physicians often require it.

antepartum	the time interval prior to delivery of the fetus
postpartum	the time interval after delivery of the fetus
prenatal	the time interval prior to birth, synonymous with antepartum
natal	relating to birth or the date of birth
gravidity*	the number of times a woman has been pregnant
parity*	number of pregnancies carried to full term
primigravida	a woman who is pregnant for the first time
primipara	a woman who has given birth to her first child
multigravida	a woman who has been pregnant more than once
nulligravida	a woman who has not been pregnant
multipara	a woman who has delivered more than one baby
nullipara	a woman who has yet to deliver her first child
grand multipara	a woman who has delivered at least seven babies
gestation	period of time for intrauterine fetal development

*The gravidity and parity of a woman is expressed in the following "shorthand": G4P2. "G" refers to the gravidity, and "P" refers to the parity. The woman in this example would have had four pregnancies and two births.

Cultural Considerations

The Importance of Prenatal Care. Women have delivered babies without any form of medical assistance for thousands of years. The introduction of obstetric practice and prenatal care has made it safe. Prenatal care should be started as soon as the pregnancy is known. It includes screening for diseases, nutritional guidance, parenting skills education, and preparations for delivery and postnatal care. Prenatal care also will help to identify potential problems early and has served to lower the infant mortality rate in industrialized countries where it is provided. For example, the island nation of Cuba has a comprehensive prenatal care system and now is able to boast an infant mortality rate that is lower than that of the United States.

The United States is still a land of opportunity, and EMS systems along the border with Mexico encounter patients who have come into this country to deliver their babies. Often, these women are economic refugees and have had limited or no prenatal care. Thus, they are at higher risk of developing complications related to their pregnancy. Several national and international organizations offer programs that provide low-cost or no-cost prenatal care and are open to patients no matter what their citizenship status.

gestation, and the estimated due date, if known. In addition, you should determine whether the patient has had any cesarean sections or any gynecologic or obstetric complications in the past. It is also important to ascertain whether the patient has had any prenatal care. Determine what type of health care professional (physician or nurse midwife) is providing her care and when she was last evaluated. Ask the patient whether a sonogram examination was done. A sonogram reveals the age of the fetus, the presence of more than one fetus, abnormal presentations, and certain birth defects. A general overview of the patient's current state of health is important. Pay particular attention to current medications and drug and/or medication allergies.

Preexisting or Aggravated Medical Conditions

Pregnancy aggravates many preexisting medical conditions and may trigger new ones.

DIABETES Previously diagnosed diabetes can become unstable during pregnancy owing to altered insulin requirements. Diabetics are at increased risk of developing preeclampsia and hypertension (discussed later in this chapter). Pregnancy may also accelerate the progression of vascular disease complications of diabetes. It is not uncommon for pregnant diabetics to have problems with fluctuating blood sugar levels, causing hypoglycemic or hyperglycemic episodes. In addition, many patients develop diabetes during pregnancy (*gestational diabetes*). Pregnant diabetics cannot be managed with oral hypoglycemic agents because these drugs tend to cross the placenta and affect the fetus. Therefore, all pregnant diabetics are placed on insulin if their blood sugar levels cannot be controlled by diet alone. It has been shown that maintaining careful control of the mother's blood sugar between 70 and 120 mg/dL reduces risks to the mother and fetus.[1]

Diabetes also affects the infant. Infants of diabetic mothers, especially those with poorly controlled blood sugar levels, tend to be large. This complicates delivery. Such infants also may have trouble maintaining body temperature after birth and may be subject to hypoglycemia. Babies born to diabetic mothers are also at increased risk of congenital anomalies (birth defects).

HEART DISEASE During pregnancy, cardiac output increases up to 30 percent. Patients who have serious preexisting heart disease may develop congestive heart failure in pregnancy. When confronted by a pregnant patient in obvious or suspected heart failure, inquire about preexisting heart disease or murmurs. It is important to be aware, however, that most patients develop a quiet systolic flow murmur during pregnancy. This is caused by increased cardiac output and is rarely a source of concern.

HYPERTENSION Hypertension is also aggravated by pregnancy. Generally, blood pressure is lower in pregnancy than in the nonpregnant state. However, women who were borderline hypertensive before becoming pregnant may become dangerously hypertensive when pregnant. Furthermore, many common blood pressure medications cannot be used during pregnancy. In addition, preeclampsia (discussed later in this chapter) may contribute to maternal hypertension. Persistent hypertension may adversely affect the placenta, thus compromising the fetus as well as placing the mother at increased risk for stroke, seizure, or renal failure.

SEIZURE DISORDERS Most women with a history of seizure disorders controlled by medication have uneventful pregnancies and deliver healthy babies. However, women who have poorly controlled seizure disorders are likely to have increased seizure activity during pregnancy. Medications to control seizures are commonly administered throughout the pregnancy.

NEUROMUSCULAR DISORDERS Disabilities associated with neuromuscular disorders, such as multiple sclerosis, may be aggravated by pregnancy. However, it is more common that pregnant women enjoy remission of symptoms during pregnancy and a slight increase in relapse rate during the postpartum period. The strength of uterine contractions is not diminished in these patients. Also, their subjective sensation of pain is often less than that seen in other patients.

Pain

If the patient is in pain, try to determine when the pain started and whether its onset was sudden or slow. Also, attempt to define the character of the pain—its duration, location, and radiation, if any. It is especially important to determine whether the pain is occurring on a regular basis.

Vaginal Bleeding

The presence of vaginal bleeding or spotting is a major concern in an obstetric patient. Ask about events immediately prior to the start of bleeding. You also need to gain information about the color, amount, and duration of bleeding. To assess the amount of bleeding, count the number of sanitary pads or tampons used. If your patient is passing clots or tissue, save this material for evaluation. In addition, question the patient about the presence of other vaginal discharges, as well as the color, amount, and duration.

Active Labor

When confronted with a patient in active labor, assess whether the mother feels the need to push or has the urge to move her bowels. Determine whether the patient thinks her membranes have ruptured. Patients often sense this as a dribbling of water or, in some cases, a true gush of water.

Physical Examination

Physical examination of the obstetric patient is essentially the same as that for any emergency patient. However, you should be particularly careful to protect the patient's modesty as well as to maintain her dignity and privacy.

When examining a pregnant patient, first estimate the date of the pregnancy by measuring the *fundal height*. The fundal height is the distance from the pubic symphysis to the top of the uterine fundus. Each centimeter of fundal height roughly corresponds to a week of gestation. For example, a woman with a fundal height of 24 centimeters has a gestational age of approximately 24 weeks. If the fundus is just palpable above the pubic symphysis, the pregnancy is about 12 to 16 weeks' gestation. When the uterine fundus reaches the umbilicus, the pregnancy is about 20 weeks. As pregnancy reaches term, the fundus is palpable near the xiphoid process. If fetal movement is felt when the abdomen is palpated, the pregnancy is at least 20 weeks. Fetal heart tones can be heard by stethoscope at approximately 18 to 20 weeks. The normal fetal heart rate ranges from 140 to 160 beats per minute.

Generally, vital signs in the pregnant patient should be taken with the patient lying on her left side. As noted earlier, as pregnancy progresses, the uterus increases in size. Ultimately, when the patient is supine, the weight of the uterus compresses the inferior vena cava, severely compromising venous blood return from the lower extremities. Turning the patient to her left side alleviates this problem. Occasionally, it may be helpful to check orthostatic vital signs. First, obtain the blood pressure and pulse rate after the patient has rested for 5 minutes in the left lateral recumbent position. Then repeat the vital signs with the patient sitting up or standing. A drop in the blood pressure level of 15 mmHg or more, or an increase in the pulse rate of 20 beats per minute or more, is considered significant and should be reported and documented. When performing this maneuver, it is always important to be alert for syncope. This procedure should *not* be performed if the patient is in obvious shock.

You may need to examine the genitals to evaluate any vaginal discharge, the progression of labor, or the presence of a *prolapsed cord,* an umbilical cord that comes out of the uterus ahead of the fetus. This can be accomplished simply by looking at the perineum. If, during the physical examination, the patient reports that she feels the need to push, or if she feels as though she must move her bowels, examine her for crowning. **Crowning** is the bulging of the fetal head past the opening of the vagina during a contraction. Crowning is an indication of impending delivery. Examine for crowning only during a contraction. *Do not perform an internal vaginal examination in the field.*

General Management of the Obstetric Patient

The first consideration for managing emergencies in obstetric patients is to remember that you are, in fact, caring for two patients—the mother and the fetus. Fetal well-being is dependent on maternal well-being. Also keep in mind that your calm, professional demeanor and caring attitude will go a long way in reducing the emotional stress during any obstetric emergency. Remember to protect your patient's privacy and maintain her modesty.

The physiologic priorities for obstetric emergencies are identical to those for any other emergency situation. Focus your efforts on maintaining the airway, breathing, and circulation. Administer oxygen, if needed, to correct hypoxia. Initiate intravenous access by using a large-bore catheter in a large vein and consider fluid resuscitation based on your local protocols. If your patient is bleeding or showing signs of shock, establish two IV lines. Cardiac monitoring is also appropriate. Place your patient in a position of comfort, but remember that the left lateral recumbent position is preferred after the 24th week.

If pain is the primary complaint, administer analgesics such as morphine. However, analgesics should be used with caution, as they can alter your ability to assess a deteriorating condition as well as other changes in patient status and may negatively affect the fetus. Nitrous oxide is the preferred analgesic in pregnancy, but narcotics are acceptable.

When transport is indicated, transport immediately to a hospital that is capable of managing emergency obstetric and neonatal care. Report the situation to the receiving hospital prior to your arrival, as emergency department personnel may want to summon obstetrics department staff to assist with patient care.

Complications of Pregnancy

Pregnancy is a normal process. However, women who are pregnant are not immune from injury or other health problems. There may also be complications associated with the pregnancy itself.

Trauma

Paramedics frequently receive calls to help a pregnant woman who has been in a motor vehicle accident or who has sustained a fall. In pregnancy, syncope occasionally occurs (studies show that between 5 and 30 percent of pregnant women experience syncope). The syncope of pregnancy often results from compression of the inferior vena cava, as described earlier, or from normal changes in the cardiovascular system associated with pregnancy. Also, the weight of the gravid uterus alters the patient's balance, making her more susceptible to falls.

Pregnant victims of major trauma are more susceptible to life-threatening injury than are nonpregnant victims because of the increased vascularity of the gravid uterus. Trauma is the most frequent nonobstetric cause of death in pregnant women. Some form of trauma, usually a motor vehicle crash or a fall and even physical abuse, can occur in 6 to 7 percent of all pregnancies. Because the primary cause for fetal mortality is maternal mortality, the pregnant trauma patient presents a unique challenge. The later in the pregnancy, the larger the uterus and the greater the likelihood of injury. All patients at 20 weeks' (or more) gestation with a history of direct or indirect injury should be transported for evaluation by a physician.

Paramedics should *anticipate* the development of shock based on the mechanism of injury rather than waiting for overt signs and symptoms. Because of the cardiovascular changes of pregnancy, overt signs of shock are late and inconsistent. Trauma significant enough to cause maternal shock is associated with a 70 to 80 percent fetal mortality. In the face of acute blood loss, significant vasoconstriction will occur in response to catecholamine release, resulting in maintenance of a normotensive state for the mother. However, this causes significant uterine hypoperfusion (20 to 30 percent decrease in cardiac output) and fetal bradycardia.

Generally, the amniotic fluid cushions the fetus from blunt trauma fairly well. However, in direct abdominal trauma, the pregnant patient may suffer premature separation of the placenta from the uterine wall, premature labor, abortion, uterine rupture, and possibly fetal death. The presence of vaginal bleeding or a tender abdomen in a pregnant patient should increase your suspicion of serious injury. Fetal death may result from death of the mother, separation of the placenta from the uterine wall, maternal shock, uterine rupture, or fetal head injury. Any pregnant patient who has suffered trauma should be immediately transported to the emergency department and evaluated by a physician. Trauma management essentials include the following:

- Apply a C-collar to provide cervical stabilization and immobilize on a long backboard.
- Administer oxygen if the patient is hypoxic.
- Initiate two large-bore IVs for crystalloid administration per protocol.
- Transport tilted to the left to minimize supine hypotension.
- Reassess frequently.
- Monitor the fetus.

Medical Conditions

The pregnant patient is subject to all the medical problems that occur in the nonpregnant state. Abdominal pain is a common complaint. It is often caused by the stretching of the ligaments (e.g., round ligament) that support the growing uterus. However, appendicitis and cholecystitis can also occur. Pregnant women are at increased risk of developing gallstones as a result of hormonal influences that delay emptying of the gallbladder. In pregnancy, the abdominal organs are displaced because of the increased mass of the gravid uterus in the abdomen, which makes assessment more difficult. The pregnant patient with appendicitis may complain of right upper quadrant pain or even back pain. The symptoms of acute cholecystitis may also differ from those in nonpregnant patients. Any pregnant patient with abdominal pain should be evaluated by a physician.

Bleeding in Pregnancy

Vaginal bleeding may occur at any time during pregnancy. Bleeding is usually due to abortion, but can also occur with ectopic pregnancy, placenta previa, or abruptio placentae. Generally, the exact etiology of vaginal bleeding during pregnancy cannot be determined in the field. Refer to the earlier discussion in this chapter and your own local protocols for management of obstetric emergencies. Vaginal bleeding is associated with potential fetal loss. Keep in mind that this is an emotional and stressful situation for your patient, so a professional, caring demeanor is imperative.

CONTENT REVIEW

➤ Causes of Bleeding during Pregnancy
- Abortion
- Ectopic pregnancy
- Placenta previa
- Abruptio placentae

Abortion

Abortion, the expulsion of the fetus prior to 20 weeks' gestation, is the most common cause of bleeding in the first and second trimesters of pregnancy. The terms *abortion* and *miscarriage* can be used interchangeably. Generally, abortion is considered to be termination of pregnancy at maternal request and miscarriage is considered to be an accident of nature. Medically, the term *abortion* applies to both kinds of fetal loss. Spontaneous abortion, the naturally occurring termination of pregnancy that is often called miscarriage, is most commonly seen between 12 and 14 weeks' gestation. It is estimated that 10 to 20 percent of all pregnancies end in spontaneous abortion. If the pregnancy has not yet been confirmed, the mother often assumes she is merely having a period with unusually heavy flow.

About half of all abortions are the result of fetal chromosomal anomalies. Other causes include maternal reproductive system abnormalities, maternal use of drugs, placental defects, or maternal infections. Although many people believe that trauma and psychological stress can cause abortion, research does not support that belief.

ASSESSMENT The patient experiencing an abortion is likely to report cramping abdominal pain and a backache. She is also likely to report vaginal bleeding, which is often accompanied by the passage of clots and tissue. If the abortion was not recent, then frank signs and symptoms of infection may be present. In addition to your routine emergency assessments, assess for orthostatic vital sign changes and ascertain the amount of vaginal bleeding.

MANAGEMENT Place the patient who is experiencing an abortion in a position of comfort. Treat for shock with oxygen therapy (if hypoxic) and IV access for fluid resuscitation. As mentioned earlier, any tissue or large clots should be retained and given to emergency department personnel. If the abortion occurs during the late first trimester or later, a fetus may be passed. Often, the placenta does not detach, and the fetus is suspended by the umbilical cord. In such a case, place the umbilical clamps from the OB kit on the cord and cut it. Carefully wrap the fetus in linen or other suitable material and transport it to the hospital with the mother.

An abortion is generally a very sad occurrence. Provide emotional support to the parents. This can be a devastating psychological experience for the mother, so avoid saying trite but inaccurate phrases meant to provide comfort. Inappropriate remarks include "You can always get pregnant again" or "This is nature's way of dealing with a defective fetus." Parents who wish to view the fetus should be allowed to do so. Occasionally, Roman Catholic parents may request baptism of the fetus. You can perform this by making the sign of a cross and stating, "I baptize you in the name of the father, the son, and the holy spirit. Amen."

Classifications of Abortion

Because you will be interacting with other health care professionals, you must be familiar with the variety of terms used to describe the classifications of abortion.

complete abortion	An abortion in which all the uterine contents, including the fetus and placenta, have been expelled.
incomplete abortion	An abortion in which some, but not all, fetal tissue has been passed. Incomplete abortions are associated with a high incidence of infection.
threatened abortion	A potential abortion characterized by unexplained vaginal bleeding during the first half of pregnancy, in which the cervix is slightly open and the fetus remains in the uterus and is still alive. In some cases of threatened abortion, the fetus still can be saved.
inevitable abortion	A potential abortion, characterized by vaginal bleeding accompanied by severe abdominal cramping and cervical dilation, in which the fetus has not yet passed from the uterus, but the fetus cannot be saved.
spontaneous abortion	Naturally occurring expulsion of the fetus prior to viability, generally as a result of chromosomal abnormalities. Most spontaneous abortions occur before week 12 of pregnancy. Many occur within two weeks after conception and are mistaken for menstrual periods. Commonly called a *miscarriage.*
elective abortion	An abortion in which the termination of pregnancy is desired and requested by the mother. Elective abortions during the first and second trimesters of pregnancy have been legal in the United States since 1973. Most elective abortions are performed during the first trimester. Some clinics perform second-trimester abortions. Second-trimester abortions have a higher complication rate than first-trimester abortions. Third-trimester elective abortions are generally illegal in this country.
criminal abortion	Intentional termination of a pregnancy under any condition not allowed by law. It is usually the attempt to destroy a fetus by a person who is not licensed or permitted to do so. Criminal abortions often are attempted by amateurs and they are rarely performed in aseptic surroundings.
therapeutic abortion	Termination of a pregnancy deemed necessary by a physician, usually to protect maternal health and well-being.
missed abortion	An abortion in which fetal death occurs but the fetus is not expelled. This poses a potential threat to the life of the mother if the fetus is retained beyond six weeks.
habitual abortion	Spontaneous abortions that occur in three or more consecutive pregnancies.

Ectopic Pregnancy

As you learned earlier, the fertilized egg normally is implanted in the endometrial lining of the uterine wall. The term *ectopic pregnancy* refers to the abnormal implantation of the fertilized egg outside the uterus. Approximately 95 percent are implanted in the fallopian tube. Occasionally (< 1 percent), the egg is implanted in the abdominal cavity. Current research indicates that the incidence of ectopic pregnancy is 1 in 44 live births. Improved diagnostic technology is credited with an increased incidence, as most are detected between the 2nd and 12th week. Ectopic pregnancy accounts for approximately 10 percent of maternal mortality.

Predisposing factors in the development of ectopic pregnancy include scarring of the fallopian tubes due to pelvic inflammatory disease (PID), a previous ectopic pregnancy, or previous pelvic or tubal surgery, such as a tubal ligation. Other factors include endometriosis or use of an intrauterine device (IUD) for birth control.[2]

ASSESSMENT Ectopic pregnancy most often presents as abdominal pain, which starts out as diffuse tenderness and then localizes as a sharp pain in the lower abdominal quadrant on the affected side. This pain is due to rupture of the fallopian tube when the fetus outgrows the available space. The woman often reports that she missed a period or that her LMP occurred four to six weeks earlier, but with decreased menstrual flow that was brownish in color and of shorter duration than usual. As the intraabdominal bleeding continues, the abdomen becomes rigid and the pain intensifies and is

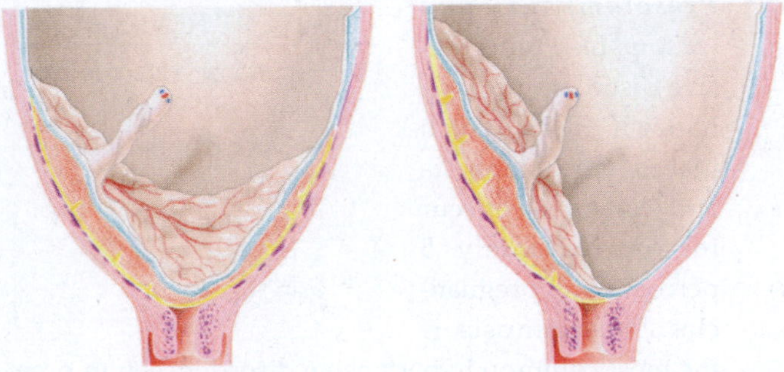

FIGURE 2-9 Placenta previa (abnormal implantation).

often referred to the shoulder on the affected side. The pain is often accompanied by syncope, vaginal bleeding, and shock.

Assume that any woman of childbearing age with lower abdominal pain is experiencing an ectopic pregnancy.

MANAGEMENT Ectopic pregnancy poses a significant life threat to the mother. Transport this patient immediately, as surgery is often required to resolve the situation. Interim care measures should include oxygen therapy (if the patient is hypoxic) and IV access for fluid resuscitation.

Placenta Previa

Placenta previa occurs as a result of abnormal implantation of the placenta on the lower half of the uterine wall, resulting in partial or complete coverage of the cervical opening (Figure 2-9). Vaginal bleeding, which may initially be intermittent, occurs after the 7th month of the pregnancy as the lower uterus begins to contract and dilate in preparation for the onset of labor. This process pulls the placenta away from the uterine wall, causing bright red vaginal bleeding. Placenta previa occurs in about 1 in 250 live births. It is classified as complete, partial, or marginal, depending on whether the placenta covers all or part of the cervical opening or is merely in close proximity to the opening.

Although the exact cause of placenta previa is unknown, certain predisposing factors are commonly seen. These factors include a previous history of placenta previa, multiparity, or increased maternal age. Other factors include the presence of uterine scars from Caesarean sections, a large placenta, or defective development of blood vessels in the uterine wall.

ASSESSMENT The patient with placenta previa is usually a multigravida in her third trimester of pregnancy. She may have a history of prior placenta previa or of bleeding early in the current pregnancy. She may report a recent episode of sexual intercourse or vaginal examination just before vaginal bleeding began, or she may not bleed until the onset of labor. The onset of painless bright red vaginal bleeding, which may occur as spotting or recurrent hemorrhage, is the hallmark of placenta previa. In fact, any painless bleeding in pregnancy is considered placenta previa until proven otherwise. The bleeding may or may not be associated with uterine contractions. The uterus is usually soft, and the fetus may be in an unusual presentation. *Vaginal examination should never be attempted, as an examining finger can puncture the placenta, causing fatal hemorrhage.*

The presence of placenta previa may already have been diagnosed with an ultrasound during prenatal care, in which case the mother is anticipating the onset of symptoms. The prognosis for the fetus is dependent on the extent of the previa. Obviously, in profuse hemorrhage the fetus is at risk of severe hypoxia and the viability of the placenta is compromised. You should perform your assessment and physical exam as discussed earlier in this chapter.

MANAGEMENT If the placenta previa was previously diagnosed, your patient may already have been managed by placing her on bed rest. Because of the potential for profuse hemorrhage, you should treat for shock. Administer oxygen as needed and initiate intravenous access. Additionally, continue to monitor the maternal vital signs and fetal heart tones (FHTs). Because the definitive treatment is delivery of the fetus by Caesarean section, it is imperative to transport the patient to a hospital with obstetric surgical capability.

Abruptio Placentae

Abruptio placentae, or the premature separation (abruption) of a normally implanted placenta from the uterine wall, poses a potential life threat for both mother and fetus (Figure 2-10).

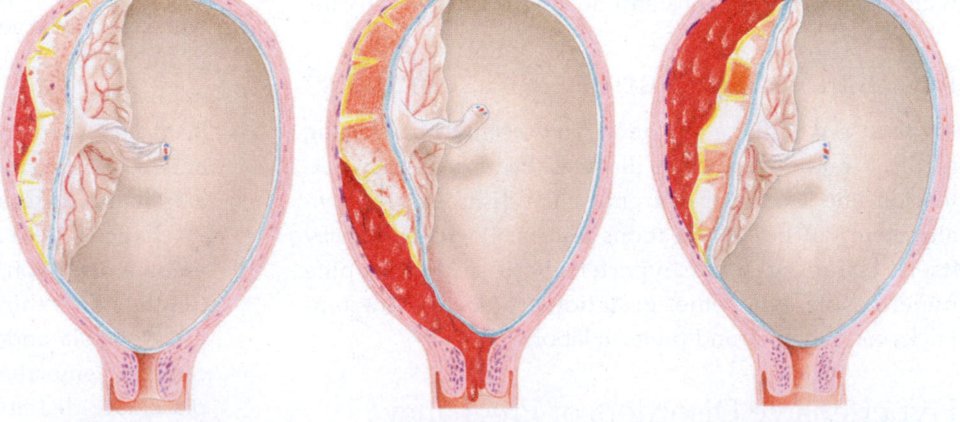

FIGURE 2-10 Abruptio placentae (premature separation).

CONTENT REVIEW

- Medical Complications of Pregnancy
  - Hypertensive disorders of pregnancy
  - Supine hypotensive syndrome
  - Gestational diabetes

The incidence of abruptio placentae is 1 in 120 live births. It is associated with 20 to 30 percent fetal mortality, which rises to 100 percent in cases in which the majority of the placenta has separated. Maternal mortality is relatively uncommon, although it rises markedly if shock is inadequately treated. Abruptio placentae is classified as marginal (or partial), central (severe), or complete, as explained next.

Although the cause of abruptio placentae is unknown, predisposing factors include multiparity, maternal hypertension, trauma, cocaine use, increasing maternal age, and history of abruption in a previous pregnancy.

ASSESSMENT The presenting signs and symptoms of abruptio placentae vary depending on the extent and character of the abruption. Partial abruptions can be marginal or central. Marginal abruption is characterized by vaginal bleeding but no increase in pain. In central abruption, the placenta separates centrally and the bleeding is trapped between the placenta and the uterine wall, or "concealed," so there is no vaginal bleeding. However, there is a sudden sharp, tearing pain and development of a stiff, boardlike abdomen. In complete abruptio placentae, there is massive vaginal bleeding and profound maternal hypotension. If the patient is in labor at the time of the abruption, separation of the placenta from the uterine wall will progress rapidly, with fetal distress versus fetal demise dependent on percentage of separation.

MANAGEMENT Abruptio placentae is a life-threatening obstetric emergency. Immediate intervention to maintain maternal oxygenation and perfusion is imperative. Immediately place two large-bore intravenous lines and begin fluid resuscitation. Position your patient in the left lateral recumbent position. Transport immediately to a hospital with available surgical obstetric and high-risk neonatal care.

Medical Complications of Pregnancy

As discussed earlier, pregnancy can exacerbate preexisting medical conditions such as diabetes, heart disease, hypertension, and seizure or neuromuscular disorder. Additionally, there may be complications associated with pregnancy itself, including some hypertensive disorders, supine hypertensive syndrome, gestational diabetes, Braxton-Hicks contractions, and preterm labor.

Hypertensive Disorders of Pregnancy

The American College of Obstetricians and Gynecologists has identified four classifications of *hypertensive disorders of pregnancy* (formerly called "toxemia of pregnancy").[3] They are:

CONTENT REVIEW

- Hypertensive Disorders of Pregnancy
  - Chronic hypertension
  - Pregnancy-induced hypertension
  - Preeclampsia
  - Eclampsia

- ***Preeclampsia and eclampsia.*** Hypertensive disorders of pregnancy (HDP), which include preeclampsia and eclampsia, occur in approximately 5 percent of all pregnancies. Preeclampsia is the most common hypertensive disorder seen in pregnancy. There is a higher incidence among primigravidas, particularly if they are teenagers or over age 35. Others at increased risk are diabetics, women with a history of preeclampsia, and those who are carrying multiple fetuses.

  Preeclampsia is a progressive disorder that is usually categorized as mild or severe. Seizures (or coma) develop in its most severe form, known as eclampsia. Preeclampsia is defined as an increase in systolic blood pressure by 30 mmHg and/or a diastolic increase of 15 mmHg over baseline on at least two occasions at least 6 hours apart. Remember that maternal blood pressure normally drops during pregnancy, so a woman may be hypertensive at 120/80 if her baseline in early pregnancy was 90/66. If there is no baseline blood pressure available, a reading of 140/90 or higher is considered to be hypertensive.

  Preeclampsia is most commonly seen in the last 10 weeks of gestation, during labor, or in the first 48 hours postpartum. The exact cause of preeclampsia is unknown. It is thought to be caused by abnormal vasospasm, which results in increased maternal blood pressure and other associated symptoms. Additionally, the vasospasm causes decreased placental perfusion, contributing to fetal growth retardation and chronic fetal hypoxia.

  Mild preeclampsia is characterized by hypertension, edema, and protein in the urine. Severe preeclampsia progresses rapidly, with maternal blood pressures reaching 160/110 mmHg or higher, while the edema becomes generalized and the amount of protein in the urine increases significantly. Other commonly seen signs and symptoms in the severe state include headache, visual disturbances, hyperactive reflexes, and the development of pulmonary edema, along with a dramatic decrease in urine output.

  Patients who are preeclamptic have intravascular volume depletion, because a great deal of their body fluid is in the third space. Those who develop severe preeclampsia and eclampsia are at increased risk for cerebral hemorrhage, pulmonary embolism, abruptio placentae, disseminated intravascular coagulopathy (DIC), and the development of renal failure.

- Eclampsia, the most serious manifestation of the hypertensive disorders of pregnancy, is characterized by generalized tonic–clonic (major motor) seizure activity. Eclampsia is often preceded by visual disturbances, such as flashing lights or spots before the eyes. The development of epigastric pain or pain in the right upper abdominal quadrant often indicates impending seizure. Eclampsia can often be distinguished from epilepsy by the history and physical appearance of the patient. Patients who become eclamptic are usually grossly edematous and have markedly elevated blood pressure, whereas epileptics usually have a prior history of seizures and are usually taking anticonvulsant medications. If eclampsia develops, death of the mother and fetus frequently results. The risk of fetal mortality increases by 10 percent with each maternal seizure.

- ***Chronic hypertension.*** Hypertension is considered chronic when the blood pressure is 140/90 mmHg or higher before pregnancy or prior to the 20th week of gestation, or if it persists for more than 42 days postpartum. As a general rule, if the diastolic pressure exceeds 80 mmHg during the second trimester, chronic hypertension is likely. The cause of chronic hypertension is unknown. The goal of management is to prevent the development of preeclampsia.
- ***Chronic hypertension superimposed with preeclampsia.*** It is not uncommon for the chronic hypertensive patient who develops preeclampsia to progress rapidly to eclampsia even prior to the 30th week of gestation. The same diagnostic criteria for preeclampsia are used (systolic blood pressure increases >30 mmHg over baseline, edema, and protein in the urine).
- ***Transient hypertension.*** Transient hypertension is defined as a temporary rise in blood pressure that occurs during labor or early in postpartum and normalizes within 10 days.

ASSESSMENT Obtaining an accurate history is extremely important when you suspect one of the hypertensive disorders of pregnancy (HDP). Question the patient about excessive weight gain, headaches, visual problems, epigastric or right upper quadrant abdominal pain, apprehension, or seizures. On physical exam, patients with HDP or preeclampsia are usually markedly edematous. They are often pale and apprehensive. The reflexes are hyperactive. The blood pressure, which is usually elevated, should be taken after the patient has rested for 5 minutes in the left lateral recumbent position.

MANAGEMENT Definitive treatment of the hypertensive disorders of pregnancy is delivery of the fetus. However, in the field, use the following management tactics to prevent dangerously high blood pressures or seizure activity.

- ***Hypertension.*** Closely monitor the patient who is pregnant and has elevated blood pressure without edema or other signs of preeclampsia. Record the fetal heart tones and the mother's blood pressure level.
- ***Preeclampsia.*** The patient who is hypertensive and shows other signs and symptoms of preeclampsia, such as edema, headaches, and visual disturbances, should be treated quickly. Keep the patient calm and dim the lights. Place the patient in the left lateral recumbent position and quickly carry out the primary assessment. Begin an IV of normal saline. Transport the patient rapidly, without lights or sirens. If the blood pressure is dangerously high (diastolic >110 mmHg), medical direction may request the administration of hydralazine (Apresoline) or similar antihypertensives that are safe for use in pregnancy. If the transport time is long, the administration of magnesium sulfate may also be ordered.
- ***Eclampsia.*** If the patient has already suffered a seizure or a seizure appears to be imminent, then, in addition to the preceding measures, administer oxygen (if the patient is hypoxic) and manage the airway appropriately. Administer a bolus dose of magnesium sulfate (2 to 5 g diluted in 50 to 100 mL slow IV push) to control the seizures. If you are unable to control the seizures with magnesium sulfate, consider diazepam (Valium) or another sedative. It is important to keep calcium gluconate available for use as an antidote to magnesium sulfate. Also monitor your patient closely for signs (vaginal bleeding or abdominal rigidity) of abruptio placentae or developing pulmonary edema. Transport immediately to a hospital with surgical obstetric and neonatal care availability.

Supine Hypotensive Syndrome

Supine hypotensive syndrome usually occurs in the third trimester of pregnancy. Also known as *vena caval syndrome*, supine hypotensive syndrome occurs when the gravid uterus compresses the inferior vena cava when the mother lies in a supine position (Figure 2-11).

ASSESSMENT Supine hypotensive syndrome usually occurs in a patient late in her pregnancy who has been supine for a period of time. The patient may complain of dizziness, which results from the decrease in venous return to the right atrium and consequent lowering of the patient's blood pressure. Question the patient about prior episodes of a similar nature and about any recent hemorrhage or fluid loss. Direct the physical examination at determining whether the patient is volume depleted.

MANAGEMENT If there are no indications of volume depletion, such as decreased skin turgor or thirst, place the patient in the left lateral recumbent position or elevate her right hip. Monitor the fetal heart tones and maternal vital

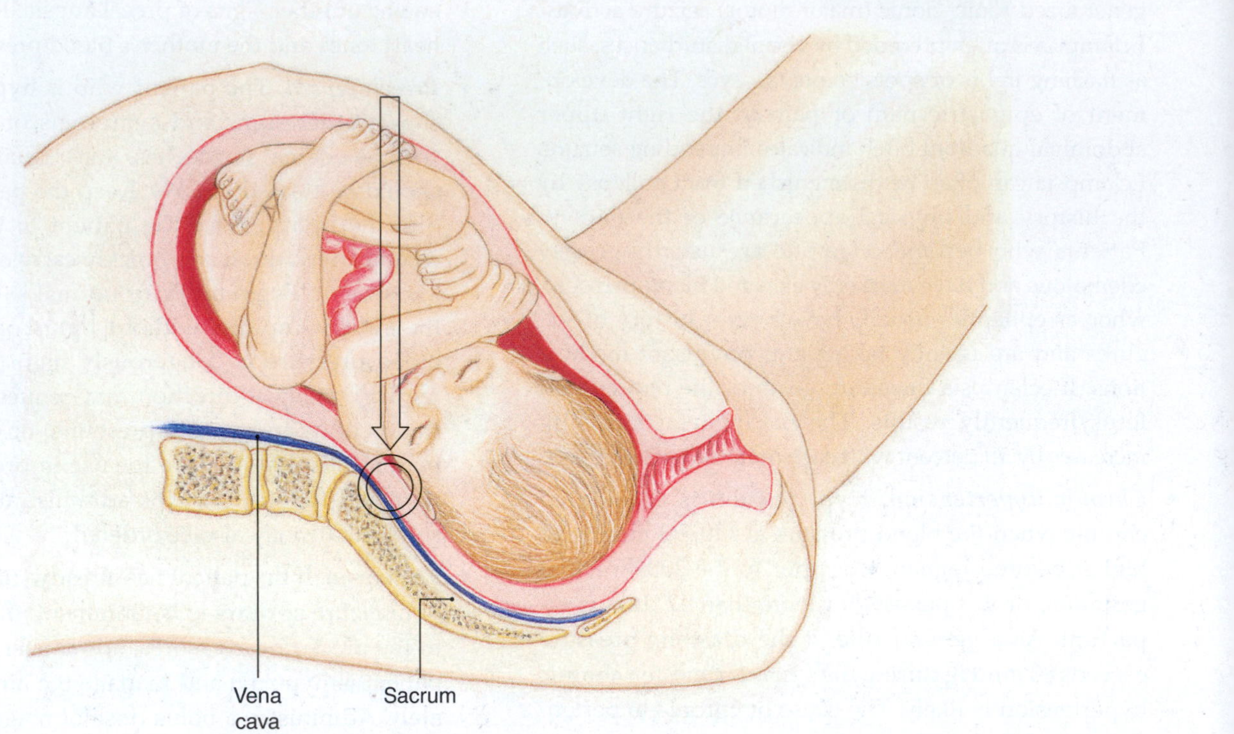

FIGURE 2-11 Supine hypotensive syndrome results from compression of the inferior vena cava by the gravid uterus.

signs frequently. If there is clinical evidence of volume depletion, administer oxygen (if the patient is hypoxic) and start an IV of normal saline. Check for orthostatic changes (a decrease in blood pressure and increase in heart rate when rising from the supine position) and place electrodes for cardiac monitoring. Transport the patient promptly in the left lateral recumbent position.

Gestational Diabetes

Diabetes mellitus occurs in approximately 4 percent of all pregnancies. Hormonal influences cause an increase in insulin production, as well as an increased tissue response to insulin, during the first 20 weeks of gestation. However, during the last 20 weeks, placental hormones cause an increased resistance to insulin and a decreased glucose tolerance. This causes catabolism (the "breaking down" phase of metabolism) between meals and during the night. At these times, ketones may be present in the urine because fats are metabolized more rapidly. Further, maternal glucose stores are used up, as they are the sole source of glucose to meet the energy needs of the growing fetus. This is known as the *diabetogenic* (diabetes-causing) *effect of pregnancy.* Gestational diabetes usually subsides after pregnancy.

Routine prenatal care includes screening to detect diabetes throughout the pregnancy. Women who are considered to be at high risk for developing gestational diabetes are given a glucose tolerance test at their first prenatal visit. High risk is associated with maternal age (over 35), obesity, hypertension, family history of diabetes, and history of prior stillbirth.

Management of gestational diabetes requires good prenatal care. The mother will be instructed on diabetes management and the importance of balancing diet and exercise, as well as how to monitor her glucose levels and administer insulin. Fetal development will be monitored on an ongoing basis throughout the pregnancy.

ASSESSMENT When you encounter a pregnant patient with an altered mental status, consider hypoglycemia as a likely cause. Remember that the clinical signs and symptoms of hypoglycemia are many and varied. An abnormal mental status is the most important. Physical signs may include diaphoresis and tachycardia. If the blood sugar falls to a critically low level, the patient may sustain a hypoglycemic seizure or become comatose, which poses a potential life threat to the mother and fetus. Obtaining an accurate history of associated signs and symptoms, such as nausea, vomiting, abdominal pain, increased urination, or a recent infection, will allow you to ascertain whether diabetic ketoacidosis might be the cause of your patient's altered mental status. Determine the blood glucose level in addition to obtaining baseline vital signs and FHTs.

MANAGEMENT If the blood glucose level is noted to be less than 60 mg/dL, draw a red-top tube of blood and start an IV of normal saline. Next, administer 50 to 100 mL (25–50 g) of 50 percent dextrose intravenously. If the patient is conscious and able to swallow, complete glucose administration with orange juice, sugared soft drinks, or commercially available glucose pastes.

If the blood glucose level is in excess of 200 mg/dL, draw a red-top tube (or the tube specified by local protocols) of blood and then establish IV access to administer 1 to 2 L of 0.9 percent sodium chloride per protocol. If transport time is lengthy, medical direction may request intravenous or subcutaneous administration of regular insulin.

Braxton-Hicks Contractions

It is occasionally difficult to determine the onset of labor. As early as the 13th week of gestation, the uterus contracts intermittently, thus conditioning itself for the birth process. It is also believed that these contractions enhance placental circulation. These painless, irregular contractions are known as *Braxton-Hicks contractions*. As the EDC approaches, these contractions become more frequent. Ultimately, the contractions become stronger and more regular, signaling the onset of labor. Labor consists of uterine contractions that cause the dilation and **effacement** (thinning and shortening) of the cervix. The contractions of labor are firm, fairly regular, and quite painful. Prior to the onset of labor Braxton-Hicks contractions, occasionally called *false labor,* increase in intensity and frequency but do not cause cervical changes.

It is virtually impossible to distinguish false labor from true labor in the field. Distinguishing the two requires repeated vaginal examinations, over time, to determine whether the cervix is effacing and dilating. *Remember: Internal vaginal exams should not be performed in the field.* Therefore, all patients with uterine contractions should be transported to the hospital for additional evaluation.

Braxton-Hicks contractions do not require treatment by the paramedic aside from reassurance of the patient and, if necessary, transport for evaluation by a physician.

Preterm Labor

As you have already learned, normal gestation is 40 weeks and, in terms of fetal development, the fetus is not considered to be full term until the 38th week. True labor that begins before the 38th week of gestation is called *preterm labor* and frequently requires medical intervention. A variety of maternal, fetal, or placental factors may cause this potentially life-threatening situation for the mother and fetus.

- Maternal factors
  - Cardiovascular disease
  - Renal disease
  - Pregnancy-induced hypertension (PIH)
  - Diabetes
  - Abdominal surgery during gestation
  - Uterine and cervical abnormalities
  - Maternal infection
  - Trauma, particularly blows to the abdomen
  - Contributory factors: history of preterm birth, smoking, and cocaine abuse
- Placental factors
  - Placenta previa
  - Abruptio placentae
- Fetal factors
  - Multiple gestation
  - Excessive amniotic fluid
  - Fetal infection

In many cases, physicians attempt to stop preterm labor to give the fetus additional time to develop in the uterus. Prematurity is the primary neonatal health problem in the nation and occurs in 7 to 10 percent of all live births. All of the preterm infant's organ systems are immature to some degree, but lung development is of greatest concern. Although technological advances in the care of preterm infants have improved the prognosis dramatically, the consequences of a preterm birth can last a lifetime.

ASSESSMENT When confronted by a patient with uterine contractions, first determine the approximate gestational age of the fetus. If it is less than 38 weeks, then suspect preterm labor. If gestational age is greater than 38 weeks, treat the patient as a term patient, as described later in this chapter.

After determining gestational age, obtain a brief obstetric history. Then question the mother about the urge to push or the need to move her bowels or urinate. Also ask if her membranes have ruptured. Any sensation of fluid leakage or "gushing" from the vagina should be interpreted as ruptured membranes until proven otherwise. Next, palpate the contractions by placing your hand on the patient's abdomen. Note the intensity and length of the contractions, as well as the interval between contractions.

Commonly reported signs and symptoms of preterm labor include contractions that occur every 10 minutes or less, low abdominal cramping that is similar to menstrual cramps, or a sensation of pelvic pressure. Other complaints, such as low backache, changes in vaginal discharge, and abdominal cramping with or without diarrhea, may also be reported. Rupture of the membranes is confirmatory for preterm labor.

MANAGEMENT Preterm labor, especially if quite early in the pregnancy, should be stopped if possible. The process of stopping labor, or **tocolysis**, is frequently practiced in obstetrics. However, it is infrequently done in the field.

There are three general approaches to tocolysis. The first is to sedate the patient, often with narcotics or barbiturates, thus allowing her to rest. Often, after a period of rest, the contractions stop on their own. The second approach is to administer a fluid bolus intravenously. The administration of approximately 1 liter of fluid intravenously increases the intravascular fluid volume, thus inhibiting ADH secretion from the posterior pituitary. Because oxytocin and ADH are secreted from the same area of the pituitary gland, the inhibition of ADH secretion also inhibits oxytocin release, often causing cessation of uterine contractions. Ultimately, if the previous methods fail, magnesium sulfate or a beta-agonist, such as terbutaline or ritodrine, may be administered to stop labor by inhibiting uterine smooth muscle contraction. Current research in tocolysis includes the administration of calcium channel blockers, such as nifedipine, and prostaglandin inhibitors, such as indomethacin. You may also find that a patient with preterm labor has been given corticosteroids to accelerate fetal lung maturity.

As a rule, tocolysis in the field is limited to sedation and hydration, especially if transport time is long. Paramedics may, however, transport a patient from one medical facility to another with beta-agonist administration under way. You should therefore be familiar with its use. Commonly associated side effects include being jittery; tachycardia, usually described by the patient as palpitations; and, occasionally, abdominal pain. You will, of course, want to transport your patient to the nearest facility that has neonatal intensive care capabilities. Careful and frequent monitoring of maternal vital signs and FHTs is imperative during tocolysis.

The Puerperium

The **puerperium** is the time period surrounding the birth of the fetus. Childbirth generally occurs in a hospital or similar facility with appropriate equipment. Occasionally, prehospital personnel may be called on to attend a delivery in the field. Therefore, you should be familiar with the birth process and some of the complications that may be associated with it.

Labor

Childbirth, or the delivery of the fetus, is the culmination of pregnancy. The process by which delivery occurs is called **labor**, the physiologic and mechanical process in which the baby, placenta, and amniotic sac are expelled through the birth canal. The duration of labor is widely variable.

Prior to the onset of true labor, the head of the fetus descends into the bony pelvis area. The frequency and intensity of the Braxton-Hicks contractions increase in preparation for true labor. Increased vaginal secretions and softening of the cervix occur. Bloody show—pink-tinged secretions—is generally considered a sign of imminent labor as the mucus plug is expelled from the cervix. Labor then usually begins within 24 to 48 hours. Many people also consider the rupture of the membranes as a sign of impending labor. If labor does not begin spontaneously within 12 to 24 hours after rupture, labor will likely require induction because of the risk of infection.

Pressure exerted by the fetus on the cervix causes changes that lead to the subsequent expulsion of the fetus. Muscular uterine contractions increase in frequency, strength, and duration. You can assess the frequency and duration of contractions by placing one hand on the fundus of the uterus. Time contractions from the beginning of one contraction until the beginning of the next. It is important to note whether the uterus relaxes completely between contractions. It is also desirable to monitor fetal heart tones during and between contractions. Occasional fetal bradycardia occurs during contractions, but the heart rate should increase to a normal rate (120–160) after the contraction ends. Failure of the heart rate to return to normal between contractions is a sign of fetal distress.

CONTENT REVIEW

➤ Stages of Labor
- Stage one: dilation
- Stage two: expulsion
- Stage three: placental

Labor is generally divided into three stages (Figure 2-12):

- ***Stage one (dilation stage).*** The first stage of labor begins with the onset of true labor contractions and ends with the complete dilation and effacement of the cervix. Early in pregnancy the cervix is quite thick and long, but after complete *effacement* it is short and paper thin. Effacement usually begins several days before active labor ensues. *Dilation* is the progressive stretching of the cervical opening. The cervix dilates from its closed position to 10 centimeters, which is considered complete dilation. This stage lasts approximately 8 to 10 hours for the woman in her first labor, the nullipara, and about 5 to 7 hours in the woman who has given birth previously, the multipara. Early in this stage the contractions are usually mild, lasting for 15 to 20 seconds with a frequency of 10 to 20 minutes. As labor progresses, the contractions increase in intensity and occur approximately every 2 to 3 minutes, with a duration of 60 seconds each.
- ***Stage two (expulsion stage).*** The second stage of labor begins with the complete dilation of the cervix and ends with the delivery of the fetus. In the nullipara, this stage lasts 50 to 60 minutes, whereas it takes about half that amount of time for the multipara. The contractions are very strong, occurring every 2 minutes and lasting for 60 to 75 seconds. Often, the patient feels pain in her lower back as the fetus descends into the pelvis. The urge to push or "bear down" usually begins in the second stage. The membranes usually rupture at this time, if they have not ruptured previously. Crowning during contractions is evident as the delivery of the fetus nears. Crowning occurs when the head (or other presenting part of the fetus) is visible at the vaginal opening during a contraction and is the definitive sign that birth is imminent. The most common presentation is for the infant to be delivered head first, face down (vertex position).
- ***Stage three (placental stage).*** The third and final stage of labor begins immediately after the birth of the infant and ends with the delivery of the placenta. The placenta generally delivers within 5 to 20 minutes. There is no need to delay transport to wait for its delivery. Classic signs of placental separation include a gush of blood from the vagina; a change in size, shape, or con-

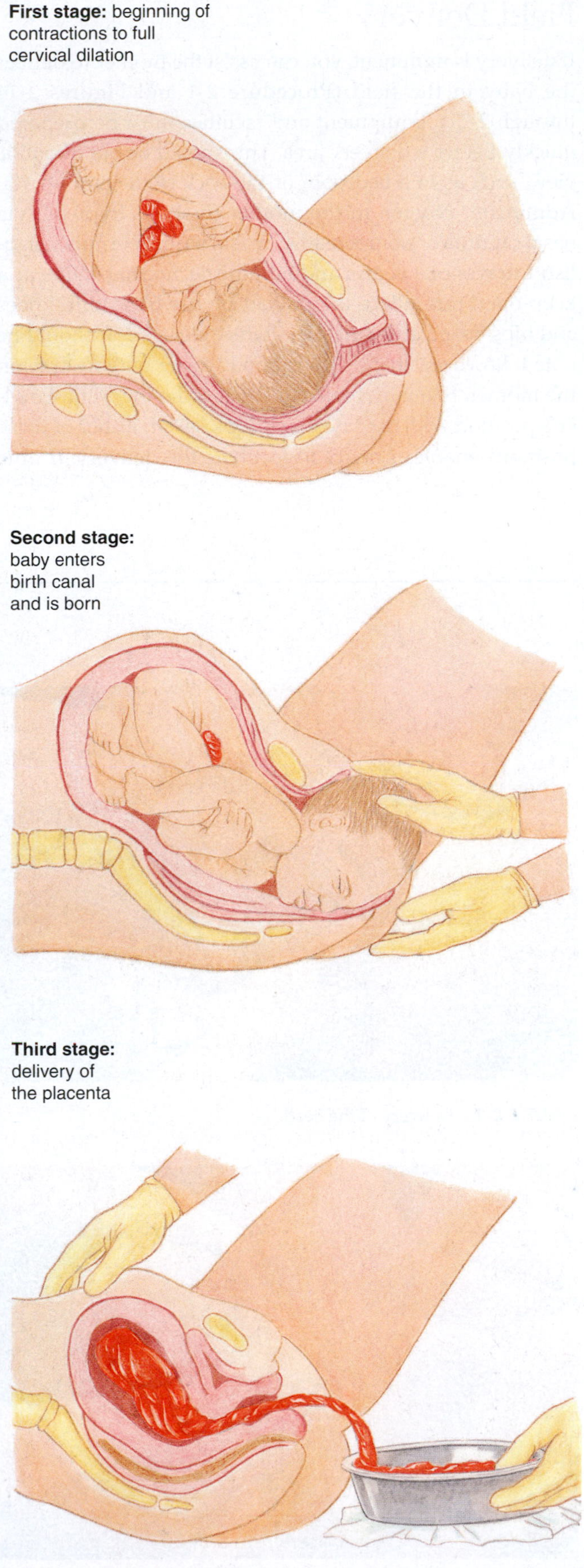

FIGURE 2-12 Stages of labor.

sistency of the uterus; lengthening of the umbilical cord protruding from the vagina; and the mother's report that she has the urge to push. There will be a continued vaginal discharge called **lochia** that contains blood, mucus, and placental tissue. It will often continue for four to six weeks after delivery.

Management of a Patient in Labor

Probably one of the most important decisions you must make with a patient in labor is whether to attempt to deliver the infant at the scene or to transport the patient to the hospital (Figure 2-13). It is generally preferable to transport the mother unless delivery is imminent. Several factors must be taken into consideration when making this decision. They include the patient's number of previous pregnancies, the length of labor during the previous pregnancies, the frequency of contractions, the maternal urge to push, and the presence of crowning. Some women have rapid labors and may be completely dilated in a short period of time. Also, as mentioned, multiparas generally have shorter labors than nulliparas. The maternal urge to push or the presence of crowning indicates that delivery is imminent. In such cases, the infant should be delivered at the scene or in the ambulance.

Traditionally, a woman who had previously delivered by a cesarean section was advised to deliver all subsequent infants by cesarean sections. However, current thinking encourages women to attempt vaginal birth after Caesarean (VBAC). If your patient has had prenatal care during this pregnancy, she has probably already discussed this with her health care provider. The only absolute contraindication

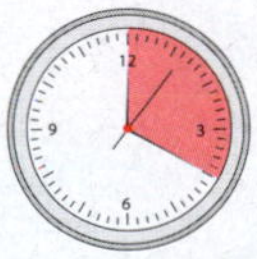

If contractions are 2 to 3 minutes apart and delivery doesn't occur within 20 minutes, transport without further delay.

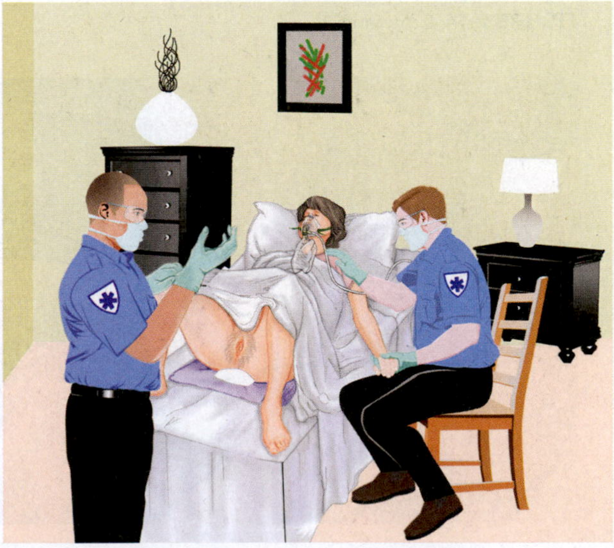

FIGURE 2-13 The decision to deliver at the scene or to attempt transport is often a difficult one.

for VBAC is a classic vertical uterine incision. However, most Caesarean sections done today are done using a low transverse uterine incision. (Note that a horizontal skin incision does not ensure that the uterine incision is horizontal.) A labor patient who is opting for VBAC requires no more special care than any other labor patient does.

However, certain factors should prompt immediate transport, despite the threat of delivery. These include prolonged rupture of membranes (>24 hours), as prolonged time between rupture and delivery often leads to fetal infection; abnormal presentation, such as breech or transverse; prolapsed cord; or fetal distress, as evidenced by fetal bradycardia or meconium staining (the presence of meconium, the first fetal stools, in the amniotic fluid). The presence of multiple fetuses may also contribute to your decision to transport. You will read more about these conditions later in this chapter.

Field Delivery

If delivery is imminent, you can assist the mother to deliver the baby in the field (Procedure 2-1 and Figures 2-14 through 2-21). Equipment and facilities must be prepared quickly. Set up a delivery area. This should be out of public view, such as in a bedroom or the back of the ambulance. Administer oxygen to the mother (if she is hypoxic) via nasal cannula or nonrebreather mask. If time permits, establish intravenous access and administer normal saline at a keep-open rate. Place the patient on her back with knees and hips flexed and buttocks slightly elevated. It should be noted, however, that this position is easier on you than on the mother. She may prefer to squat or lie in a semi-Fowler's position with her knees and hips flexed. Either of these positions enables gravity to facilitate the delivery. If time

Procedure 2-1 Normal Delivery

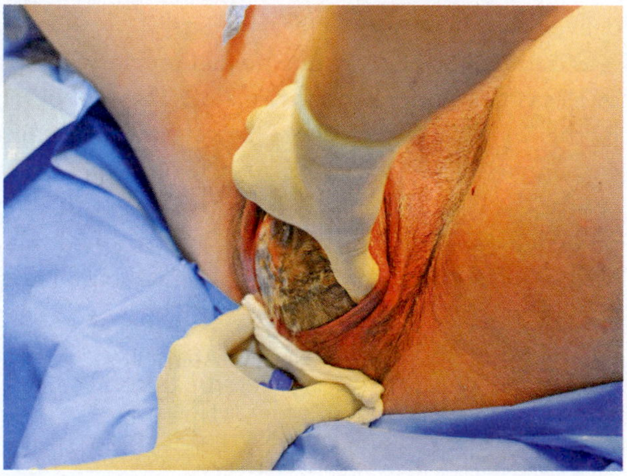

FIGURE 2-14 Crowning.

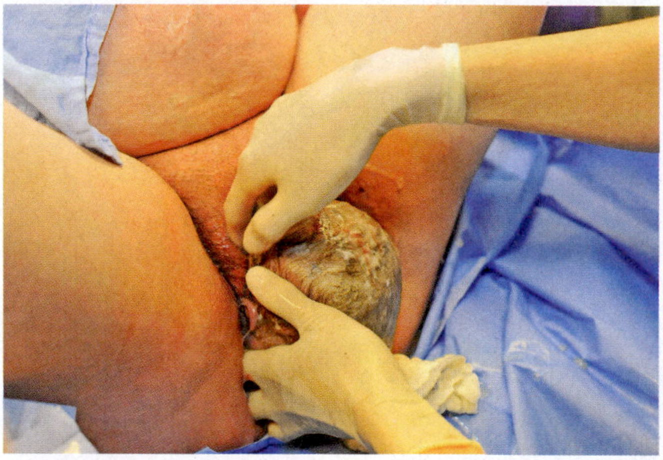

FIGURE 2-15 Delivery of the head.

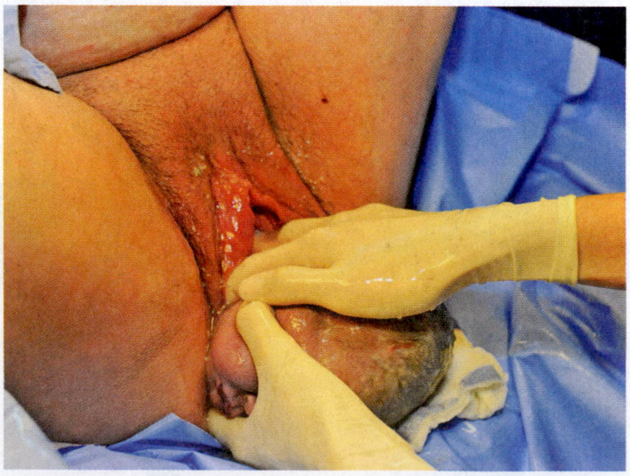

FIGURE 2-16 External rotation of the head.

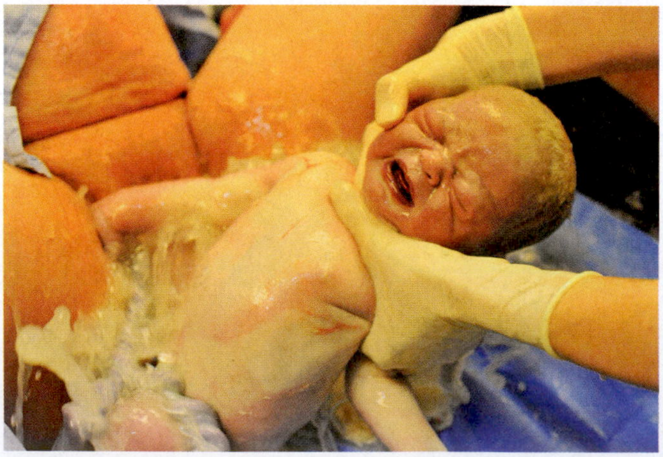

FIGURE 2-17 Delivery of the torso.

(Continued)

Procedure 2-1 *Continued*

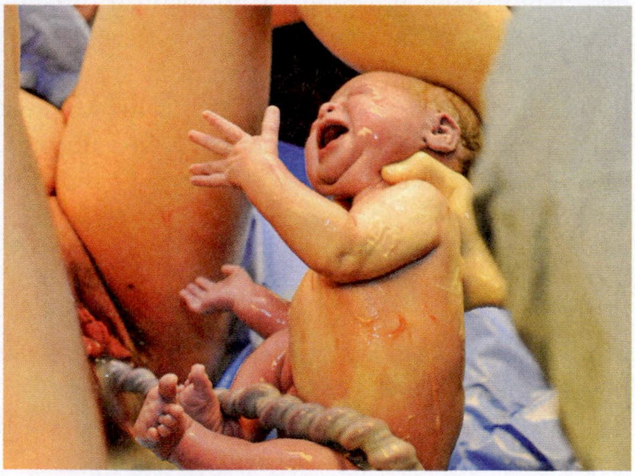

FIGURE 2-18 Complete delivery of the infant.

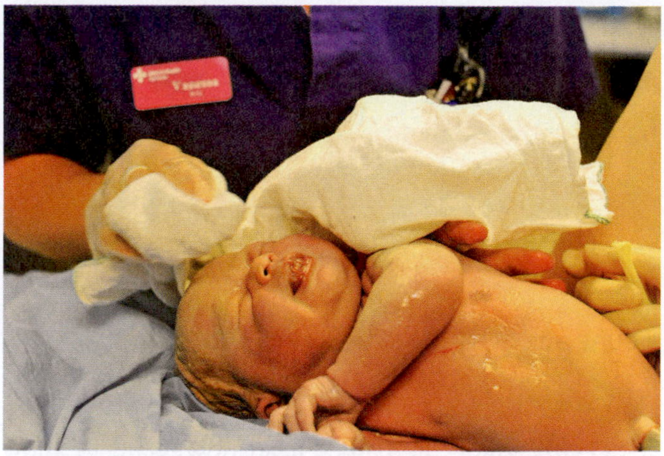

FIGURE 2-19 Dry the infant.

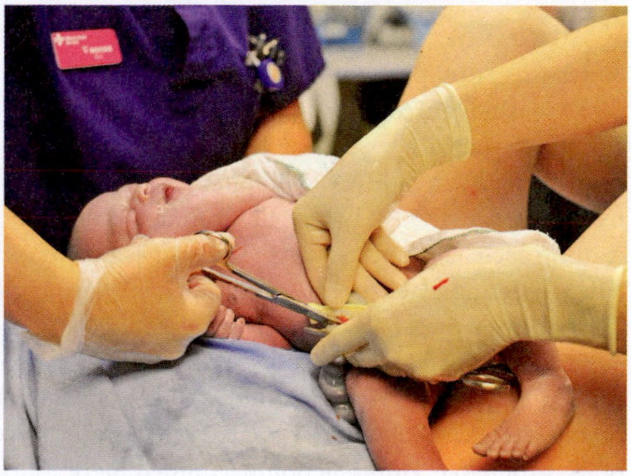

FIGURE 2-20 Place the infant on the mother's stomach and cut the umbilical cord.

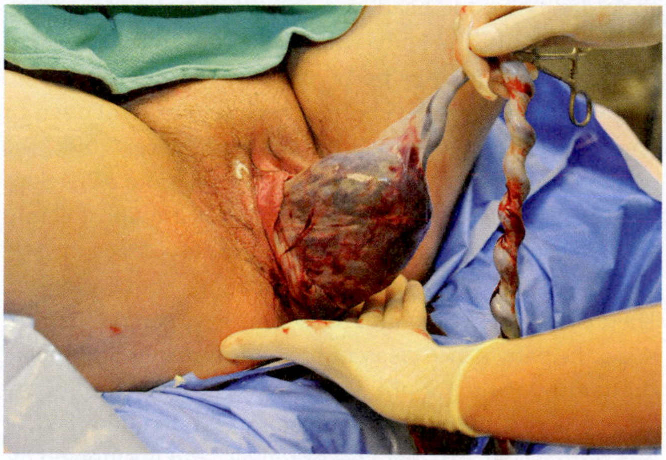

FIGURE 2-21 Deliver the placenta and save it for transport with the mother and infant.

permits, drape the mother with toweling from the OB kit. Place one towel under the buttocks, another below the vaginal opening, and another across the lower abdomen.

Until delivery, the fetal heart rate should be monitored frequently. A drop in the fetal heart rate to less than 90 beats per minute indicates fetal distress and requires prompt immediate transport with the mother in the left lateral recumbent position. Coach the mother to breathe deeply between contractions and to push with contractions. If the baby does not deliver after 20 minutes of contractions every 2 to 3 minutes, *transport immediately*.

Prepare the OB equipment and don sterile gloves, gown, and a face shield or goggles. If time permits, wash your hands and forearms prior to gloving. As the head crowns, control it with gentle pressure. Providing support to the head and perineum decreases the likelihood of vaginal and perineal tearing and decreases the potential for rapid expulsion of the baby's skull through the birth canal, which may cause intracranial injury. Support the head as it emerges from the vagina and begins to turn. If it is still enclosed in the amniotic sac, tear the sac open to permit escape of the amniotic fluid and enable the baby to breathe.

Gently slide your finger along the head and neck to ensure that the umbilical cord is not wrapped around the baby's neck. If it is, try to gently slip it over the shoulder and head. If this cannot be done and it is wrapped so tightly that it inhibits labor, carefully place two umbilical cord clamps approximately 2 inches apart and cut the cord between the clamps. As soon as the infant's head is clear of the vagina, instruct the mother to stop pushing. Then tell the mother to resume pushing, while you support the infant's head as it rotates. Although it was once a common practice, suctioning of the nasopharynx in neonates without obvious obstruction is no longer recommended.

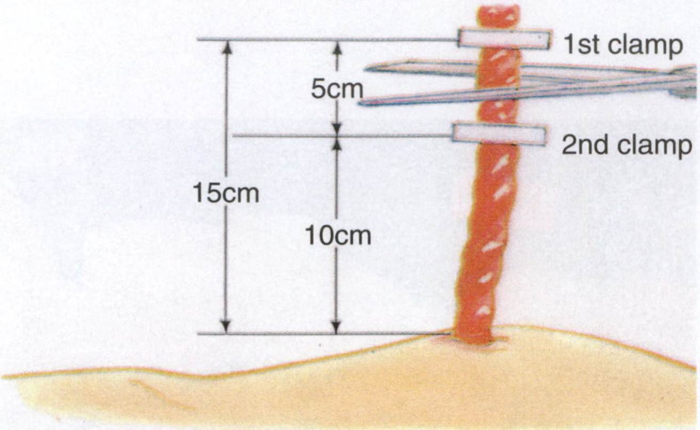

FIGURE 2-22 Clamp and cut the cord.

Gently guide the baby's head downward to allow delivery of the upper shoulder. Do not pull! Gently guide the baby's body upward to allow delivery of the lower shoulder. Once the head and shoulders have been delivered, the rest of the body will follow rapidly. Be prepared to support the infant's body as it emerges. Remember to keep the baby at the level of the vagina to prevent over- or undertransfusion of blood from the cord. Never "milk" the cord. Clamp and cut the cord as follows (Figure 2-22): Supporting the baby's body, place the first umbilical clamp approximately 10 centimeters from the baby. Place the second clamp approximately 5 centimeters above the first. Then carefully cut the umbilical cord between the clamps. Wipe the baby's face clean of blood and mucus and repeat suctioning of the mouth and nose, if necessary, until the airway is clear. Dry the infant thoroughly and then cover him with warm, dry blankets or towels, and position on his side. Record the time of birth.

Usual maternal blood loss with delivery is 1 pint (about 500 mL). Following delivery, if the uterus is contracting normally, the fundus should be at the level of the umbilicus and have the size and consistency of a grapefruit. After birth, the mother's vagina should continue to ooze blood. Do not pull on the umbilical cord. Eventually, the cord will appear to lengthen, which indicates separation of the placenta. The placenta should be delivered and transported with the mother to the hospital. If it does deliver, place it in a plastic biohazard bag and bring it to the hospital for evaluation. Retained placenta may cause maternal hemorrhage or become a source of infection. However, there is no need to delay transport for delivery of the placenta. At this time, massage the uterine fundus by placing one hand immediately above the pubic symphysis and the other on the uterine fundus. Cup the uterus between the two hands and support it as it is massaged. Continue massage until the uterus assumes a woody hardness. Avoid overmassage. Putting the baby to the mother's breast also stimulates uterine contractions, which will further decrease bleeding.

Following delivery, inspect the mother's perineum for tears. If any tears are present, apply direct pressure. Continuously monitor vital signs. Note the presence of continued hemorrhage and report it to medical direction. In some systems, paramedics may administer oxytocin (Pitocin) to facilitate uterine contraction in the control of postpartum hemorrhage. Oxytocin should be administered only *after* delivery of the placenta has been confirmed. Following stabilization, transport the mother and infant to the hospital.

Neonatal Care

Care of the neonate is discussed in detail in the chapter "Neonatology." Initial care of the neonate has been described in the preceding section. Several additional important considerations regarding routine care of the neonate, APGAR scoring, and neonatal resuscitation are discussed briefly in the following sections.

Routine Care of the Neonate

Newborns are slippery and will require both hands to support the head and torso. Position yourself so you can work close to the surface where you have placed the infant.

Maintain warmth! Cold infants rapidly become distressed infants. Quickly dry the infant with towels, discarding each as it becomes wet. Then cover the infant with a dry receiving blanket or use a commercial warming blanket made of a material such as Thinsulate®.

Clearing the airway. Routine suctioning of the neonate, especially when the amniotic fluid is clear, is no longer recommended, as it has been associated with bradycardia and other problems. Thus, suctioning immediately following birth should be reserved for neonates with obvious obstruction to spontaneous breathing. Generally, drying and tactile stimulation will stimulate respirations, crying, and activity.[4] This should cause the infant to "pink up." (Do not be alarmed if the extremities remain dusky. This is known as *acrocyanosis* and is very common in the first hours of life.) If this is not effective, you may try flicking your finger against the soles of the feet or rubbing gently in a circular motion in the middle of the back (Figure 2-23).

Assess the neonate as soon as possible after birth. The normal neonatal respiratory rate should average 30 to 60 breaths per minute, whereas the heart rate should be 100 to 180 beats per minute. If resuscitation is not indicated, assign APGAR scores. Do not, however, delay resuscitative efforts and transport in order to complete APGAR scoring.

APGAR Scoring

Named for Dr. Virginia Apgar, who developed the assessment tool, the APGAR scoring system is a means of evaluating the status of a newborn's vital functions at 1 minute and 5 minutes after delivery. There are five parameters;

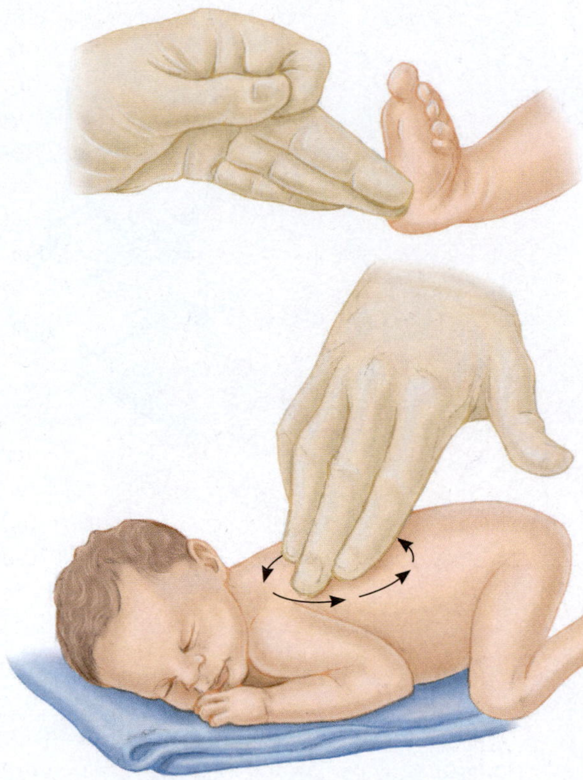

FIGURE 2-23 Stimulate the infant as required.

each is given a score from a low value of 0 to a normal value of 2. APGAR is an acronym for the names of the five parameters, which are appearance (skin color), pulse rate, grimace (irritability), activity (muscle tone), and respiratory effort (Table 2-2).

Most infants are healthy and active and have total scores between 7 and 10, requiring only routine care. Infants scoring between 4 and 6 are moderately depressed and require oxygen and stimulation to breathe. Infants scoring 0 to 3 are severely depressed and require immediate ventilatory and circulatory assistance. By repeating the score at 1 and 5 minutes, it is possible to determine whether intervention has caused a change in infant status.

Neonatal Resuscitation

It is estimated that approximately 6 percent of all neonates born in a hospital require resuscitation. It is likely that this percentage is higher for out-of-hospital deliveries, although the exact numbers are not available. Factors that contribute to the need for resuscitation include prematurity, pregnancy and delivery complications, maternal health problems, or inadequate prenatal care.

If tactile stimulation does not increase the neonate's respiratory rate, immediately assist ventilations using a pediatric bag-valve mask with room air initially. If the respiratory rate is now within normal limits, assess the heart rate. If not, continue ventilations.

Assess the heart rate using a stethoscope to auscultate the apical pulse, by feeling the pulse at the base of the umbilical cord, or by palpating the brachial or femoral artery. The heart rate should normally be between 100 and 180 beats per minute, with a range of 140 to 160 beats per minute being optimal. If the pulse is 100 or greater with spontaneous respirations, continue your assessment. If the rate is less than 100, continue positive pressure ventilations. Initiate chest compressions if the heart rate is less than 60 beats per minute and is not responding to ventilations. Continue to reassess respiratory status and heart rate frequently.

Make every effort to expedite transport to a facility capable of providing neonatal intensive care while you continue resuscitative efforts. If you have a long transport time, it may be necessary to initiate vascular access to administer medications or fluid resuscitation. The most logical (and easiest) access is the umbilical vein. If this is not feasible, consider peripheral veins or an intraosseous access. During transport, continue to maintain warmth while supporting ventilations, oxygenation, and circulation. Refer to the "Neonatology" chapter for more detailed information regarding neonatal resuscitation.

CONTENT REVIEW

➤ Abnormal Deliveries
- Breech presentation
- Prolapsed cord
- Limb presentation
- Occiput posterior

Table 2-2 The APGAR Score

Element	0	1	2	Score
Appearance (skin color)	Body and extremities blue, pale	Body pink, extremities blue	Completely pink	
Pulse Rate	Absent	Below 100/min	100/min or above	
Grimace (irritability)	No response	Grimace	Cough, sneeze, cry	
Activity (muscle tone)	Limp	Some flexion of extremities	Active motion	
Respiratory Effort	Absent	Slow and irregular	Strong cry	
			TOTAL SCORE =	

Abnormal Delivery Situations

Breech Presentation

Most infants present head first and face down, which is called the *vertex position*. *Breech presentation* is the term used to describe the situation in which either the buttocks or both feet present first. This occurs in approximately 4 percent of all live births. In such presentations, there is an increased risk for delivery trauma to the mother, as well as an increased potential for cord prolapse, cord compression, or anoxic insult for the infant. Although the cause is unknown, breech presentations are most commonly associated with preterm birth, placenta previa, multiple gestation, and uterine and fetal anomalies.

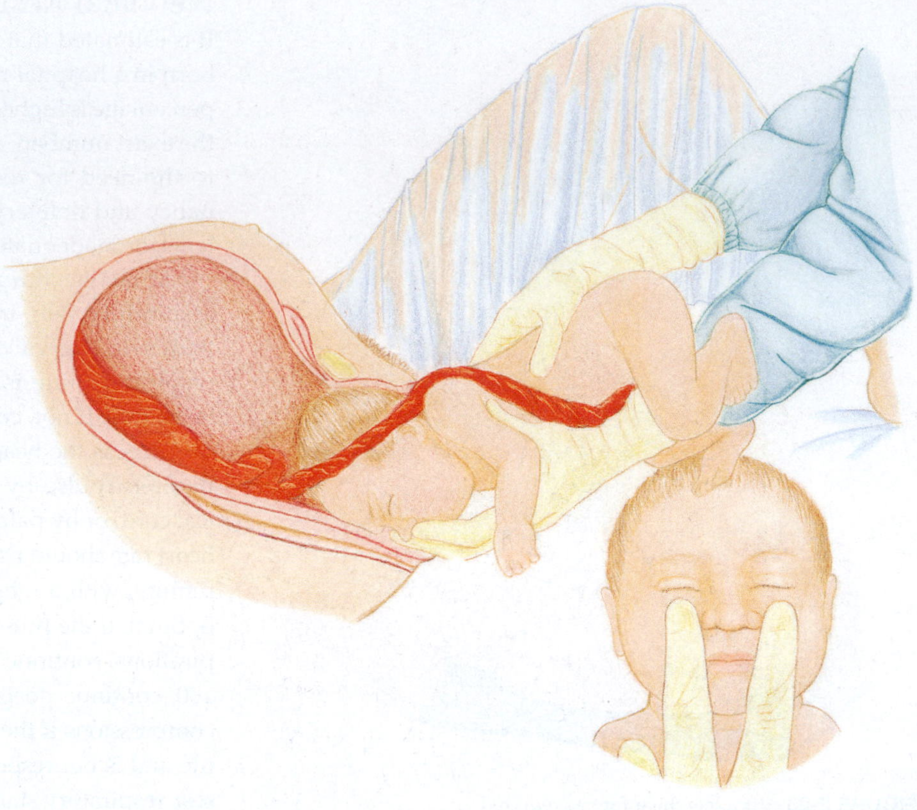

FIGURE 2-25 Placement of the fingers to maintain the airway in a breech birth.

MANAGEMENT Because Caesarean section is often required, delivery of an infant with breech presentation is best accomplished at the hospital. However, if field delivery is unavoidable, the following maneuvers are recommended. First, position the mother with her buttocks at the edge of a firm bed. Ask her to hold her legs in a flexed position. She will often require assistance in doing this. As the infant delivers, do not pull on the infant's legs. Simply support them. Allow the entire body to be delivered with contractions while you merely continue to support the infant's body (Figure 2-24).

As the head passes the pubis, apply gentle upward traction until the mouth appears over the perineum. If the head does not deliver, and the baby begins to breathe spontaneously with its face pressed against the vaginal wall, place a gloved hand in the vagina with the palm toward the infant's face. Form a "V" with the index and middle fingers on either side of the infant's nose, and push the vaginal wall away from the infant's face to allow unrestricted respiration (Figure 2-25). If necessary, continue during transport.

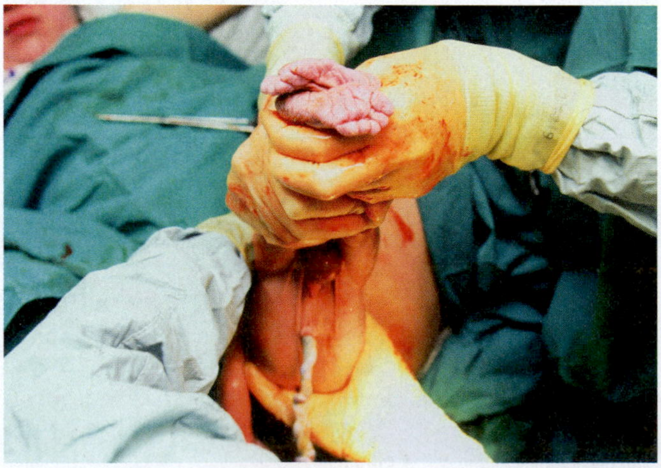

FIGURE 2-24 Breech delivery.

(© Eddie Lawrence/Science Photo Library)

Alternatively, you may find that the shoulders, not the head, are the most difficult part to deliver. In that case, allow the body to deliver to the level of the umbilicus. Support the infant's body in your palm while gently extracting approximately 4 to 6 inches of umbilical cord. Be very careful that you do not compress the cord during this extraction. Gently rotate the infant's body so that the shoulders are now in an anterior–posterior position. Apply gentle traction to the body until the axillae become visible. Guide the infant's body upward to deliver the posterior shoulder. Then, guide the neonate downward to facilitate delivery of the anterior shoulder. Now gently ease the head through the birth canal. Continue your care of the mother and infant as you would with a normal delivery.

Prolapsed Cord

A *prolapsed cord* occurs when the umbilical cord precedes the fetal presenting part. This causes the cord to be compressed between the fetus and the bony pelvis, shutting off fetal circulation (Figure 2-26). This occurs once in every 250

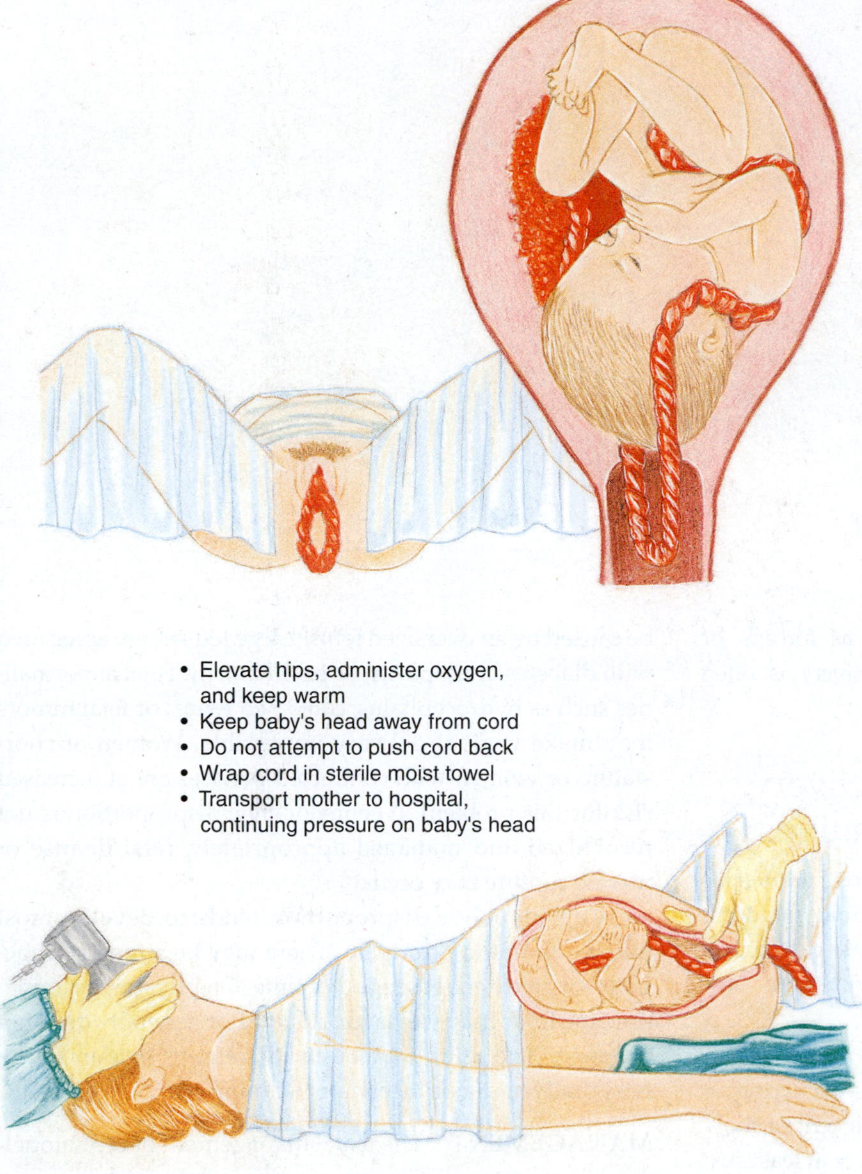

FIGURE 2-26 Prolapsed cord.

deliveries. Predisposing factors include prematurity, multiple births, and premature rupture of the membranes before the head is fully engaged. It is a serious emergency, and fetal death will occur quickly without prompt intervention.

MANAGEMENT If the umbilical cord is seen in the vagina, insert two fingers of a gloved hand to raise the presenting part of the fetus off the cord. At the same time, gently check the cord for pulsations, but take great care to ensure that you do not compress the cord. Place the mother in a Trendelenburg or knee–chest position (Figure 2-27). Administer oxygen (if the mother is hypoxic) and transport her immediately, with the fingers continuing to hold the presenting part off the umbilical cord. If assistance is available, apply a dressing moistened with sterile saline to the exposed cord. *Do not attempt delivery. Do not pull on the cord. Do not attempt to push the cord back into the vagina.*

Limb Presentation

Sometimes, if the baby is in a transverse lie across the uterus, an arm or leg is the presenting part protruding from the vagina. This is seen in less than 1 percent of births and is more commonly associated with preterm birth and multiple gestation.

MANAGEMENT When examination of the perineum reveals a single arm or leg protruding from the birth canal, a Caesarean section is necessary. Under no circumstances should you attempt a field delivery. Do not touch the extremity, as to do so may stimulate the infant to gasp, risking inhalation and aspiration of amniotic fluid. *Do not pull on the extremity or attempt to push it back into the vagina.*

Assist the mother into a knee–chest position, as is also done when there is a prolapsed cord, and administer oxygen (if the mother is hypoxic). Provide reassurance to the mother. Transport immediately (still in the knee–chest position) for an emergency Caesarean section.

Other Abnormal Presentations

Other abnormal presentations can complicate delivery. One of the most common is the *occiput posterior position*. Normally, as the infant descends into the pelvis, its face is turned posteriorly. This is important, as extension of the head assists delivery. However, if the infant descends facing forward, or occiput posterior, its passage through the pelvis is delayed. This presentation occurs most frequently in primiparas. In multiparas it usually resolves spontaneously.

The presenting part may also be the face or brow, rather than the crown of the head. Occasionally, during these presentations, the face or brow can be seen high in the pelvis during a contraction. Usually, vaginal delivery is impossible in these cases.

As described earlier for a limb presentation, the fetus can lie transversely in the uterus. In such a case, the fetus cannot enter the pelvis for delivery. If the membranes rupture, the umbilical cord can prolapse, or an arm or leg can enter the vagina. Vaginal delivery is impossible.

MANAGEMENT Early recognition of an abnormal presentation is important. If one is suspected, the mother should be reassured, placed on oxygen (if hypoxic), and transported

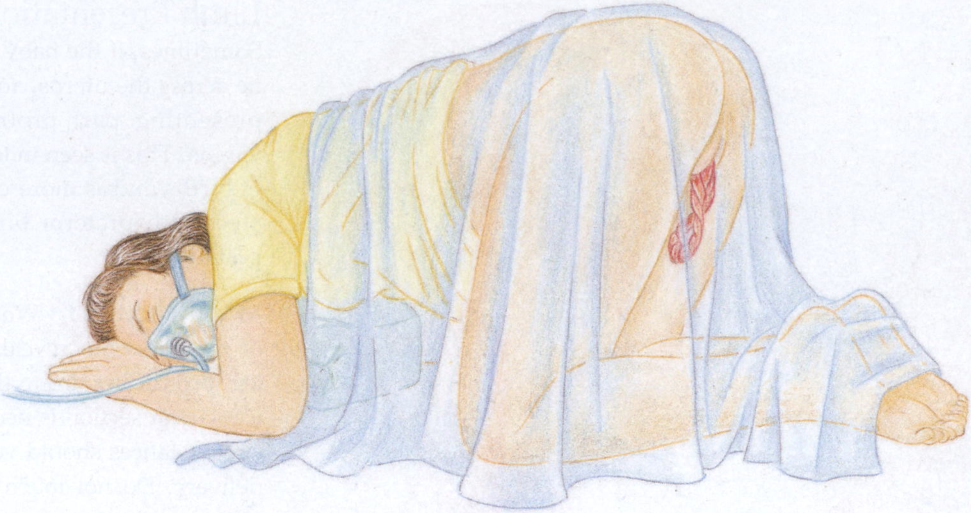

FIGURE 2-27 Patient positioning for prolapsed cord.

immediately, as forceps or Caesarean delivery is often required.

CONTENT REVIEW

- Other Delivery Complications
  - Multiple births
  - Cephalopelvic disproportion
  - Precipitous delivery
  - Shoulder dystocia
  - Meconium staining

Other Delivery Complications

Although most deliveries proceed without incident, complications can arise. Therefore, you should be prepared to deal with them.

Multiple Births

Multiple births are fairly rare, with twins occurring in approximately 1 in 90 deliveries, about 40 percent of those being preterm. Usually, the mother knows of, or at least suspects, the presence of more than one fetus. Multiple births should also be suspected if the mother's abdomen remains large after delivery of one baby and labor continues.

MANAGEMENT Manage this situation with the normal delivery guidelines, recognizing that you will need additional personnel and equipment to manage a multiple birth. In twin births, labor often begins earlier than expected, and the infants are generally smaller than babies born singly. Usually, one twin presents vertex and the other breech. There may be one shared placenta or two placentas. After delivery of the first baby, clamp and cut the cord. Then deliver the second baby. Because prematurity is common in multiple births, low birth weight is common and prevention of hypothermia is even more crucial.

Cephalopelvic Disproportion

Cephalopelvic disproportion occurs when the infant's head is too big to pass through the maternal pelvis easily. This may be caused by an oversized fetus. Large fetuses are associated with diabetes, multiparity, or postmaturity. Fetal abnormalities such as hydrocephalus, conjoined twins, or fetal tumors may make vaginal delivery impossible. Women of short stature or women with contracted pelvises are at increased risk for this problem. If cephalopelvic disproportion is not recognized and managed appropriately, fetal demise or uterine rupture may occur.

Cephalopelvic disproportion tends to develop most frequently in the primipara. There may be strong contractions for an extended period of time. On physical examination, the fetus may feel large. Also, labor generally does not progress. The fetus may be in distress, as evidenced by fetal bradycardia or meconium staining.

MANAGEMENT The usual management of cephalopelvic disproportion is Caesarean section. Administer oxygen to the mother (if she is hypoxic) and establish intravenous access. Transport should be immediate and rapid.

Precipitous Delivery

A *precipitous delivery* is a delivery that occurs after less than 3 hours of labor. This type of delivery occurs most frequently in the grand multipara and is associated with a higher-than-normal incidence of fetal trauma, tearing of the umbilical cord, or maternal lacerations.

MANAGEMENT The best way to handle precipitous delivery is to be prepared. Do not turn your attention from the mother. Be ready for a rapid delivery, and attempt to control the infant's head. Once delivered, the baby may have some difficulty with temperature regulation and must be kept warm.

Shoulder Dystocia

A *shoulder dystocia* occurs when the infant's shoulders are larger than the head. This occurs most frequently with

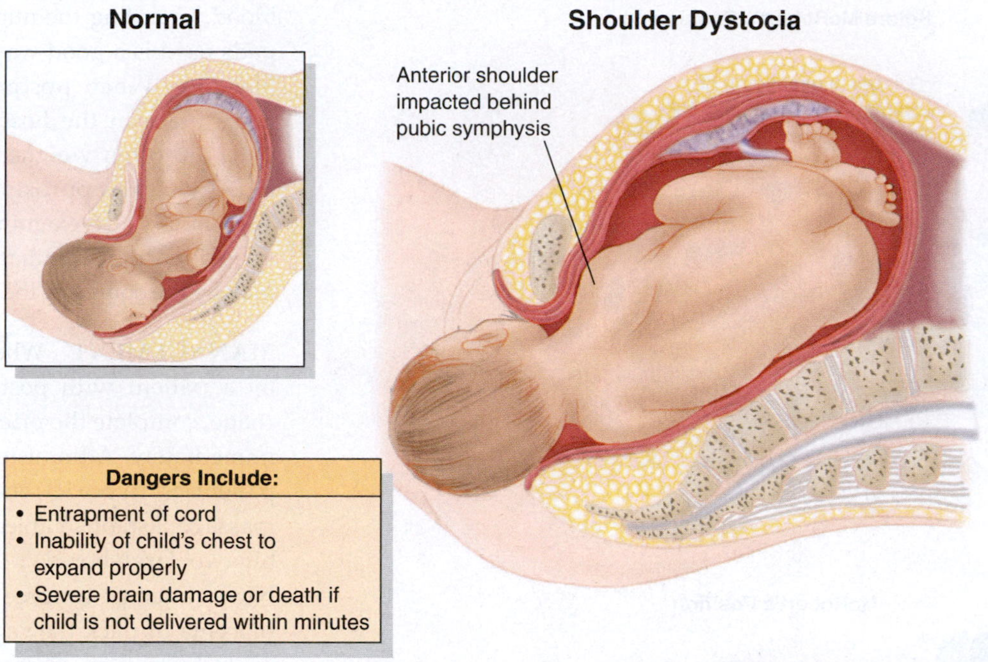

FIGURE 2-28 Shoulder dystocia.

diabetic and obese mothers and in postterm pregnancies. In shoulder dystocia, labor progresses normally and the head is delivered routinely. However, immediately after the head is delivered, it retracts back into the perineum because the shoulders are trapped between the pubic symphysis and the sacrum ("turtle sign") (Figure 2-28).

MANAGEMENT If a shoulder dystocia occurs, *do not pull on the infant's head.* Administer oxygen to the mother (if she is hypoxic) and have her drop her buttocks off the end of the bed. Then flex her thighs upward to facilitate delivery and apply firm pressure with an open hand immediately above the pubic symphysis (McRobert's maneuver). If delivery does not occur, transport the patient immediately (Figure 2-29).

Meconium Staining

Meconium staining occurs when the fetus passes feces into the amniotic fluid. Between 10 and 30 percent of all deliveries have meconium-stained fluid. It is always indicative of a fetal hypoxic incident. Hypoxia causes an increase in fetal peristalsis along with relaxation of the anal sphincter, causing meconium to pass into the amniotic fluid. In addition to the stress that caused the incident, there is a risk of aspiration of the meconium-stained fluid.

Meconium staining is often associated with prolonged labor but may be seen in term, postterm, and low-birthweight infants. The incident may occur a few days prior to delivery or during labor. Some meconium staining is virtually always associated with breech deliveries as a result of vagal stimulation, which occurs as a result of the pressure of the contracting uterus on the fetus's head.

Evidence of meconium staining is readily observable. Normally the amniotic fluid is clear or possibly light-straw colored. When meconium is present, the color varies from a light yellowish-green to light green or, worst case, dark green, which is sometimes described as "pea soup." As a rule, the thicker and darker the color, the higher the risk of fetal morbidity.

MANAGEMENT As noted earlier, bulb suctioning is no longer recommended. If the meconium is thin and light colored, no further treatment is generally required and you should continue with the delivery and routine care. However, if the meconium is thick, visualize the glottis and suction the hypopharynx and trachea using an endotracheal tube until you have cleared all of the meconium from the newborn's airway. Failure to do so will cause the meconium to be pushed farther into the airway and down into the lungs during the delivery process.

Maternal Complications of Labor and Delivery

Several maternal problems can arise during and after delivery. These include postpartum hemorrhage, uterine rupture, uterine inversion, and pulmonary embolism.

CONTENT REVIEW

➤ Maternal Complications
- Postpartum hemorrhage
- Uterine rupture
- Uterine inversion
- Pulmonary embolism

Postpartum Hemorrhage

Postpartum hemorrhage is the loss of more than 500 mL of blood immediately follow-

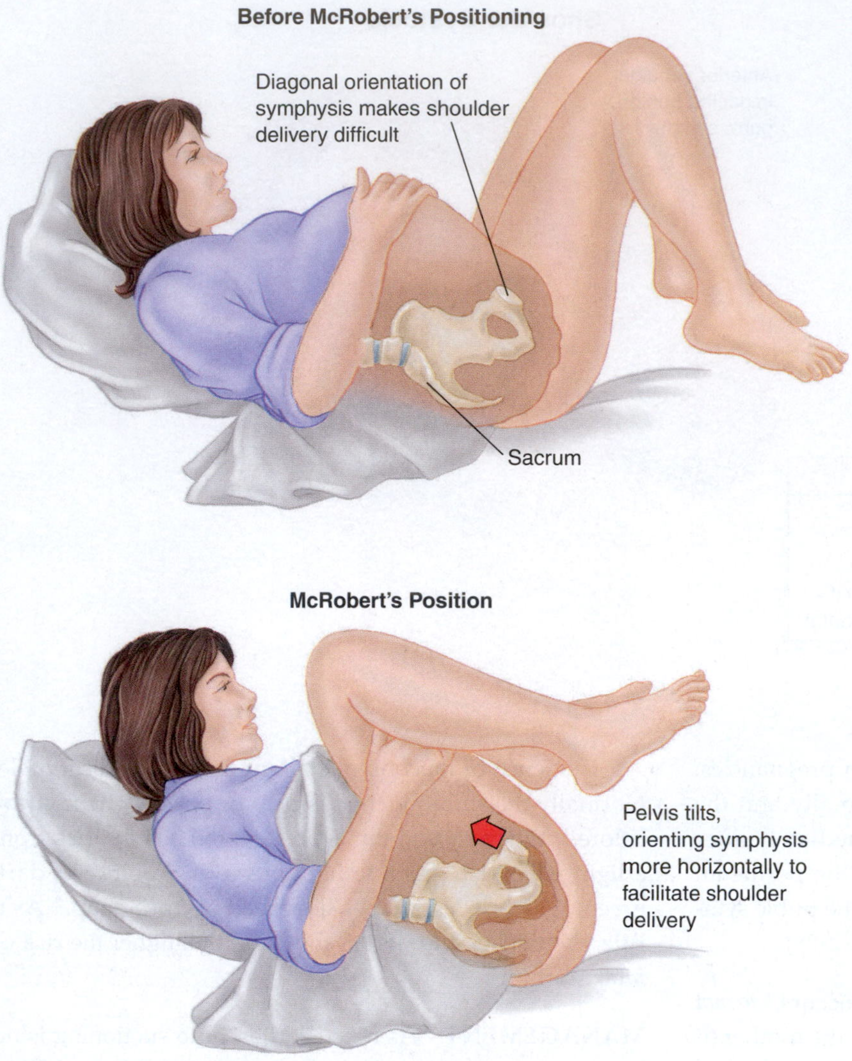

FIGURE 2-29 McRobert's maneuver for shoulder dystocia.

ing delivery. It occurs in approximately 5 percent of deliveries. The most common cause of postpartum hemorrhage is *uterine atony*, or lack of uterine muscle tone. This tends to occur most frequently in the multigravida and is most common following multiple births or births of large infants. Uterine atony also occurs after precipitous deliveries and prolonged labors. In addition to uterine atony, postpartum hemorrhage can be caused by placenta previa, abruptio placentae, retained placental parts, clotting disorders in the mother, or vaginal and cervical tears. Occasionally, the uterus fails to return to its normal size during the postpartum period, and postpartum hemorrhage occurs long after the birth, potentially as much as two weeks postpartum.

Assessment of the patient with postpartum hemorrhage should focus on the history and the predisposing factors as described. You must rely heavily on the clinical appearance of the patient and her vital signs. Often, the uterus will feel boggy and soft on physical examination. Vaginal bleeding is usually obvious as a steady, free flow of blood. Counting the number of sanitary pads used is a good way to monitor the bleeding. When postpartum bleeding takes place in the hospital setting the pads are often weighed, as 500 mL of blood weighs approximately 1 pound. You should also examine the perineum for evidence of traumatic injury, which may be the source of the bleeding.

MANAGEMENT When confronted by a patient with postpartum hemorrhage, complete the primary assessment immediately. Administer oxygen (if the patient is hypoxic) and begin fundal massage. Establish at least one, preferably two, large-bore IVs of normal saline. Never attempt to force delivery of the placenta or pack the vagina with dressings. In severe cases, medical direction may request the administration of oxytocin (Pitocin). The usual dose is 10 to 20 USP units oxytocin in 1 liter of normal saline to run at 125 mL/hour titrated to response. If IV access cannot be obtained, an alternative therapy is to administer 10 USP units intramuscularly.

Uterine Rupture

Uterine rupture is the actual tearing, or rupture, of the uterus. It usually occurs with the onset of labor. However, it can also occur before labor, as a result of blunt abdominal trauma. During labor, it often results from prolonged uterine contractions or a surgically scarred uterus, such as that which occurs from previous Caesarean sections, especially in those with the classic vertical incision. It can also occur following a prolonged or obstructed labor, as in the case of cephalopelvic disproportion or in conjunction with abnormal presentations. Although it is a rare occurrence, it carries with it an extremely high maternal and fetal mortality rate.

The patient with uterine rupture will complain of excruciating abdominal pain and will often be in shock. Uterine rupture is virtually always associated with the cessation of labor contractions. If the rupture is complete, the pain usually subsides. On physical examination, there is often profound shock without evidence of external hemorrhage, although it is sometimes associated with vaginal bleeding. Fetal heart tones are absent. The abdomen is often tender and rigid and may exhibit rebound tenderness. It is often possible to palpate the uterus as a separate hard mass found next to the fetus.

MANAGEMENT Management is the same as for any patient in shock. Administer oxygen at high concentration. Next, establish two large-bore IVs with normal saline and begin fluid resuscitation. Monitor vital signs and fetal heart tones continuously. Transport the patient rapidly. If the fetus is still viable, the definitive treatment is Caesarean section with subsequent repair or removal of the uterus.

Uterine Inversion

Uterine inversion is a rare emergency, occurring only once in every 2,500 live births. It occurs when the uterus turns inside out after delivery and extends through the cervix. When uterine inversion occurs, the supporting ligaments and blood vessels supplying blood to the uterus are torn, usually causing profound shock. The average blood loss associated with uterine inversion ranges from 800 to 1,800 mL. Uterine inversion usually results from pulling on the umbilical cord while awaiting delivery of the placenta or from attempts to express the placenta when the uterus is relaxed.

MANAGEMENT If uterine inversion occurs, you must act quickly. First, place the patient in a supine position and begin oxygen administration (if the patient is hypoxic). *Do not* attempt to detach the placenta or pull on the cord. Initiate two large-bore IVs of normal saline and begin fluid resuscitation. Make one attempt to replace the uterus, using the following technique: With the palm of the hand, push the fundus of the inverted uterus toward the vagina. If this single attempt is unsuccessful, cover the uterus with towels moistened with saline and transport the patient immediately.

Pulmonary Embolism

Pulmonary embolism is the presence of a blood clot in the pulmonary vascular system (see the chapter titled "Pulmonology"). It can occur after pregnancy, usually as a result of venous thromboembolism. It is one of the most common causes of maternal death and appears to occur more frequently following Caesarean section than vaginal delivery. Pulmonary embolism may occur at any time during pregnancy. There is usually a sudden onset of severe dyspnea, accompanied by sharp chest pain. Some patients also report a sense of impending doom. On physical examination, the patient may show tachycardia, tachypnea, jugular vein distention, and, in severe cases, hypotension.

MANAGEMENT Management of pulmonary embolism consists of administration of high-concentration oxygen and ventilatory support as needed. Establish an IV of normal saline at a keep-open rate. Initiate cardiac monitoring and carefully monitor the patient's vital signs and oxygen saturation while transporting her immediately.

Cardiac Arrest in Pregnancy

CONTENT REVIEW

- Considerations for Cardiac Arrest in Pregnancy
  - Estimation of gestational age
  - Chest compressions
  - Manual lateral uterine displacement
  - Defibrillation
  - Airway management
  - Use of emergency drugs
  - Transport decisions

Cardiac arrest in the setting of pregnancy can be quite challenging. In essence, you are resuscitating two patients. In 2015, the American Heart Association issued the first-ever guidelines for resuscitation of the pregnant patient.[5] These guidelines highlight important patient care strategies that are different for the pregnant patient when compared to those who are not pregnant.

Estimation of Gestational Age

It is important, when treating a pregnant patient in cardiac arrest, to try to estimate the gestational age. This is best accomplished by comparing the uterine fundal height to the mother's symphysis pubis. Typically, each centimeter in height between the symphysis pubis and the uterine fundus corresponds to one week of gestation. This is less accurate if the patient is beyond 36 weeks gestation. Generally speaking, if the uterine fundus is palpable at the symphysis pubis, then the pregnancy is approximately 12 weeks. If the uterine fundus is palpable at the umbilicus, then the pregnancy is typically 20 weeks. If the uterine fundus is present at the xiphoid, then the pregnancy is at least 36 weeks. Although these are simply estimates, they are a good guide for emergency care procedures.

Chest Compressions in Pregnancy

High-quality chest compressions are essential in the management of the pregnant cardiac arrest patient (Figure 2-30). For compressions to be effective, the patient should be on a hard surface and the compressions should be of the proper rate and depth. Any interruptions must be minimized. Chest compressions should be performed at a rate of at least 100 per minute and at a depth of at least 2 inches (5 centimeters). Full recoil should be allowed before the next compression (to enhance ventricular filling). Interruptions should be minimized. Ventilations should be provided at a compression to ventilation ratio of 30:2. Mechanical chest compression devices should not be used in pregnancy.

Aortocaval Compression

Several factors can adversely affect the quality of chest compressions of the pregnant patient. Among these is **aortocaval compression**. In the pregnant patient, the large gravid uterus can compress the aorta and the vena cava when the patient is supine. To facilitate optimal CPR, the uterus must be manually moved off the aorta and vena

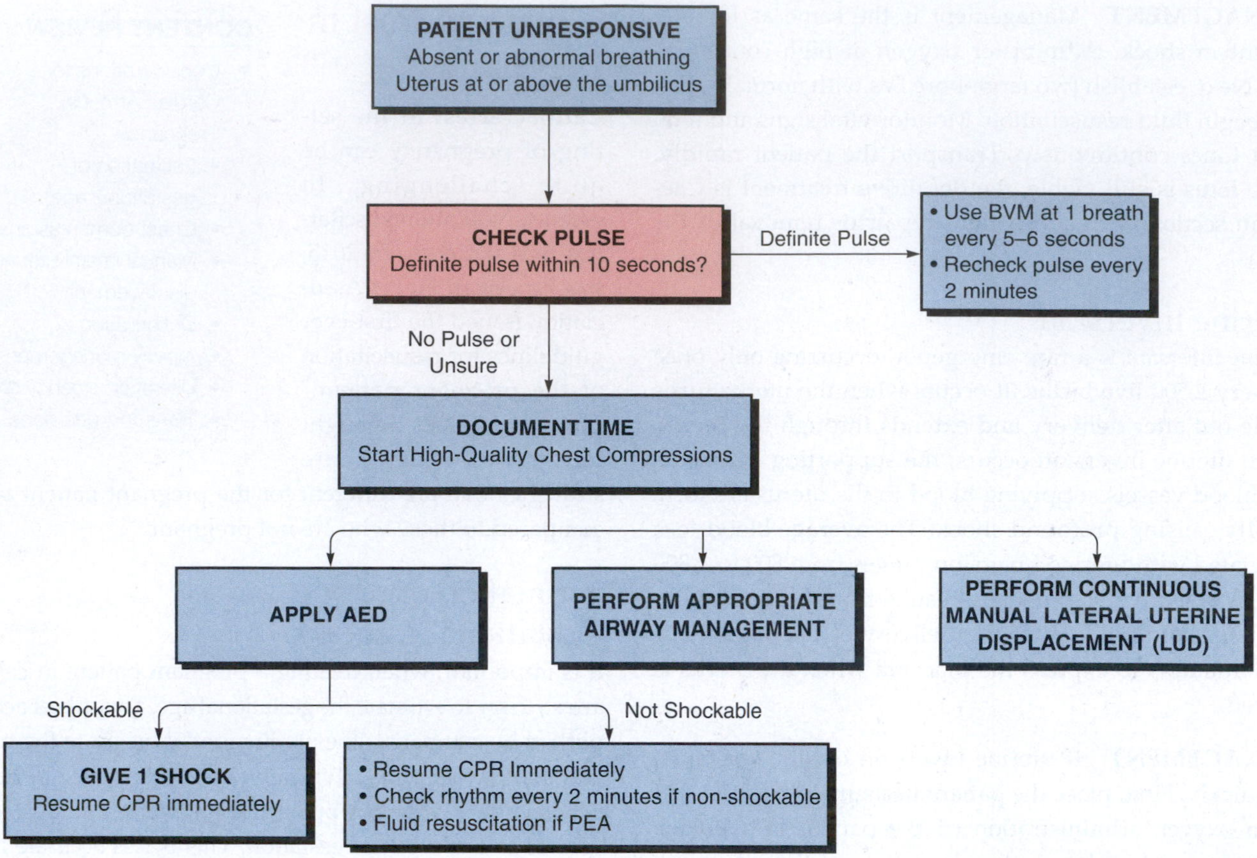

FIGURE 2-30 Pregnant cardiac arrest treatment strategy.

cava to allow adequate blood return to the heart. Placing a patient in a position other than the supine position (e.g., tilted 30 degrees to the left) may compromise the effectiveness of CPR. Because of this, it is now recommended that all pregnant patients in cardiac arrest with an estimated gestational age of 20 weeks or greater receive a procedure called **manual lateral uterine displacement (LUD)**. If the uterus is difficult to assess, as can occur in the morbidly obese patient, then LUD should be provided if technically feasible. Manual LUD can be accomplished from either side of the patient, using one or both hands to move the uterus upward and leftward off the maternal blood vessels (Figures 2-31 and 2-32. The rescuer must be careful not to inadvertently push down, which would actually increase vena caval compression.

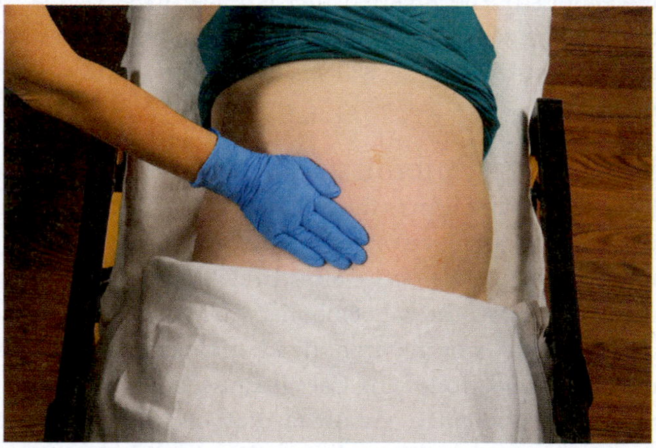

FIGURE 2-31 Manual LUD performed with one-handed technique.

Defibrillation in Pregnancy

In cases of cardiac arrest that are due to ventricular fibrillation or pulseless ventricular tachycardia, survival is most likely when rapid defibrillation is provided. The same is true for the pregnant patient who sustains one of these two potentially fatal arrhythmias. There is no significant evidence that defibrillation or cardioversion shocks to the mother pass a significant amount of electrical energy to the fetus. Thus, defibrillation and cardioversion are generally considered safe in all stages of pregnancy. The same defibrillation protocol used in nonpregnant patients should be used in pregnant patients, without modification.

Airway Management in Pregnancy

Because of the changes in maternal physiology associated with pregnancy, hypoxia develops much more quickly in the pregnant patient than in those who are not pregnant.

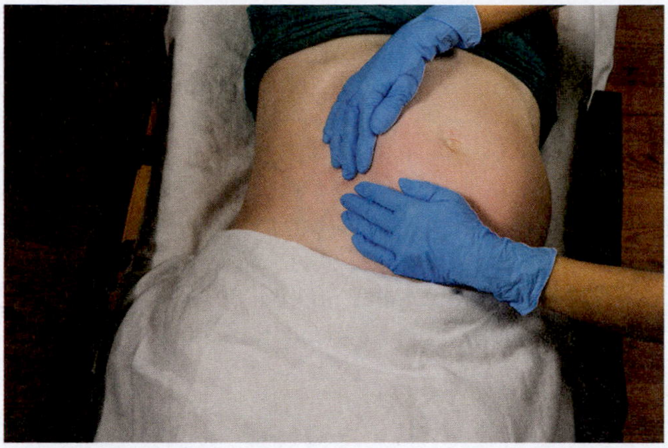

FIGURE 2-32 Manual LUD performed with two-handed technique.

Because of this, rapid high-quality airway management techniques and mechanical ventilation are essential. In addition, the pregnant patient should be provided early bag-valve-mask ventilation with 100 percent supplemental oxygen, if possible. As with nonpregnant cardiac arrest, hyperventilation should be avoided. The pregnant patient has limited oxygen reserves, so supplemental oxygen should be provided early in resuscitation. During endotracheal intubation, consider the use of passive oxygenation techniques. When intubating the pregnant patient, start with an endotracheal tube size of 6.0 to 7.0 mm. Ideally, no more than two attempts at intubation should be made. If an endotracheal tube cannot be readily placed, a extraglottic airway is the preferred device. Cricoid pressure is not recommended. Continuous waveform capnography is also essential in maintaining proper ventilation rates and should be readily applied in all resuscitations.

Use of Emergency Drugs in the Pregnant Cardiac Arrest Patient

Pharmacologic therapy for cardiac arrest in the pregnant patient differs little from that for patients who are not pregnant. Medication doses should not be altered because of pregnancy. Epinephrine, administered at a 1 mg dose IV or IO every 3 to 5 minutes, should be considered in the pregnant cardiac arrest patient. Epinephrine is preferred over vasopressin because of the effects of vasopressin on the gravid uterus. For refractory (shock-resistant) ventricular fibrillation or ventricular tachycardia, a rapid infusion of 300 mg of amiodarone should be provided with repeat 150 mg doses as needed. In cardiac arrest, no medicines should be withheld from the emergency treatment regimen out of concerns about fetal damage. Other ACLS medications should be provided at the standard nonpregnant dosage.

Transport Destinations for the Pregnant Cardiac Arrest Patient

The pregnant cardiac arrest patient should be transported to a hospital that has the appropriate staffing and capabilities to manage this type of emergency. This includes the possible performance of a perimortem Caesarean delivery (PMCD). In addition, personnel and equipment must be available for resuscitation and stabilization of the potential neonate. The purpose of the PMCD is to facilitate resuscitation of the mother by relieving aortocaval compression and evacuating the uterus. Both these measures can significantly improve resuscitation efforts. In addition, PMCD allows for early delivery of the baby and, hopefully, protection from anoxia. Even in cases where the mother is not salvageable, such as with severe trauma or prolonged pulselessness, timely delivery of the fetus is essential. PMCD should not be considered a prehospital skill.

Summary

Childbirth is a normal process, and obstetric emergencies are fairly uncommon. However, all pregnant patients are at risk for developing complications, and it is impossible to predict which ones will actually occur. It is therefore important to recognize these complications and act accordingly. Luckily for us, if the mother has been seeing her obstetrician regularly for prenatal care, she will have a good idea of her situation and will be able to provide important information about the placenta's location and baby positioning. Unfortunately, though, the vast majority of EMS responses for obstetric emergencies are to a population of patients who do not seek prenatal care and wait until the last minute to summon EMS for help. In these cases, you will barely have enough time to introduce yourself before being presented with the second patient.

Keep in mind that in all obstetric calls, you are caring for two patients, including one whom you are unable to monitor until birth. Whenever possible, it is always best to deliver in a facility that has the ability to monitor the baby and protect him. However, there will be times when a field delivery is necessary.

One of the most important things you can do following delivery is to keep the baby warm. A general rule of thumb is that you should be sweating in the back of the ambulance. Remember, the average room temperature is 68°F to 72°F but the baby should be kept at a balmy 98°F.

Field delivery can be an exciting and nerve-racking experience. As long as you remember the priorities of patient care, the situation should go smoothly. Relax and enjoy the opportunity to help bring a new life into the world. This is one of the few times when paramedics get to participate in a positive medical scenario.

You Make the Call

It is 9 A.M. and you and your partner are participating in an in-station drill when you are dispatched for a "possible stroke." You soon arrive at a garden apartment, where you are met by a very anxious man. He reports that he just arrived home from working the night shift and found his pregnant wife semiconscious on the living room floor. He says that he talked to her about an hour earlier and she was "fine."

Your assessment reveals a 25-year-old pregnant woman who responds to verbal stimuli with incoherent muttering. Her airway is patent and her respirations are nonlabored at a rate of 20 per minute. Lung sounds are clear bilaterally. Her pulse is strong and regular at 96 per minute. Her flushed skin is warm to the touch. She is diaphoretic. You observe that her ankles are markedly edematous. Her blood pressure is 158/100 mmHg. There are no obvious signs of traumatic injury.

Your partner places a saline lock. He also checks her blood glucose level and finds that it is >120 mg/dL. You obtain her obstetric history, learning that she is a G1P0 who is at 32 weeks' gestation. She has had good prenatal care and is scheduled for an appointment today at 4 P.M. Her husband tells you that she has been taking prenatal vitamins with iron throughout her pregnancy. He denies any other medical problems other than the fact that her doctor has been "watching" her blood pressure for the past couple of months. He denies any alcohol or recreational drug use by his wife.

1. What is your first priority?
2. What do you suspect is the likely cause of the patient's signs and symptoms?
3. Your patient's husband is very concerned about the well-being of his wife and baby. What should you tell him?
4. How should this patient be transported to the hospital?

See Suggested Responses at the back of this book.

Review Questions

1. The first two weeks of the menstrual cycle are dominated by which hormone, which causes the endometrium to thicken and become engorged with blood?
   a. Pitocin
   b. Estrogen
   c. Epinephrine
   d. Progesterone

2. In which week of gestation is the gender of the fetus typically able to be determined ?
   a. 10
   b. 12
   c. 14
   d. 16

3. A woman who has given birth to her first child is termed ______________
   a. multipara.
   b. primipara.
   c. primigravida.
   d. multigravida.
4. During transport of a woman in her third trimester, vital signs should be obtained with the patient in which position?
   a. Sitting upright
   b. Lying on her right side
   c. Lying on her left side
   d. Lying flat on her back
5. Although it is not always available in the ambulance, what is the preferred analgesic in pregnancy?
   a. Fentanyl
   b. Ibuprofen
   c. Morphine sulfate
   d. Nitrous oxide
6. Intentional termination of a pregnancy under any condition not allowed by law is termed _____
   a. missed abortion.
   b. elective abortion.
   c. criminal abortion.
   d. therapeutic abortion.
7. Which third-trimester emergency can occur as a result of abnormal implantation of the placenta on the lower half of the uterine wall, resulting in partial or complete coverage of the cervical opening?
   a. Placenta previa
   b. Ectopic pregnancy
   c. Abruptio placentae
   d. Incomplete abortion
8. An abortion in which fetal death occurs but the fetus is not expelled is termed ____________
   a. missed abortion.
   b. criminal abortion.
   c. habitual abortion.
   d. incomplete abortion.
9. Which stage of labor begins with the complete dilation of the cervix and ends with the delivery of the fetus?
   a. First
   b. Second
   c. Third
   d. Dilation
10. Infants scoring _____ on the one-minute APGAR scoring system are termed moderately depressed and require oxygen and stimulation to breathe.
    a. 0–3
    b. 4–6
    c. 6–9
    d. 7–10
11. What type of delivery presentation is related to preterm birth, multiple gestation, or uterine anomalies?
    a. Occiput anterior
    b. Occiput posterior
    c. Vertex
    d. Breech
12. What should you do if, during delivery of a baby, the umbilical cord is the presenting part out of the birth canal?
    a. Place a dry dressing over the exposed umbilical cord.
    b. Administer high-flow oxygen to the mother.
    c. Place the patient in a knee–chest position.
    d. Initiate an infusion of TXA to inhibit excessive blood loss.
13. Which birthing emergency may require you to perform McRobert's maneuver?
    a. Exposed umbilical cord
    b. Vertex presentation
    c. Meconium staining
    d. Shoulder dystocia
14. In which of the following situations should you provide manual lateral uterine displacement?
    a. Maternal cardiac arrest after 20 weeks' gestation
    b. After visualizing any soft tissue trauma in a suspected rape victim
    c. Only when cardiac compressions have failed to result in ROSC after 10 minutes
    d. Prior to placing the patient in a knee–chest position for a breech delivery

See Answers to Review Questions at the end of this book.

References

1. American Diabetes Association. "Executive Summary: Standards of Medical Care in Diabetes—2011." *Diabetes Care* 34 (Suppl 1) (2011): S4–S10.
2. Nama, V. and I. Manyonda. "Tubal Ectopic Pregnancy: Diagnosis and Management." *Arch Gynecol Obstet* 279 (2009): 443–453.
3. Leeman, L. and P. Fontaine. "Hypertensive Disorders of Pregnancy." *Am Fam Physician* 78 (2008): 93–100.
4. Wyckoff, M. H., K. Aziz, M. B. Escobedo, et al. "Part 13: Neonatal Resuscitation: 2015 American Heart Association Guidelines for Cardiopulmonary Resuscitation and Emergency Cardiovascular Care." *Circulation* 132 (2015): S543–S560.
5. Jeejeebhoy, F. M., C. M. Zelop, S. Lipman, et al. "Cardiac Arrest in Pregnancy: A Scientific Statement from the American Heart Association." *Circulation* 132 (2015):1747-1773.

Further Reading

Cunningham, F., K. Loveno, S. Bloom, J. Hauth, D. Rouse, and C. Spong. *Williams Obstetrics.* 24th ed. New York: McGraw Hill, 2014.

Gruenber, B. N. *Essentials of Prehospital Maternity Care.* Upper Saddle River, NJ: Pearson/Prentice Hall, 2006.

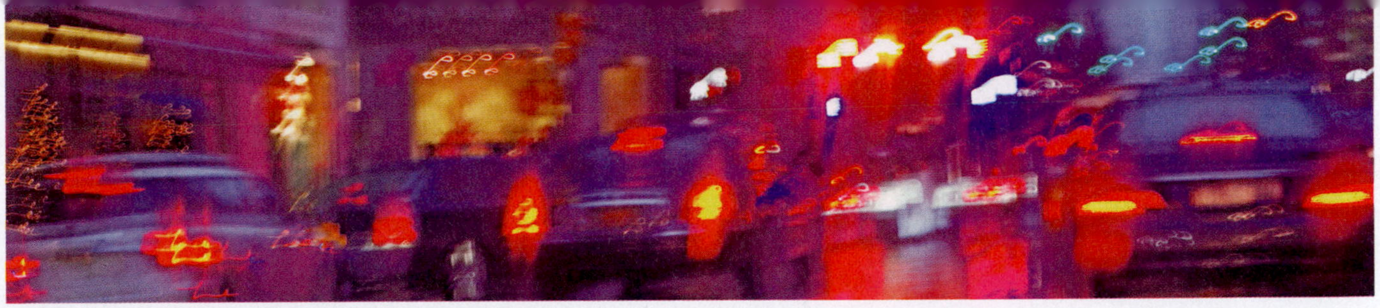

Chapter 3 Neonatology

Bryan Bledsoe, DO, FACEP, FAAEM, EMT-P

STANDARD

Special Patient Populations (Neonatal Care)

COMPETENCY

Integrates assessment findings with principles of epidemiology and pathophysiology and knowledge of psychosocial needs to formulate a field impression and implement a comprehensive treatment/disposition plan for patients with special needs.

Learning Objectives

Terminal Performance Objective: After reading this chapter, you should be able to integrate patient assessment findings, patient history, and knowledge of anatomy, physiology, pathophysiology, and basic and advanced life support interventions to recognize and manage problems in neonatal patients.

Enabling Objectives: To accomplish the terminal performance objective, you should be able to:

1. Define key terms introduced in this chapter.
2. Identify basic epidemiology findings regarding neonatology and the risk factors that can indicate possible complications in newborns.
3. Discuss the physiology of the neonate as he shifts from intrauterine to extrauterine life.
4. Identify and discuss the pathophysiology and assessment findings of various congenital anomalies that may be encountered at birth.
5. Use a process of clinical reasoning to guide and interpret the patient assessment and management process for normal and distressed neonatal patients, according to the neonatal resuscitation algorithm.
6. List the components of and describe how to use the APGAR scoring system with neonates.
7. Identify how to recognize and manage neonatal problems such as meconium aspiration, apnea, respiratory distress, heart rate disorders, prematurity, seizures, birth injuries, and others, as appropriate.
8. Given various neonatal scenarios, discuss how the paramedic should assess and manage these emergencies in the prehospital environment.

KEY TERMS

acrocyanosis, p. 74
antepartum, p. 55
APGAR score, p. 61
birth injury, p. 75
choanal atresia, p. 59
cleft lip, p. 59
cleft palate, p. 59
delayed cord clamping (DCC) , p. 63
diaphragmatic hernia, p. 59
ductus arteriosus, p. 55
extrauterine, p. 55
glottic function, p. 67
herniation, p. 71
hyperbilirubinemia, p. 63
intrapartum, p. 55
isolette, p. 70
meconium, p. 62
meningomyelocele, p. 59
nasogastric tube/orogastric tube, p. 67
neonatal abstinence syndrome (NAS), p. 75
neonate, p. 54
newborn, p. 54
omphalocele, p. 59
PEEP, p. 67
persistent fetal circulation, p. 55
phototherapy, p. 75
Pierre Robin syndrome, p. 59
polycythemia, p. 63
thyrotoxicosis, p. 75
vagal stimulation, p. 75

Case Study

A storm rages outside, making travel dangerous. Around midnight, you receive a call from the dispatcher. A woman has just gone into labor. She lives about 20 minutes from the hospital, but her husband is worried about the weather conditions and requests help from your EMS unit.

On arrival, you find a 24-year-old woman who is about to deliver her second baby. You quickly determine that there is not enough time to transport the patient to the hospital. You and your partner begin to prepare the equipment needed for a field delivery.

The delivery goes beautifully, and you announce the arrival of the couple's new daughter. Following the birth, however, the baby remains blue and limp—even after you quickly dry the baby and then wrap her in a dry blanket. You stimulate the baby by rubbing her back and flicking the soles of her feet gently.

When the baby stays blue and limp, you push aside a very normal urge to panic and deliver breaths using a bag-valve-mask unit and room air. The baby "pinks up" almost immediately and begins to cry.

Using the pulse oximeter, you determine that the oxygen saturation is 95 percent and increasing. You prepare the baby for transport, making sure her head is covered. You ask the mother to hold her new daughter and then load both of your patients into the ambulance.

En route to the hospital, you continue to monitor the infant and assign a 5-minute APGAR score of 9. The trip is uneventful. The baby leaves the hospital only one day after the mother. The parents later pay a surprise visit to your EMS unit and proudly introduce their healthy baby daughter!

Introduction

Babies pass through stages of physical and emotional development. This chapter concerns itself with babies 1 month old and under. Babies less than 1 month old are called **neonates**. Recently born neonates—those in the first few hours of their lives—may also be called **newborns** or *newly born infants* (Figure 3-1).

After an unscheduled delivery in the field, you have two patients to manage—the mother and the baby. You can review information on care of the mother in the "Obstetrics" chapter. The present chapter will describe the initial care of newborns, focusing on the special needs of distressed and premature newborns.

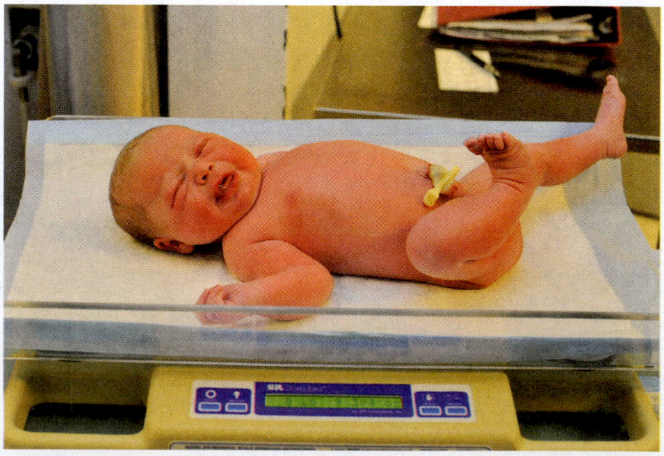

FIGURE 3-1 Term newborn.

General Pathophysiology, Assessment, and Management

The care of newborns follows the same priorities as for all patients. Complete the primary assessment first. Correct any problems detected during the primary assessment before proceeding to the next step. The vast majority of newborns require no resuscitation beyond suctioning the airway, mild stimulation, and maintenance of body temperature. However, for newborns who require additional care, your quick actions can make the difference between life and death.

Epidemiology

Approximately 10 percent of newborns require some assistance to begin breathing at birth, whereas less than 1 percent require extensive resuscitative measures.[1,2] Medications are rarely indicated in newborn resuscitation. The incidence of complications increases as the birth weight decreases. About 80 percent of newborns weighing less than 1,500 grams (3 pounds, 5 ounces) at birth require resuscitation. Determine whether newborns are at risk by considering the **antepartum** and **intrapartum** factors that may indicate complications at the time of delivery (Table 3-1).

Your success in resuscitating at-risk infants increases with training, ongoing practice, and proper stocking of equipment on board the ambulance. Make sure your ambulance carries a basic OB kit and resuscitation equipment for newborns of various sizes. (See the list in the Resuscitation section later in this chapter.)

Plan transport in advance. Know the types of facilities available in your locality, and the local protocols governing use of these facilities. A nearby neonatal intensive care unit (NICU) makes the best choice for at-risk newborns. However, if you must transport to a distant NICU, determine whether it might be in the best interests of the infant to transport him to the nearest facility for stabilization. Follow local protocols and consult medical direction as needed.

Table 3-1 Risk Factors Indicating Possible Complications in Newborns

Antepartum Factors	Intrapartum Factors
Multiple gestation	Premature labor
Inadequate prenatal care	Meconium-stained amniotic fluid
Mother's age (<16 or >35)	Rupture of membranes more than 24 hours prior to delivery
History of perinatal morbidity or mortality	Use of narcotics within 4 hours of delivery
Postterm gestation	Abnormal presentation
Drugs/medications	Prolonged labor or precipitous delivery
Toxemia, hypertension, diabetes	Prolapsed cord or bleeding

Pathophysiology

Upon birth, dramatic changes occur within the newborn to prepare it for **extrauterine** life. The respiratory system, which is essentially nonfunctional when the fetus is in the uterus, must suddenly initiate and maintain respirations. While in the uterus, fetal lung fluid fills the fetal lungs. The capillaries and arterioles of the lungs are closed. Most blood pumped by the heart bypasses the nonfunctional respiratory system by flowing through the **ductus arteriosus**.

Approximately one-third of fetal lung fluid is removed through compression of the chest during vaginal delivery. Under normal conditions, the newborn takes his first breath within the first few seconds after delivery. The timing of the first breath is unrelated to the cutting of the umbilical cord. Factors that stimulate the baby's first breath include:

- Mild acidosis
- Initiation of stretch reflexes in the lungs
- Hypoxia
- Hypothermia

With the first breaths, the lungs rapidly fill with air, which displaces the remaining fetal fluid. The pulmonary arterioles and capillaries open, decreasing pulmonary vascular resistance. At this point, the resistance to blood flow in the lungs is now less than the resistance of the ductus arteriosus. Because of this pressure difference, blood flow is diverted from the ductus arteriosus to the lungs, where it picks up oxygen for transport to the peripheral tissues (Figure 3-2).

Soon, there is no need for the ductus arteriosus, and it eventually closes and becomes the *ligamentum arteriosum*. However, if hypoxia or severe acidosis occurs, the pulmonary vascular bed may constrict again and the ductus may reopen. This will retrigger fetal circulation, with its attendant shunting and ongoing hypoxia. (This condition is called **persistent fetal circulation**.) To help the newborn make the transition to extrauterine life, it is very important for the paramedic to facilitate the first few breaths and to prevent ongoing hypoxia and acidosis.

Remain alert at all times to signs of respiratory distress. Infants are susceptible to hypoxemia, which can lead to permanent brain damage. After initial hypoxia, the

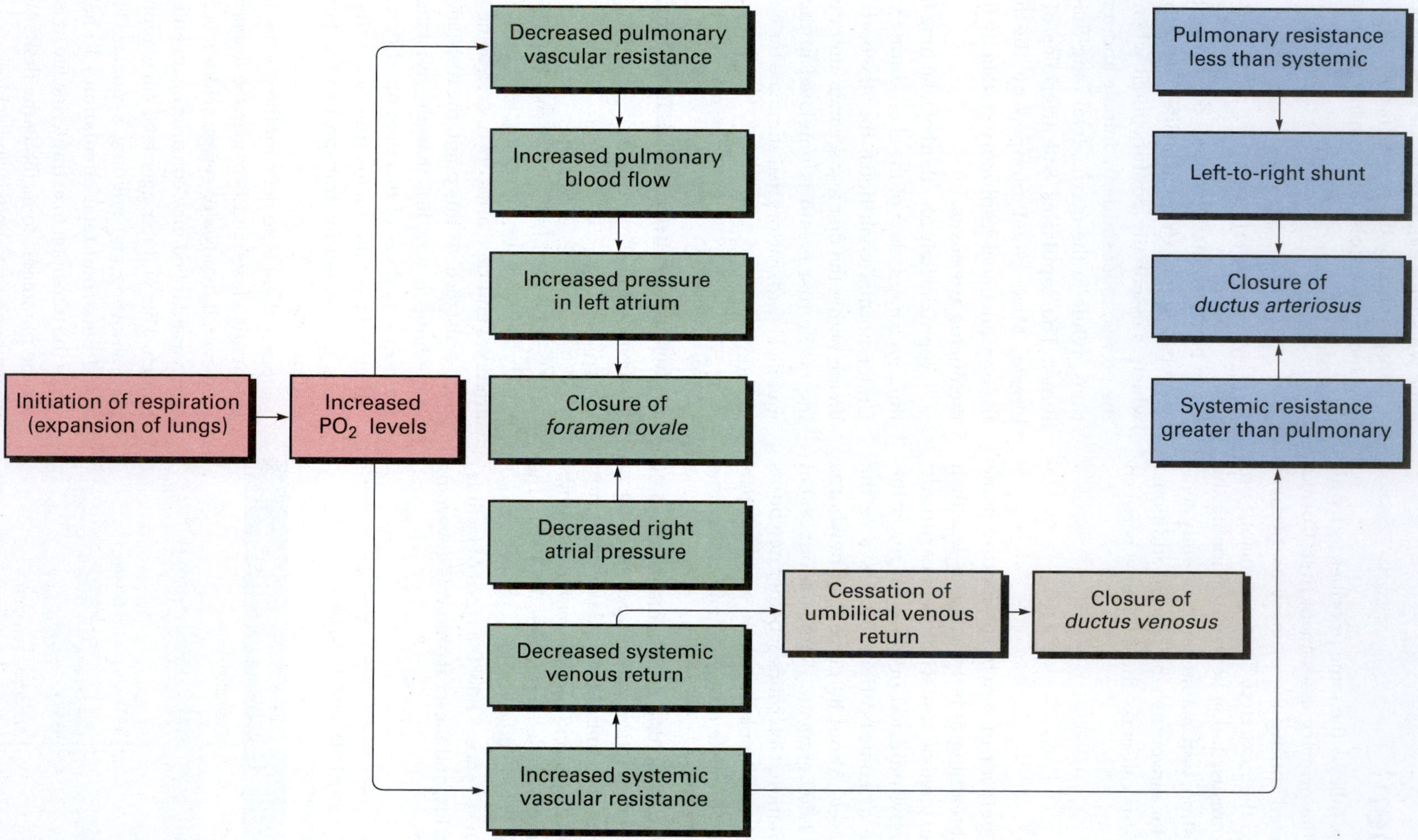

FIGURE 3-2 Hemodynamic changes in the newborn at birth.

infant rapidly gasps for breath. If the asphyxia continues, respiratory movements cease altogether, the heart rate begins to fall, and neuromuscular tone gradually diminishes. The infant then enters a period of apnea known as *primary apnea*. In most cases, simple stimulation and exposure to oxygen will reverse bradycardia and assist in the development of pulmonary perfusion.

With ongoing asphyxia, however, the infant will enter a period known as *secondary apnea*. During secondary apnea, the infant takes several last deep gasping respirations. The heart rate, blood pressure, and oxygen saturation in the blood continue to fall. The infant becomes unresponsive to stimulation and will not spontaneously resume respiration on his own. Death will occur unless you promptly initiate resuscitation. For this reason, always assume that apnea in the newborn is secondary apnea and rapidly treat it with ventilatory assistance and, when appropriate, chest compressions.

Many of the structures necessary for intrauterine life change following birth. The ductus arteriosus becomes the ligamentum arteriosum. The *foramen ovale* closes and becomes the *fossa ovalis*. The *ductus venosus* becomes the *ligamentum venosum*. The umbilical vein becomes the *ligamentum teres*. The umbilical arteries constrict although the proximal portions persist (Figure 3-3).

Congenital Anomalies

Approximately 2 percent of infants are born with some sort of congenital problem. Congenital problems typically arise from a problem in fetal development. Most fetal development occurs during the first trimester of pregnancy. It is during this time that the developing fetus is most sensitive to environmental factors and substances that can affect normal development.

There are many types of congenital anomalies. These may affect a single organ or structure or may affect many organs or structures. Congenital anomalies are the leading cause of death in infants, causing approximately one-quarter of infant deaths. Several recognized patterns, called *syndromes*, occur. It is not within the scope of this text to discuss all of the various congenital anomalies. However, a few of the congenital anomalies may make resuscitation of the neonate more difficult.

Among the congenital anomalies encountered, congenital heart defects are among the most common. The cause of these is largely unknown. Congenital heart defects are often classified by whether or not they increase pulmonary blood flow, decrease pulmonary blood flow, or obstruct blood flow.

Some congenital heart problems result in increased pulmonary blood flow. These include cases where the ductus arteriosus fails to close, a condition referred to as *patent ductus arteriosus* (also called a *persistent ductus arteriosus*) (Figure 3-4). Septal defects (a hole in the wall between the atria or the ventricles) can also result in increased pulmonary blood flow. With *atrial septal defect*, a hole between the atria allows the commixing of blood (Figure 3-5). With a *ventricular septal defect*, a hole between the two ventricles allows commixing of blood (Figure 3-6). The increase in pulmonary blood flow that results from either type of septal defect can lead to congestive heart failure.

Other congenital cardiac anomalies can lead to decreased pulmonary blood flow, which decreases the

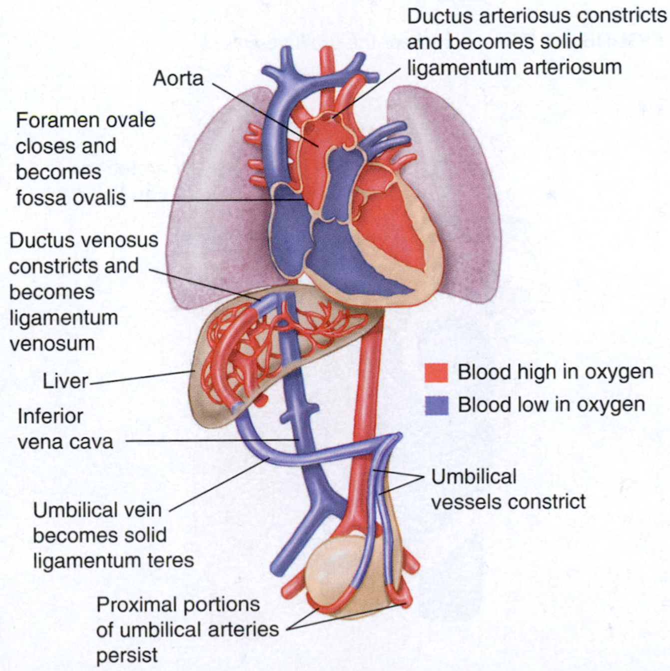

FIGURE 3-3 Major changes in the newborn's circulatory system.

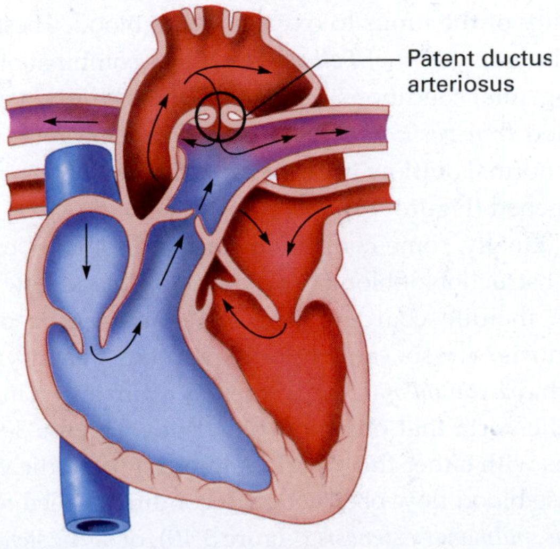

FIGURE 3-4 Patent ductus arteriosus (PDA).

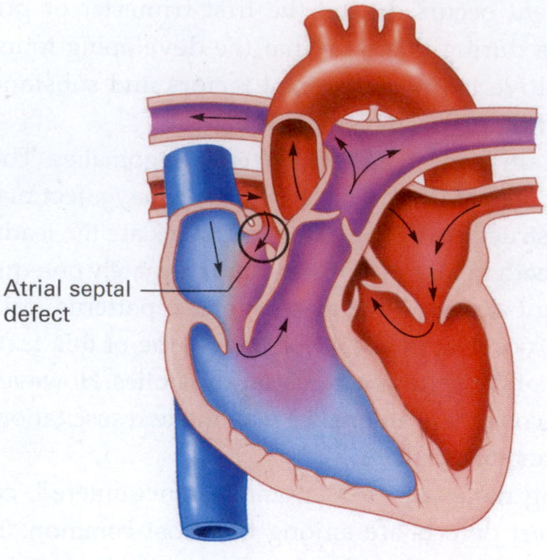

FIGURE 3-5 Atrial septal defect (ASD).

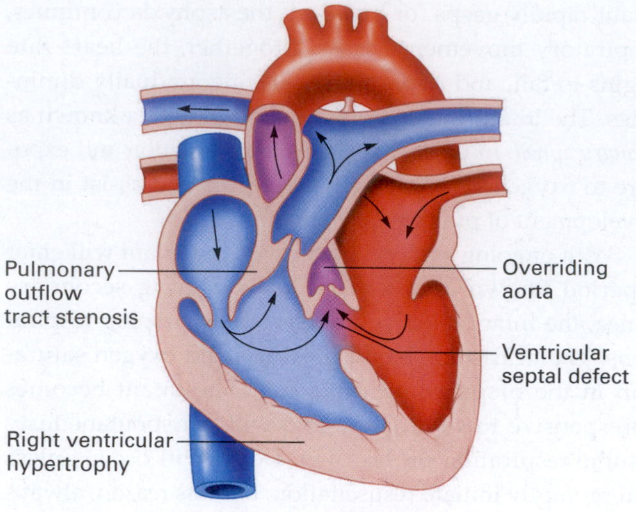

FIGURE 3-7 Tetralogy of Fallot.

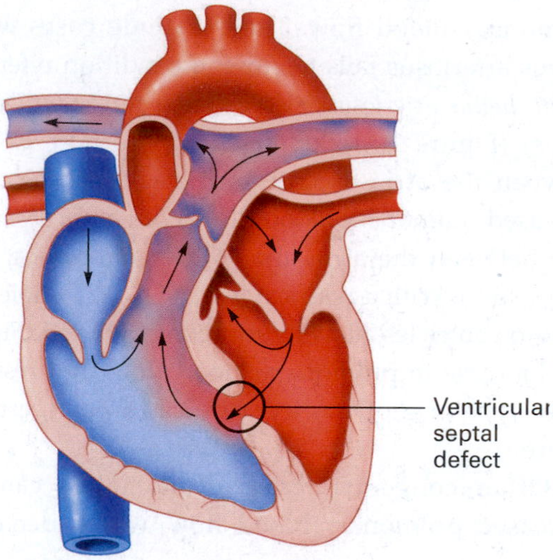

FIGURE 3-6 Ventricular septal defect (VSD).

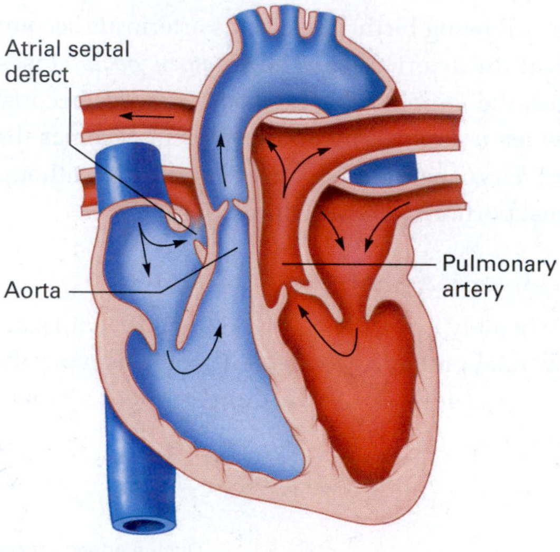

FIGURE 3-8 Transposition of the great vessels.

ability of the lungs to oxygenate the blood. These defects include *tetralogy of Fallot*, which is a combination of four congenital conditions (Figure 3-7). In addition, a condition called *transposition of the great vessels* can occur, whereby the normal outflow tracts of the right and left ventricles are switched (Figure 3-8).

Finally, some congenital cardiac anomalies can result in obstruction of blood flow. Causes of blood flow obstruction include coarctation of the aorta, aortic or mitral stenosis/atresia, and hypoplastic left heart syndrome. With *coarctation of the aorta*, there is a narrowing in the arch of the aorta that obstructs blood flow (Figure 3-9). Problems with either the mitral, pulmonary, or aortic valve can cause blood flow obstruction, a condition called *mitral stenosis, pulmonary stenosis* (Figure 3-10), or *aortic stenosis* (Figure 3-11). With *hypoplastic left heart syndrome*, the left side of

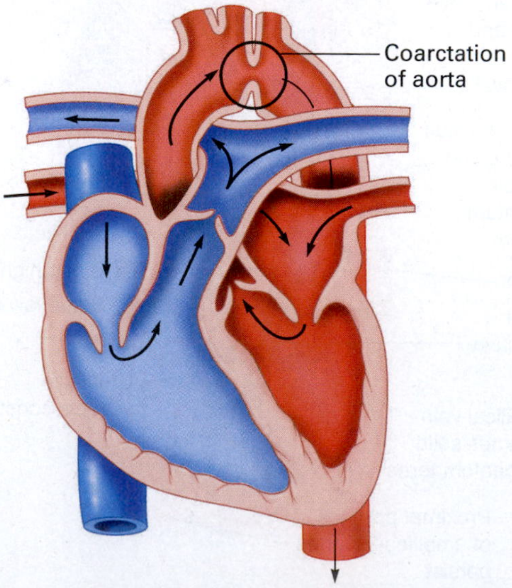

FIGURE 3-9 Coarctation of the aorta.

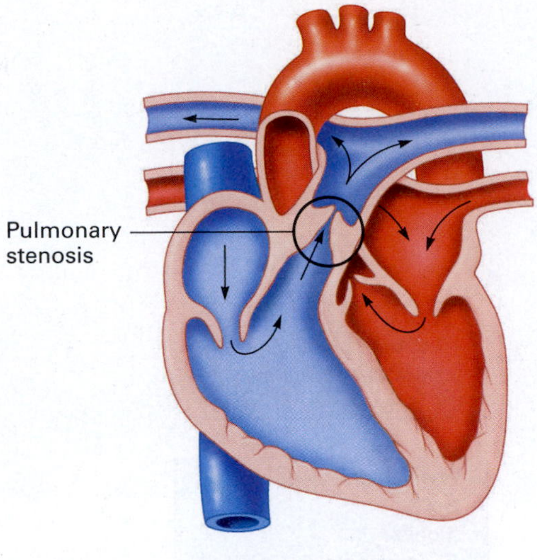

FIGURE 3-10 Pulmonary stenosis.

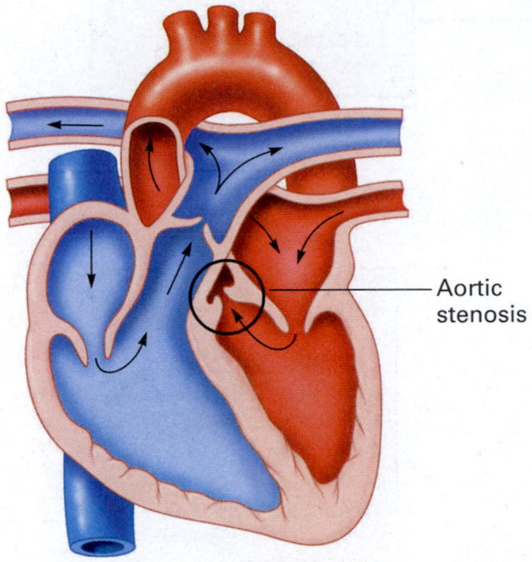

FIGURE 3-11 Aortic stenosis.

the heart is underdeveloped, a condition that is usually fatal by 1 month of age if untreated.

There are some noncardiac congenital anomalies of note. For example, some children may be born with a defect in the diaphragm that allows some of the abdominal contents to enter the chest through the defect. This abnormality is referred to as a **diaphragmatic hernia**. If you suspect a diaphragmatic hernia, do not treat the infant with bag-valve-mask ventilation. If there is a diaphragmatic hernia, bag-valve-mask or other positive-pressure ventilation will cause stomach distention, which will cause the stomach to protrude into the chest cavity, thus decreasing ventilatory capacity. Instead, immediately intubate the infant. Diaphragmatic hernia is discussed in more detail later in this chapter.

Some infants are born with a defect in the spinal cord. In some cases, the spinal cord and associated structures may be exposed. This abnormality is called a **meningomyelocele**. Infants born with a meningomyelocele should not be placed on the back. Instead, place them on the stomach or side and conduct resuscitation in this position, if possible. Cover the spinal defect with sterile gauze pads soaked in warm sterile saline and inserted in a plastic covering.

A newborn may exhibit a defect in the area of the umbilicus. In some cases, the abdominal contents will fill this defect, resulting in an **omphalocele**. If you encounter a newborn with an omphalocele, cover the defect with an occlusive plastic covering to decrease water and heat loss.

Because newborns are obligate nose breathers, **choanal atresia** can cause upper airway obstruction and respiratory distress. Choanal atresia is the most common birth defect involving the nose and is caused by the presence of a bony or membranous septum between the nasal cavity and the pharynx. Suspect this condition if you are unable to pass a catheter through either naris into the oropharynx. An oral airway will usually bypass the obstruction.

A fairly common congenital anomaly is cleft lip and cleft palate. During fetal development, the lip and palate come together in the middle, forming the oral cavity. Failure of the palate to completely close during fetal development can result in a defect known as **cleft palate**. Cleft palate may also be associated with failure of the upper lip to close. This condition, referred to as **cleft lip**, can make it difficult to obtain an adequate seal for effective mask ventilation. If a child with a cleft lip or cleft palate will require more than brief mechanical ventilation, you should place an endotracheal tube.

Pierre Robin syndrome is a congenital condition characterized by a small jaw and large tongue in conjunction with a cleft palate. In this condition, the tongue is likely to obstruct the upper airway. A nasal or oral airway usually bypasses the obstruction. If the obstruction cannot be bypassed with a simple airway, then intubation will be necessary, although intubation can be very difficult to carry out on newborns with this condition.

Assessment

Assess the newborn immediately after birth (Figure 3-12). (Ideally, if two paramedics are available, one paramedic will attend the mother while the other attends the newborn.) Make a mental note of the time of birth and then quickly obtain vital signs.

CONTENT REVIEW

➤ Normal Newborn Vital Signs
- Respirations: 30–60
- Heart rate: 100–180
- Blood pressure: 60–90 systolic
- Temperature 36.7°C–37.8°C (98°F–100°F)

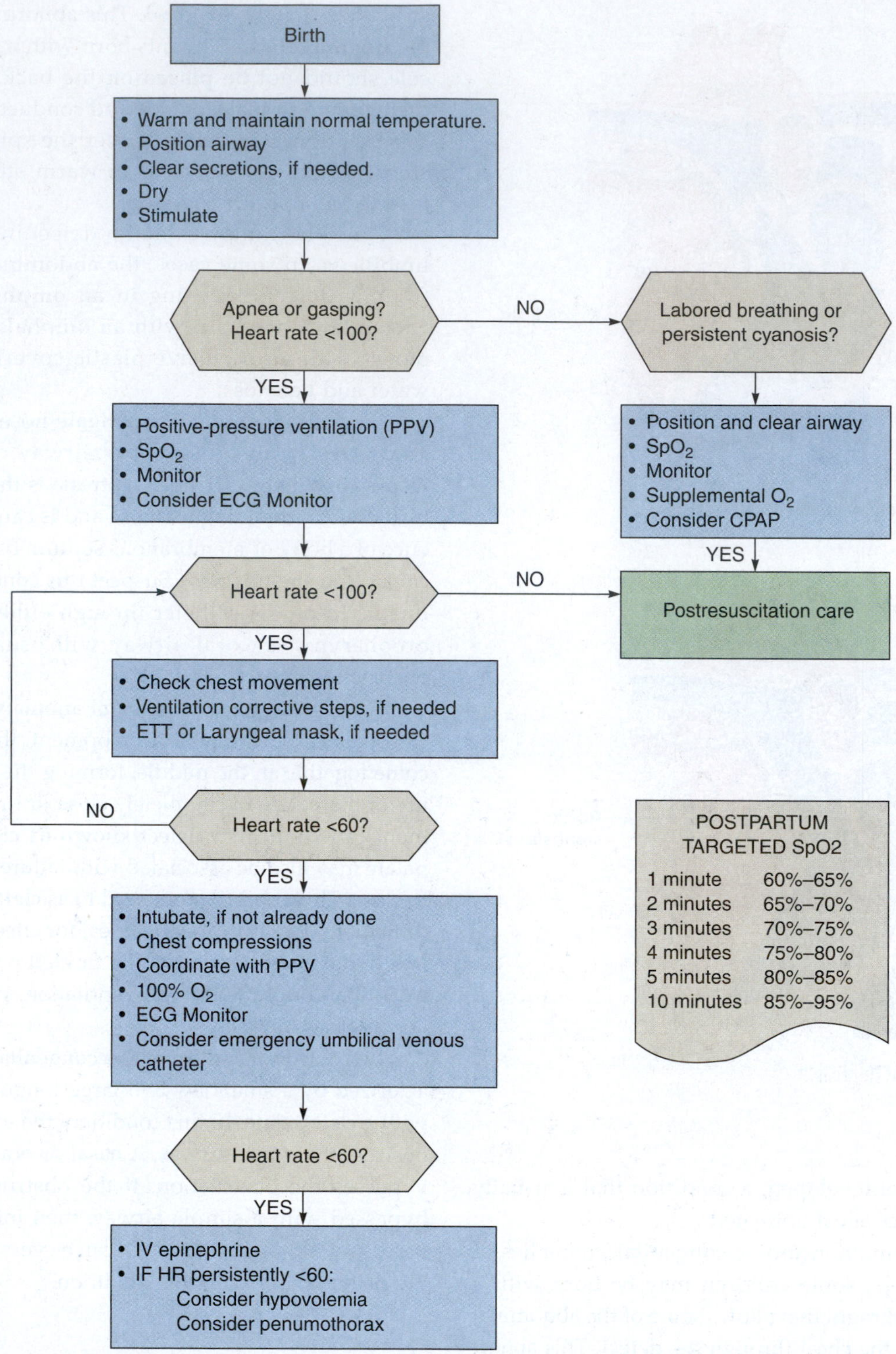

FIGURE 3-12 Neonatal resuscitation algorithm.

Remember that newborns are slippery and will require both hands to support the head and torso. Position yourself so you can work close to the surface where you have placed the infant.

The newborn's respiratory rate should average 40 to 60 breaths per minute. If respirations are not adequate or if the newborn is gasping, immediately start positive-pressure ventilation.

Expect a normal heart rate of 150 to 180 beats per minute at birth, slowing to 130 to 140 beats per minute thereafter. A pulse rate of less than 100 beats per minute indicates distress and requires emergency intervention.

CONTENT REVIEW

➤ Newborn Assessment Parameters
- Respiratory effort
- Heart rate
- Color
- APGAR score

Table 3-2 Targeted Predicted Oxygen Saturation (SpO_2) Levels after Birth

Time after Birth	Predicted SpO_2 Levels
1 minute	60–65%
2 minutes	65–70%
3 minutes	70–75%
4 minutes	75–80%
5 minutes	80–85%
10 minutes	85–95%

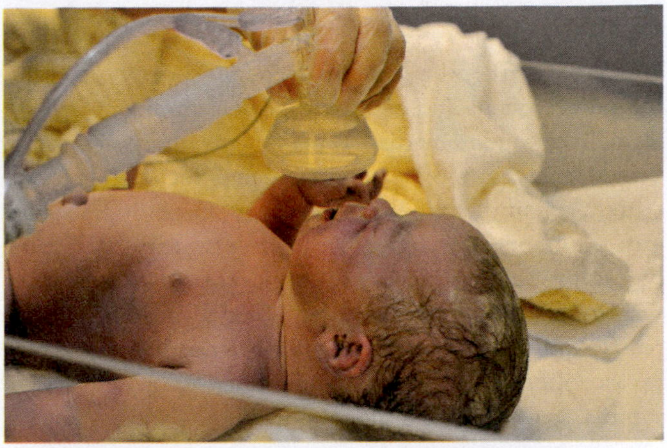

FIGURE 3-13 Administer supplemental oxygen if central cyanosis is present.

Evaluate the skin color as well. Some cyanosis of the extremities is common immediately after birth. Unfortunately, cyanosis is a poor indicator of oxygen saturation in newborns. Pulse oximetry is a better indicator of oxygen saturation. It is important to remember that neonatal oxygen saturations do not reach normal levels until approximately 10 minutes after birth. They are initially in the 70 to 80 percent range (Table 3-2).[3] Supplemental oxygen should be provided only in cases in which oxygen saturation levels are lower than those detailed in Table 3-2. If needed, administer only enough oxygen to maintain the oxygen saturation levels as detailed.[4,5]

The APGAR Score

As soon as possible, assign the newborn an **APGAR score** (Table 3-3). Ideally, try to do this at 1 and 5 minutes after birth. However, if the newborn is not breathing, *do not* withhold resuscitation to determine the APGAR score.

The APGAR scoring system helps distinguish between newborns who need only routine care and those who need greater assistance. The system also predicts long-term survival. An anesthesiologist named Dr. Virginia Apgar developed the system in 1952, and her name forms an acronym for its parameters.[6,7] The parameters for APGAR scoring include:

- Appearance
- Pulse rate
- Grimace
- Activity
- Respiratory effort

CONTENT REVIEW

➤ APGAR
- Appearance
- Pulse rate
- Grimace
- Activity
- Respiratory effort

A score of 0, 1, or 2 is given for each of these parameters. The minimum total score is 0 and the maximum is 10. A score of 7 to 10 indicates an active and vigorous newborn who requires only routine care. A score of 4 to 6 indicates a moderately distressed newborn who requires oxygenation and stimulation (Figure 3-13). Severely distressed newborns—those with APGAR scores of less than 4—require immediate resuscitation. By determining the APGAR score at 1 and 5 minutes, you can determine whether intervention has caused a change in the newborn's status.

Table 3-3 The APGAR Score

				Score	
Sign	**0**	**1**	**2**	**1 min**	**5 min**
Appearance (skin color)	Blue, pale	Body pink, extremities blue	Completely pink		
Pulse Rate (heart rate)	Absent	Below 100	Above 100		
Grimace (irritability)	No response	Grimace	Cries		
Activity (muscle tone)	Limp	Some flexion of extremities	Active motion		
Respiratory Effort	Absent	Slow and irregular	Strong cry		
			TOTAL SCORE =		

Treatment

Treatment starts prior to delivery. Begin care by preparing the environment and assembling the equipment needed for delivery and immediate care of the newborn. The initial care of a newborn follows the same priorities as care for all patients. Complete the primary assessment first. Correct any problems detected during the primary assessment before proceeding to the next step. The vast majority of term newborns—approximately 80 percent—require no resuscitation. Newly born infants who do not require resuscitation can be generally identified upon delivery by rapidly answering the following three questions:

- Is this a term gestation?
- Does the infant exhibit good tone?
- Is the infant breathing or crying?

If the answer to all three questions is "yes," the infant may stay with the mother for routine care. Routine care means the infant is dried, placed skin to skin with the mother, and covered with dry linen to maintain a normal temperature. Observation of breathing, activity, and color should be ongoing.

If the answer to any of these assessment questions is "no," the infant should receive one or more of the following four actions in sequence:

- Initial steps in infant stabilization (warm and maintain normal temperature, position, clear secretions only if copious and/or obstructing the airway, dry, stimulate)
- Ventilation and oxygenation
- Initiation of chest compressions, and/or
- Administration of epinephrine and/or fluid volume

Establishing the Airway

Airway management is one of the most critical steps in caring for the newborn. During delivery, fluid is forced out of the baby's lungs, into the oropharynx, and out through the nose and mouth. Fluid drainage occurs independently of gravity. Immediately following delivery, maintain the newborn in the "sniffing position" with the head at the same level as the mother's vagina.

Bulb suctioning during delivery and following delivery was once a common practice. However, it has been found to be relatively ineffective and can actually cause neonatal bradycardia. It is no longer recommended. Thus, if the amniotic fluid is clear, suctioning (either bulb or otherwise) is indicated only in babies with an obstruction to spontaneous breathing or who require positive-pressure ventilation. If **meconium** is present, especially thick meconium, proceed with initiation of ventilations within the first minute of life in nonbreathing or ineffectively breathing infants. Appropriate interventions to support ventilation and oxygenation should be initiated as indicated for each individual infant. This may include intubation and suctioning if the airway is obstructed.

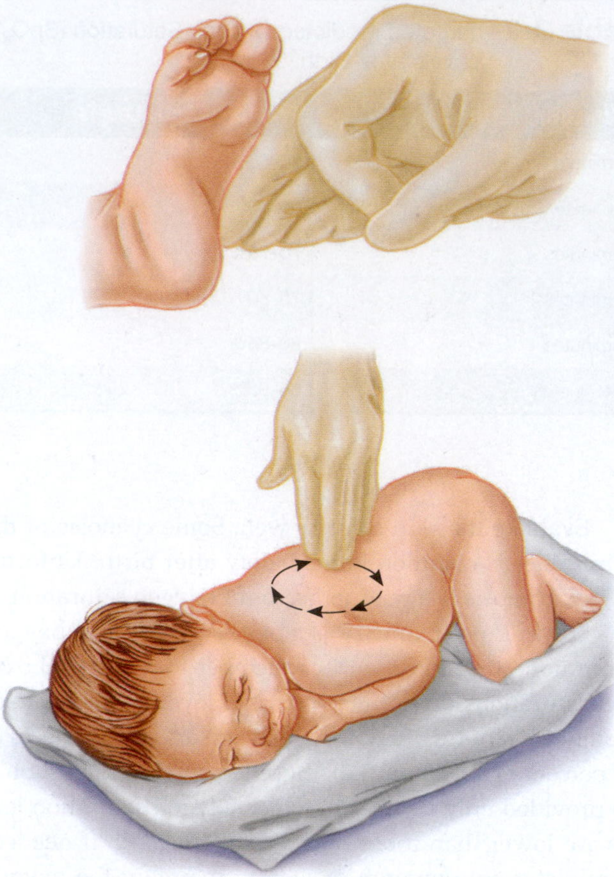

FIGURE 3-14 Stimulate the newborn as required.

Drying and tactile stimulation usually produce enough stimulation to initiate respirations in most newborns. If the newborn does not cry immediately, stimulate him by flicking the soles of his feet or gently rubbing his back (Figure 3-14). *Do not* spank or vigorously rub a newborn.

Preventing Heat Loss

Heat loss can be a life-threatening condition in newborns. Cold infants quickly become distressed infants. Heat loss occurs through evaporation, convection, conduction, and radiation. Most heat loss in newborns results from evaporation. The newborn comes into the world wet, and the amniotic fluid quickly evaporates. Immediately after birth, the newborn's core temperature can drop 1°C (1.8°F) or more from his birth temperature of 38°C (100.4°F).

Loss of heat can also occur through convection, depending on the temperature of the room and the movement of the air around the newborn. The newborn can lose additional heat through contact with surrounding surfaces (convection) or by radiating heat to colder objects nearby.

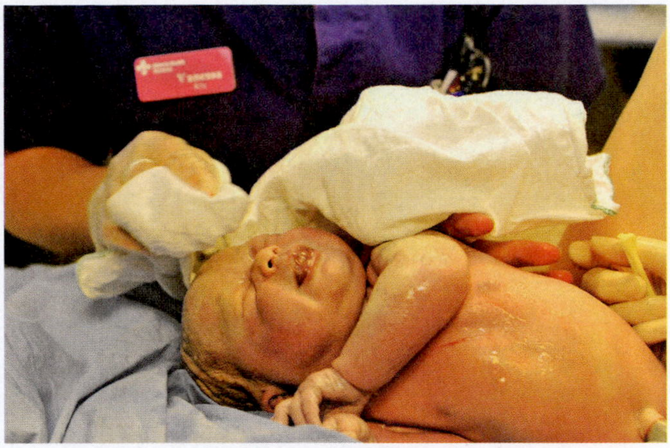

FIGURE 3-15 Dry the infant to prevent loss of evaporative heat.

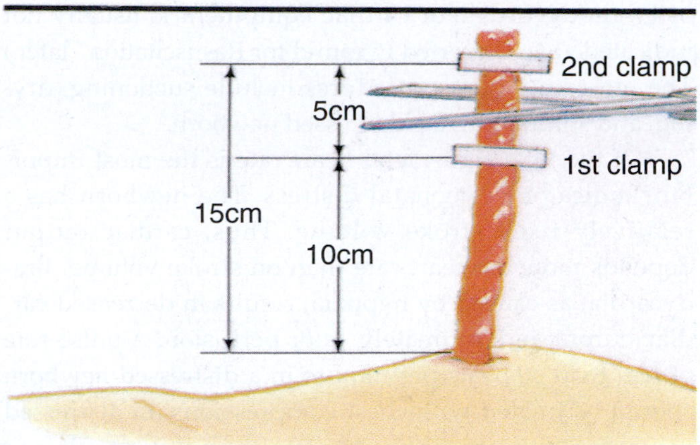

FIGURE 3-16 Clamping and cutting the cord.

To prevent heat loss, take these steps:

- Dry the newborn immediately to prevent evaporative cooling (Figure 3-15).
- Maintain the ambient temperature—the temperature in the delivery room or ambulance—at a *minimum* of 23°C to 24°C (74°F–76°F).
- Close all windows and doors.
- Discard the towel used to dry the newborn and swaddle the infant in a warm, dry receiving blanket or other suitable material. Cover the head.
- The maintenance of body temperature and the prevention of hypothermia in the out-of-hospital environment during the first 1 to 2 hours of life in well newborn infants can be achieved by use of a clean food-grade plastic bag up to the level of the neck and swaddling after drying. Another option that may be reasonable is to have the mother nurse the newborn with skin-to-skin contact.
- In colder areas, place well-insulated water bottles or rubber gloves filled with warm water (40°C [104°F]) around the newborn to help maintain a warm body temperature. To avoid burns, do not place these items against the skin. Be sure the newborn is wrapped in a blanket and place the water bottle or rubber glove against the blanket.

Cutting the Umbilical Cord

It had been a common practice to clamp the umbilical cord soon after birth to allow for additional neonatal care and stabilization. More recent evidence has demonstrated that **delayed cord clamping (DCC)** might be beneficial for infants who do not require immediate resuscitation at birth. DCC may minimize the likelihood of intraventricular hemorrhage. As a result, immediately after birth, infants who are breathing and crying may undergo DCC. Infants who are not breathing or crying should have the cord clamped so that resuscitation measures can begin.

You can prevent over- and undertransfusion of blood by maintaining the baby at the same level as the mother's vagina, as previously described. Do not "milk" or strip the umbilical cord, as this increases blood viscosity, or **polycythemia**, and can lead to maternal–fetal transfusion. Polycythemia can cause cardiopulmonary problems. It can also contribute to excessive red blood cell destruction, which may in turn lead to **hyperbilirubinemia**—an increased level of bilirubin in the blood, which causes jaundice.

If umbilical cord clamping is indicated, apply the umbilical clamps within 30 to 45 seconds after birth. Place the first clamp approximately 10 cm (4 inches) from the newborn. Place the second clamp about 5 cm (2 inches) farther away than the first. Then cut the cord between the two clamps (Figure 3-16). After the cord is cut, inspect it periodically to make sure there is no additional bleeding.

The Distressed Newborn

The distressed newborn can be either full term or premature. (See the "Prematurity" section later in this chapter.) The presence of fetal meconium at birth indicates that fetal distress has occurred at some point during pregnancy. If the newborn is simply meconium stained, then distress may have occurred at a remote time. If you see *particulate* meconium, however, distress may have occurred recently and the newborn should be managed accordingly.

Aspiration of meconium can cause significant respiratory problems. (More will be said about this topic in the "Meconium-Stained Amniotic Fluid" section later.) Be sure to report the presence of meconium to the medical direction physician.

The most common problem experienced by newborns during the first minutes of life is ventilation. For this reason, resuscitation usually consists of ventilation and, if needed, oxygenation. Except in special situations, the use of IV fluids, drugs, or cardiac equipment is usually not indicated. (See "Inverted Pyramid for Resuscitation" later.) The most important procedures include suctioning, drying, and stimulating the distressed newborn.

Of the vital signs, fetal heart rate is the most important indicator of neonatal distress. The newborn has a relatively fixed stroke volume. Thus, cardiac output depends more on heart rate than on stroke volume. Bradycardia, as caused by hypoxia, results in decreased cardiac output and, ultimately, poor perfusion. A pulse rate of less than 60 beats per minute in a distressed newborn should be treated with chest compressions. In distressed newborns, monitor the heart rate with an ECG monitor or pulse oximetry.

Resuscitation

The vast majority of newborns do not require resuscitation beyond stimulation, maintenance of the airway, and maintenance of body temperature. Unfortunately, it is difficult to predict which newborns ultimately will require resuscitation. Each EMS unit, therefore, should carry a neonatal resuscitation kit that contains the following items:

- Neonatal bag-valve-mask unit
- Bulb syringe
- Laryngoscope with size 0 and 1 blades
- Uncuffed endotracheal tubes (2.5, 3.0, 3.5, 4.0) with appropriate suction catheters
- Endotracheal tube stylet
- Tape or device to secure endotracheal tube
- Laryngeal mask airway
- Umbilical catheter and 10-mL syringe
- Three-way stopcock
- 20-mL syringe and 8-French (Fr.) feeding tube for gastric suction
- Glucometer
- Assorted syringes and needles
- Towels (sterile)
- Medications:
    - Epinephrine 1:10,000 and 1:1,000
    - Volume expander (lactated Ringer's solution or saline)

Inverted Pyramid for Resuscitation

Resuscitation of the newborn follows an inverted pyramid (Figure 3-17). As this pyramid indicates, most distressed newborns respond to relatively simple maneuvers. Few require CPR or advanced life support measures.

The following are steps for the initial care of the newborn (also see Procedure 3-1).

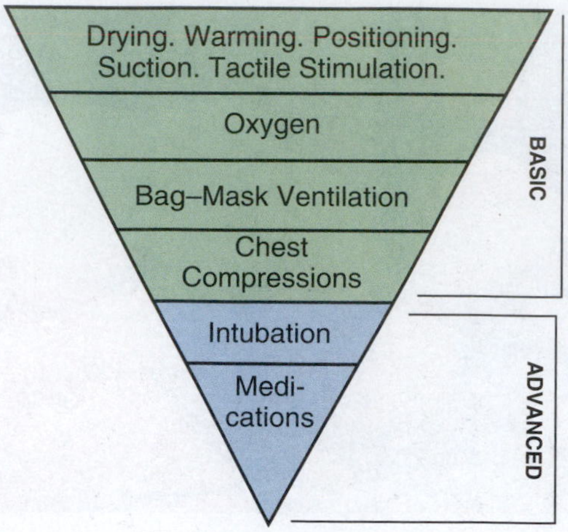

FIGURE 3-17 The inverted pyramid of neonatal resuscitation, showing approximate relative frequencies of neonatal care and resuscitative efforts. Most infants respond to the simple measures noted at the top, wide part of the pyramid.

STEP 1: DRYING, WARMING, POSITIONING, SUCTIONING, AND TACTILE STIMULATION Resuscitation begins with drying, warming, positioning, and stimulating the newborn. Immediately upon delivery, minimize heat loss by drying the newborn. Next, place the newborn in skin-to-skin contact with the mother. If this is not possible, consider a warm, dry blanket. Make sure the environment is warm and free of drafts.

If further resuscitation is required, such as ventilations or chest compressions, clamp and cut the cord and move the infant to an appropriate area for resuscitation. Place him on his back with his head in the "sniffing position." (Figure 3-18). Place a small blanket, folded to a 2-cm (0.75-inch) thickness, under the newborn's shoulders to help maintain this position.

After carrying out the preceding procedures, assess the newborn as noted here:

Newborn Assessment Parameters

- ***Respiratory effort.*** The rate and depth of the newborn's breathing should increase immediately with tactile stimulation. If the respiratory response is adequate, evaluate the heart rate next. If the respiratory rate is inadequate, begin positive-pressure ventilation (see Step 2).
- ***Heart rate.*** As noted earlier, heart rate is critical in the newborn. In previous treatment guidelines, auscultation of the precordium was recommended as the preferred physical examination method for assessing heart rate. Pulse oximetry was recommended as an adjunct to provide a noninvasive, rapid, and continuous assessment of heart rate during resuscitation. Now, both 3-lead ECG monitoring and pulse oximetry are recommended as useful in measuring neonatal

Procedure 3-1 Resuscitation of the Distressed Newborn

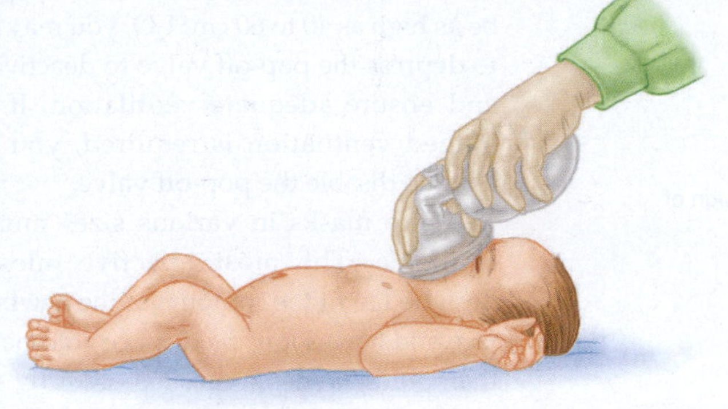

3-1a Ventilate for 15–30 seconds.

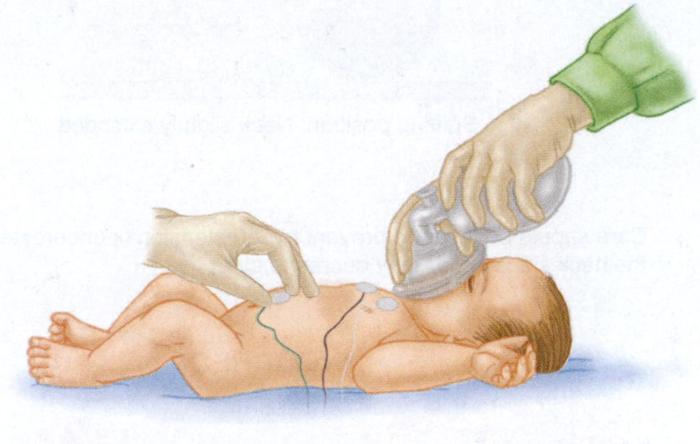

3-1b Evaluate the heart rate.

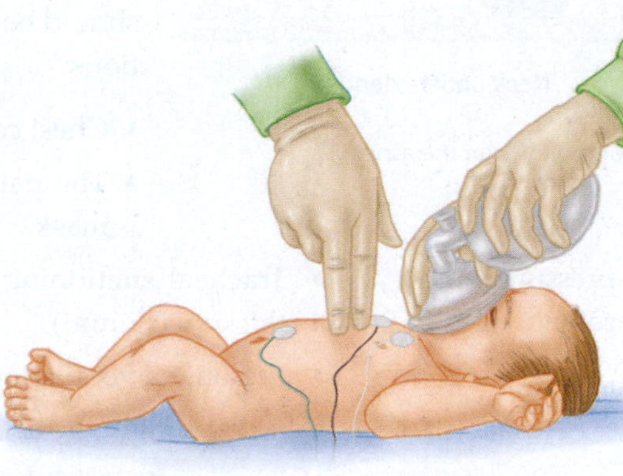

3-1c Initiate chest compressions if the heart rate is less than 60.

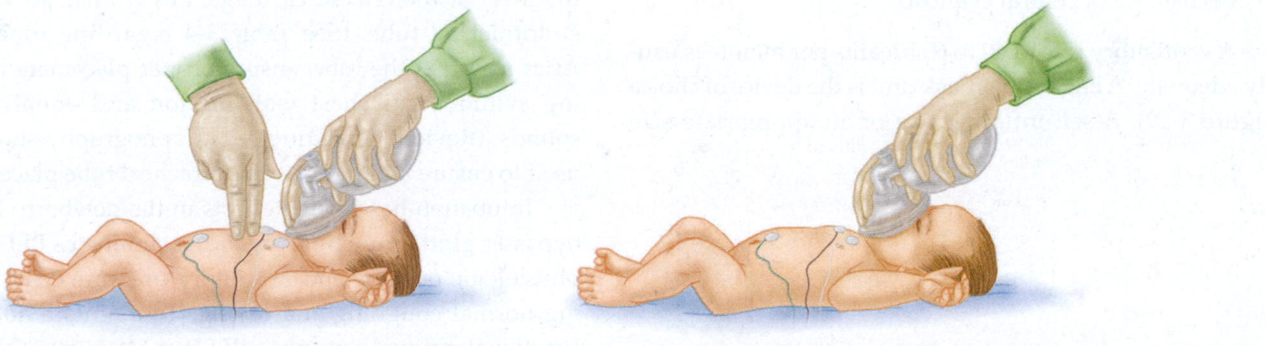

3-1d Evaluate the heart rate: below 60—continue chest compressions; 60 or above—discontinue chest compressions.

heart rate. If the heart rate is greater than 100 and spontaneous respirations are present, continue the assessment. If the heart rate is less than 100, immediately begin positive-pressure ventilation (see Step 2).

- ***Color.*** A newborn may be cyanotic despite a heart rate greater than 100 and spontaneous respirations. If you note central cyanosis, or cyanosis of the chest and abdomen, in a newborn with adequate ventilation and a pulse rate greater than 100, assess oxygen saturation and administer supplemental oxygen as needed to maintain appropriate oxygen saturation, as detailed in Table 3-2 (see Step 3). Newborns with peripheral cyanosis do not usually need supplemental oxygen *unless* the cyanosis is prolonged.
- ***APGAR score.*** Unless resuscitation is required, obtain 1- and 5-minute APGAR scores.

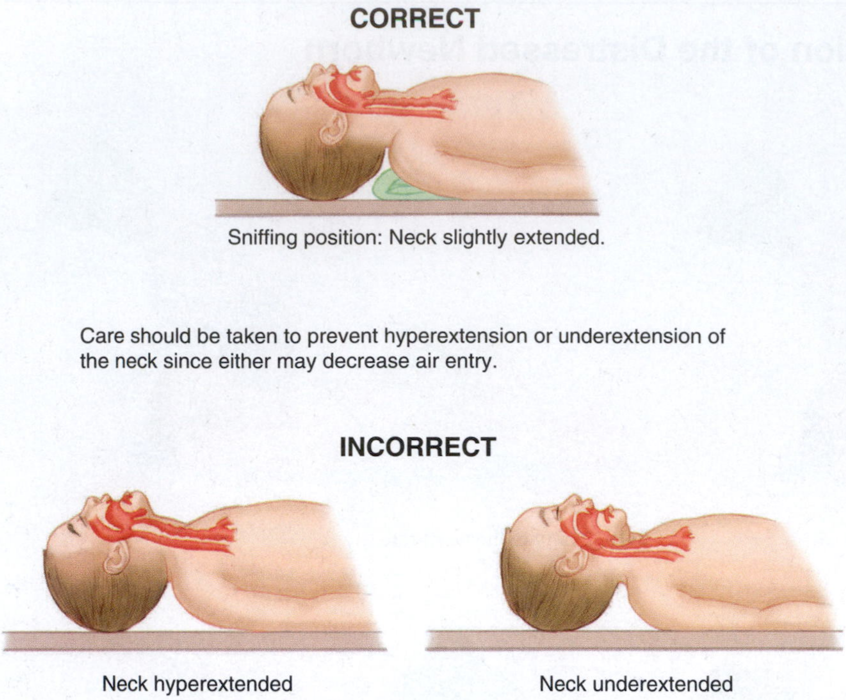

FIGURE 3-18 Place the newborn in the sniffing position to open the airway.

STEP 2: VENTILATION Begin positive-pressure ventilation if *any* of the following conditions is present:

- Heart rate less than 100 beats per minute
- Apnea
- SpO_2 less than expected for post-birth values (Review Table 3-2)
- Persistence of central cyanosis

A ventilatory rate of 40 to 60 breaths per minute is usually adequate. A bag-valve-mask unit is the device of choice (Figure 3-19). A self-inflating bag of an appropriate size (450 mL is optimal) should be used. Many self-inflating bags have a pressure-limiting pop-off valve that is preset at 30 to 45 cmH_2O. However, because the initial pressures required to ventilate a newborn may be as high as 40 to 60 cmH_2O, you may have to depress the pop-off valve to deactivate it and ensure adequate ventilation. If prolonged ventilation is required, you may have to disable the pop-off valve.

Face masks in various sizes must be available. The most effective ones are designed to fit the contours of the newborn's face and have a low dead space volume (less than 5 mL). When a mask is correctly sized and positioned, it covers the newborn's nose and mouth, but not the eyes.

Endotracheal intubation of a newborn should be carried out in the following situations:

- Chest compressions are performed.
- The patient cannot be ventilated with a mask.
- Tracheal suctioning is required (such as in cases of thick meconium).
- Prolonged ventilation will be required.
- A diaphragmatic hernia is suspected.
- Inadequate respiratory effort is found.

Because of the narrowness of the neonatal airway at the level of the cricoid cartilage, always use an *uncuffed* endotracheal tube. (See Table 3-4 regarding tube size.) After inserting the tube, ensure proper placement by noting symmetrical chest wall motion and equal breath sounds. (Review Procedure 3-2.) Capnography should be used to ensure and monitor endotracheal tube placement.

Intubation has several effects in the newborn. First, it bypasses **glottic function**. Second, it eliminates **PEEP**—the physiologic positive end-expiratory pressure created during normal coughing and crying. To maintain adequate functional residual capacity, a PEEP of 2 to 4 cmH_2O should be provided when mechanical ventilation is initiated by adding a magnetic-disk PEEP valve to the bag-valve outlet.

Gastric distention, caused by a leak around an uncuffed endotracheal tube, may compromise ventilation of a newborn. This can be minimized by using a properly sized endotracheal tube. If significant gastric distention is present, a **nasogastric tube or orogastric tube** should be inserted (through the nose or mouth, respectively, then through the esophagus into the stomach) as soon as the airway is controlled. The endotracheal tube should be placed before the gastric tube is placed to avoid misplacing the gastric tube into the trachea.

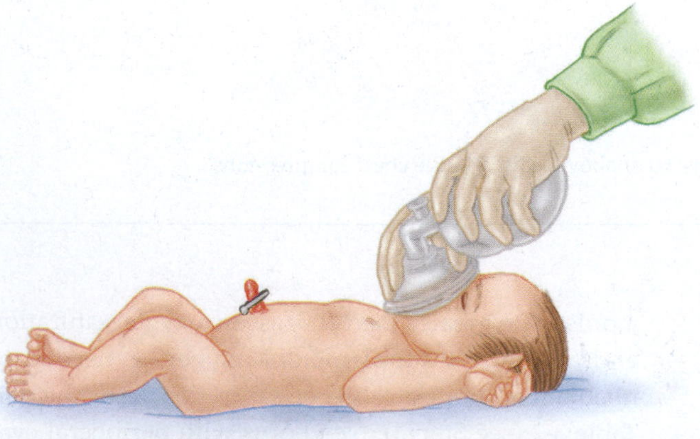

FIGURE 3-19 Use of a bag-valve-mask unit to provide positive-pressure ventilation. Maintain a good mask seal and use just enough force to raise the infant's chest. Ventilate at a rate of 60 per minute for 30 seconds, then reassess.

Table 3-4 Guidelines for Tracheal Tube Sizes and Depth of Insertion in the Newborn

Tube Size (mm ID)	Depth of Insertion from Upper Lip (cm)	Weight (g)	Gestation (wk)
2.5	6.5–7	<1000	<28
3.0	7–8	1000–2000	28–34
3.5	8–9	2000–3000	34–38
3.5–4.0	>9	>3000	>38

Make sure the newborn is well ventilated before attempting to insert a gastric tube. To determine the depth of insertion, measure a nasogastric tube from the tip of the nose, around the ear, to below the xiphoid process. Measure an orogastric tube from the lips to below the xiphoid process. Lubricate the end of the tube and pass it gently along the nasal floor or the mouth and into the esophagus. Confirm that the tube is in the stomach by injecting 10 mL of air into the tube and auscultating a bubbling sound, or sound of rushing air, over the epigastrium.

STEP 3: SUPPLEMENTAL OXYGEN If central cyanosis is present or if SpO_2 levels are less than expected (see Table 3-2), administer only enough supplemental oxygen to maintain the SpO_2 within the normal range. Avoid both hypoxia and hyperoxia. Hyperoxia has been associated with numerous adverse outcomes in neonates and should be avoided to the same degree that we avoid hypoxia. Generally, supplemental oxygen will usually be provided in conjunction with mechanical ventilation. If possible, the oxygen should be warmed and humidified. Continue oxygen administration until the newborn's color has improved or the SpO_2 is maintained at target levels.[8]

STEP 4: CHEST COMPRESSIONS Initiate chest compressions if the heart rate is less than 60 beats per minute.[9] Perform chest compressions by following these steps:

- Encircle the newborn's chest, placing both of your thumbs on the lower third of the sternum. If the newborn is very small, you may need to overlap your thumbs. If the newborn is very large, you may need to place the ring and middle fingers of one hand just below the nipple line and perform two-finger compression (Figure 3-20).
- Compress the lower half of the sternum at a compressions-to-ventilation ratio of 3:1. It is recommended that compressions and ventilations be coordinated to avoid simultaneous delivery. The chest should be allowed to re-expand fully during relaxation, and the rescuer's thumbs should not leave the chest. Use a 3:1 ratio of compressions to ventilation at 90 compressions and 30 breaths per minute to achieve approximately 120 events per minute. This serves to maximize ventilation at an achievable rate. Thus, each event will take approximately a half of a second with exhalation occurring during the first compression after each ventilation. A 3:1 compressions-to-ventilation ratio is used for neonatal resuscitation in which compromise of gas exchange is almost always the primary cause of cardiovascular collapse.
- Reassess heart rate, respiration, and color every 30 seconds. Coordinate with chest compressions and ventilation.
- Discontinue compressions if the spontaneous heart rate exceeds 80 per minute.

STEP 5: MEDICATIONS AND FLUIDS Most cardiopulmonary arrests in newborns result from hypoxia. Because of this, initial therapy consists of ventilation and oxygenation. However, when these measures fail, fluids and medications should be administered. They may also be necessary in cases of persistent bradycardia, hypovolemia, respiratory depression secondary to narcotics, and metabolic acidosis.

Vascular access for the administration of fluids and drugs can be managed most readily by using the umbilical vein. The umbilical cord contains three vessels—two arteries and one vein. The vein is larger than the arteries and has a thinner wall (Figure 3-21).

To establish venous access, follow these procedures:

- Trim the umbilical cord with a scalpel blade to 1 cm above the abdomen. Be sure to save enough of the umbilical cord stump in case neonatal personnel have to place additional lines.
- Insert a 5-Fr. umbilical catheter into the umbilical vein. Connect the catheter to a three-way stopcock and fill it with saline.
- Insert the catheter until the tip is just below the skin and you note the free flow of blood. (If the catheter is inserted too far, it may become wedged against the liver, and it will not function.)
- After the catheter is in place, secure it with umbilical tape.

If an umbilical vein catheter cannot be placed, some medications can be given via the endotracheal tube. Other options for vascular access are peripheral vein cannulation and intraosseous cannulation. Fluid therapy should consist of 10 mL/kg of saline or lactated Ringer's solution given by syringe as a slow IV push.

Procedure 3-2 Intubation and Tracheal Suctioning in the Newborn

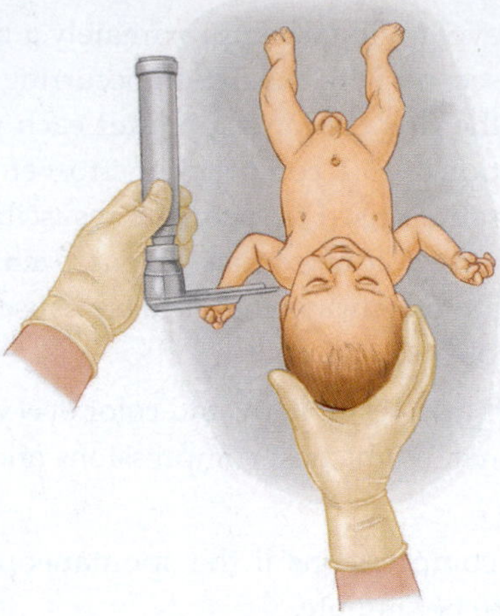

3-2a Position the infant.

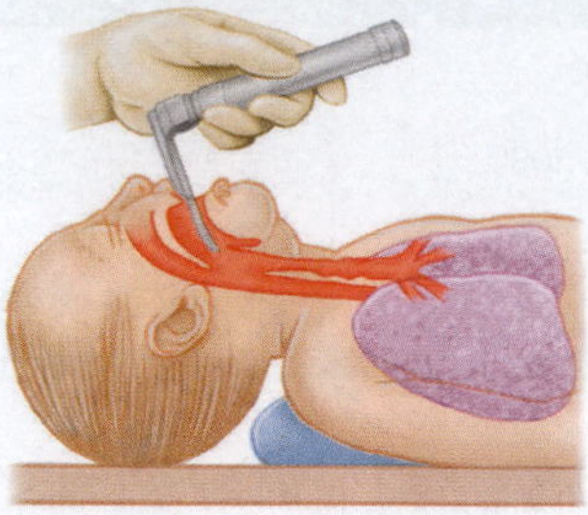

3-2b Insert the laryngoscope.

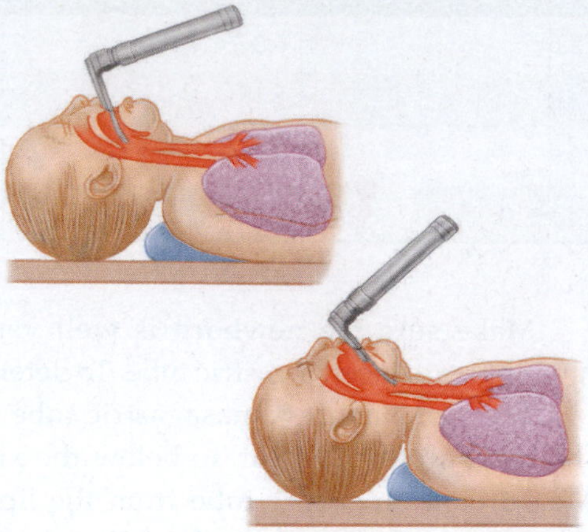

3-2c Elevate the epiglottis by lifting.

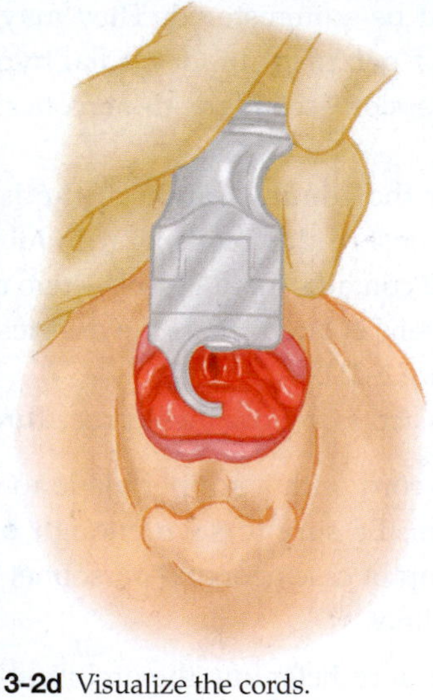

3-2d Visualize the cords.

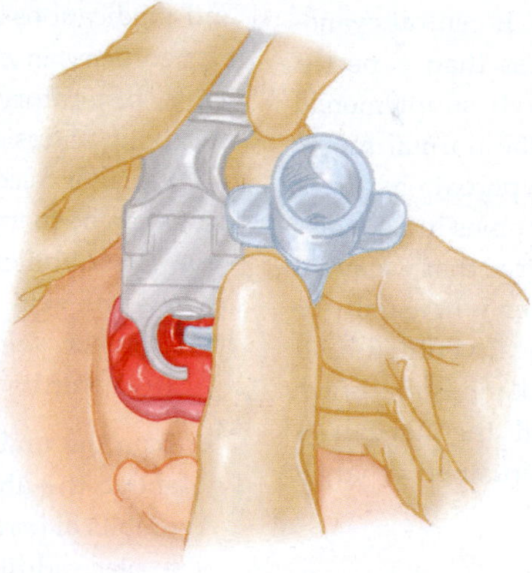

3-2e Insert a fresh tube for ventilation.

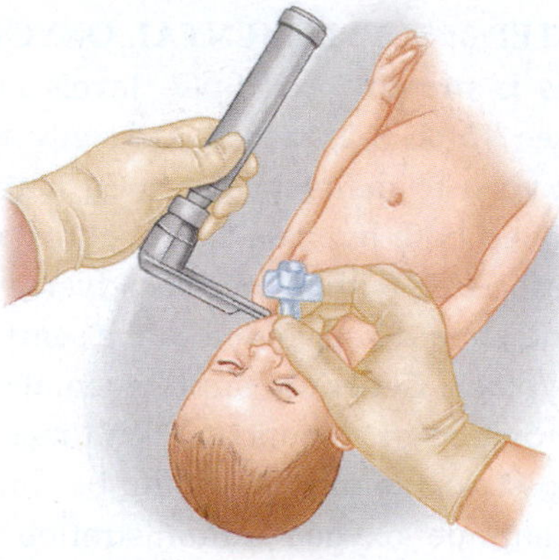

3-2f Remove the laryngoscope.

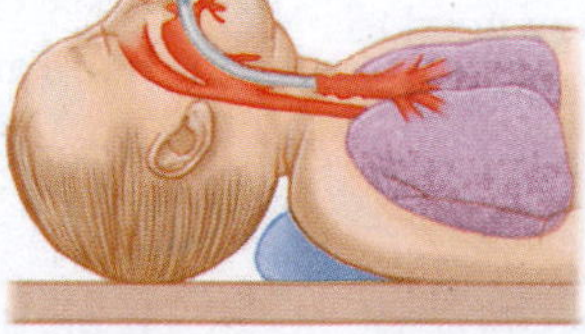

3-2g Check proper tube placement.

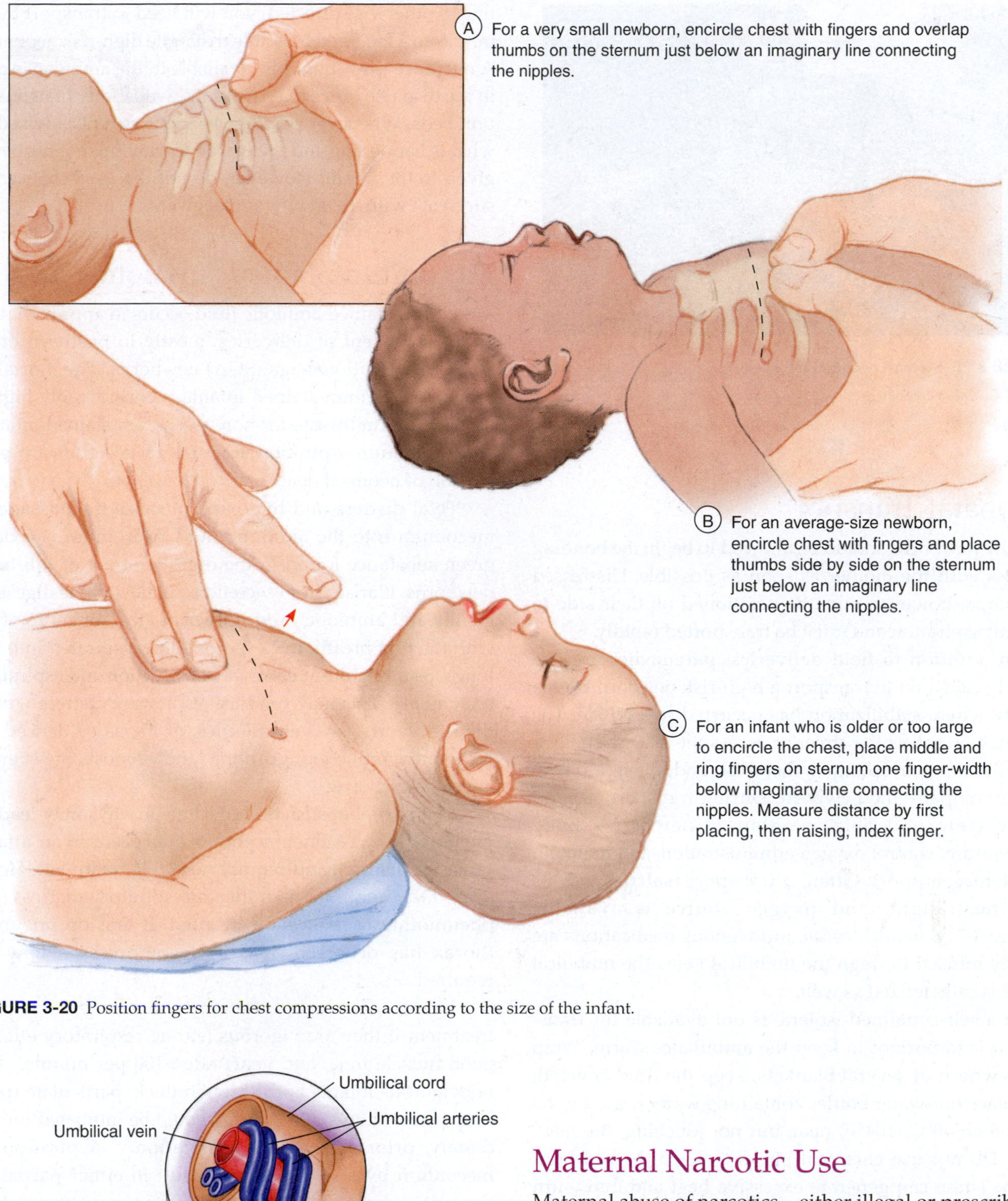

FIGURE 3-20 Position fingers for chest compressions according to the size of the infant.

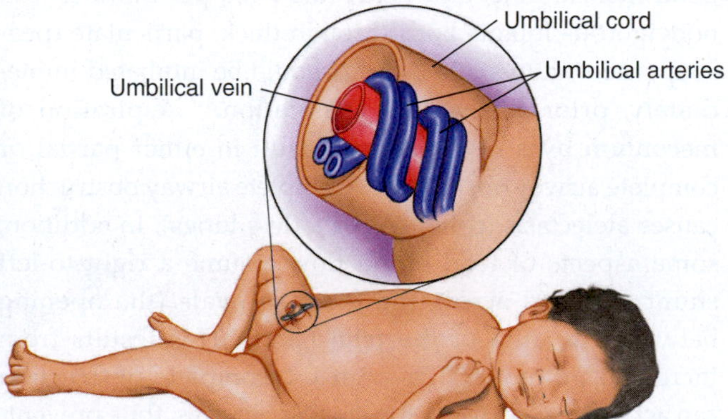

FIGURE 3-21 The umbilical cord contains two arteries and one vein. The umbilical vein can be accessed for vascular administration of fluids and drugs. The vein is larger than the arteries and has a thinner wall.

Maternal Narcotic Use

Maternal abuse of narcotics—either illegal or prescribed—can complicate field deliveries. Maternal narcotic use has been shown to produce low-birth-weight infants. Such infants may demonstrate withdrawal symptoms—tremors, startles, and decreased alertness. They also face a serious risk of respiratory depression at birth. Although formerly used, the narcotic antagonist naloxone (Narcan) is not indicated in neonatal resuscitation. As with other newborns, continue all resuscitative measures until the newborn is resuscitated or until the emergency staff assumes care.

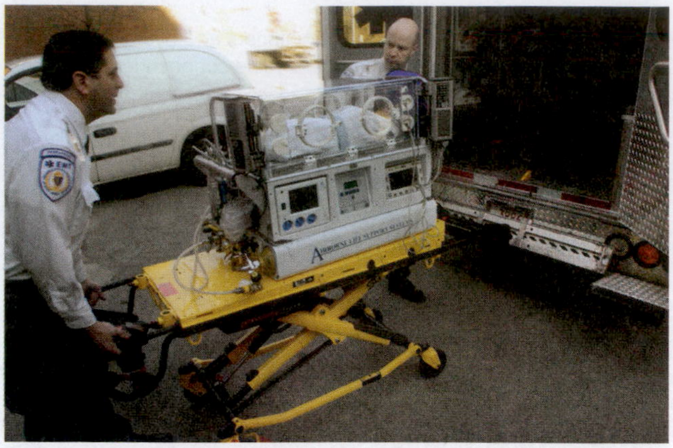

FIGURE 3-22 Modern neonatal transport.

(© Mark C. Ide/Science Source)

Neonatal Transport

Healthy newborns should be allowed to begin the bonding process with the mother as soon as possible. Distressed newborns, however, must be positioned on their side to prevent aspiration and must be transported rapidly.

In addition to field deliveries, paramedics are frequently called on to transport a high-risk newborn from a facility where stabilization has occurred to a NICU. The trip may be across the street or across the state. Usually a pediatric nurse, respiratory therapist, and, often, a physician accompany the newborn. During transport, a paramedic crew will help maintain a newborn's body temperature, control oxygen administration, and maintain ventilatory support. Often, a transport **isolette** with its own heat, light, and oxygen source is available (Figure 3-22). In such cases, intravenous medications are usually infused through the umbilical vein. The umbilical artery is catheterized as well.

If a self-contained isolette is not available for transport, it is important to keep the ambulance warm. Wrap the newborn in several blankets, keep the head covered, and place hot-water bottles containing water heated to no more than 40°C (104°F) near, but not touching, the newborn. Do not use chemical packs to keep the newborn warm. These can generate excessive heat and may burn the infant.

Specific Neonatal Situations

Rapid assessment and treatment of a distressed newborn are the keys to the infant's survival. The following information will help you to formulate treatment plans for specific emergencies involving newborns. Remember that, unless otherwise directed, you will need to transport these infants to a facility that is able to handle high-risk neonates. A reference card should be available in the ambulance and in the dispatch office that tracks the availability of neonatal unit beds. Whenever possible, keep the parents advised of what is happening and the reason for any treatments being given to the infant. However, do not discuss "chances of survival" with the family or caregivers.

Meconium-Stained Amniotic Fluid

Meconium-stained amniotic fluid occurs in approximately 10 to 15 percent of deliveries, mostly in postterm or in small-for-gestational-age (SGA) newborns. The mortality rate for meconium-stained infants is considerably higher than the mortality rate for non–meconium-stained infants, and meconium aspiration accounts for a significant proportion of neonatal deaths.

Fetal distress and hypoxia can cause the passage of meconium into the amniotic fluid. Meconium is a dark green substance found in the digestive tract of full-term newborns. It arises from secretions of the various digestive glands and amniotic fluid. Either *in utero*, or more often with the first breath, thick meconium is aspirated into the lungs, resulting in small-airway obstruction and aspiration pneumonia. This may produce respiratory distress within the first hours, or even minutes, of life as evidenced by tachypnea, retraction, grunting, and cyanosis in severely affected newborns.

The partial obstruction of some airways may lead to pneumothorax. A pneumothorax may occur in an infant, cause no distress, and require no active treatment. However, if the infant has significant respiratory distress, the pneumothorax must be evacuated. If tension pneumothorax has occurred, needle decompression may be required.

Infants born through thin meconium may not require treatment if they are vigorous (strong respiratory efforts, good muscle tone, and heart rate >100 per minute), but nonvigorous infants born through thick, particulate (pea-soup) meconium-stained fluid should be intubated immediately, prior to the first ventilation.[10] Aspiration of meconium by a newborn can result in either partial or complete airway obstruction. Complete airway obstruction causes atelectasis (collapsed or airless lungs). In addition, some aspects of fetal blood flow resume a right-to-left shunt of blood across the foramen ovale (the opening between the atria of the fetal heart). This results from increased pulmonary pressures. Incomplete obstruction can act as a ball-valve in the smaller airways, thus preventing exhalation. The newborn is also at increased risk of developing a pneumothorax.

Before stimulating the infant to breathe, apply suction with a meconium aspirator attached to an endotracheal tube. Connect to suction at 100 cmH_2O or less to remove meconium from the airway. Withdraw the endotracheal tube as suction is applied.

Repeat intubation and suction until the meconium clears, usually not more than two times. Once the airway is clear and the infant is able to breathe on his own, ventilate and provide supplemental oxygen as needed to maintain target SpO_2 levels for age. If the infant is found to be hypotensive, consider a fluid challenge. Remember to warm the infant to prevent hypothermia. The parents will probably question the treatment being performed on the infant. Explain what you are doing and why, without discussing chances of survival. Stress the need for rapid transport to a facility able to handle high-risk infants.

Apnea

Apnea is a common finding in preterm infants, infants weighing less than 1,500 grams (3 pounds, 5 ounces), infants exposed to drugs, or infants born after prolonged or difficult labor and delivery. Typically, the infant fails to breathe spontaneously after stimulation, or the infant experiences respiratory pauses of more than 20 seconds.

Although apnea is usually the result of hypoxia or hypothermia, there may be other causative factors. These include:

- Narcotic or central nervous depressants
- Weakness of the respiratory muscles
- Sepsis
- Metabolic disorders
- Central nervous system disorders

Begin management of apnea with tactile stimulation. Flick the soles of the infant's feet or gently rub his back. If necessary, ventilate using a bag-valve-mask unit with the pop-off valve disabled, as explained earlier. If the infant still does not breathe on his own, or if he has a heart rate of less than 60 with adequate ventilation and chest compressions, perform tracheal intubation with direct visualization. Gain circulatory access, and monitor the heart rate continuously. Generally, neonatal naloxone is no longer recommended.[11]

Early and aggressive treatment of apnea usually results in a good outcome. Throughout treatment, keep the infant warm to prevent hypothermia. Also explain to parents the procedures and the need for rapid transport.

Diaphragmatic Hernia

Diaphragmatic hernias rarely occur. They are seen in approximately 1 out of every 2,200 live births. When they do appear, the **herniation** takes place most often in the posterolateral segments of the diaphragm, and most commonly (90 percent) on the left side. The defect is caused by the failure of the pleuroperitoneal canal (foramen of Bochdalek) to close completely. The survival rate for infants who require mechanical ventilation in the first 18 to 24 hours is approximately 50 percent. However, if there is no respiratory distress in the first 24 hours of life, the survival rate approaches 100 percent.

CONTENT REVIEW

➤ Causes of Apnea in Newborns
- Hypoxia
- Hypothermia
- Narcotics
- Respiratory muscle weakness
- Septicemia
- Metabolic disorder
- Central nervous system disorder

Protrusion of abdominal viscera through the hernia into the thoracic cavity occurs in varying degrees. In severe cases, the stomach and a large part of the intestines and the spleen, liver, and kidneys displace the lungs and heart to the opposite side. The lung on the affected side is compressed, causing diminished total lung volume. In at least one-third of patients, pulmonary hypertension is present. With a patent ductus arteriosus, severe right-to-left shunting may occur, further aggravating tissue hypoxia.

Assessment findings may include the following:

- Little to severe distress present from birth
- Dyspnea and cyanosis unresponsive to ventilations
- Small, flat (scaphoid) abdomen
- Bowel sounds in the chest
- Heart sounds displaced to the right

As soon as you suspect a diaphragmatic hernia, position the infant with his head and thorax higher than the abdomen and feet (Figure 3-23). This will help facilitate the downward displacement of the abdominal organs. Place a nasogastric or orogastric tube and apply low, intermittent suctioning. This will decrease the entrapment of air and fluid within the herniated viscera and will reduce the degree of ventilatory compromise. *Do not* use bag-valve-mask ventilation, which can worsen this condition by causing gastric distention. If necessary, cautiously administer positive-pressure ventilation through an endotracheal tube.

This condition usually requires surgical repair. Explain the possible need for surgery to the parents, assuring them that their newborn child will be transported quickly to the facility best able to handle this procedure.

Bradycardia

Bradycardia in the newborn is most commonly caused by hypoxia. However, it may also be caused by several other factors, including increased intracranial pressure, hypothyroidism, or acidosis.

In cases of hypoxia, the infant experiences minimal risk if the hypoxia is corrected quickly. In providing

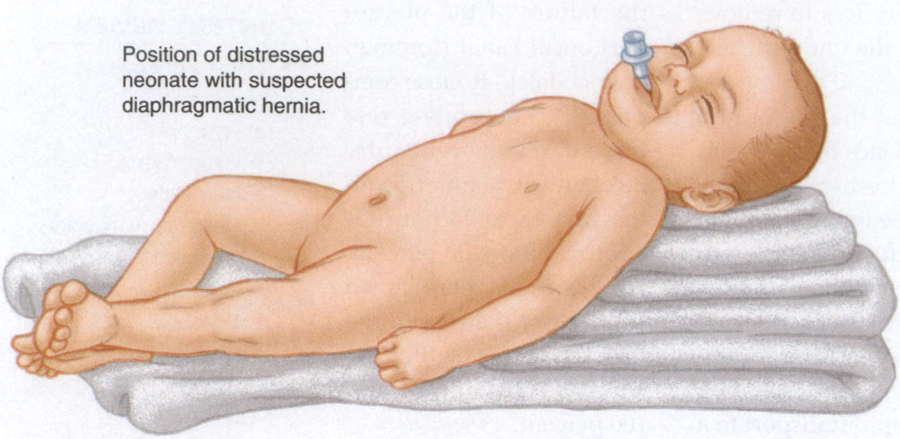

FIGURE 3-23 If a diaphragmatic hernia is suspected, position the infant with the head and thorax higher than the abdomen and feet to facilitate downward displacement of abdominal organs.

treatment, follow the procedures in the inverted pyramid, as discussed earlier. Check for secretions in the airway, check tongue and soft tissue positioning, and check for possible foreign body obstruction. Resist the inclination to treat the bradycardia with pharmacological measures alone. Although epinephrine may be necessary, in all likelihood you will be able to correct the problem with ventilation and supplemental oxygen (if needed). Throughout treatment, keep the newborn warm and transport to the nearest facility.

Prematurity

A premature newborn is an infant born prior to 37 weeks of gestation or with weight ranging from 0.6 to 2.2 kg (1 pound, 5 ounces to 4 pounds, 13 ounces). Healthy premature infants weighing more than 1,700 grams (3 pounds, 12 ounces) have a survivability and outcome approximately equal to that of full-term infants. The mortality rate decreases weekly as the gestational age surpasses the age of fetal viability. With the technology currently available, fetal viability is considered to be 23 to 24 weeks of gestation.

Premature newborns are at greater risk of respiratory suppression, head or brain injury caused by hypoxemia, changes in blood pressure, intraventricular hemorrhage, and fluctuations in serum osmolarity. They are also more susceptible to hypothermia than full-term newborns. Reasons premature newborns lose heat more readily include the following:

- The premature newborn has a relatively large body surface area and comparatively small weight.
- The premature newborn has not sufficiently developed the various control mechanisms needed to regulate body temperature.
- The premature newborn has smaller subcutaneous stores of insulating fat.
- Newborns cannot shiver and must maintain body temperature through other mechanisms.

The degree of immaturity determines the physical characteristics of a premature newborn (Figure 3-24). Premature newborns often appear to have a larger head relative to body size. They may have large trunks and short extremities, transparent skin, and few wrinkles.

Prematurity should not be a factor in short-term treatment. Resuscitation should be attempted if there is any sign of life, and the measures of resuscitation should be the same as those for newborns of normal weight and maturity. Maintain a patent airway and avoid potential aspiration of gastric contents. Medical direction may advise administration of epinephrine. Throughout treatment, maintain the newborn's body temperature and transport to a facility with special services for low-birth-weight newborns.

Respiratory Distress/Cyanosis

Prematurity is the single most common factor causing respiratory distress and cyanosis in the newborn. The problem occurs most frequently in infants weighing less than 1,200 grams (2 pounds, 10 ounces) and who are born at less than 30 weeks' gestation. Premature infants have an immature central respiratory control center and are easily affected by environmental or metabolic changes. Multiple gestations or prenatal maternal complications may also increase the risk of respiratory distress and cyanosis.

The severely ill newborn with respiratory distress and cyanosis presents a difficult diagnostic challenge. Contributing factors include lung or heart disease, central nervous

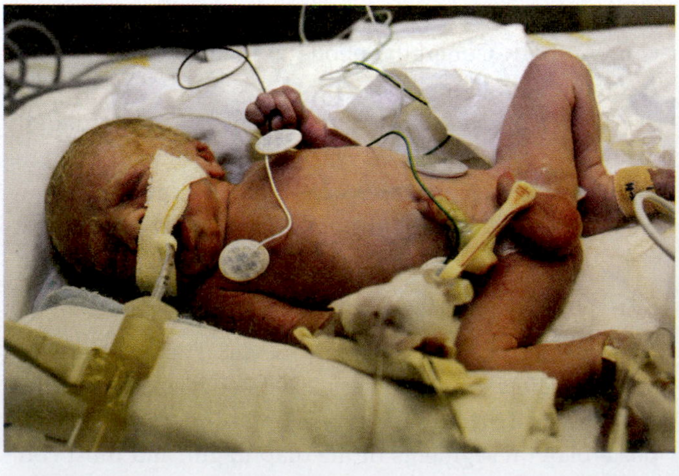

FIGURE 3-24 The premature newborn.

system disorders, meconium aspiration, metabolic problems, obstruction of the nasal passages, shock and sepsis, diaphragmatic hernia, and more. Assessment findings include:

- Tachypnea
- Paradoxical breathing
- Intercostal retractions
- Nasal flaring
- Expiratory grunt

Follow the inverted pyramid of treatment (Figure 3-17), paying particular attention to airway and ventilation. Suction as needed and provide high-concentration oxygen. Ventilate, as needed, with a bag-valve-mask unit. If prolonged ventilation will be required, consider placing an endotracheal tube. Perform chest compressions, if indicated. Sodium bicarbonate may be helpful for prolonged resuscitation. Consider dextrose ($D_{10}W$ or $D_{25}W$) solution if the newborn is hypoglycemic. Maintain body temperature and transport. Be sure to keep the parents informed and provide needed psychological support.

Hypovolemia

Hypovolemia is the leading cause of shock in newborns. It may result from dehydration, hemorrhage, or third-spacing of fluids. Dehydration is by far the most common cause. Signs of hypovolemia include:

- Pale color
- Cool skin
- Diminished peripheral pulses
- Delayed capillary refill, despite normal ambient temperature
- Mental status changes
- Diminished urination (oliguria) as evidenced by dark urine or dry diaper

When you observe these signs, administer a fluid bolus and assess the infant's response. If signs of shock continue, administer a second bolus. Additional boluses should be infused as indicated by repeated assessments. A hypovolemic infant may often need 40 to 60 mL/kg of fluid during the first hour of resuscitation.

Fluid bolus resuscitation consists of 10 mL/kg of an isotonic crystalloid solution, such as Ringer's lactate or normal saline. Administer the bolus over 5 to 10 minutes as soon as intravascular or intraosseous access is obtained. Do not use solutions containing dextrose, because they can produce hypokalemia or worsen ischemic brain injury. Avoid giving volume expanders too rapidly, as rapid infusion of large volumes of fluid has been associated with brain (intraventricular) hemorrhage.

Seizures

Although seizures occur in a very small percentage of all newborns, they usually indicate a serious underlying abnormality and represent a medical emergency. Prolonged and frequent multiple seizures may result in metabolic changes and cardiopulmonary difficulties.

Neonatal seizures differ from seizures in a child or an adult, because generalized tonic-clonic convulsions normally do not occur during the first month of life. Seizures in neonates include these types:

- ***Subtle seizures.*** These seizures consist of chewing motions, excessive salivation, blinking, sucking, swimming movements of the arms, pedaling movements of the legs, apnea, and changes in color.
- ***Tonic seizures.*** These seizures are characterized by rigid posturing of the extremities and trunk. They are sometimes associated with fixed deviation of the eyes. They occur more commonly in premature infants, especially those with an intraventricular hemorrhage.
- ***Focal clonic seizures.*** These seizures consist of rhythmic twitching of muscle groups, particularly in the extremities and face. They may occur in both full-term and premature infants.
- ***Multifocal seizures.*** These seizures are similar to focal clonic seizures, except that multiple muscle groups are involved. Clonic activity randomly migrates. These seizures occur primarily in full-term newborns.
- ***Myoclonic seizures.*** These seizures involve brief focal or generalized jerks of the extremities or parts of the body that tend to involve distal muscle groups. They may occur singly or in a series of repetitive jerks.

Causes of neonatal seizures include sepsis, fever, hypoglycemia, hypoxic–ischemic encephalopathy, metabolic disturbances, meningitis, developmental abnormalities, or drug withdrawal. Assessment findings include a decreased level of consciousness and seizure activities such as those just described. Treatment focuses on airway management and oxygen saturation. With medical direction, consider administration of an anticonvulsant. You might also administer a benzodiazepine (usually lorazepam) for status epilepticus or dextrose ($D_{10}W$ or $D_{25}W$) for hypoglycemia. As with all distressed newborns, maintain body temperature and transport rapidly.

Fever

The average normal temperature in a newborn is 37.5°C (99.5°F). A rectal temperature of 38.0°C (100.4°F) or higher is considered fever. Neonates do not develop fever as readily as older children do. Thus, any fever in a neonate requires extensive evaluation because it may be caused by life-threatening conditions such as pneumonia, sepsis, or meningitis. Fever may be the only sign of meningitis in a neonate. Because of their immature development, neonates do not develop the classic symptoms such as a stiff neck. Thus, any neonate with a fever should be considered to have meningitis or sepsis until proven otherwise.

In assessing a neonate with fever, remember that infants have a limited ability to control their body temperature. As a result, fever can be a serious problem. Assessment findings will probably include the following:

- Mental status changes (irritability/somnolence)
- Decreased feeding
- Skin warm to the touch
- Rashes or petechiae (small, purplish, hemorrhagic spots on the skin)

Full-term infants may produce beads of sweat on their brow but not on the rest of their body. Premature infants will have no visible sweat at all.

Treatment of a neonate with fever will, for the most part, be limited to ensuring a patent airway and adequate ventilation. Do not use cold packs, which may drop the temperature too quickly and may also cause seizures. If the newborn becomes bradycardic, provide chest compressions. In the prehospital setting, administration of an antipyretic agent to a neonate is of questionable benefit and should be avoided. Select the appropriate treatment facility and explain the need for transport to the parents or caregivers.

Hypothermia

As previously noted, hypothermia presents a common and life-threatening condition for newborns. Adults sometimes fail to realize that a newborn may die because of exposure to temperatures that adults find comfortable. The increased surface-to-volume relationship in newborns makes them extremely sensitive to environmental temperatures, especially right after delivery when they are wet. As a result, it is important to control the four methods of heat loss: evaporation, conduction, convection, and radiation.

In treating hypothermia—a body temperature below 35°C (95°F)—keep in mind that it can also be an indicator of sepsis in the newborn. Regardless of the cause, the increased metabolic demands created by hypothermia can produce a variety of related conditions, including metabolic acidosis, pulmonary hypertension, and hypoxemia.

In assessing hypothermic newborns, remember that they do not shiver. Instead, expect these findings:

- Pale color
- Skin cool to the touch, particularly in the extremities
- **Acrocyanosis**
- Respiratory distress
- Possible apnea
- Bradycardia
- Central cyanosis
- Initial irritability
- Lethargy in later stages

Management focuses on ensuring adequate ventilations and oxygenation. Chest compressions may be performed, if necessary. With medical direction, you might administer warm fluids through an IV fluid heater. Do not microwave fluids, because great variations in fluid temperature can result. Dextrose ($D_{10}W$ or $D_{25}W$) may also be given if the newborn is hypoglycemic. Above all, the newborn must be kept warm. Set the ambulance temperature at 24°C to 26°C (75.2°F–78.8°F). Also remember to warm your hands before touching the newborn. Select the appropriate receiving facility and transport rapidly.

Hypoglycemia

Newborns are the only age group that can develop severe hypoglycemia and not have diabetes mellitus. Hypoglycemia may be caused by inadequate glucose intake or increased glucose utilization. Stress and other factors can also cause the blood sugar to fall, sometimes to a critical level.

Hypoglycemia is more common in premature or small-for-gestational-age (SGA) infants, the smaller twin, and newborns of a diabetic mother, because these infants often have decreased glycogen stores. Hypoglycemia can also develop as a result of increased glucose utilization. Causes include respiratory illnesses, hypothermia, toxemia, CNS hemorrhage, asphyxia, meningitis, and sepsis. In an older infant, hypoglycemia may be caused by an inadequate glucose intake or increased utilization of glucose. Infants receiving glucose infusions can develop hypoglycemia if the infusion is suddenly stopped.

Infants with hypoglycemia may be asymptomatic or they may exhibit symptoms such as apnea, color changes, respiratory distress, lethargy, seizures, acidosis, and poor myocardial contractility.

Persistent hypoglycemia can have catastrophic effects on the brain. The normal newborn's glycogen stores are sufficient to meet glucose requirements for only 8 to 12 hours. This time frame is diminished in infants with decreased glycogen stores or the presence of other problems in which glucose utilization increases. As a result, you should determine the blood glucose level on all sick infants. A blood glucose screening test of less than 45 mg/dL indicates hypoglycemia.

In response to hypoglycemia, the newborn's body will release counterregulatory hormones such as glucagon, epinephrine, cortisol, and growth hormone. These hormones help raise the blood glucose level by mobilizing glucose stores. In fact, this hormone response may cause transient symptoms of hyperglycemia that can last for several hours. However, when the infant's glucose stores are depleted, the glucose level will again fall.

In assessing hypoglycemic newborns, expect these findings:

- Twitching or seizures
- Limpness
- Lethargy
- Eye rolling
- High-pitched cry
- Apnea
- Irregular respirations
- Possible cyanosis

Treatment begins with management of the airway and ventilations. Ensure adequate oxygenation. Perform chest compressions, if indicated. With medical direction, administer dextrose ($D_{10}W$ or $D_{25}W$). Maintain a normal body temperature in the newborn and transport to the appropriate facility.

Vomiting

Vomiting in a neonate may result from a variety of causes and rarely presents as an isolated symptom. Vomiting (a forceful ejection of stomach contents) is uncommon during the first weeks of life and may be confused with regurgitation (a simple backflow of stomach contents into the mouth, or "spitting up"). Vomiting in the neonate usually occurs because of an anatomic abnormality such as a tracheoesophageal fistula or upper gastrointestinal obstruction. More often, it may be a symptom of a serious disorder, such as increased intracranial pressure or an infection. Vomitus containing dark blood often signals a life-threatening illness. Keep in mind, however, that vomiting of mucus, which may occasionally be blood streaked, in the first few hours after birth is not uncommon.

Assessment findings may include a distended stomach, signs of infection, increased intracranial pressure, or drug withdrawal. Because vomitus can be aspirated, management considerations focus on ensuring a patent airway. If you detect respiratory difficulties or obstruction of the airway, suction or clear vomitus from the airway and ensure adequate oxygenation. Fluid administration may be needed to prevent dehydration. Also remember that, as with older patients, **vagal stimulation** may cause bradycardia in the neonate.

After you have protected the airway, place the infant on his side and transport to an appropriate facility. As with all other situations involving distressed neonates, advise parents or caregivers of the steps taken and why.

Diarrhea

Diarrhea in a neonate can cause severe dehydration and electrolyte imbalances. Although diarrhea may be harder to assess in neonates than in other patients, consider five to six stools per day as normal, especially in breast-fed infants.

Causes of diarrhea in a neonate include:

- Bacterial or viral infection
- Gastroenteritis
- Lactose intolerance
- **Phototherapy**
- **Neonatal abstinence syndrome (NAS)**
- **Thyrotoxicosis**
- Cystic fibrosis

In treating neonates with diarrhea, remember to take Standard Precautions, just as you would do in any situation involving body fluids. Expect to find loose stools, decreased urinary output, and other signs of dehydration, such as prolonged capillary refill time, cool extremities, and listlessness or lethargy. It is often difficult for the parents to estimate the number of stools. In such cases, it might be better to inquire about the number of diapers the baby is using.

Management consists of maintenance of airway and ventilations, adequate oxygenation, and chest compressions, if indicated. With medical direction, you might also consider fluid therapy. Explain all treatments to parents or caregivers, and transport the neonate to a facility able to handle high-risk infants.

Common Birth Injuries

A **birth injury** occurs in an estimated 2 to 7 of every 1,000 live births in the United States. About 5 to 8 of every 100,000 infants die of birth trauma and 25 of every 100,000 die of anoxic injuries. Such injuries account for 2 to 3 percent of infant deaths. Risk factors for birth injury include the following:

- Prematurity
- Postmaturity
- Cephalopelvic disproportion
- Prolonged labor
- Breech presentation
- Explosive delivery

- Shoulder dystocia
- Diabetic mother

Birth injuries take various forms. Cranial injuries may include molding of the head and overriding of the parietal bones, erythema (reddening of the skin), abrasions, ecchymosis (black-and-blue discoloration) and subcutaneous fat necrosis, subconjunctival and retinal hemorrhage, subperiosteal hemorrhage, and fracture of the skull. Intracranial hemorrhage may result from trauma or asphyxia. Often the infant will develop a large scalp hematoma during the birth process. This injury, called *caput succedaneum*, will usually resolve over a week's time. Damage to the spine and spinal cord may occur as a result of strong traction exerted when the spine is hyperextended or there is a lateral pull. Other birth injuries include peripheral nerve injury, injury to the liver, rupture of the spleen, adrenal hemorrhage, fractures of the clavicle or extremities, and, of course, hypoxia/ischemia.

Assessment findings may include:

- Diffuse, sometimes ecchymotic, edematous swelling of soft tissues around the scalp
- Paralysis below the level of the spinal cord injury
- Paralysis of the upper arm with or without paralysis of the forearm
- Diaphragmatic paralysis
- Movement on only one side of the face when crying
- Inability to move the arm freely on the side of the fractured clavicle
- Lack of spontaneous movement of the affected extremity
- Hypoxia
- Shock

Management of a newborn with birth injuries usually centers on protection of the airway, provision of adequate ventilation and oxygen, and, if needed, chest compressions. With medical direction, you may administer medications or take other nonpharmacological steps to support the specific injury. Newborns with birth injuries usually require treatment at specialized facilities. As in the management of other neonatal emergencies, provide professional and compassionate communication to parents or caregivers.

Cultural Considerations

When Parents Request Baptism. *Occasionally, prehospital childbirth may result in the delivery of a stillborn infant. The reasons for the infant's demise may be obvious or the infant may appear otherwise normal. Some Christian families may request that the infant be baptized as soon as possible after birth. In fact, in some faiths, failure to baptize the infant might "deny a child the priceless grace of becoming a child of God." Infant baptism is primarily a practice of the Roman Catholic Church, although similar faiths (Episcopalian, Anglican) also often practice the rite. If you are asked to baptize an infant, remember that, despite your own personal religious beliefs, this is very important to the parents and they have put a great deal of trust in you. According to the Catechism of the Catholic Church, dip your finger into a bowl of water and make a sign of the cross on the infant's forehead. Then say, "I baptize you in the name of the Father and of the Son and of the Holy Spirit. Amen." Even if you are not baptized, in an emergency you may baptize an infant if that is the parents' wish, provided you act in the spirit of church teaching. Most parents will appreciate the act. Sometimes, even in this era of sophisticated medical technology, there is little we can do other than provide support to the survivors.*

Cardiac Resuscitation, Postresuscitation, and Stabilization

The incidence of neonatal cardiac arrest is related primarily to hypoxia. As explained previously, the outcome will be poor unless you immediately initiate appropriate interventions. As you might expect, cases involving cardiac arrest have an increased chance of brain and organ damage. Risk factors for cardiac arrest in newborns include:

- Bradycardia
- Intrauterine asphyxia
- Prematurity
- Drugs administered to or taken by the mother
- Congenital neuromuscular diseases
- Congenital malformations
- Intrapartum hypoxemia

Cardiac arrest can be caused by primary or secondary apnea, bradycardia, persistent fetal circulation, or pulmonary hypertension. Assessment findings may include peripheral cyanosis, inadequate respiratory effort, and ineffective or absent heart rate.

In managing neonatal cardiac arrest, follow the inverted pyramid for resuscitation (Figure 3-17). Administer drugs or fluids according to medical direction. Maintain normal body temperature while you transport the distressed newborn to the appropriate facility. This situation will require delicate handling of the parents or caregivers. Explain what is being done for the infant, without discussing the possibilities of survival.

CONTENT REVIEW

➤ Causes of Neonatal Cardiac Arrest
- Primary or secondary apnea
- Bradycardia
- Persistent fetal circulation
- Pulmonary hypertension

Summary

After a woman gives birth, you must care for two patients—the mother and her newborn child. The newborn has several special needs, the most important of which are protection of the airway and support of ventilations. The most important aspects of newborn care, aside from airway and ventilation, are preventing heat loss and warming the newborn, who must be kept warm at all times.

If assessment reveals a distressed newborn, you should initiate ventilatory support, stimulation, and, if required, CPR. Keep in mind that it is not uncommon for the newborn to require a little oxygen and even ventilatory support following birth. Generally, oxygen therapy and ventilatory support will dramatically improve the majority of poorly presenting infants. Remember to start simply (blow-by oxygen) and progress to the more invasive procedures (CPR) when the newborn presents with a low APGAR score. When possible, newborns born away from a facility should be transported to a facility with an NICU.

You Make the Call

You are called to assist an EMT unit with a difficult delivery. When you arrive at the scene, the EMTs report that the patient is a 35-year-old woman who is two weeks past full term. Her amniotic sac has just ruptured, and thick meconium staining is observed. The infant is crowning. Just after your arrival at the scene, the mother begins to scream that the baby is coming.

1. Should you stimulate this baby to breathe as soon as it is delivered? Why or why not?
2. What is the major danger associated with this type of problem?
3. Once you have stabilized this infant, where should he be transported?

See Suggested Responses at the back of this book.

Review Questions

1. Most neonates who weigh less than ____________ at birth require resuscitation.
   a. 1,500 grams
   b. 5 pounds, 6 ounces
   c. 2,500 grams
   d. 3 pounds, 8 ounces
2. Factors that stimulate the baby's first breath include all of the following *except* ____________
   a. hypoxia.
   b. hyperthermia.
   c. mild acidosis.
   d. initiation of stretch reflexes in the lungs.
3. Most fetal development occurs during the ____________ trimester of pregnancy.
   a. first
   b. second
   c. third
   d. last
4. The newborn's respiratory rate should average ____________ breaths per minute and the heart rate should fall within the range of ____________ beats per minute moments after birth.
   a. 20–30, 90–110
   b. 25–35, 100–110
   c. 30–40, 120–140
   d. 40–60, 150–180
5. The maximum APGAR score is ____________.
   a. 6
   b. 7
   c. 8
   d. 10
6. Most heat loss in newborns results from ____________
   a. radiation.
   b. convection.
   c. conduction.
   d. evaporation.

7. What is the name of the condition in which the newborn has an excessively high level of red blood cells?
   a. Choanal atresia
   b. Polycythemia
   c. Omphalocele
   d. Pierre Robin syndrome
8. Bulb suctioning of a newborn __________
   a. should take less than 5 seconds.
   b. should be done only by a physician.
   c. is no longer routinely recommended.
   d. is done for every neonate.
9. In the newborn, vascular access for the administration of fluids and drugs can most readily be managed by using which vein?
   a. Cephalic
   b. Brachial
   c. Umbilical
   d. Saphenous
10. A premature newborn is an infant born prior to __________ weeks of gestation or with weight ranging from 0.6 to 2.2 kg.
   a. 40
   b. 39
   c. 38
   d. 37
11. A blood glucose level less than __________ in a neonate constitutes hypoglycemia.
   a. 75 mg/dL
   b. 65 mg/dL
   c. 55 mg/dL
   d. 45 mg/dL
12. You are going to administer a fluid bolus to a neonate. What is the dosage for this bolus?
   a. 30 mL/kg
   b. 20 mL/kg
   c. 10 mL/kg
   d. 5 mL/kg

See Answers to Review Questions at the end of this book.

References

1. Perlman, J. M., and R. Risser. "Cardiopulmonary Resuscitation in the Delivery Room: Associated Clinical Events." *Arch Pediatr Adolesc Med* 149 (1995): 20–25.
2. Barber, C. A. and M. H. Wyckoff. "Use and Efficacy of Endotracheal versus Intravenous Epinephrine during Neonatal Cardiopulmonary Resuscitation in the Delivery Room." *Pediatrics* 118 (2006): 1028–1034.
3. Toth, B., A. Becker, and B. Seelbach-Gobel. "Oxygen Saturation in Healthy Newborn Infants Immediately after Birth Measured by Pulse Oximetry." *Arch Gynecol Obstet* 266 (2002): 105–107.
4. Davis, P. G., A. Tan, C. P. O'Donnell, and A. Schulze. "Resuscitation of Newborn Infants with 100% Oxygen or Air: A Systematic Review and Meta-Analysis." *Lancet* 364 (2004): 1329–1333.
5. Rabi, Y., D. Rabi, and W. Yee. "Room Air Resuscitation of the Depressed Newborn: A Systematic Review and Meta-Analysis." *Resuscitation* 72 (2007): 353–363.
6. Apgar, V. "A Proposal for a New Method of Evaluation of the Newborn Infant." *Anesth Analg* 32 (1953): 260–267.
7. Mieczyslaw, F. and M. Wood. "The APGAR Score Has Survived the Test of Time." *Anesthesiology* 102 (2005): 855–857.
8. Wyckoff, M. H., K. Aziz, M. B. Escobedo, et al. "Part 13: Neonatal Resuscitation: 2015 American Heart Association Guidelines for Cardiopulmonary Resuscitation and Emergency Cardiovascular Care." *Circulation* 132 (2015): S543–S560.
9. Atkins, D. L., S. Berger, J. P. Duff, et al. "Part 11: Pediatric Basic Life Support: 2015 American Heart Association Guidelines for Cardiopulmonary Resuscitation and Emergency Cardiovascular Care." *Circulation* 132 (2015): S519–S525.
10. Roggensack, A., A. L. Jeffries, D. Farine, et al. "Management of Meconium at Birth." *J Obstet Gynaecol Can* 31 (2009): 355–357.
11. Raghuveer, T. S. and A. J. Cox. "Neonatal Resuscitation: An Update." *Am Family Physician* 83 (2011): 911–918.

Further Reading

American Heart Association. *2015 American Heart Association Guidelines for CPR and ECC.* Dallas: American Heart Association, 2015.

American Heart Association and American Academy of Pediatrics. *PALS Provider Manual.* 6th ed. Dallas: American Heart Association, 2011.

Braner, D., J. Kattwinkel, S. Denson, and S. Niermeyer, eds. *Neonatal Resuscitation.* 5th ed. Elk Grove Village, IL: American Academy of Pediatrics, 2011.

DeBoer, J. L. *Emergency Newborn Care: The First Minutes of Life.* Chicago: ACM Publications, 2004.

Kleigman, R. M., et al. *Nelson Textbook of Pediatrics.* 20th ed. Philadelphia: W. B. Saunders, 2015.

Tintinalli, J. E., J. Stapczynski, O. John Ma, D. Cline, and R. Cydulka. *Emergency Medicine: A Comprehensive Study Guide.* 7th ed. New York: McGraw-Hill, 2013.

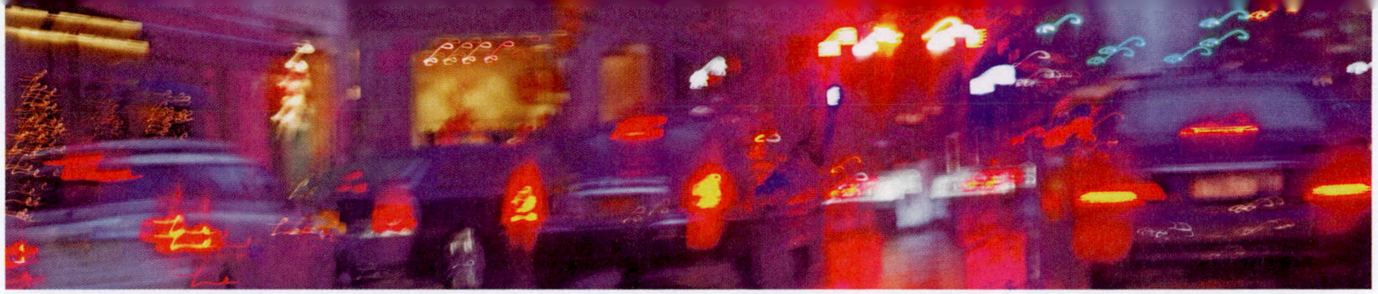

Chapter 4
Pediatrics

Bryan Bledsoe, DO, FACEP, FAAEM, EMT-P
David Nelson, MD, FAAP, FAAEM

STANDARD
Special Patient Populations (Pediatrics)

COMPETENCY
Integrates assessment findings with principles of epidemiology and pathophysiology and knowledge of psychosocial needs to formulate a field impression and implement a comprehensive treatment/disposition plan for patients with special needs.

Learning Objectives

Terminal Performance Objective: After reading this chapter, you should be able to integrate patient assessment findings, patient history, and knowledge of anatomy, physiology, pathophysiology, and basic and advanced life support interventions to recognize and manage emergencies in pediatric patients.

Enabling Objectives: To accomplish the terminal performance objective, you should be able to:

1. Define key terms introduced in this chapter.
2. Identify the basic epidemiological findings as they relate to the pediatric patient, and the role of the paramedic in pediatric care.
3. Relate the differences of children of various ages to adaptations in communication, assessment, and management of pediatric patients, and the psychosocial needs of the parents or caregivers.
4. Discuss the evolving physiology of pediatrics from newborns to adolescents as it relates to anatomy, physiology, and pathophysiology.
5. Identify how to adapt the scene size-up, primary assessment, patient history, secondary assessment, vital sign values, and use of monitoring technology to guide clinical reasoning.
6. Use a process of clinical reasoning to guide and interpret the patient assessment and management process for pediatric patients.
7. Discuss the general management of pediatric patients regarding airway management, ventilation, oxygenation, vascular access, fluid and medication administration, and cardiac arrest management.
8. Based on assessment findings, discuss how to delineate and individually manage respiratory distress, respiratory failure, and respiratory arrest.

9. Relate the pathophysiology of traumatic and medical pediatric emergencies to the priorities of patient assessment and management by the paramedic.
10. Describe special considerations in management and documentation of situations involving SIDS, ALTE, abuse, and neglect.
11. Discuss the process of assessing and managing special needs pediatric patients who are dependent on medical technology.
12. Apply the JumpSTART triage method to multiple-casualty incidents involving children.
13. Given various pediatric scenarios, discuss how the paramedic should integrate assessment and management of these emergencies in the prehospital environment.

KEY TERMS

asthma, p. 121
bacterial tracheitis, p. 120
bend fractures, p. 139
bronchiolitis, p. 122
buckle fractures, p. 139
cardiogenic shock, p. 124
central IV line, p. 144
congenital, p. 125
croup, p. 118
diabetic ketoacidosis, p. 132
distributive shock, p. 125
Emergency Medical Services for Children (EMSC), p. 81
epiglottitis, p. 119
febrile seizures, p. 129
foreign body airway obstruction (FBAO), p. 84
greenstick fractures, p. 139
growth plate, p. 89
hyperglycemia, p. 132
hypoglycemia, p. 131
hypovolemic shock, p. 124
noncardiogenic shock, p. 124
shunt, p. 145
status epilepticus, p. 129
stoma, p. 144
sudden infant death syndrome, p. 140
tracheostomy, p. 143

Case Study

Three tones sound on the paramedic radios in the ED. A message crackles: "LA Fifty-Four, I need you to be in-service." The crew of LA 54 transfers care of the patient in Bed 6 to the hospital staff. Within 60 seconds, they depart the hospital parking lot. En route to the emergency, they review information provided by the dispatcher. They will be treating a 5-month-old girl who is described as "not breathing" by her father.

The response time is 4 minutes. On arrival, the parents lead the paramedics into the patient's bedroom. The little girl is lying in a crib. Immediately, paramedics note that she has pale, cool, clammy skin. Her anterior fontanelle is noticeably sunken. The respiratory rate and quality are 20 and shallow. Upon mild painful stimuli, the infant cries vigorously, increasing her tidal rate and volume. However, no tears appear. After taking Standard Precautions, the paramedics check the diaper and find that it is dry. "She hasn't kept any food down for three days," explains the mother. "She hasn't wet her diaper in hours."

The crew administers supplemental oxygen via a nonrebreather mask. The infant responds to the mask by crying. Capillary refill is borderline (2.5 seconds). The paramedics prepare to transport the infant to the ED, informing the parents of all the steps that will be taken to help their daughter.

En route to the hospital, the crew establishes an IV and administers a fluid bolus of 20 mL/kg of normal saline. By the time they pull up to the ambulance ramp at the ED, the patient's color and respiratory rate have improved greatly. Capillary refill time and pulse rate move toward normal limits. The ED staff evaluates the patient and admits her for 24-hour observation and IV fluid therapy. She returns home the following day. The paramedics later learn that she had contracted a viral gastroenteritis that was going around her day care center. Within 48 hours she was back to her usual playful self.

CONTENT REVIEW

- Top Causes of Pediatric Deaths
  - Motor vehicle crashes
  - Burns
  - Drownings
  - Suicides
  - Homicides

Introduction

The ill or injured child presents special concerns for prehospital personnel. Current research indicates that more than 20,000 pediatric deaths occur each year in the United States. The leading causes of death are age specific. They include motor vehicle collisions, burns, drownings, suicides, and homicides. These alarming facts become even more troublesome when experts theorize that many of them could have been prevented by early intervention. Tragedies involving children—neonates to adolescents—account for some of the most stressful incidents that you will encounter in EMS practice.[1]

Treatment of pediatric patients presents a number of challenges for the paramedic. Children, especially young ones, often cannot describe what is bothering them or what has happened to them. In addition to the child patient, you must deal with the parents or caregivers. Finally, a child's size often makes routine procedures more difficult. Keep in mind that children are not simply small adults. They have special considerations and needs. This chapter will present the topic of pediatric emergencies as it applies to advanced prehospital care.

Role of Paramedics in Pediatric Care

When considering the reduction of pediatric morbidity and mortality, your role as a paramedic centers around two key concepts. First, you must realize that pediatric injuries have become a major health concern. Second, you should remember that children are at a higher risk of injury than adults and that they are more likely to be adversely affected by the injuries that they suffer.

Numerous factors account for the high pediatric injury rates. Some factors, such as geography and weather, cannot be altered. However, other factors, particularly dangers within the home and community, can be eliminated or minimized. As health care professionals, we must all get involved in identifying and implementing methods and mechanisms that prevent injuries to infants and children. Those of us who deliver prehospital care must do more than simply enter the picture after an injury has taken place.

In addition to treating pediatric injuries, paramedics are often responsible for treating the ill child. Many aspects of disease and disease processes are unique to children. It is important that the paramedic be familiar with these, because early intervention is often the key to reduced morbidity and mortality.

Continuing Education and Training

Your role in improving the health care offered to pediatric patients begins with your own training. Because you will encounter pediatric patients less frequently than adult patients, you have a professional responsibility to maintain and improve on your pediatric knowledge, particularly your clinical skills.[2] Continuing education programs include:

- Pediatric Advanced Life Support (PALS)
- Pediatric Education for Paramedic Professionals (PEPP)
- Advanced Pediatric Life Support (APLS)
- Prehospital Pediatric Care (PPC)

In addition to these programs, you can also attend regional conferences and seminars designed to increase your knowledge of pediatric care. These are often conducted by regional children's hospitals. You can further enhance your clinical skills by spending time in pediatric emergency departments, pediatric hospitals, or pediatric departments in local hospitals. You might also visit the offices of pediatricians or talk with pediatric nurse practitioners—registered nurses who provide primary health care to children.

Improved Health Care and Injury Prevention

Funding for a significant amount of prehospital pediatric education comes largely from a program known as **Emergency Medical Services for Children (EMSC)**.[3] This federally funded program falls under the management of the Maternal and Child Health Bureau, an agency of the U.S. Department of Health and Human Services. The EMSC was formed for the express purpose of improving the health of pediatric patients who suffer potentially life-threatening illnesses or injuries. This nationally coordinated effort has identified a number of pediatric health care concerns, including:

- Community education
- Data collection
- Quality improvement
- Injury prevention
- Access
- Prehospital care
- Emergency care
- Definitive care
- Finance
- Rehabilitation
- A systems approach to pediatric care
- Ongoing health care from birth to young adulthood

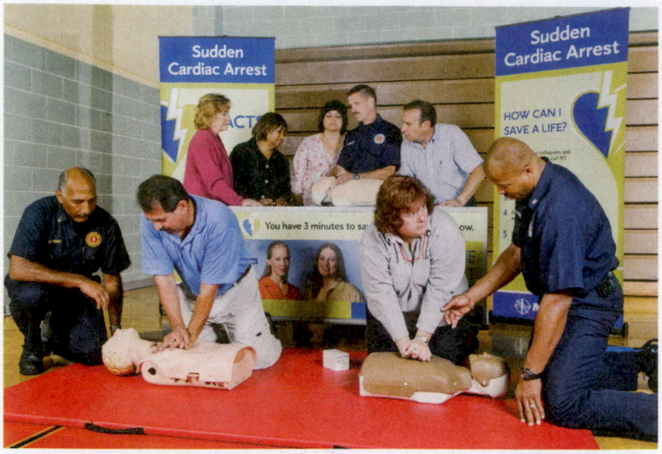

FIGURE 4-1 It is important to organize or participate in programs that educate the public about injury prevention and health care.

As a paramedic, you can take part in this national effort by actively participating in programs that promote injury prevention. Let's face it—as prehospital care providers, we see the consequences of pediatric trauma all too often. You can help reduce the rate of injury by taking advantage of opportunities to share "teaching points" in your daily life, both personally and professionally. Take part in, or offer to organize, school or community programs in injury prevention or health care (Figure 4-1). Engage student interest in the EMS profession by volunteering to speak at "career days," emphasizing those aspects of your job that relate to young people. Use nonurgent ambulance calls as a chance to educate family members or caregivers on the importance of "childproofing" a home or neighborhood. Work with appropriate agencies in initiating or conducting safety inspections, block watches, and more.

Increased effort has been made to identify the severity and nature of prehospital pediatric emergencies. Many regions now have both pediatric and trauma registries. These, in addition to standard epidemiological research conducted by local health departments, are dependent on quality prehospital documentation. If your area is participating in a registry program or research study, be sure to obtain and record all required data. Information gained from these registries will help identify the need for more or specialized resources.

Advanced Life Support Skills in Pediatrics

Several recent research studies have shown that up to 85 percent of children treated by EMS personnel need nothing more than basic life support skills.[4] These include such things as bandaging and splinting, oxygen administration, and similar fundamental skills. In addition, only a limited percentage of EMS transports involve children. Thus, it is fairly rare that a paramedic will be called on to perform an advanced life support (ALS) skill such as intubation, IV access, or drug administration in a child. Because these skills are used infrequently in EMS, it is difficult for paramedics to remain proficient in them. For this reason, several large EMS systems have abandoned the practice of pediatric endotracheal intubation in favor of simple bag-valve-mask (BVM) ventilation. A large study comparing endotracheal intubation versus BVM ventilation in children in the prehospital setting has also concluded that BVM ventilation leads to equal or better outcomes for children.[5]

Regardless of how your system operates, it is important to remember that the less frequently a skill is used, the more frequently it should be practiced. Certain ALS skills can be lifesaving when properly applied. Thus, it is incumbent on each paramedic to realize that pediatric ALS skills will be needed infrequently. When they are needed, however, they must be applied competently.

General Approach to Pediatric Emergencies

The approach to the pediatric patient varies with the age of the patient and with the problem being treated. Foremost in approaching any pediatric emergency is consideration of the patient's emotional and physiologic development. Care also involves the family members or caregivers responsible for the child. They will demand information, express fears, and, ultimately, give or refuse consent for treatment and/or transport.

Communication and Psychological Support

Treatment of an infant, child, or teenager begins with communication and psychological support. Interaction with pediatric patients and related adults continues throughout assessment and management. When obtaining the medical history of the pediatric patient, you should gather information as quickly and as accurately as possible. The parents and caregivers are often the primary source of information, especially in the case of infants. However, as children become older, they can also be a good source of information. Older children, for example, can often give accurate descriptions of symptoms or other details.

Treat pediatric patients with respect, allowing them to express opinions and ask questions. Your listening skills will play an important role in alleviating the fears of child patients. You can even communicate a calm and caring attitude to infants, who respond to touch and voice just like any other human being.

Responding to Patient Needs

As previously mentioned, a child's response to an emergency will vary, depending on the age and emotional maturity of the child. The child's most common response to illness or injury is fear. Common fears of children include:

- Fear of being separated from the parents or caregivers
- Fear of being removed from a family place, such as home, and never returning
- Fear of being hurt
- Fear of being mutilated or disfigured
- Fear of the unknown

These fears may be intensified if the child detects fear or anxiety from the parents or caregivers. The general chaos and panic that often surround pediatric emergency situations may further distress the child.

Remember that children have the right to know what is being done to them. You should be as honest as possible with them. If a procedure such as an IV needle stick will hurt, tell them so—but tell them immediately before performing a procedure. Do not say that a procedure will be painful and then take 5 minutes to prepare the equipment, allowing time for the child's anticipation of pain to build.

Always use language that is appropriate for the age of the child. Medical and anatomic terms that we routinely use may be completely foreign to children. Telling a child that you are going to "apply a cervical collar" means nothing. Instead, tell the child: "I'm going to put this collar around your neck to keep it from moving." "Try to hold your head still." "Tell me if it is too tight." Communication such as this will involve children in their own care and reduce their feelings of helplessness.

Responding to Parents or Caregivers

As you might expect, the reactions of parents or caregivers to a pediatric emergency will vary. Initial reactions might include shock, grief, denial, anger, guilt, fear, or complete loss of control. Their behavior may change during the course of the emergency. Communication is the key. Preferably, only one paramedic will speak with adults at the scene. This will reduce any chance of providing conflicting information and will allow a second paramedic to focus on the child. If parents or caregivers sense your confidence and professionalism, they will regain control and trust your suggestions for care. As with the child, most parents and caregivers feel overwhelmed by fear. They often express their fears in questions such as the following:

"Is my child going to die?"

"Did my child suffer brain damage?"

"Is my child going to be all right?"

"What are you doing to my child?"

"Will my child be able to walk?"

It may be difficult to answer these questions in the prehospital setting. However, the following actions may help allay parents' fears:

- Tell them your name and qualifications.
- Acknowledge their fears and concerns.
- Reassure them that it is all right to feel the way they do.
- Redirect their energies toward helping you care for the child.
- Remain calm and appear in control of the emergency.
- Keep the parents or caregivers informed as to what you are doing.
- Don't "talk down" to them.
- Assure parents or caregivers that everything possible is being done for their child.

If conditions permit, you should allow one of the parents or caregivers to remain with the child at all times. Some family members may be extremely emotional in emergency situations. The child will react more positively to a family member who appears calm and reassuring. If a parent or caregiver is "out of control," have another person take him or her away from the immediate area to settle down. Maintain a reasonable level of suspicion if a child shows a pattern of injuries, some old and some new. In such cases, the parent or caregiver may try to cover up what may be an abusive situation. They may also try to block examination and treatment. (Potential abuse or neglect will be discussed in more detail later in this chapter.)

Growth and Development

Children progress through developmental stages on their way to adulthood. You should tailor your approach to the developmental level of your pediatric patient, as discussed in the following segments.

Newborns (First Hours after Birth)

Although the terms *newborn* and *neonate* are often used interchangeably, *newborn* refers to a baby in the first hours of extrauterine life. The term *neonate* describes infants from birth to one month of age. The method most frequently used to assess newborns is the APGAR scoring system, which was described in the chapter "Neonatology." Resuscitation of the newborn generally follows the inverted pyramid described in that chapter and the guidelines established in the Neonatal Advanced Life Support (NALS) curriculum.

Neonates (Birth to 1 Month)

The neonate, as just noted and as described in the chapter "Neonatology," is an infant up to one month of age. This is a major stage of development. Soon after birth, the neonate typically loses up to 10 percent of his birth weight as he adjusts to extrauterine life. This lost weight, however, is ordinarily recovered within 10 days. Gestational age affects early growth. Children born at term (40 weeks) should follow accepted developmental guidelines. Infants born prematurely will not be as developed, either neurologically or physically, as their full-term counterparts.

The neonatal stage of development centers on reflexes. The neonate's personality also begins to form. The infant is close to the mother and may stare at faces and smile. The mother, and occasionally the father, can comfort and quiet the child. Common signs and symptoms in this age group include jaundice, vomiting, and respiratory distress. Serious illnesses, such as meningitis, are difficult to distinguish from minor illnesses in neonates. Often, fever is the only sign, although the majority of neonates with fever have minor illnesses. The few who are seriously ill can be easily missed. For this reason, any fever in a neonate requires extensive evaluation.

The approach to this age group should include several factors. First, the child should always be kept warm. Observe skin color, tone, and respiratory activity. The absence of tears when crying may indicate dehydration. The lungs should be auscultated early during the exam, while the infant is quiet. You might find it helpful to have the child suck on a pacifier during the examination. Allowing the infant to remain in a parent's or caregiver's lap may help keep the child calm. Obviously, the history must be obtained from the parents or caregivers. However, it is also important to observe the child.

Infants (Ages 1 to 5 Months)

Infants should have doubled their birth weight by five to six months of age. They should be able to follow the movements of others with their eyes. Muscle control develops in a cephalocaudal progression. This means, literally, that development of muscular control begins at the head (cephalo) and moves toward the tail (caudal). Muscular control also spreads from the trunk toward the extremities during this period. The infant's personality at this stage still centers closely on the parents or caregivers. The history must be obtained from these individuals, with close attention to possible illnesses and accidents, including sudden infant death syndrome (SIDS), vomiting, dehydration, meningitis, child abuse, and household accidents.

Concentrate on keeping these patients warm and comfortable. Allow the infant to remain in the parent's or caregiver's lap. A pacifier or bottle can be used to help keep the baby quiet during the examination.

Infants (Ages 6 Months to 1 Year)

Infants in this age group may stand or even walk with assistance. They are quite active and enjoy exploring the world with their mouths. In this stage of development, the risk of **foreign body airway obstruction (FBAO)** becomes a serious concern.

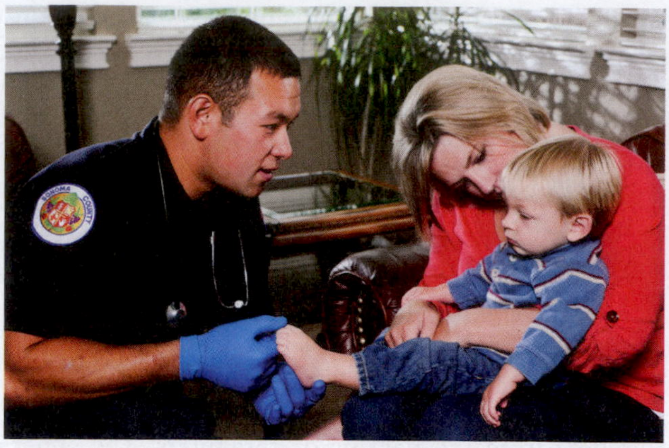

FIGURE 4-2 Infants and young children should be allowed to remain in their mothers' arms.

Infants six months of age and older have more fully formed personalities and express themselves more readily. They have considerable anxiety toward strangers. They do not like lying on their backs. Children in this age group tend to cling to the mother, although the father "will do" in many cases. Common illnesses and accidents include febrile seizures, vomiting, diarrhea, dehydration, bronchiolitis, car crashes, croup, child abuse, poisonings, falls, and airway obstructions.

These children should be examined while sitting in the lap of the parent or caregiver (Figure 4-2). The exam should progress in a toe-to-head order, because starting at the face may upset the child. If time and conditions permit, allow the child to become familiar with you before beginning the examination.

Toddlers (Ages 1 to 3 Years)

Great strides occur in gross motor development during this stage. Children tend to run underneath or stand on almost everything. They seem to always be on the move. As they grow older, toddlers become braver and more curious or stubborn. They begin to stray away from the parents or caregivers more frequently. These remain the only people who can comfort them quickly, however, and most children will cling to a parent or caregiver if frightened.

At ages one to three years, language development begins. Often children can understand better than they can speak. Therefore, the majority of the medical history will still come from the parents or caregivers. Remember, however, that you can ask toddlers simple and specific questions.

Accidents of all types are the leading cause of injury deaths in pediatric patients ages 1 to 15 years. Common accidents in this age group include motor vehicle collisions, homicides, burn injuries, drownings, and pedestrian collisions. Common illnesses and injuries in the toddler age group include vomiting, diarrhea, febrile seizures, poisonings, falls, child abuse, and croup. Keep in mind that FBAO is still a high risk for toddlers.

Be cautious when treating toddlers. Approach toddlers slowly and try to gain their confidence. Conduct the exam in a toe-to-head order. The child may be difficult to examine and may resist being touched. Speak quietly and use only simple words. Avoid asking questions that allow the child to say "no." If the situation permits, allow toddlers to hold transitional objects such as a favorite blanket or toy. Be sure to tell the child if something will hurt. If at all possible, avoid procedures on the dominant arm/hand, which the child will try to pull away.

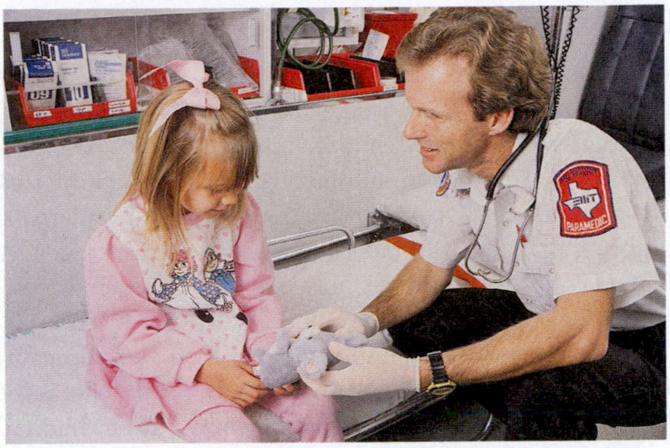

FIGURE 4-3 A small toy may calm a child in the six- to ten-year age range.

Preschoolers (Ages 3 to 5 Years)

Children in this age group show a tremendous increase in fine and gross motor development. Language skills increase greatly. Children in this age group know how to talk. However, if frightened, they often refuse to speak, especially to strangers. They often have vivid imaginations and may see monsters as part of their world. Preschoolers may have tempers and will express them. During this stage of development, children fear mutilation and may feel threatened by treatment. Avoid frightening comments, but also avoid misleading comments, such as saying "This won't hurt" when it will hurt.

Preschoolers often run to a particular parent or caregiver, depending on the occasion. They stick up for the people they love and are openly affectionate. They still seek support and comfort from within the home.

When evaluating children in this age group, question the child first, keeping in mind that imagination may interfere with the facts. The child often has a distorted sense of time; thus, you must rely on the parents or caregivers to fill in the gaps. Common illnesses and injuries in this age group include croup, asthma, poisonings, auto collisions, burns, child abuse, ingestion of foreign bodies, drownings, and febrile seizures.

Treatment of preschoolers requires tact. Avoid baby talk. If time and situation permit, give the child health care choices. Often, the use of a doll or stuffed animal will assist in the examination. Allow the child to hold a piece of equipment, such as a stethoscope, and to use it. Let the child sit on your lap. Start the examination with the chest and evaluate the head last. Avoid misleading comments. You must speak in very basic terms. Do not trick or lie to the child and always explain what you are going to do.

School-Age Children (Ages 6 to 12 Years)

Children in this age group are active and carefree. Growth spurts sometimes lead to clumsiness. The personality continues to develop. School-age children are protective and proud of their parents or caregivers and seek their attention. They value peers, but also need home support.

When examining school-age children, give them the responsibility of providing the history. However, remember that children may be reluctant to provide information if they sustained an injury while doing something forbidden. The parents or caregivers can fill in the pertinent details. When assessing children in this age group, it is important to respect their modesty. Be honest and tell the child what is wrong. A small toy may help to calm the child (Figures 4-3 and 4-4). Common illnesses and injuries for this age group include asthma, drownings, auto collisions, bicycle accidents, falls, fractures, sports injuries, child abuse, and burns.

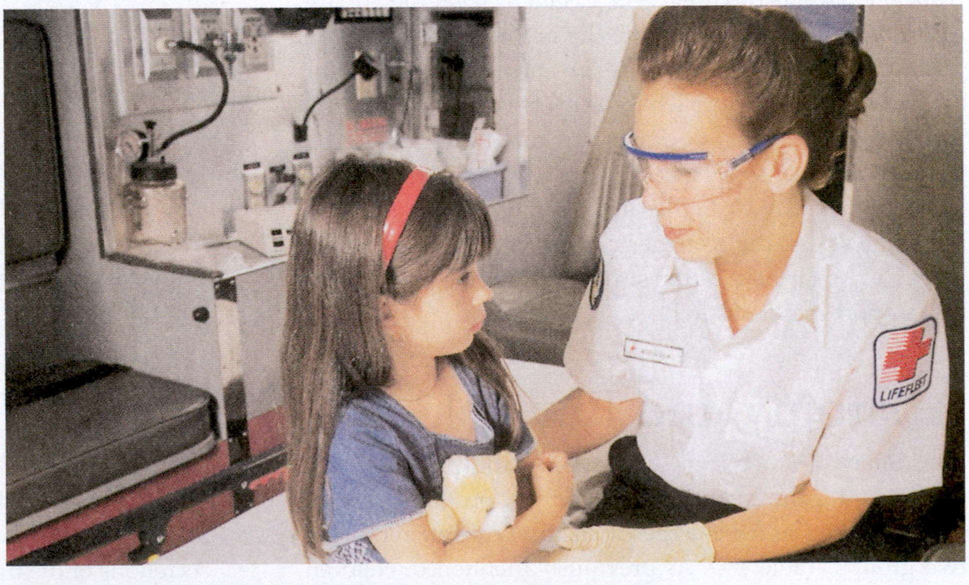

FIGURE 4-4 The approach to the pediatric patient should be gentle and slow.

Adolescents (Ages 13 to 18 Years)

Adolescence covers the period from the end of childhood to the start of adulthood (age 18). It begins with puberty, roughly age 13 for male children and age 11 for female children. (For this reason, adolescence is often defined as including ages 11 to 18, rather than 13 to 18.) Puberty is highly child specific and can begin at various ages. A female child, for example, may experience her first menstrual period as early as age 7 or 8.

Adolescents vary significantly in their development. Those over age 15 are physically nearer to adults in terms of their vital signs, but emotionally they may still be children. Regardless of physical maturity, remember that teenagers as a group are "body conscious." They worry about their physical image more than any other pediatric age group. You should tactfully address their stated concerns about body integrity or disfigurement. The slightest possibility of a lasting scar may be a tremendous issue to the adolescent patient.

Although patients in this age group are not yet legally adults, most consider themselves to be grown up. They take offense at the use of the word "child." They have a strong desire to be liked by their peers and to be included. Relationships with parents and caregivers may, at times, be strained as the adolescent demands greater independence. They value the opinions of other adolescents. Generally, these patients make good historians. Do not be surprised, however, if their perception of events differs from that of their parents or caregivers.

Common illnesses and injuries in this age group include mononucleosis, asthma, auto collisions, sports injuries, drug and alcohol problems, suicide gestures, and sexual abuse. Remember that pregnancy is also possible in female adolescents. When assessing teenagers, remember that their vital signs will approach those of adults. In gathering a history, be factual and address the patient's questions. It may be wise to interview the patient away from the parents or caregivers. Listen to what the adolescent is saying, as well as what he or she is *not* saying. If you suspect substance abuse or endangerment of the patient or others, approach the subject with tact and compassion. If you must perform a detailed physical exam, respect the teenager's sense of privacy. If the patient exhibits modesty or bodily shame, have a paramedic of the same sex as the teenager conduct the examination, if possible. Regardless of the situation, provide psychological support and reassurance.

Anatomy and Physiology

The differences between the anatomy and physiology of infants and children and those of adults form the basis for the differences in the emergency medical care offered to the two groups (Table 4-1). As previously mentioned, children are not simply small adults. They possess bodies well suited to growth. As a rule, they have healthier organs, a greater ability to compensate for most illnesses, and softer, more flexible tissues. Because you will probably have infrequent contact with pediatric patients, you need to regularly review the physical characteristics that distinguish them from the adult patients that you encounter more often (Figure 4-5).

Head

The pediatric patient's head is proportionately larger than an adult's and the occipital region is significantly larger. In comparison to their head size, most pediatric patients have small faces and flat noses, which makes it difficult to obtain a good face–mask seal.

With infants, pay special attention to the fontanelles—areas of the skull that have not yet fused. The fontanelles allow for compression of the head during childbirth and for rapid growth of the brain during early life. The posterior fontanelle generally closes by 4 months of age. The anterior fontanelle diminishes after 6 months of age and usually closes between 9 and 18 months.

During assessment, always inspect the anterior fontanelle. Normally, it should be level with the surface of the skull or slightly sunken. It also may pulsate. With increased intracranial pressure, as with meningitis or head trauma, the fontanelle may become tight and bulging, thus causing the pulsations to diminish or disappear. In the presence of dehydration, the anterior fontanelle often falls below the level of the skull and appears sunken.

The heavy head relative to body size places an infant or child at risk of blunt head trauma. In accidents, the head may be propelled more forcefully than the body, resulting in a higher incidence of brain injury. Head size also affects the airway positioning techniques you should use in treating pediatric patients. In general, follow these guidelines:

- In treating seriously injured patients less than three years of age, place a thin layer of padding under the back to obtain a neutral position. This will prevent the head from tipping forward when supine, causing flexion of the neck (Figure 4-6).
- In treating medically ill children over three years of age, place a folded sheet or towel under the occiput to obtain a sniffing position (neck flexed slightly forward, head extended slightly backward to align the pharynx and trachea).

Airway

In managing the airway of an infant or child, keep in mind these anatomic and physiologic considerations:

- Pediatric patients have narrower airways than adults at all levels, and these are more easily blocked by secretions or obstructions.

Table 4-1 Anatomic and Physiologic Characteristics of Infants and Children

Differences in Infants and Children Compared with Adults	Potential Effects That May Affect Assessment and Care
Tongue proportionately larger	More likely to block airway
Smaller airway structures	More easily blocked
Abundant secretions	Can block the airway
Deciduous (baby) teeth	Easily dislodged; can block the airway
Flat nose and face	Difficult to obtain good face mask seal
Head heavier relative to body and less-developed neck structures and muscles	Head may be propelled more forcefully than body, producing a higher incidence of head injury in trauma
Fontanelle and open sutures (soft spots) palpable on top of young infant's head	Bulging fontanelle can be a sign of increased intracranial pressure (but may be normal if infant is crying); sunken fontanelle may indicate dehydration
Thinner, softer brain tissue	Susceptible to serious brain injury
Head larger in proportion to body	Tips forward when supine; possible flexion of neck, which makes neutral alignment of airway difficult
Shorter, narrower, more elastic (flexible) trachea	Can close off trachea with hyperextension of neck
Short neck	Difficult to stabilize
Abdominal breathers	Difficult to evaluate breathing
Faster respiratory rate	Muscles fatigue easily, causing respiratory distress
Newborns breathe primarily through the nose (obligate nose breathers)	May not automatically open mouth to breathe if nose is blocked; airway more easily blocked
Larger body surface relative to body mass	Prone to hypothermia
Softer bones	More flexible, less easily fractured; traumatic forces may be transmitted to internal organs, causing injury without fracturing the ribs; lungs easily damaged with trauma
Spleen and liver more exposed	Organ injury likely with significant force to abdomen

- Infants are obligate nose breathers. If their noses are blocked by secretions, for example, they may not automatically "know" to open their mouths to breathe.
- The tongue takes up more space proportionately in a child's mouth than in an adult's and can more easily obstruct breathing in an unconscious patient.
- The trachea is softer and more flexible in a child than in an adult and can collapse if the neck and head are hyperextended.
- A child's larynx is higher (C-3–C-4) than an adult's and extends into the pharynx.
- In young children, the cricoid ring is the narrowest part of the airway (below the cords).
- Infants have an omega (horseshoe)-shaped epiglottis that extends at a 45-degree angle into the airway. Because epiglottic folds in pediatric patients have softer cartilage than in adults, they can be more floppy, especially in infants.

Take these anatomic and physiologic differences into account by following these general procedures: Always keep the nares clear in infants less than six months of age. Do not overextend the neck, which may collapse the trachea. Open the airway gently to avoid soft tissue injury. Because any device placed in the infant's or child's airway further narrows the passage's diameter and may result in localized swelling, consider use of an oral or a nasal airway only after other manual maneuvers have failed to keep the airway open. (More information on pediatric airway management is provided later in this chapter.)

Chest and Lungs

In evaluating the chest and lungs of an infant or child, remember that tissues and muscles are more immature than in adults. Chest muscles tire easily, and lung tissues are more fragile. The soft, pliable ribs offer less protection to organs. Expect the ribs to be positioned horizontally and the mediastinum to be more mobile.

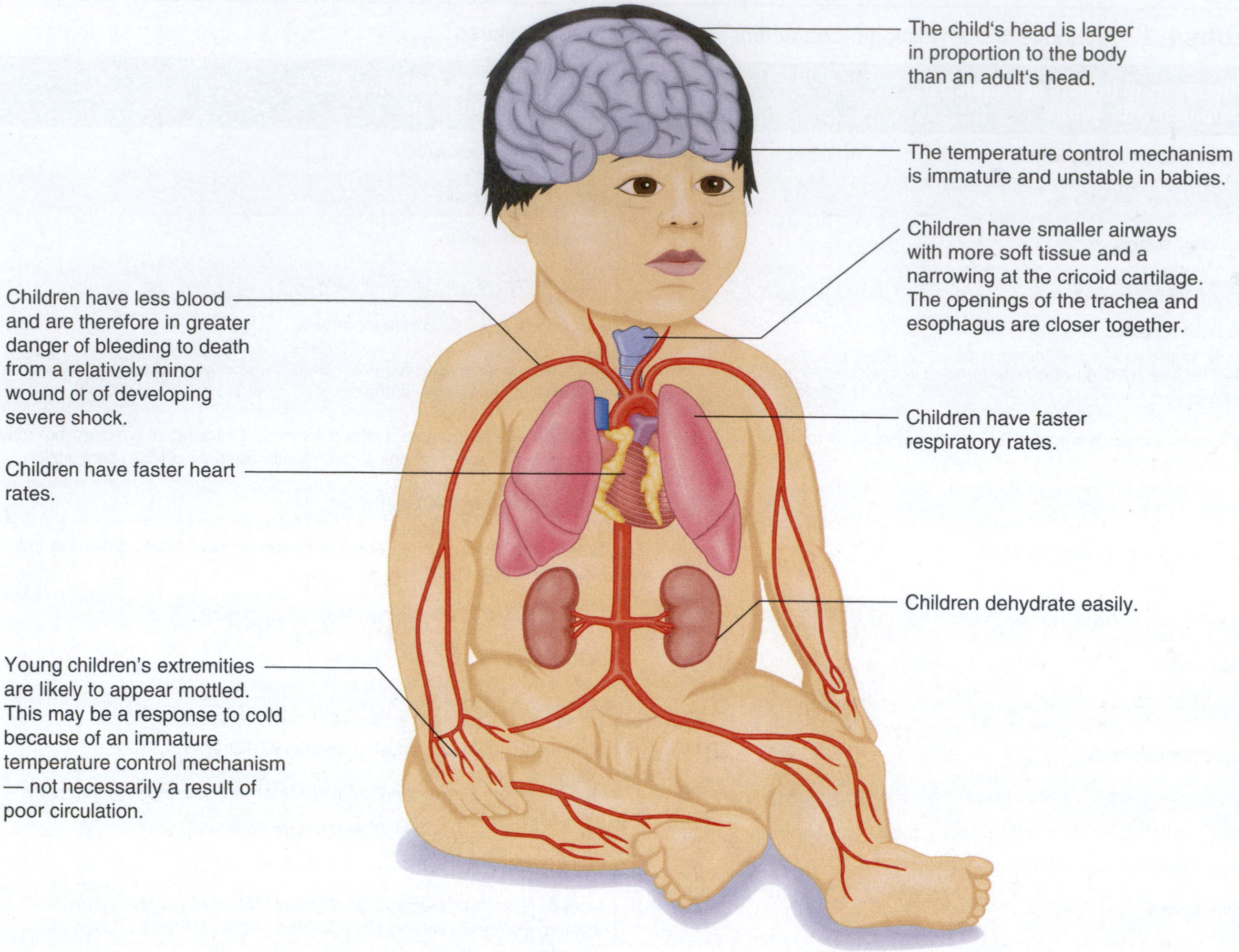

FIGURE 4-5 Anatomic and physiologic considerations in the infant and child.

Take into account the following anatomic and physiologic considerations when assessing the chest and lungs of a pediatric patient:

- Infants and children are diaphragmatic breathers.
- Pediatric patients, especially young infants, are prone to gastric distention.
- Although rib fractures occur less frequently in children, they are not uncommon in cases of child abuse.

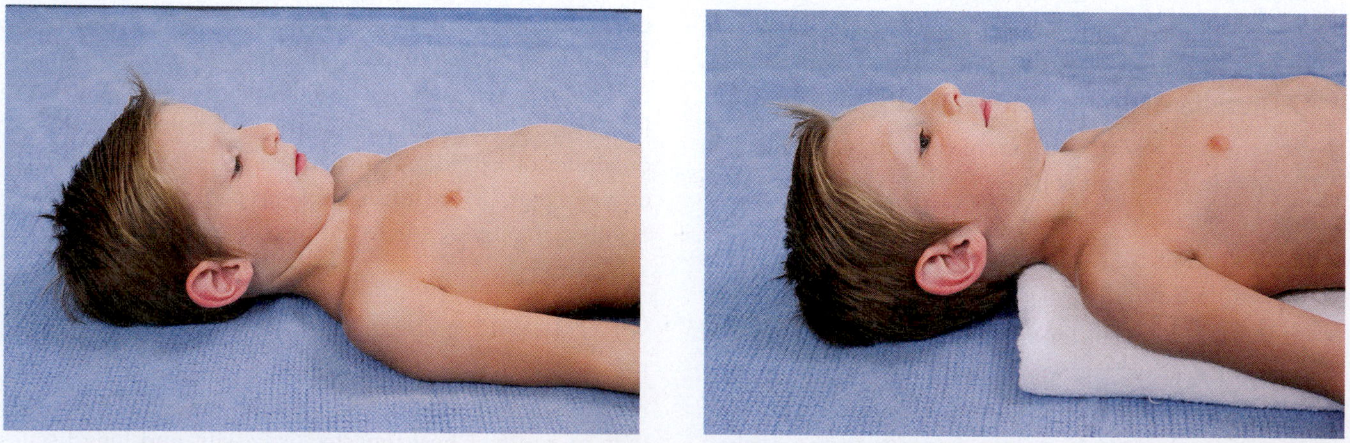

(a) (b)

FIGURE 4-6 (a) In the supine position, an infant's or child's larger head tips forward, causing airway obstruction. (b) Placing padding under the patient's back and shoulders will bring the airway to a neutral or slightly extended position.

- Because of the softness of a child's ribs, greater energy can be transmitted to underlying organs following trauma. As a result, significant internal injury can be present without external signs.
- Pulmonary contusions are more common in pediatric patients who have been subjected to major trauma.
- An infant's or child's lungs are more prone than an adult's to pneumothorax following barotrauma.
- The mediastinum of a child or infant will shift more with tension pneumothorax than in an adult.
- Thin chest walls in infants and children allow for easily transmitted breath sounds. This may result in perception of breath sounds from elsewhere in the chest, which may cause you to miss a pneumothorax or misplaced intubation.

Abdomen

The liver and spleen, both very vascular organs, are proportionately larger in the pediatric patient than in the adult patient. Abdominal organs lie closer together. Because of the immature abdominal muscles in an infant or child, expect to find more frequent damage to the liver and spleen and more multiple organ injuries than in an adult.

Extremities

Until pediatric patients reach adolescence, they have softer and more porous bones than adults. Therefore, you should treat "sprains" and "strains" as fractures and immobilize them accordingly.

During early stages of development, injuries to the **growth plate** may also disrupt bone growth. Keep this in mind when inserting an intraosseous needle, which could mistakenly pierce the plate. (Intraosseous infusion is discussed later in this chapter.)

Skin and Body Surface Area

The pediatric patient's skin and body surface area (BSA) have three distinguishing features. First, the skin of an infant or child is thinner than that of an adult. Second, infants and children generally have less subcutaneous fat. Finally, they have a larger BSA-to-weight ratio.

As a result of these features, children risk greater injury than adults do from extremes in temperature or thermal exposure. They lose fluids and heat more quickly than adults and have a greater likelihood of dehydration and hypothermia. They also burn more easily and deeply than adults, explaining why burns account for one of the leading causes of death among pediatric trauma patients.

Respiratory System

Although infants and children have a tidal volume proportionately similar to that of adolescents and adults, they require double the metabolic oxygen. They also have proportionately smaller oxygen reserves. The combination of increased oxygen requirements and decreased oxygen reserves makes infants and children especially susceptible to hypoxia.

Cardiovascular System

Cardiac output is rate dependent in infants and small children. They possess vigorous, but limited, cardiovascular reserves. Although infants and children have a circulating blood volume proportionately larger than that of adults, their absolute blood volume is smaller. As a result, they can maintain blood pressure longer than adults but still be at risk of shock (hypoperfusion). In assessing a pediatric patient for shock, keep in mind the following points:

- A smaller absolute volume of fluid/blood loss is needed to cause shock in infants and children.
- A larger proportional volume of fluid/blood loss is needed to cause shock in these same patients.
- As with all categories of patients, hypotension is a late sign of shock. In pediatric patients, it is an ominous sign of imminent cardiopulmonary arrest.
- A child may be in shock despite a normal blood pressure.
- Shock assessment in children and infants is based on clinical signs of tissue perfusion. (See the later discussion of circulation assessment.)
- Suspect shock if tachycardia is present.
- Monitor the pediatric patient carefully for the development of hypotension.

Once again, remember that children are not small adults. Bleeding that would not be dangerous in an adult may be a serious and life-threatening condition in an infant or child. Shock can develop in the small child who has a laceration to the scalp (with its many blood vessels) or in the 3-year-old who loses as little as a cup of blood. (Management of shock in pediatric patients is discussed in detail later in the chapter.)

Nervous System

The nervous system develops continually throughout childhood. Even so, the neural tissue remains more fragile than in adults. The skull and spinal column, which are softer and more pliable than in adults, offer less protection of the brain and spinal cord. Therefore, greater force can be transmitted to a child's neural tissue, with more devastating consequences. These injuries can occur without injury to the skull or to the spinal column. (Treatment of head and neck trauma is discussed later in this chapter.)

Metabolic Differences

You may have noticed the repeated emphasis on the need to keep neonatal and pediatric patients warm during treatment and transport. The emphasis on warming techniques is based on the following metabolic considerations:

- Infants and children have a limited store of glycogen and glucose.
- Pediatric patients are prone to hypothermia because of their greater BSA-to-weight ratio.
- Significant volume loss can result from vomiting and diarrhea.
- Newborns and neonates lack the ability to shiver.

To prevent heat loss, always cover the patient's head and maintain adequate temperature controls in the ambulance. Ensure that the ambulance is always stocked with an adequate supply of blankets and, if you live in a cold area, hot-water bottles.

General Approach to Pediatric Assessment

Priorities in the management of the pediatric patient, as with all patients, are established on a threat-to-life basis. If life-threatening problems are not present, you will complete each of the general steps discussed in the following sections.

Basic Considerations

Many of the components of the primary assessment can be done during a visual examination of the scene. (This is sometimes called the "assessment from the doorway," during which you quickly note signs of an ill child, such as lethargy.) Whenever possible, involve the parent or caregiver in efforts to calm or comfort the child. Depending on the situation, you may decide to allow the parent or caregiver to remain with the child during treatment and transport. As mentioned previously, the developmental stage of the patient and the coping skills of the parents or guardians will be key factors in making this decision.

When interacting with parents or other responsible adults, keep in mind the communication techniques suggested earlier. Pay attention to the way in which parents or caregivers interact with the child. Are the interactions appropriate to the emergency? Are family members concerned? Are they angry? Are they overly emotional or entirely indifferent?

From the time of dispatch, you will continually acquire information relative to the patient's condition. As with all patients, personal safety must be your first priority. In treating pediatric patients, follow the same guidelines in approaching the scene as you would with any other patient. Observe for potentially hazardous situations and make sure you take appropriate Standard Precautions. Remember that infants and young children are at especially high risk of an infectious process.

Legal Considerations

When Is a Child No Longer a Child? EMS providers face a difficult question: Legally, when is a child no longer a child? The answer varies from state to state. Children, as a rule, are considered to have reached the age of majority on their eighteenth birthday. At this point, the law allows them to make decisions for themselves, sign contracts, join the military, and provide consent for medical care. In addition, a married person—even if younger than 18 years of age—generally is considered to be able to provide consent, especially for any children he or she might have.

Some children under the age of 18 live independent of their parents. Although the laws pertaining to this vary somewhat, the true emancipated minor is one who has appealed to a court to be declared emancipated and granted the ability to make decisions for himself, including providing consent for medical care. Again, the laws vary from state to state. *Know the laws of the state or states where you work.*

When confronted with a minor seeking medical care, you must contact the parents, if possible, and obtain consent. The refusal of care by a minor is a particular problem. If the parents cannot be contacted, it is usually safest to transport the minor and have the emergency department staff or law enforcement try to locate the parents and obtain consent for treatment or a refusal-of-care declaration. Similarly, when confronted by a minor who claims to be emancipated but who cannot provide the documentation, it might be better to err on the side of transport. In any of these situations, involve your supervisor and law enforcement in the decision-making process.

Scene Size-Up

On arrival, conduct a quick scene size-up. Dispatch information received en route, as well as your own observations, can provide critical indicators of scene safety. Be aware of the increased anxiety and stress in any situation involving an infant or child. Try to set aside thoughts of your own children and adopt the professional, systematic approach to assessment necessary for scene safety and effective patient management. If you find yourself getting angry or upset, temporarily turn over care to another paramedic until you compose yourself.

As you survey the scene, look for clues to the mechanism of injury (MOI) or the nature of illness (NOI). These clues will help guide your assessment and determine appropriate interventions. Note the presence of dangerous substances (e.g., medicine bottles, household chemicals, or poisonous plants) that the child may have ingested. Spot environmental hazards such as unprotected stairwells, kerosene heaters, and so on. Identify possible causes of trauma, especially in motor vehicle collisions. Remain alert for evidence of child abuse, particularly in cases in which the injury and history do not coincide. As already mentioned, pay attention to the way parents or caregivers respond to the child and the way the child responds to them.

Keep the child in mind while conducting your scene size-up. Pace your approach to give the child time to adjust to your presence. Speak in a soft voice, using simple words. As soon as you reach the child, position yourself at eye level with the patient and make every effort to win his trust. If the child bonds more readily with one member of the team than another, allow that person to remain with the child and, if possible, allow him to conduct most of the secondary assessment.

Primary Assessment

The patient's condition determines the course of your primary assessment. An active and alert child will allow for a more comfortable approach, with more time spent on communication with the child and appropriate adults. A critically ill or injured child, however, may require quick intervention and rapid transport. Your choice of action depends on your general impression of the patient. (For a summary of the primary assessment of a pediatric patient, see Figure 4-7.)

General Impression

The major points in forming your general impression are outlined in an assessment tool called the *pediatric assessment triangle* (PAT, included in Figure 5-7). Many experts recommend this assessment tool as a way of quickly evaluating the level of severity and the need for immediate intervention.[5,6] It is a rapid "eyes-open, hands-on" approach that allows you to detect a life-threatening situation without the use of a stethoscope, blood pressure cuff, pulse oximeter, or other medical device. The triangle's three components are:

- ***Appearance***—focuses on the child's mental status and muscle tone
- ***Breathing***—directs attention to respiratory rate and respiratory effort
- ***Circulation***—uses skin signs and color as well as capillary refill as indicators of the patient's circulatory status

CONTENT REVIEW

➤ Pediatric Assessment Triangle
- Appearance
- Breathing
- Circulation

Vital Functions

After quickly applying the pediatric assessment triangle to form a general impression, you will evaluate vital functions—mental status (level of consciousness) and the ABCs—as they apply to infants and children. Although assessment steps are basically the same as for adults, certain modifications must be made to collect accurate data.

LEVEL OF CONSCIOUSNESS Employ the AVPU method (*A*lert, responds to *V*erbal stimuli, responds to *P*ainful stimuli, *U*nresponsive) to evaluate the pediatric patient's level of consciousness. Adjust the techniques for the child's age. With an infant, you may need to shout to elicit a response (perhaps crying) to verbal stimulus. An infant should withdraw from a noxious stimulus. *Never shake an infant or child.*

AIRWAY Assess the airway using the techniques shown in Figures 4-8 through 4-11. If at any point the patient shows little or no movement of air, intervene immediately. Keep this fact in mind: *Airway and respiratory problems are the most common cause of cardiac arrest in infants and young children.*

As you inspect the airway, ask yourself the following questions:

- Is the airway patent?
- Is the airway maintainable with head positioning, suctioning, or airway adjuncts?
- Is the airway *not* maintainable? If so, what action is required? (Airway management techniques are discussed later in this chapter.)

BREATHING In assessing the breathing of a pediatric patient, recall the CPR certification courses in which you learned to "look, listen, and feel." *Look* at the patient's chest and abdomen for movement. *Listen* for breath sounds—both normal and abnormal. *Feel* for air movement at the patient's mouth.

Keep in mind that pediatric patients have small chests. For this reason, place the stethoscope near each of the armpits to minimize transmitted breath sounds. When considering the respiratory rate, remember that pain or fear can increase a child's respiratory efforts. Tachypnea, an abnormally rapid rate of breathing, may indicate fear, pain, inadequate oxygenation, or, in the case of neonates, exposure to cold.

If you suspect trauma, check the infant or child for life-threatening chest injuries. Keep in mind that even a minor injury to the chest can interfere with a child's breathing efforts. A chest injury can also interfere with your effort to provide adequate oxygenation or ventilation.

Your goal is to identify any evidence of compromised breathing (Figure 4-12). Evaluation of breathing includes assessment of the following conditions:

- ***Respiratory rate.*** Tachypnea is often the first manifestation of respiratory distress in infants. Regardless of the cause, an infant breathing at a rapid rate will eventually

PEDIATRIC ASSESSMENT TRIANGLE

Initial Assessment

The basics of pediatric assessment are auditory and visual clues obtained from "across the room" without threatening an anxious child.

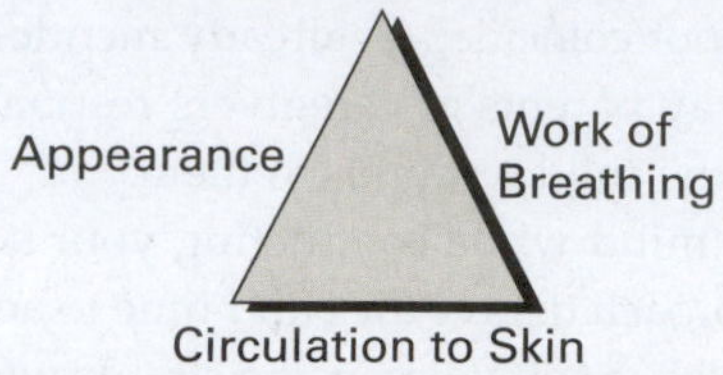

Appearance (Mental Status)

"The Tickles" (TICLS) can serve as the "AV" part of the AVPU assessment.

- Tone
- Interactiveness
- Consolability
- Look/gaze
- Speech/cry

Up close: the "PU" part of AVPU.

- Response to pain
- Unresponsiveness

Work of Breathing

PAT across-the-room observations:

- Abnormal airway/breathing sounds (hoarseness, muffled speech, grunting, wheezing, stridor, crowing)
- Abnormal body positioning (sniffing position, tripoding, refusing to lie down)
- Retractions, nasal flaring, "see-saw" breathing, head bobbing in infants

Up close after PAT observations:

- Listen with a stethoscope to both sides of the chest

Circulation to Skin

PAT across-the-room observations:

- Pallor
- Mottling
- Cyanosis

Up close after PAT observations:

- Feel for brachial, femoral, and peripheral pulses
- Check capillary refill in children 5 years or younger
- Assess blood pressure in children older than 3 years

History and Physical Exam

Common Medical Problems

- Airway obstruction
- Respiratory emergencies
- Seizures
- Altered mental status
- Fever
- Poisonings
- Shock
- Near drowning
- Sudden infant death syndrome (SIDS)

Common Trauma Situations

- Seat belt injuries
- Bicycle-related injuries
- Car vs. pedestrian injuries
- Head and neck injuries
- Burns
- Abuse and neglect

FIGURE 4-7 The basic steps in pediatric assessment.

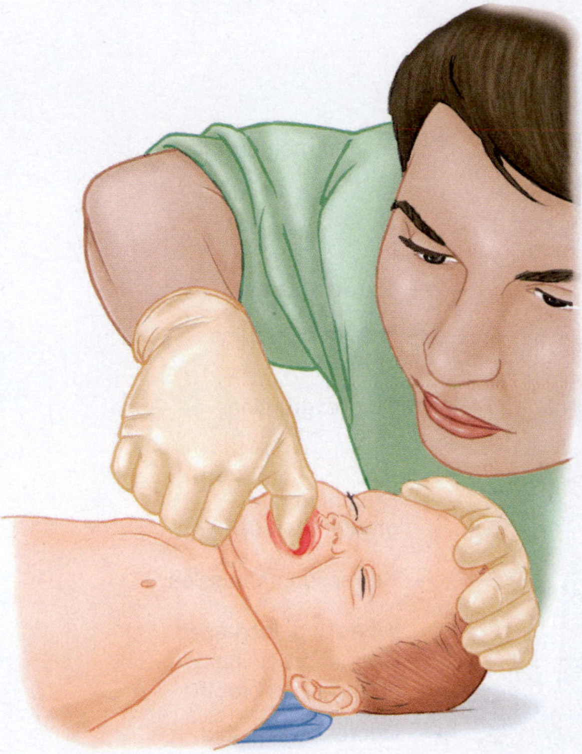

FIGURE 4-8 Opening the airway in a child.

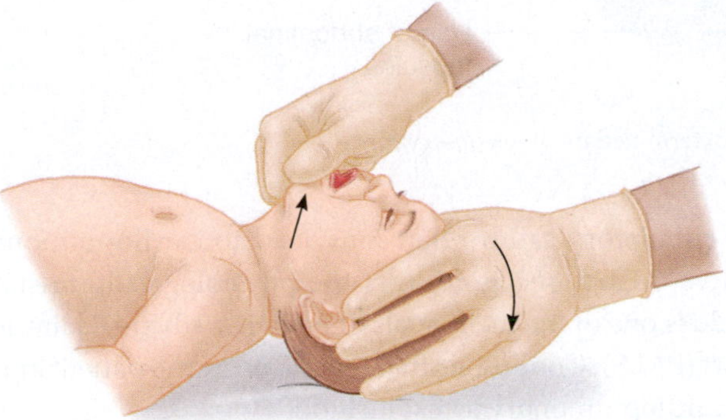

FIGURE 4-9 Head-tilt/chin-lift method.

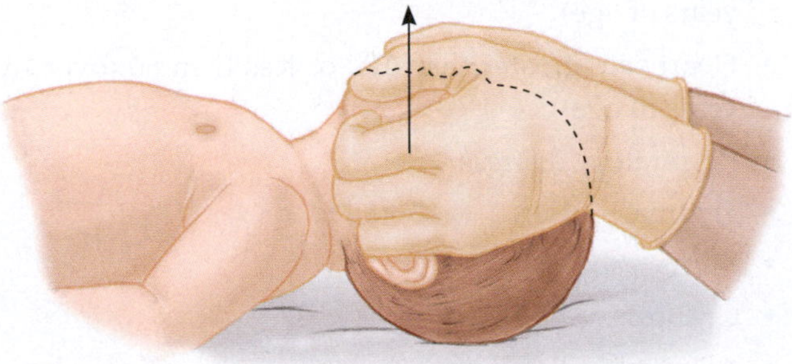

FIGURE 4-10 Jaw-thrust method.

tire. Keep in mind that a decreasing respiratory rate may be a result of tiring and is not necessarily a sign of improvement. A slow respiratory rate in an acutely ill infant or child is an ominous sign. (Normal respiratory

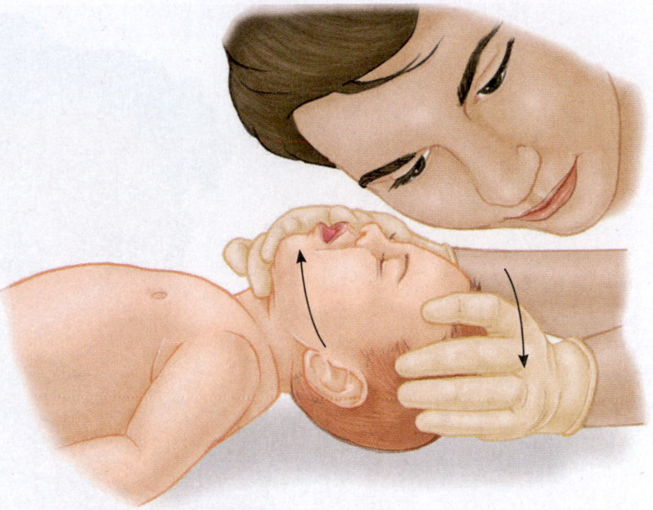

FIGURE 4-11 Assessing breathing.

rates are listed in Table 4-2.) In short, be alert for a respiratory rate that is *either* abnormally fast *or* abnormally slow.

- ***Respiratory effort.*** The quality of air entry can be assessed by observing for chest rise, breath sounds, stridor, or wheezing. An increased respiratory effort in the infant or child is also evidenced by nasal flaring and the use of accessory respiratory muscles. (Signs of respiratory effort are listed in Table 4-3.)
- ***Color.*** Cyanosis is a fairly late sign of respiratory failure and is most frequently seen in the mucous membranes of the mouth and the nail beds. Cyanosis of the extremities alone is more likely due to circulatory failure (shock) than to respiratory failure.

CIRCULATION As mentioned earlier, you should assess a pediatric patient's circulation by first checking the child's color. Keep in mind that the pediatric patient tends to become hypothermic; therefore, you should check the capillary refill time in an area of central circulation, such as the sternum or forehead. (Capillary refill time, as discussed later in this chapter, is considered reliable as a sign of perfusion, primarily in children less than six years of age.) In general, evaluate the following conditions when assessing circulation during the primary assessment:

- ***Heart rate.*** As previously mentioned, infants develop sinus tachycardia in response to stress. Thus, any tachycardia in an infant or child requires further evaluation to determine the cause. Bradycardia in a distressed infant or child may indicate hypoxia and is an ominous sign of impending cardiac arrest. (Normal heart rates are listed in Table 4-2.)
- ***Peripheral circulation.*** The presence of peripheral pulses is a good indicator of the adequacy of end-organ perfusion. Loss of central pulses is an ominous sign.

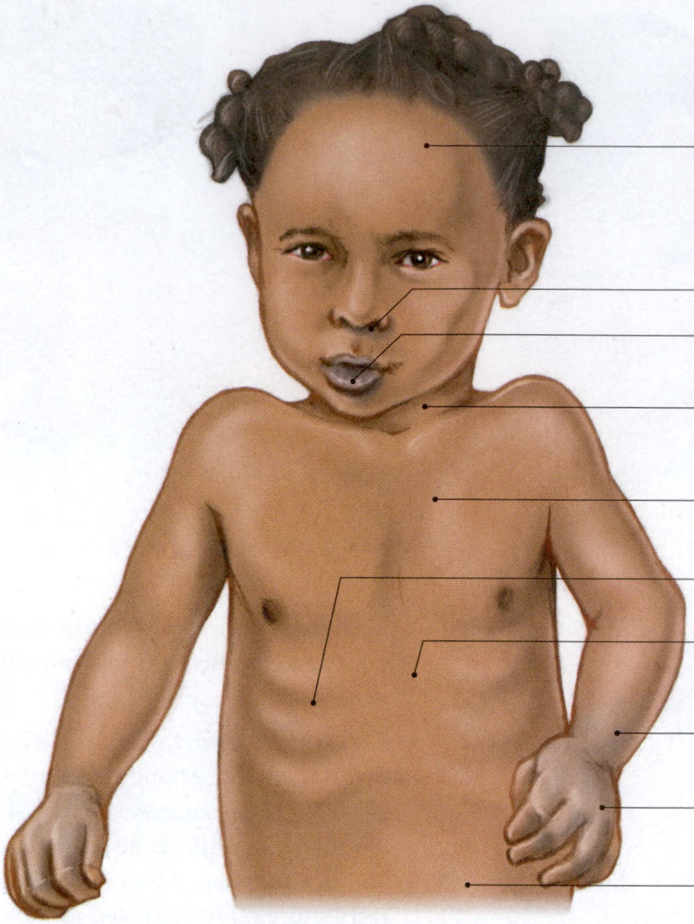

FIGURE 4-12 Signs of respiratory distress. Notice the conditions that can be determined by quick observation.

- ***End-organ perfusion.*** End-organ perfusion is most evident in the skin, kidneys, and brain. Decreased perfusion of the skin is an early sign of shock. A capillary refill time of greater than 2 seconds is indicative of low cardiac output. Impairment of brain perfusion is usually evidenced by a change in mental status. The child may become confused or lethargic. Seizures may occur. Failure of the child to recognize the parents' faces is often an ominous sign. Urine output directly relates to kidney perfusion. Normal urine output is 1 to 2 mL/kg/hr. Urine flow of less than 1 mL/kg/hr is an indicator of poor renal perfusion.

Remember that evaluation of mental status and ABCs during the primary assessment is rapid and not detailed because it is aimed at discovering and correcting immediate life threats. More thorough measurements will be performed during the secondary assessment.

Anticipating Cardiopulmonary Arrest

Your primary assessment and the repeated assessments that follow help you to recognize and prevent cardiopulmonary arrest. At each stage of evaluating vital functions, ask yourself this question: "Does this child have pulmonary or circulatory failure that may lead to cardiopulmonary arrest?" Early recognition of the physiologically unstable child is one of the main goals of pediatric advanced life support (PALS). Conditions that place a pediatric patient at risk of cardiopulmonary arrest include:

- Respiratory rate greater than 60
- Heart rate greater than 180 or less than 80 (under five years of age)
- Heart rate greater than 180 or less than 60 (over five years of age)
- Respiratory distress
- Trauma
- Burns
- Cyanosis
- Altered level of consciousness
- Seizures
- Fever with petechiae (small purple spots resulting from skin hemorrhages)

Evaluate the patient for these conditions throughout assessment and transport. Cardiopulmonary arrest in infants and children is usually not a sudden event. Instead,

Table 4-2 Normal Vital Signs: Infants and Children*

Normal Pulse Rates (Beats per Minute, at Rest)		
Newborn (0–1 month)	100–180	
Infant (1–12 months)	100–160	
Toddler (1–3 years)	80–110	
Preschooler (3–5 years)	70–110	
School age (6–10 years)	65–110	
Early adolescence (11–14 years)	60–90	
Normal Respiratory Rates (Breaths per Minute, at Rest)		
Newborn (0–1 month)	30–60	
Infant (1–12 months)	30–60	
Toddler (1–3 years)	24–40	
Preschooler (3–5 years)	22–34	
School age (6–10 years)	18–30	
Early adolescence (11–14 years)	12–26	
Normal Blood Pressure Ranges (mmHg, at Rest)		
	Systolic Approx. 90 + 2 × Age	**Diastolic Approx. 2/3 Systolic**
Preschooler (3–5 years)	Average 98 (78–116)	Average 65
School age (6–10 years)	Average 105 (80–122)	Average 69
Early adolescence (11–14 years)	Average 114 (88–140)	Average 76

*Adolescents ages 15 to 18 approach the vital signs of adults.

Note: A high pulse in an infant or child is not as great a concern as a low pulse. A low pulse may indicate imminent cardiac arrest. Blood pressure is usually not taken in a child under three years of age. In cases of blood loss or shock, a child's blood pressure will remain within normal limits until near the end, then fall swiftly.

it is the end result of progressive deterioration in respiratory and cardiac function. Therefore, you need to determine whether the patient's condition is deteriorating or improving. Any decompensation or change in the patient's status will prompt you to perform basic or advanced life support measures, as detailed in American Heart Association guidelines and system protocols.

Transport Priority

Based on your primary assessment, you will assign the patient one of the following transport priorities:

- *Urgent.* Proceed with the rapid secondary assessment, if trauma is suspected, then transport immediately with further assessment and treatment performed en route.

Table 4-3 Signs of Increased Respiratory Effort

Retraction	Visible sinking of the skin and soft tissues of the chest around and below the ribs and above the collarbone
Nasal flaring	Widening of the nostrils; seen primarily on inspiration
Head bobbing	Observed when the head lifts and tilts back as the child inhales and then moves forward as the child exhales
Grunting	Sound heard when an infant attempts to keep the alveoli open by building back pressure during expiration
Wheezing	Passage of air over mucus secretions or airway constrictions in the bronchi; heard more commonly on expiration; a low- or high-pitched sound
Gurgling	Coarse, abnormal bubbling sound heard in the airway during inspiration or expiration; may indicate an open chest wound or a foreign body in the airway
Stridor	Abnormal, musical, high-pitched sound, more commonly heard on inspiration

- *Nonurgent.* Complete the secondary assessment at the scene, then transport.

To help determine transport priority, some EMS systems use a trauma score that is modified for pediatric patients, which includes the elements of the Glasgow Coma Scale, also modified for pediatric patients (Table 4-4). These scores can help predict patient outcome and help in the decision on whether rapid transport to a trauma center is required. If used in your EMS system, your medical director and/or system protocols will determine what numerical score mandates rapid transport.

Transitional Phase

The way in which the pediatric patient is transferred to EMS care depends entirely on the seriousness of the patient's condition. A transitional phase is intended for the conscious, non-acutely ill child. This phase of assessment allows the infant or child to become familiar with you and the equipment that you will be using. When dealing with the unconscious or acutely ill patient, however, you will skip this phase and proceed directly to the treatment and transport phases of assessment. In essence, you assign the patient an "urgent" status.

Secondary Assessment

After you have prioritized patient care at the end of the primary assessment, you will perform the secondary assessment, including a history and a physical exam. If the patient has a medical illness, the history will precede the physical exam. If the patient is suffering from trauma, the physical exam will take precedence. If partners are working together, the history and physical exam may be performed simultaneously. (For a summary of conditions that may be found during the focused history and physical exam, review Figure 4-7.)

Table 4-4 Pediatric Trauma Score and Glasgow Coma Scale Score

Pediatric Trauma Score			
Score	**+2**	**+1**	**–1**
Weight	>44 lb (>20 kg)	22–44 lb (10–20 kg)	>22 lb (<10 kg)
Airway	Normal	Oral or nasal airway	Intubated, tracheostomy, invasive airway
Blood Pressure	Pulse at wrist >.90 mmHg	Carotid or femoral pulse palpable, 50–90 mmHg	No palpable pulse or >50 mmHg
Level of Consciousness	Completely awake	Obtunded or any loss of consciousness	Comatose
Open Wound	None	Minor	Major or penetrating
Fractures	None	Closed fracture	Open or multiple fractures

Pediatric Glasgow Coma Scale				
		>1 Year	**<1 Year**	
Eye Opening	4	Spontaneous	Spontaneous	
	3	To verbal command	To shout	
	2	To pain	To pain	
	1	No response	No response	
		>1 Year	**<1 Year**	
Best Motor Response	6	Obeys		
	5	Localizes pain	Localizes pain	
	4	Flexion-withdrawal	Flexion-withdrawal	
	3	Flexion-abnormal (decorticate rigidity)	Flexion-abnormal (decorticate rigidity)	
	2	Extension (decerebrate rigidity)	Extension (decerebrate rigidity)	
	1	No response	No response	
		>5 Years	**2–5 Years**	**0–23 Months**
Best Verbal Response	5	Oriented and converses	Appropriate words and phrases	Smiles, coos, cries appropriately
	4	Disoriented and converses	Inappropriate words	Cries
	3	Inappropriate words	Cries and/or screams	Inappropriate crying and/or screaming
	2	Incomprehensible sounds	Grunts	Grunts
	1	No response	No response	No response

History

Whenever a patient is identified as a priority patient, the focused history will occur en route to the hospital, after essential treatments or interventions for life-threatening conditions have been performed.

To obtain a history for a pediatric patient, you will probably need to involve a family member or caregiver. Remember, however, that school-age children and adolescents like to take part in their own care. As previously mentioned, you can elicit valuable information from even very young patients. As a general precaution, question older adolescent patients in private, especially about issues such as sexual activity, pregnancy, or illicit drug and alcohol use. If you question adolescents about these subjects in the presence of an adult, they will probably be more reticent for fear of later repercussions.

As with any patient, you will use the history to uncover additional pertinent injuries or medical conditions. The history should center on the chief complaint and past medical history.

To evaluate the nature of the chief complaint, determine each of the following:

- Nature of the illness/injury
- Length of time the patient has been sick/injured
- Presence of fever
- Effects of the illness/injury on patient behavior
- Bowel/urine habits
- Presence of vomiting/diarrhea
- Frequency of urination

The past medical history identifies chronic illnesses, use of medications, and allergies. Be sure to inquire whether the infant or child is currently under a doctor's care. If so, obtain the name of the physician and present it at the receiving hospital. In the case of trauma patients, reconsider the mechanism of injury and the results of your on-scene physical examination (which, as noted earlier, will precede the history in the case of trauma).

Physical Exam

FOCUSED EXAM Carry out the physical exam after all life-threatening conditions have been identified and addressed. If there is a significant mechanism of injury or if the patient is unresponsive, perform a complete rapid trauma assessment or rapid medical assessment. Use the toe-to-head approach with the younger child (or begin with the chest and examine the head last) and the head-to-toe approach in the older child. If the injury is minor or if the ill patient is responsive, perform a physical exam that is focused on the affected areas and systems.

Perform the physical exam as described in the chapter "Secondary Assessment." Depending on the particular situation, some or all of the following assessment techniques may be appropriate to include in the exam:

- ***Pupils.*** Inspect the patient's pupils for equality and reaction to light.
- ***Capillary refill.*** As noted earlier, this technique is valuable for pediatric patients less than six years of age. Blanch the nail bed, base of the thumb, or sole of one of the feet. Remember that normal capillary refill is 2 seconds or less. Recall that this technique is less reliable in cold environments.
- ***Hydration.*** Note skin turgor, presence of tears and saliva, and, with infants, the condition of the fontanelles.
- ***Pulse oximetry.*** Use this electronic device on injured or ill infants and children. Readings will give you immediate information regarding peripheral oxygen saturation and allow you to follow trends in the patient's pulse rate and oxygenation status. Keep in mind, however, that hypothermia or shock can affect readings.

CONTENT REVIEW

➤ Elements of the Glasgow Coma Scale
- Verbal responses
- Motor functions
- Eye movements

GLASGOW COMA SCALE In cases of trauma, you may need to apply the Glasgow Coma Scale (GCS), a scoring system for monitoring the neurologic status of patients with possible head injuries. The GCS assigns scores based on verbal responses, motor functions, and eye movements.

In using the GCS with pediatric patients, you will have to make certain modifications; the younger the patient, the more adjustments you will need to make. Verbal responses, for example, will not be possible for neonates and infants. However, motor function may be assessed in very young children by observing voluntary movement. Infants under four months of age should have a grasp reflex when an object is placed on the palmar surface of the hand. The grasp should be immediate. Children over three years of age will follow directions, when encouraged. Sensory function can be observed by the withdrawal reaction from "tickling" the patient. (Review Table 4-4 for a modified GCS for pediatric patients.)

After you score the GCS for the patient, prioritize the patient according to severity. Guidelines are:

- ***Mild***—GCS 13 to 15
- ***Moderate***—GCS 9 to 12
- ***Severe***—GCS less than or equal to 8

VITAL SIGNS Remember that poorly taken vital signs are of less value than no vital signs at all. The following guidelines will help you obtain accurate pediatric readings. (Review Table 5–2 for normal pediatric vital signs.)

- Take vital signs with the patient in as close to a resting state as possible. If necessary, allow the child to calm down before attempting vital signs. Vital signs in the field should include pulse, respiration, blood pressure, and temperature.
- Obtain blood pressure with an appropriate-sized cuff. The cuff should be two-thirds the width of the upper arm. The pulse pressure (the difference between the systolic and diastolic blood pressure) narrows as shock develops. *Note that hypotension is a late and often sudden sign of cardiovascular decompensation.* Even mild hypotension should be taken seriously and treated quickly and vigorously, because cardiopulmonary arrest is probably imminent.
- Feel for peripheral, brachial, or femoral pulses (Figures 4-13a and b). There is often a significant variation in pulse rate in children, owing to varied respirations. Therefore, it is important to monitor

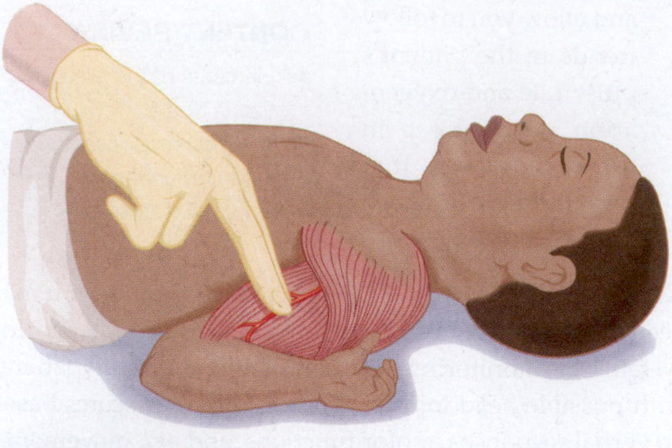

FIGURE 4-13a Taking the brachial pulse.

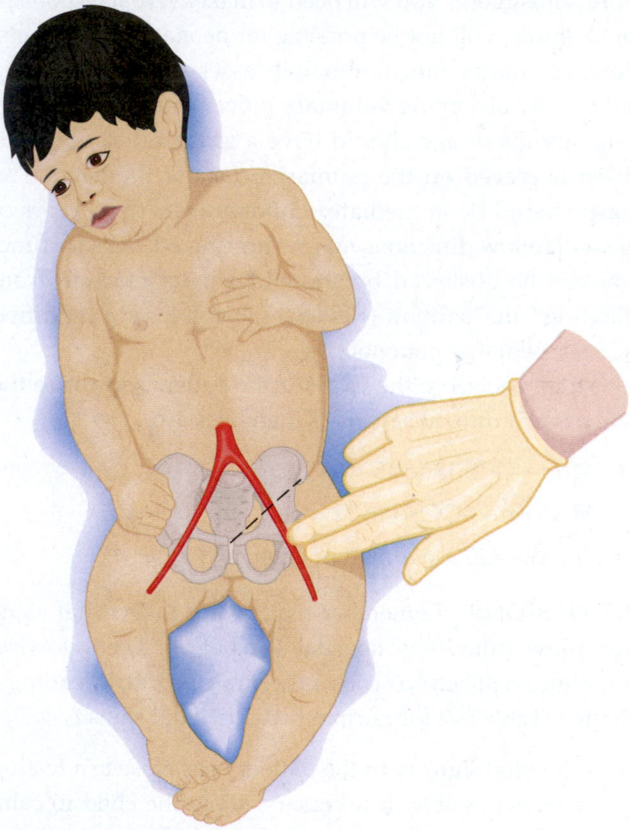

FIGURE 4-13b Taking the femoral pulse.

the pulse for at least 30 seconds, with one full minute being preferable.

- It is generally not possible to weigh the child. However, if medications are required, make a good estimate of the child's weight. Often the parents or caregivers can provide a fairly reliable weight from a recent visit to the doctor. Table 4-5 lists the average weights by age for pediatric patients. (Remember, these are only averages.)
- Observe the child's respiratory rate before beginning the examination. After the examination is started, the child will often begin to cry. It will then be impossible to determine the respiratory rate. For an estimate of

Table 4-5 Pediatric Weights and Pound–Kilogram Conversion

Age	Weight (lb)	Weight (kg)
Birth	7	3.5
3 Months	10	5
6 Months	15	7
9 Months	18	8
1 Year	22	10
2 Years	26	12
3 Years	33	15
4 Years	37	17
5 Years	40	18
6 Years	44	20
7 Years	50	23
8 Years	56	25
9 Years	60	28
10 Years	70	33
11 Years	75	35
12 Years	85	40
13 Years	98	44

the upper limit of respiratory rate, subtract the child's age from 40. It is also important to identify the respiratory pattern, as well as retractions, nasal flaring, or paradoxical chest movement.

- Measure temperature early in the patient encounter and repeat toward the end. IV fluid and exposure to the environment can cause a drop in core temperature.
- Continue to observe the child for level of consciousness. The level of consciousness and activity during treatment may vary widely.

NONINVASIVE MONITORING Modern noninvasive monitoring devices all have their applications in pediatric emergency care (Figure 4-14). These may include the pulse oximeter, capnography, automated blood pressure devices, self-registering thermometers, and ECGs.

To promote the goal of early recognition of cardiopulmonary arrest, every seriously ill or injured child should receive continuous pulse oximetry. This will provide you with essential information regarding the patient's heart rate and peripheral O_2 saturation. It will also help you monitor the effects of any medications administered. Hyperoxia can be harmful. Thus, pulse oximetry can be used to guide supplemental oxygen therapy. The goal is to maintain a SpO_2 of 95 percent or greater.

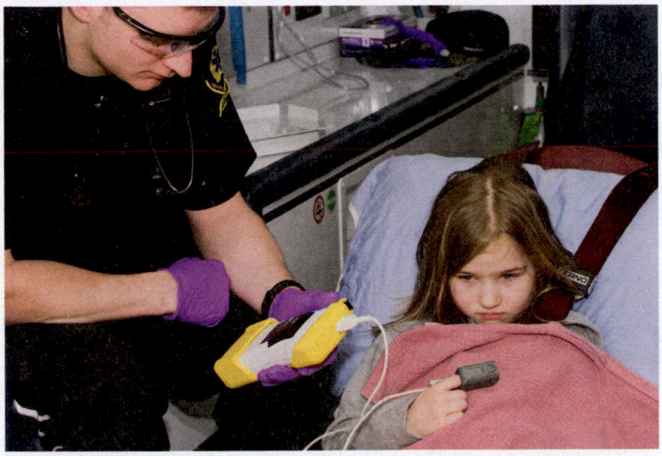

FIGURE 4-14 If available, noninvasive monitoring, including pulse oximetry and temperature measurement, should be used in prehospital pediatric care.

Capnography, also called end-tidal carbon dioxide monitoring ($EtCO_2$), is useful in pediatrics (Figure 4-15). It provides essential information about ventilation and can also provide diagnostic information. If the $EtCO_2$ is consistently greater than 10 to 15 mmHg, focus efforts on improving ventilation and ensuring that the patient does not receive excessive ventilation (hyperventilation).[7,8]

An ECG and automated blood pressure/pulse monitor should also be considered. However, these devices may frighten the child. Before applying any monitoring device, explain what you are going to do. Demonstrate the display or lights. If the monitoring device makes noise, allow the child to hear the noise before you apply it. Reassure the child that the device will not hurt him.

Reassessment

Because a pediatric patient's condition can rapidly change for the better or the worse, it is necessary to repeat relevant portions of the assessment. You should continually monitor the patient's respiratory effort, skin color, mental status, temperature, and pulse oximetry. Retake vital signs and compare them with baseline vitals. In general, reassess stable patients every 15 minutes and critical patients every 5 minutes.

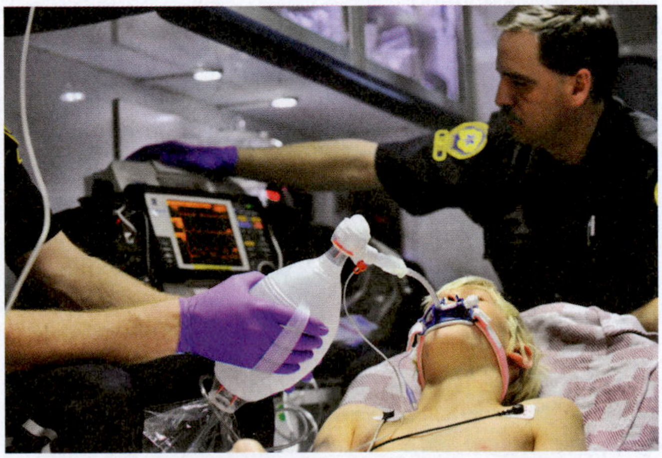

FIGURE 4-15 Capnography is an effective tool for evaluation and monitoring of pediatric patients.

General Management of Pediatric Patients

The same ABCs that guide the management of adult patients apply to pediatric patients: Your top priorities in treating an infant or child are airway, breathing, and circulation. However, because of the special anatomic and physiologic considerations that influence the management of pediatric patients, you need to practice these skills on an ongoing and regular basis.

Basic Airway Management

In treating the pediatric patient, basic life support (BLS) should be applied according to current standards and protocols. BLS should include maintenance of the airway, artificial ventilation, and, if required, chest compressions (Table 4-6). As with all patients, your priority is to ensure an open airway. The following modifications of BLS airway skills will ensure that you take into account the clinical implications of the pediatric airway.

Manual Positioning

Allow the pediatric patient to assume a position of comfort, if possible. When placing the patient in a supine position, avoid hyperextension of the neck. As previously mentioned, infants and small children risk collapsed tracheas from hyperextension of the neck. For trauma patients less than three years old, place support under the upper torso or shoulders. For supine medical patients three years old and older, provide occipital elevation.

Foreign Body Airway Obstruction

Before administering treatment, determine whether an airway obstruction is mild or severe. Infants or children with a mild airway obstruction will have a cough, hoarse voice or cry, stridor, or some other evidence that at least some air is passing through the airway. Avoid any maneuvers that will turn a mild obstruction into a severe obstruction. Instead, place the patient in a position of comfort and transport immediately.

In the case of severe airway obstruction, take one of the following age-specific maneuvers:

- ***Children.*** For children older than one year of age, perform a series of abdominal thrusts until the item is expelled or the victim becomes unresponsive (Figure 4-16). If the victim becomes unresponsive, start CPR.

Table 4-6 Summary of BLS Maneuvers in Infants and Children

Target of Maneuver	Infant (<1 Year)	Child (1 Year–Puberty)
Airway		
Open airway	Head-tilt/chin-lift (unless trauma present) Jaw thrust	Head-tilt/chin-lift (unless trauma present) Jaw thrust
Clear foreign body obstruction	Back blows/chest thrusts	Abdominal thrusts
Breathing		
Initial	2 breaths that make the chest rise	2 breaths that make the chest rise
Subsequent	1 breath every 3 seconds (12–20/minute)	1 breath every 3 seconds (12–20/minute)
Circulation		
Pulse check	Brachial/femoral	Carotid
Compression area	Lower third of sternum	Lower third of sternum
Compression width	2 or 3 fingers	Heel of one hand
Depth	Approximately ⅓ to ½ AP diameter of chest	Approximately ⅓ to ½ AP diameter of chest
Rate	At least 100/minute	100/minute
Compression-to-ventilation ratio	30:2 (1 rescuer); 15:2 (2 rescuers)	30:2 (1 rescuer); 15:2 (2 rescuers)

- ***Infants.*** For an infant, deliver a series of five back blows followed by five chest thrusts (abdominal thrusts are not recommended for infants). Inspect the infant's mouth on completion of each series (Procedure 4-1). If the infant becomes unresponsive, begin CPR.

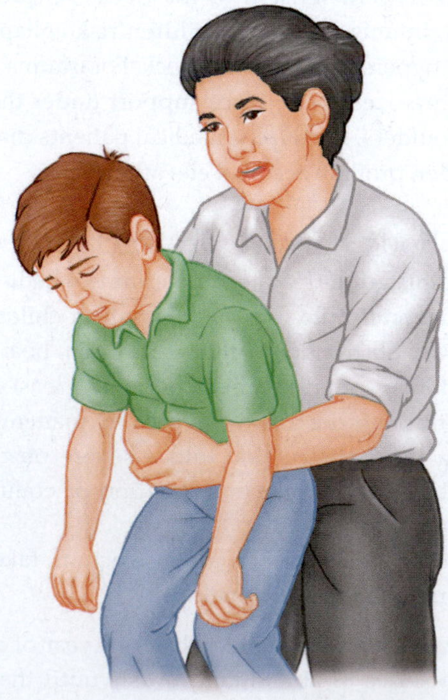

FIGURE 4-16 Delivering abdominal thrusts to a child.

As you recall from your basic CPR courses, never check a pediatric patient's mouth with blind finger sweeps.

Suctioning

Apply suctioning whenever you detect heavy secretions in the nose or mouth of a pediatric patient, especially if the patient has a diminished level of consciousness. You can use a bulb syringe, flexible suction catheter, or rigid-tip suction catheter, depending on the patient's age or size (Figure 4-17). Make sure that flexible catheters are correctly sized (Table 4-7).

Although pediatric suctioning techniques vary very little from adult suctioning techniques, keep the following modifications in mind:

- Decrease suction pressure to less than 100 mmHg in infants.
- Avoid excessive suctioning time (suction less than 10 seconds), to decrease the possibility of hypoxia.
- Avoid stimulation of the vagus nerve, which may produce bradycardia. As a general rule, suction no deeper than you can see and for no more than 10 seconds per attempt.
- Frequently check the patient's pulse. If bradycardia occurs, stop suctioning immediately and oxygenate.

Oxygenation

Adequate oxygenation is the hallmark of pediatric patient management, but excess oxygen can be harmful. When

Procedure 4-1 Clearing an Infant's Airway

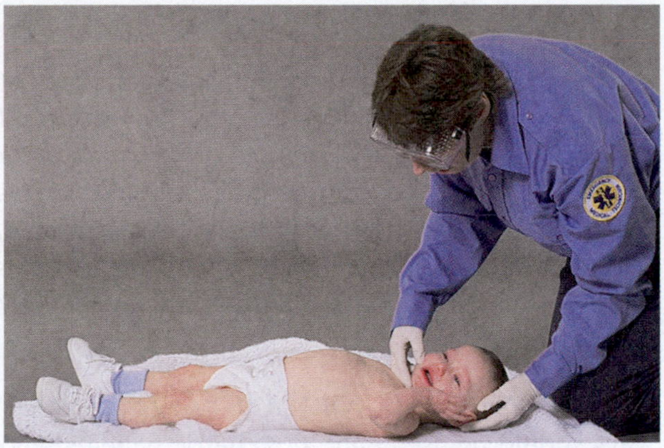

4-1a Recognize and assess for choking. Look for breathing difficulty, ineffective cough, and lack of a strong cry.

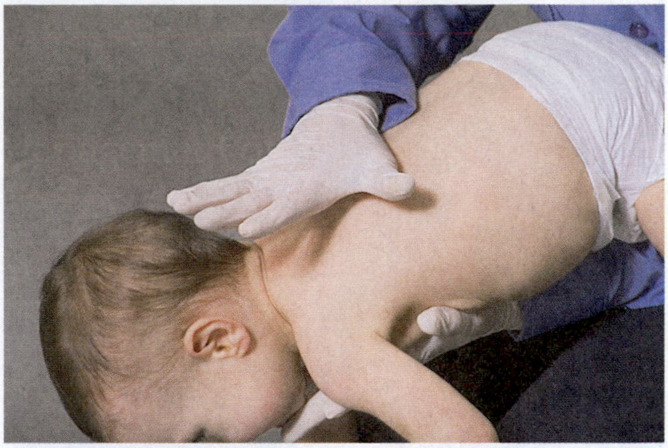

4-1b Give up to five back blows.

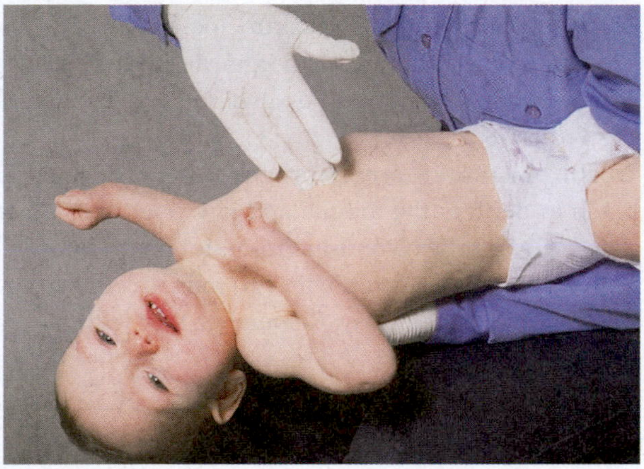

4-1c Then administer five chest thrusts.

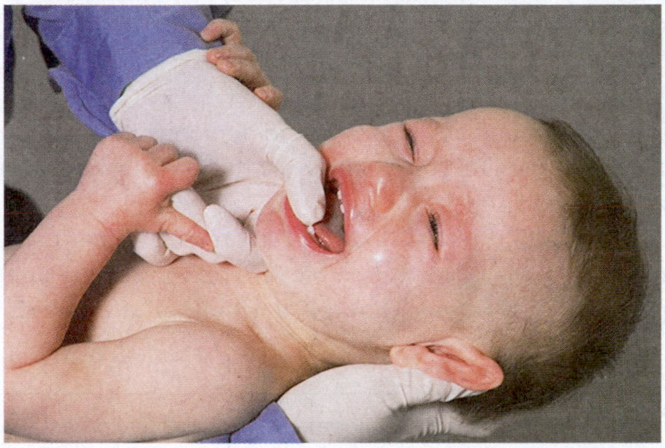

4-1d If the infant becomes unresponsive, begin CPR.

possible, use pulse oximetry to guide supplemental oxygen administration. The goal is to provide just enough oxygen to maintain a SpO_2 of 94 percent or greater. For resuscitation, use 100 percent oxygen when possible (except in newborns). Methods of oxygen delivery include "blow-by" techniques (especially for neonates) and pediatric-sized nonrebreather masks. Although nonrebreather masks provide the highest concentration of supplemental oxygen, children may resist their use. Try to overcome their fear by demonstrating the use of the mask on yourself (Figure 4-18). Better yet, enlist the support of a parent

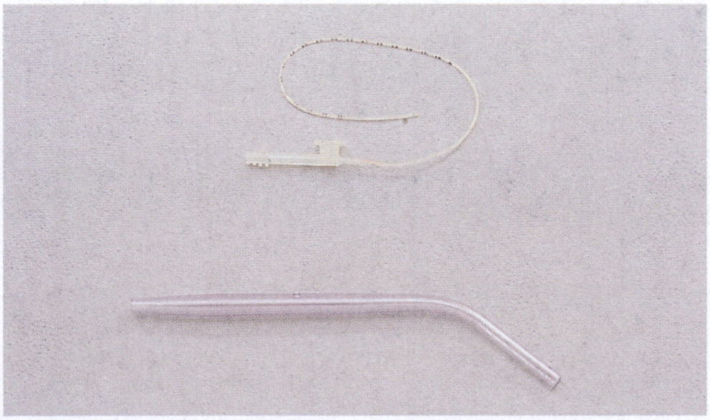

FIGURE 4-17 Pediatric-size suction catheters. Top: soft suction catheter. Bottom: rigid or hard suction catheter.

Table 4-7 Suction Catheter Sizes for Infants and Children

Age	Suction Catheter Size (French)
Up to 1 year	8
1 to 6 years	8–10
7 to 15 years	10–12
16 years	12

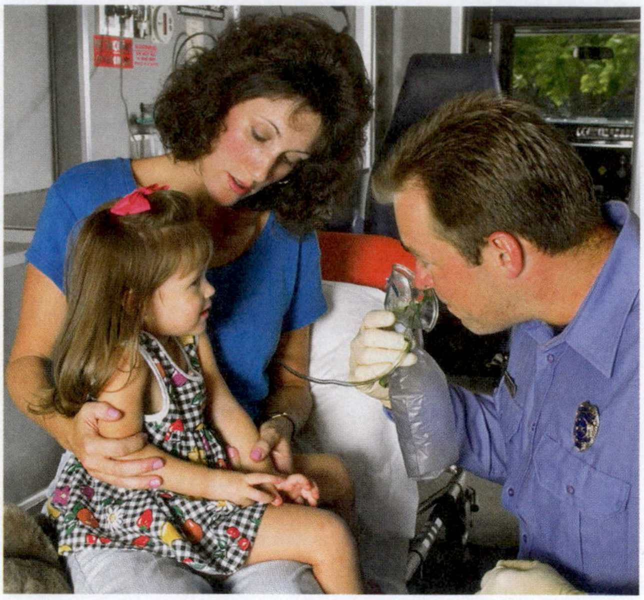

FIGURE 4-18 To overcome the child's fear of the nonrebreather mask, try it on yourself or have the parent try it on before attempting to place it on the child.

or caregiver and ask him or her to demonstrate the mask. As an alternative, you might place the mask over the face of a stuffed animal.

If the child refuses to accept the nonrebreather mask, resort to high-concentration blow-by oxygen. Some units place oxygen tubing through the bottom of a colorful paper cup and use it to deliver the blow-by supplemental oxygen. Children often find a familiar object less frightening than complicated medical equipment.

Airway Adjuncts

As a general rule, use airway adjuncts in pediatric patients only if prolonged artificial ventilations are required. There are two reasons for this. First, infants and children often improve quickly through the administration of 100 percent oxygen. Second, airway adjuncts may create greater complications in children than in adults. Pediatric patients risk soft tissue damage, vomiting, and stimulation of the vagus nerve.

OROPHARYNGEAL AIRWAYS Oropharyngeal airways should be used only in pediatric patients who lack a gag reflex. (Patients with a gag reflex risk vomiting and bradycardia.) Size the airway by measuring from the corner of the mouth to the front of the earlobe. Remember, oropharyngeal airways that are too small can obstruct breathing; ones that are too large can both block the airway and cause trauma. (For general sizing suggestions, see Table 4-8.)

In placing an oropharyngeal airway, use a tongue blade to depress the tongue and jaw (Figure 4-19). If you detect a gag reflex, continue to maintain an open airway with a manual (head-tilt/chin-lift) maneuver and consider the use of a nasal airway. Remember that with a pediatric

Table 4-8 Airway Management: Pediatric Equipment Guidelines

Equipment	Premature (1–2.5 kg; 2.2–5.5 lb*)	Neonate (2.5–4 kg; 5.5–8.8 lb)	6 Months (6–8 kg; 13.2–17.6 lb)	1–4 Years (10–14 kg; 22–30.8 lb)	5 Years (16–18 kg; 35.2–39.6 lb)	5–10 Years (24–30 kg; 52.8–66 lb)
Airway	Infant	Infant/small	Small	Small	Medium	Medium/large
Oral	(00)	(0)	(1)	(2)	(3)	(4.5)
Breathing						
O_2 ventilation mask	Premature	Newborn	Infant/child	Child	Child	Small adult
Bag-valve device	Infant	Infant	Child	Child	Child	Child/adult
Endotracheal tube	2.5–3.0 (uncuffed)	3.0–3.5 (uncuffed)	3.5–4.0	4.0–4.5	5.0–5.5	5.5–6.5
Suction/stylet (French)	6–8/6	8/6	8–10/6	10/6	14/14	14/14
Laryngoscope blade	0 (straight)	1 (straight)	1 (straight)	1–2 (straight)	2 (straight or curved)	2–3 (straight or curved)
Circulation						
Blood pressure cuff	Newborn	Newborn	Infant	Child	Child	Child/adult
Orogastric Tube (French)	5	5–8	8	10	10–12	14–18
Chest Tube (French)	10–14	12–18	14–20	14–24	20–32	28–38

Weights are the 50th percentile for the given age range.

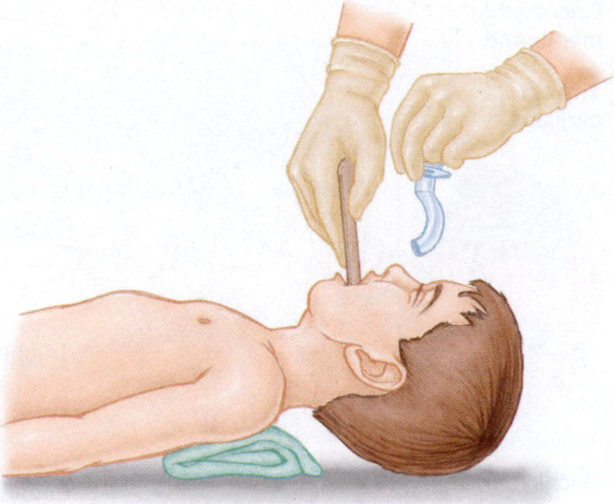

FIGURE 4-19 Inserting an oropharyngeal airway in a child with the use of a tongue blade.

patient, the oral airway is inserted with the tip pointing toward the tongue and pharynx. For a comparison with insertion in the adult patient, see Figures 4-20a and b.

NASOPHARYNGEAL AIRWAYS Use nasopharyngeal airways for children who possess a gag reflex and who require prolonged artificial ventilations. *Do not* use them on any child with midface or head trauma. You might mistakenly pass the airway through a fracture into the sinuses or the brain.

Size the pediatric nasal airway in the same fashion as for adult patients. Pay particular attention to determining proper airway diameter and length. A nasopharyngeal airway that is too short may not maintain an open airway. One that is too long may obstruct the airway. A small-diameter nasopharyngeal airway may be easily obstructed by secretions, thus requiring frequent suctioning. Use the outside diameter of the patient's little finger as a rough measure of airway diameter. Nasopharyngeal airways come in a variety of sizes, but they are not readily available for infants less than one year old. Equipment required for insertion of a nasal airway includes:

- Appropriately sized soft, flexible latex tubing
- Water-based lubricant

When inserting the nasal airway, follow the same basic method as you would in an adult patient. It is important to remember that younger children often have enlarged adenoids (lymphatic tissues in the nasopharynx), which can be easily lacerated when inserting a nasopharyngeal airway. Because of this, always use care when inserting a nasopharyngeal airway in a younger child. Gentle rotation of the airway may help it slide past obstructions. If resistance is met, do not force the airway, because significant bleeding can result.

Ventilation

Adequate tidal volume and ventilatory rate provide more than just a high oxygen saturation for your patient. Ventilation is a two-way physiologic street regarding maintenance of appropriate oxygen and carbon dioxide levels. However, you will achieve neither of these clinically important events without tailoring the ventilatory device and technique to your pediatric patient. Important points to remember include the following:

- Avoid excessive bag pressure and volume (hyperventilation). Ventilate at an age-appropriate rate, using only enough ventilation to make the chest rise.
- Use continuous waveform capnography to monitor and guide ventilation.

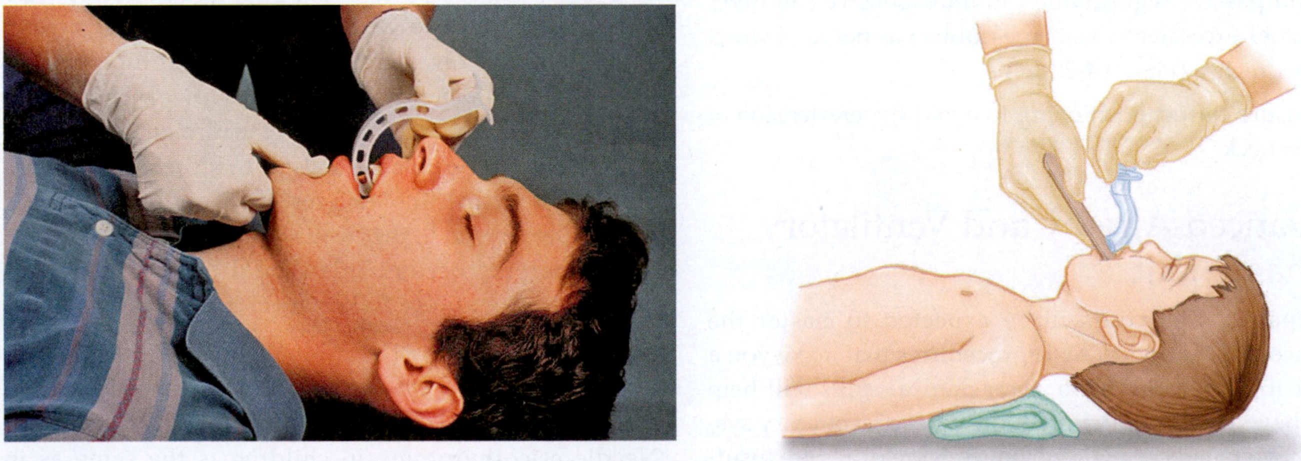

(a) (b)

FIGURE 4-20 (a) In an adult, the airway is inserted with the tip pointing to the roof of the mouth, then rotated into position. (b) In an infant or small child, the airway is inserted with the tip pointing toward the tongue and pharynx, in the same position it will be in after insertion.

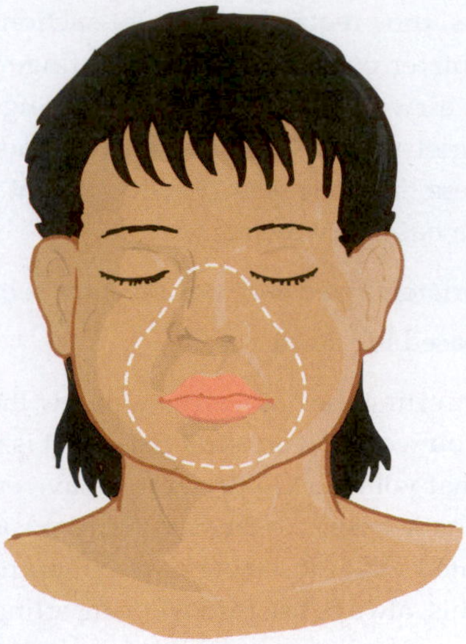

FIGURE 4-21 A mask used for a child should fit on the bridge of the nose and the cleft of the chin.

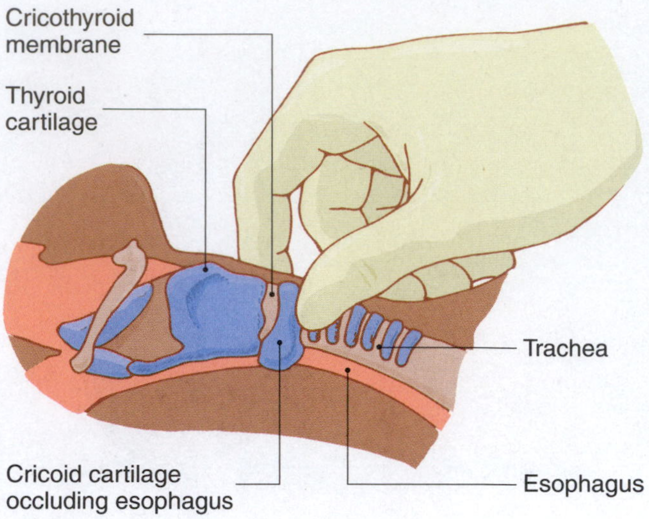

FIGURE 4-22 Cricoid pressure compresses the esophagus. This reduces regurgitation and helps bring the vocal cords into view, which is useful if intubation is to be performed.

- Use a properly sized mask to ensure a good fit. In general, the mask should fit on the bridge of the nose and the cleft of the chin (Figure 4-21).
- Obtain a chest rise with each breath.
- Allow adequate time for full chest recoil and exhalation.
- Assess bag-valve-mask (BVM) ventilation. (Provide 100 percent oxygen by using a reservoir attached to the BVM for resuscitation.)
- Remember that flow-restricted, oxygen-powered ventilation devices are contraindicated in pediatric resuscitation.
- Do not use BVMs with pop-off valves unless they can be readily occluded, if necessary. (Ventilatory pressures required during pediatric CPR may exceed the limit of the pop-off valve.)
- Apply cricoid pressure to minimize gastric inflation and passive regurgitation in unresponsive children.[9] Avoid excessive cricoid pressure so as not to obstruct the trachea (Figure 4-22).
- Ensure correct positioning to avoid hyperextension of the neck.

Advanced Airway and Ventilatory Management

As a paramedic, you will be expected to master the advanced life support (ALS) procedures that make you a leader in the EMS system. Your clinical skills will help save the lives of pediatric patients whose respiratory systems have failed so severely that BLS measures are insufficient. When signs of impending cardiopulmonary arrest have been identified (as discussed earlier), you may be called on to implement the following pediatric advanced life support (PALS) techniques, either in your own unit or in a transfer of care from a BLS unit. The success of these techniques requires knowledge of the procedures that set pediatric skills apart from the ALS skills used on adults. (Review the advanced airway skills for adults discussed in the chapter "Airway Management and Ventilation.")

Foreign Body Airway Obstruction

One advantage of being able to perform endotracheal intubation is that it gives you another treatment modality for children with foreign body airway obstructions. If a child's airway cannot be cleared by basic airway procedures, visualize the airway with the laryngoscope. Often, the obstructing foreign body can be seen. Once it is visualized, grasp the foreign body with Magill forceps and remove it. If you cannot remove the foreign body with Magill forceps, try to intubate around the obstruction. This often requires using an endotracheal tube smaller than you would normally choose. However, this will provide an adequate airway until the foreign body can be removed at the hospital. Finally, if the foreign body cannot be removed with Magill forceps and it is impossible to intubate around it, then you should consider placing a cricothyrotomy needle. This should only be done as a last resort. Be sure to follow local protocols regarding needle cricothyrotomy.

Needle Cricothyrotomy

Needle cricothyrotomy in children is the same as in adult patients (as discussed in the chapter "Airway Management and Ventilation"). It is important to remember that the anatomic landmarks are smaller and more difficult to identify. For years, it was taught that needle cricothyrotomy was contraindicated in children less than one year of age. However, current thinking is that the possible benefit (life) exceeds the risks (bleeding, local tissue damage). Remember, the only indication for cricothyrotomy is failure to obtain an airway by any other method.

Endotracheal Intubation

Endotracheal intubation allows direct visualization of the lower airway through the trachea, bypassing the entire upper airway. It is the most effective method of controlling a patient's airway, whether the patient is an adult or a child. However, endotracheal intubation is not without complications. It is an invasive technique with little room for error. A tube that is mistakenly sized or misplaced, especially in an apneic patient, can quickly lead to hypoxia and death.

Pediatric endotracheal intubation has come under increasing scrutiny in EMS. Several studies have questioned the effectiveness of prehospital pediatric endotracheal intubation.[5] Bag-mask ventilation can be as effective as, and may be safer than, endotracheal tube ventilation for short periods during prehospital resuscitation.[10]

ANATOMIC AND PHYSIOLOGIC CONCERNS Although endotracheal intubation of a child and an adult follow the same basic procedures, the special features of the pediatric airway complicate placement of any orotracheal tube. In fact, variations in the airway size of children preclude the use of certain airways, including esophageal obturator airways (EOAs), pharyngeotracheal lumen airways (PtLs), and esophageal–tracheal combitubes (ETCs). Properly sized laryngeal mask airways (LMAs) may be used in children but do not protect the airway from aspiration. In using an endotracheal tube, keep in mind these points:

- In infants and small children, it is often more difficult to create a single clear visual plane from the mouth, through the pharynx, and into the glottis. A straight-blade laryngoscope is preferred, as it provides greater displacement of the tongue and better visualization of the relatively cephalad and anterior glottis. For larger children, a curved blade may sometimes be used. (Review Table 4-8.)
- Variations in the sizes of pediatric airways, coupled with the fact that the narrowest portion of the airway is at the level of the cricoid ring, make proper sizing of the endotracheal tube crucial. To determine correct size, apply any of the following methods:
    - Use a resuscitation tape, such as the Broselow™ tape, to estimate tube size based on height.
    - Estimate the correct tube size by using the diameter of the patient's little finger or the diameter of the nasal opening.
    - Calculate the correct tube size by using this simple numerical formula: (Patient's age in years + 16) ÷ 4 = tube size.
- The depth of insertion can be estimated based on age (Table 4-9). However, the best method of determining depth is direct visualization. Because of the distance between the mouth and the trachea, a stylet is rarely needed to position the tube properly. When a stylet is used, select a malleable yet rigid style. Make sure the tip of the stylet does not extend out of the end of the tube where it could possibly injure the soft tissues of the trachea.
- Either cuffed or uncuffed endotracheal tubes can be used in children (but not in neonates). In certain conditions, a cuffed tube may be superior, but cuff pressure should be limited to 20 cmH_2O. If using a cuffed endotracheal tube, it may be necessary to select a tube that is 0.5 mm smaller than an uncuffed tube.
- Infants and small children may have greater vagal response than adults. Therefore, laryngoscopy and passage of an endotracheal tube are likely to cause a vagal response, dramatically slowing the child's heart rate and decreasing the cardiac output and blood pressure. As a result, pediatric intubations must be carried out swiftly, accurately, and with continuous monitoring.

INDICATIONS The indications for endotracheal intubation in a pediatric patient are the same as those for an adult. They include:

- Need for prolonged artificial ventilations
- Inadequate ventilatory support with a BVM
- Cardiac or respiratory arrest
- Control of an airway in a patient without a cough or gag reflex
- Need to provide a route for drug administration
- Need to gain access to the airway for suctioning

Table 4-9 Infant/Child Endotracheal Tubes

Age of Patient	Measurement of the Endotracheal Tube at the Teeth to the Midtrachea (cm)
6 Months to 1 year	12
2 Years	14
4–6 Years	16
6–10 Years	18
10–12 Years	20

Procedure 4-2 Endotracheal Intubation in the Child

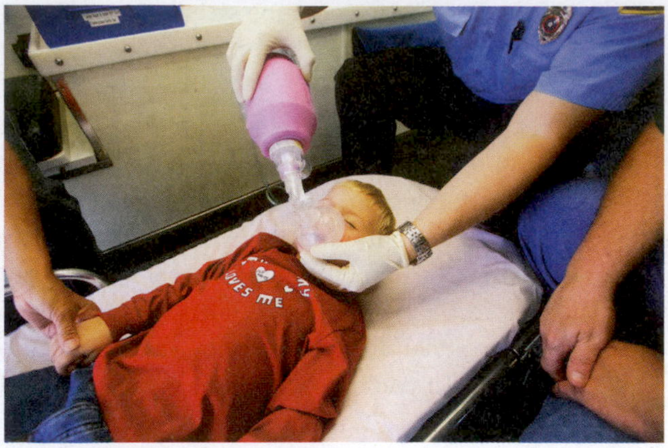

4-2a Hyperventilate the child.

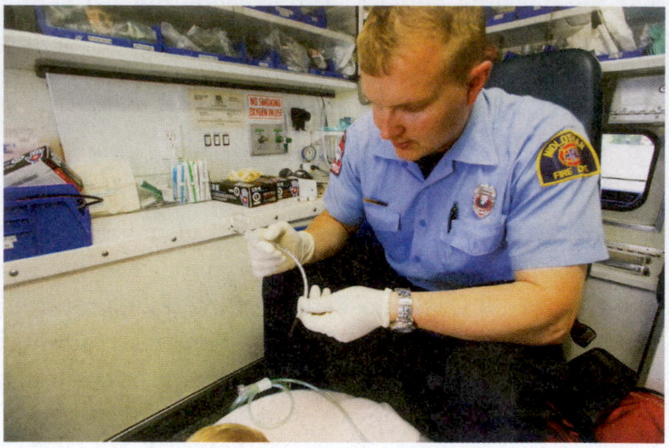

4-2b Prepare the equipment.

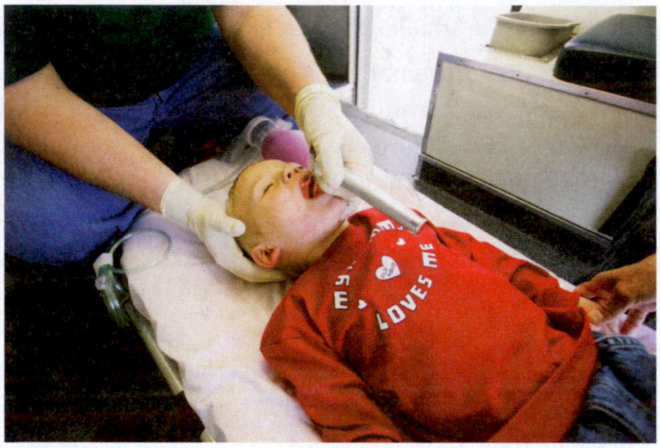

4-2c Insert the laryngoscope.

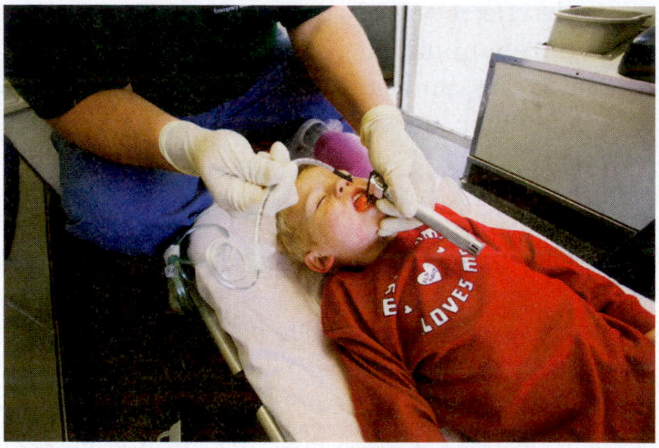

4-2d Visualize the child's larynx and insert the ETT.

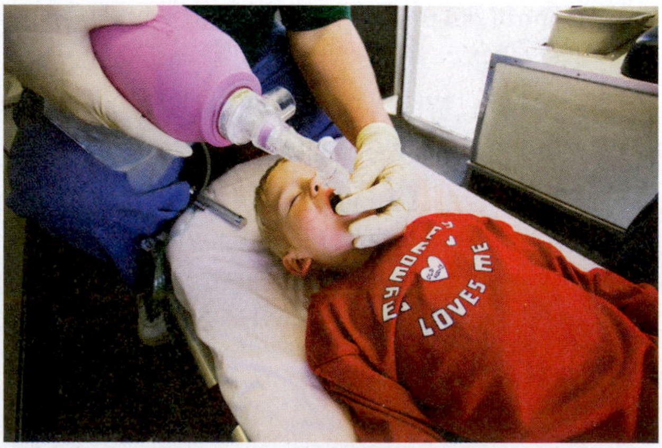

4-2e Ventilate, inflate the ETT cuff (if it is a cuffed tube), and auscultate.

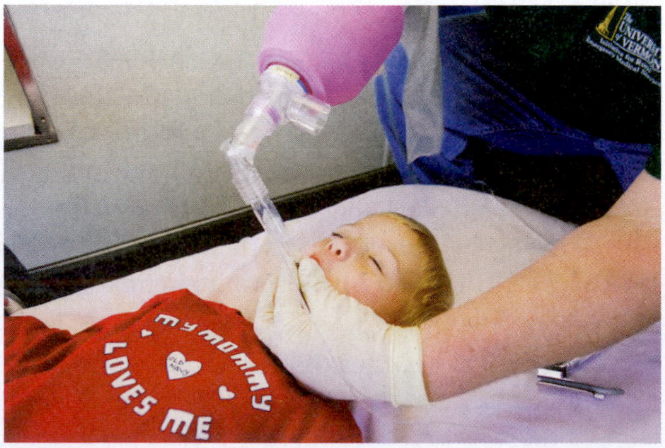

4-2f Confirm placement with an $ETCO_2$ detector or waveform capnography.

(Continued)

Procedure 4-2 *Continued*

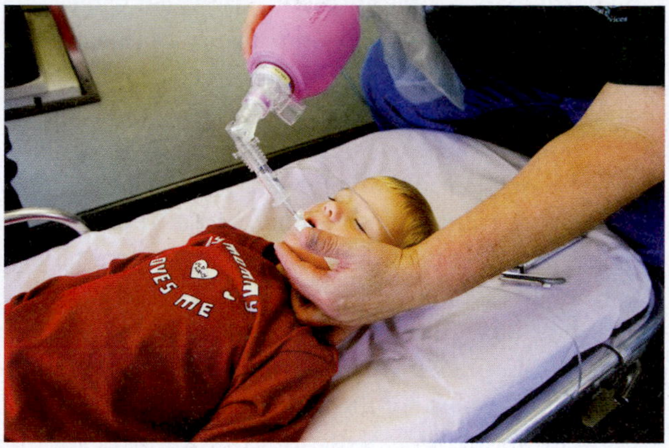

4-2g Secure the tube.

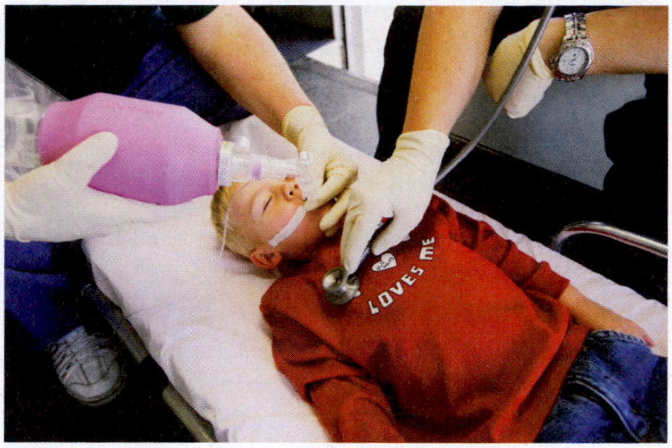

4-2h Reconfirm proper ETT placement.

TECHNIQUES FOR PEDIATRIC INTUBATION To perform endotracheal intubation on a pediatric patient, follow the basic steps shown in Procedure 4-2. Detailed steps are as follows:

1. Assemble and check your equipment. As stated earlier, a straight-blade laryngoscope is preferred. Assorted sizes of endotracheal tubes, both cuffed and uncuffed, should be stocked in the pediatric kit aboard your ambulance.
2. While maintaining ventilatory support, ventilate the patient with 100 percent oxygen. If time allows, ventilate for a full 2 minutes.
3. Place the patient's head and neck into an appropriate position. With a pediatric patient, the head should be maintained in a sniffing position.
4. Hold the laryngoscope in your left hand.
5. Insert your laryngoscope blade into the right side of the patient's mouth. With a sweeping action, displace the tongue to the left.
6. Move the blade slightly toward the midline, then advance it until the distal end is positioned at the base of the tongue (Figure 4-23).
7. Look for the tip of the epiglottis, and place the laryngoscope blade into its proper position. Keep in mind that a child—particularly an infant—has a shorter airway and a higher glottis than an adult. Because of this, you will see the cords much sooner than you may expect.
8. With your left wrist straight, use your shoulder and arm to lift the mandible and tongue at a 45-degree

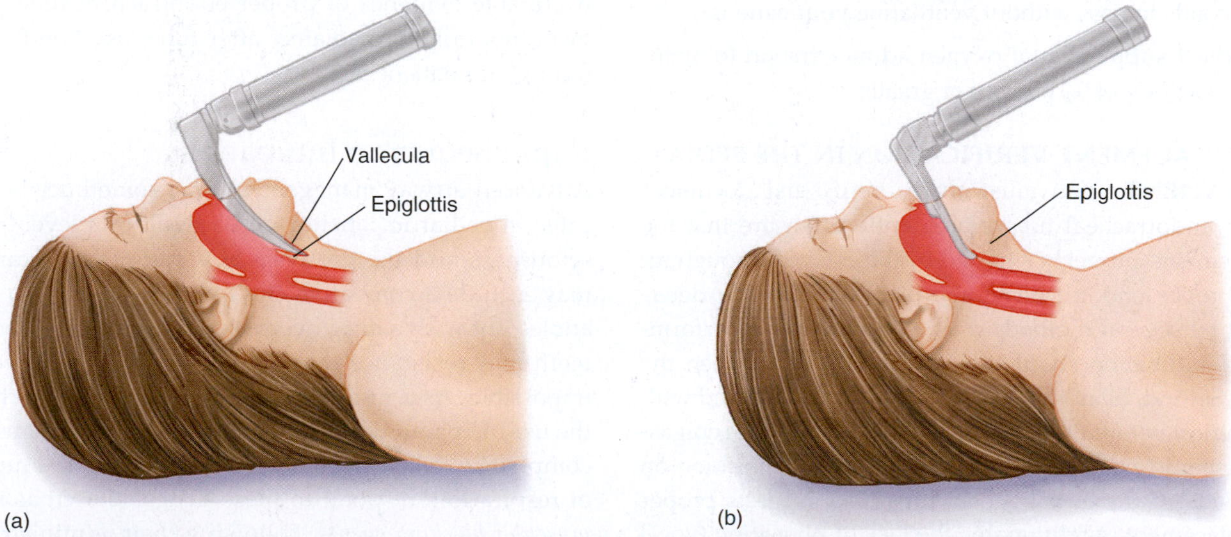

FIGURE 4-23 Placement of the laryngoscope: (a) MacIntosh (curved) blade and (b) Miller (straight) blade.

angle to the floor until the glottis is exposed. Use the little finger of your left hand to apply gentle downward pressure to the cricoid cartilage. This will permit easier visualization of the cords.

9. Grasp the endotracheal tube in your right hand. To pass the tube into your patient's mouth, it may be helpful to hold it so that its curve is in a horizontal plane (bevel sideways). Insert the tube through the right corner of the child's mouth.
10. Under direct observation, insert the endotracheal tube into the glottic opening and pass it through until its distal cuff disappears past the vocal cords—approximately 5 to 10 cm. As a tube is advanced, it should be rotated into the proper plane. In some cases, it will be difficult to advance an endotracheal tube at the level of the cricoid. *Do not* force the tube through this region, because it can cause laryngeal edema.
11. Hold the tube in place with your left hand. Attach an infant- or child-size bag-valve device to the 15/22-mm adapter and deliver several breaths.
12. Check for proper tube placement. Watch for chest rise and fall with each ventilation and listen for equal, bilateral breath sounds. There should also be an absence of sounds over the epigastrium with ventilations. Confirm placement with capnography.
13. If the tube has a distal cuff, inflate it with the recommended amount of air.
14. Recheck for proper placement of the tube and ventilate the patient with 100 percent oxygen.
15. Secure the endotracheal tube with umbilical tape while maintaining ventilatory support.
16. Continue supporting the tube manually while maintaining ventilations. Check periodically to ensure proper tube position. As with adults, allow no more than 30 seconds to pass without ventilating your patient.
17. Adjust supplemental oxygen administration to maintain a SpO_2 of 94 percent or greater.

TUBE PLACEMENT VERIFICATION IN THE PEDIATRIC PATIENT You must *always* verify and document proper endotracheal tube placement and ensure that the tube remains properly situated in the trachea throughout care. Proper endotracheal tube placement can be determined by several methods. First, the paramedic performing the intubation should see the tube pass between the cords. Second, bilateral chest rise should be observed with mechanical ventilation, and breath sounds over the epigastrium should be absent. The presence of condensation on the inside of the endotracheal tube also suggests proper tube placement. Additionally, the lack of phonation (vocal sounds) indicates that the tube is properly placed into the trachea. Esophageal detector devices are sometimes used in prehospital care to confirm proper tube placement. However, it is important to use these devices with caution in pediatric patients because you might get a false-positive finding even if the tube is improperly placed. This is particularly true when uncuffed endotracheal tubes have been used. The preferred method of endotracheal tube verification is through the use of capnography with either a colorimetric detector or waveform capnography. (Esophageal detector devices and end-tidal carbon dioxide detection devices are discussed in the chapter "Airway Management and Ventilation.")

It is not uncommon for an endotracheal tube to become displaced during patient care, movement, or transport. Because of this, paramedics must be extremely vigilant about repeatedly or continuously monitoring proper endotracheal tube placement. Monitoring can be accomplished through repeated assessments or through the use of continuous waveform capnography. Continuous waveform capnography provides breath-to-breath verification of proper tube placement and will rapidly alert providers of a problem with ventilation or with endotracheal tube placement. The mnemonic DOPE will help in remembering the possible causes of deterioration in an intubated child:

- *D*isplacement of the endotracheal tube from the trachea
- *O*bstruction of the tube
- *P*neumothorax
- *E*quipment failure

Problems with endotracheal tube placement remain a major malpractice risk for EMS personnel. For this reason, it is essential that proper endotracheal tube placement is not only verified *but also documented* by at least three methods. Continuous waveform capnography is rapidly becoming a standard of care and, if properly used, becomes irrefutable evidence of proper endotracheal tube placement, not only immediately after tube insertion but also throughout patient care.

Rapid Sequence Intubation

Advanced airway management may sometimes be indicated in pediatric patients with a significant level of consciousness and the presence of a gag reflex. Examples may include a combative child with head trauma or an adolescent with a drug overdose. In such cases, clenched teeth and resistance may make intubation difficult or impossible. As a result, medical direction may authorize the use of "paralytics" to induce a state of neuromuscular compliance. All skeletal muscles, including the muscles of respiration, respond to these drugs, known as *neuromuscular blocking agents*. Following their administration, the patient will require mechanical ventilation.

An example of a commonly used neuromuscular blocker is succinylcholine (Anectine). Typically, it is administered at 1 to 2 mg/kg IV push. It acts in 60 to 90 seconds and lasts approximately 3 to 5 minutes. Remember that succinylcholine has no effect on consciousness or pain. Thus, a sedative agent must be used for all children except those who are unconscious. Commonly used drugs include midazolam (Versed), diazepam (Valium), thiopental, and fentanyl. A bite block should be placed to prevent the patient from biting the endotracheal tube. Medical direction may authorize sedation to minimize the emotional trauma to the patient, or drugs such as pancuronium or vecuronium if longer paralysis is required.

Extraglottic Airways

Endotracheal intubation has long been regarded as the "gold standard" for airway management. However, the use of alternative airways has become more common. This same trend is also occurring in pediatric airway management. The laryngeal mask airway (LMA) and the King LT-D are available in pediatric sizes and are now routinely used in several EMS systems for prehospital airway management.[11] The LMA is easy to insert and requires less education and practice than endotracheal intubation (Figure 4-24).

Nasogastric Intubation

If gastric distention is present in a pediatric patient, you may consider placing a nasogastric (NG) tube. In infants and children, gastric distention may result from overly aggressive artificial ventilations or from air swallowing. Placement of an NG tube will allow you to decompress the stomach and proximal bowel of air. An NG tube can also be used to empty the stomach of blood or other substances. Indications for use of a nasogastric intubation include:

- Inability to achieve adequate tidal volumes during ventilation due to gastric distention
- Presence of gastric distention in an unresponsive patient

As with nasopharyngeal airways, an NG tube is contraindicated in pediatric patients who have sustained head or facial trauma. Because the NG tube might migrate into the cranial sinuses, consider the use of an orogastric tube instead. Other contraindications include soft tissue injuries of the nose. Sometimes, insertion of an NG tube can stimulate the gag reflex and induce vomiting.

Equipment for placing an NG tube includes:

- Age-appropriate NG tubes
- 20-mL syringe
- Water-soluble lubricant
- Emesis basin
- Tape
- Suctioning equipment
- Stethoscope

In sizing the NG tube, keep in mind the following recommended guidelines:

- Newborn/infant: 8.0 French
- Toddler/preschooler: 10 French
- School-age children: 12 French
- Adolescents: 14–16 French

In determining the correct length, measure the tube from the tip of the nose, over the ear, to the tip of the xiphoid process. The steps in Procedure 4-3 can be followed for inserting the tube. Keep in mind, as you examine these steps, that many experts believe that an NG tube should be inserted only when an endotracheal tube is in place. This precaution will prevent misplacement of the tube into the trachea instead of the esophagus. Consult protocols in your area on the use of NG tubes.

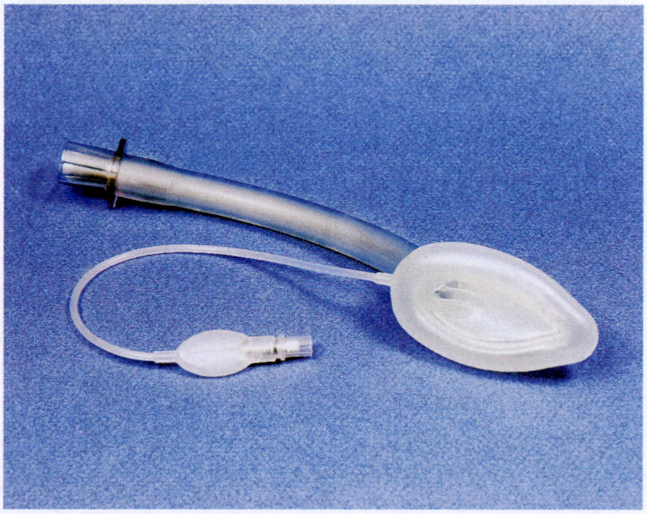

FIGURE 4-24 Pediatric laryngeal mask airway (LMA).

Circulation

As mentioned earlier, the respiratory and cardiovascular systems are interdependent. In pediatrics, you are encouraged to look at the total child. You should assess the child by assessing the various body systems. For example, instead of simply checking a pulse, you should look for end-organ changes that indicate the effectiveness of respiratory and cardiovascular function. These include such things as mental status, skin color, skin temperature, urine output, and others.

Two problems lead to cardiopulmonary arrest in children: shock and respiratory failure. Both must be identified and corrected early. The following section will address assessment of the cardiovascular system. Particular emphasis is placed on venous access and fluid resuscitation, because these are essential skills for prehospital ALS personnel who treat pediatric patients.

Procedure 4-3 Nasogastric Intubation in the Child

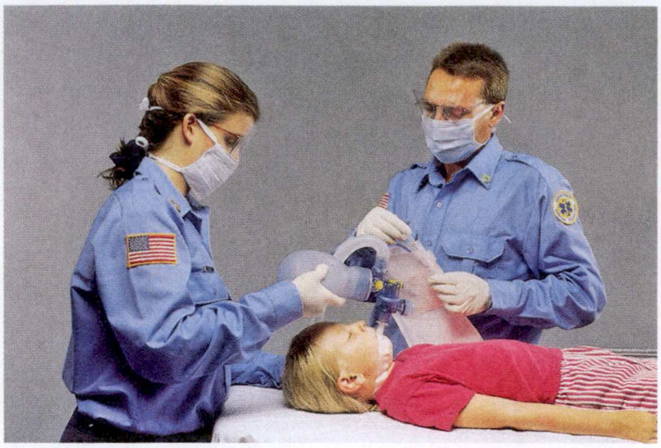

4-3a Oxygenate and continue to ventilate, if possible.

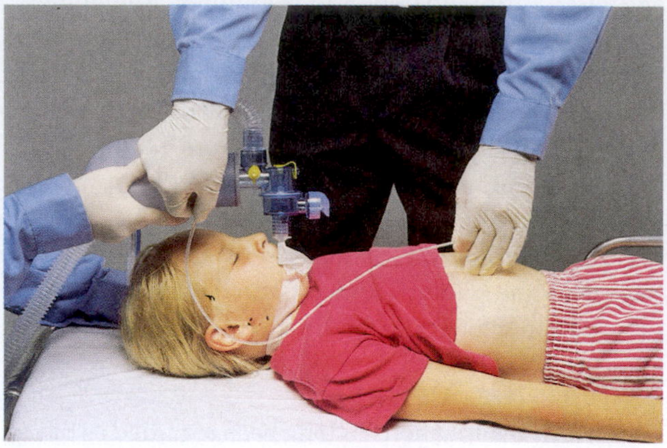

4-3b Measure the NG tube from the tip of the nose, over the ear, to the tip of the xiphoid process.

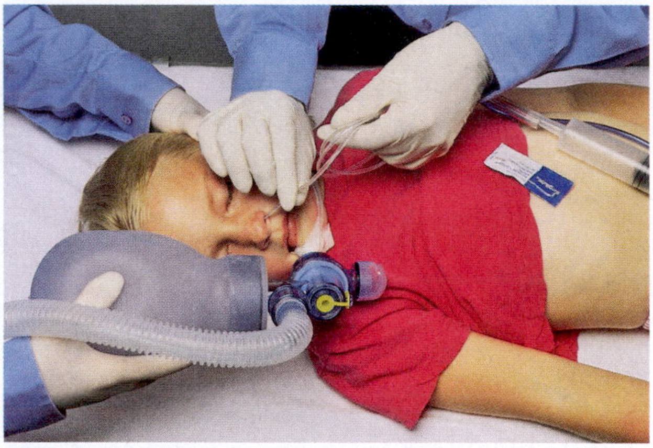

4-3c Lubricate the end of the tube. Then pass it gently downward along the nasal floor to the stomach.

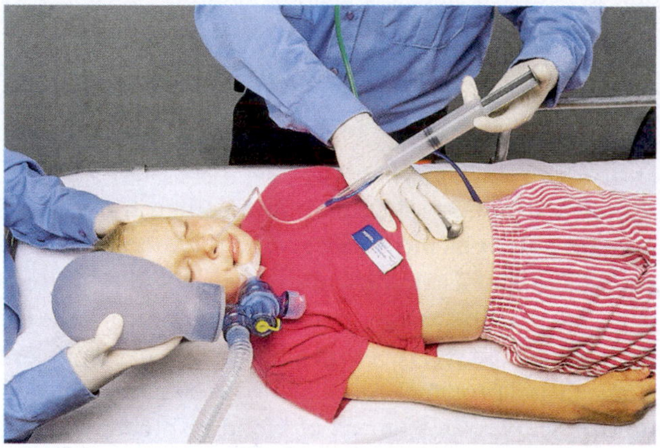

4-3d Auscultate over the epigastrium to confirm correct placement. Listen for bubbling while injecting 10–20 cc of air into the tube.

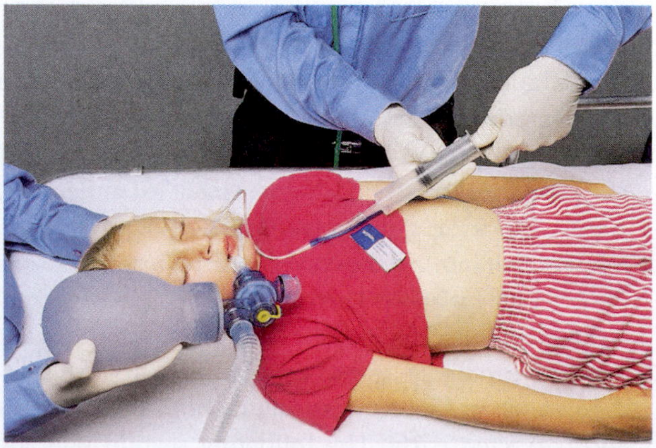

4-3e Use suction to aspirate stomach contents.

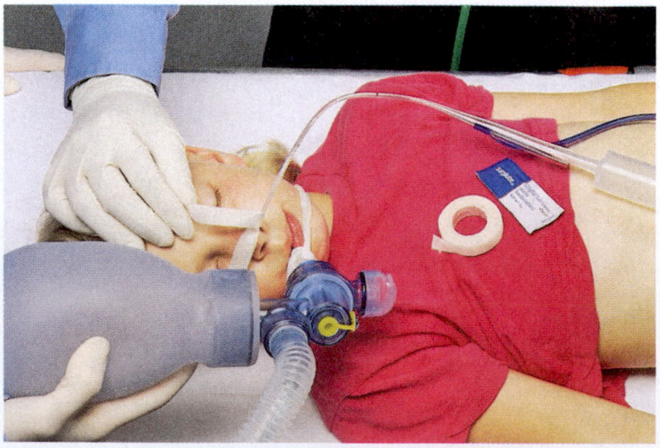

4-3f Secure the tube in place.

Vascular Access

Intravenous techniques for children are basically the same as for adults (see the chapter "Intravenous Access and Medication Administration"). However, additional veins may be accessed in the infant. These include veins of the neck and scalp as well as those of the arms, hands, and feet. The external jugular vein, however, should be used only for life-threatening situations.

Intraosseous Infusion

The use of intraosseous (IO) infusion has become popular in treating pediatric patients (Figure 4-25a). This is especially true when large volumes of fluid must be administered, as occurs in hypovolemic shock, and when other means of venous access are unavailable. Certain medications can be administered intraosseously, including epinephrine, atropine, dopamine, lidocaine, sodium bicarbonate, and dobutamine. Indications for IO infusion include:

- Existence of shock or cardiac arrest
- An unresponsive patient
- Suspected sepsis
- Unsuccessful attempts at peripheral IV insertion

The primary contraindications for IO infusion include:

- Presence of a fracture in the bone chosen for infusion
- Fracture of the pelvis or extremity fracture in the bone proximal to the chosen site

In performing IO perfusion, you can use a standard 16- or 18-gauge needle (either hypodermic or spinal). However, an intraosseous needle is preferred and is significantly better (Figure 4-25b). The anterior surface of the leg below the knee should be prepped with antiseptic solution. The needle is then inserted, in a twisting fashion, 1 to 3 cm below the tuberosity. Insertion should be slightly inferior in direction (to avoid the growth plate) and perpendicular to the skin (Figure 4-26). Placement of the needle into the marrow cavity can be determined by noting a lack of resistance as the needle passes through the bony cortex. Other indications include the needle standing upright without support, the ability to aspirate bone marrow into a syringe, or free flow of the infusion without infiltration into the subcutaneous tissues. Several intraosseous devices, such as the EZ-IO® and the Bone Injection Gun (B.I.G.), are approved for usage in children. (See also the discussion of intraosseous infusion in the chapter "Intravenous Access and Medication Administration.")

Fluid Therapy

The accurate dosing of fluids in children is crucial. Too much fluid can result in heart failure and pulmonary edema. Too little fluid can be ineffective. The primary dosage of fluid in hypovolemic shock should be 20 mL/kg of an isotonic solution such as lactated Ringer's or normal saline as soon as IV access is obtained. After the infusion, the child should be reassessed. If perfusion is still diminished, then a second bolus of 20 mL/kg should be administered. A child with hypovolemic shock may require 40 to 60 mL/kg, whereas a child with septic shock may require at least 60 to 80 mL/kg. Fluid therapy should be guided by the child's clinical response.

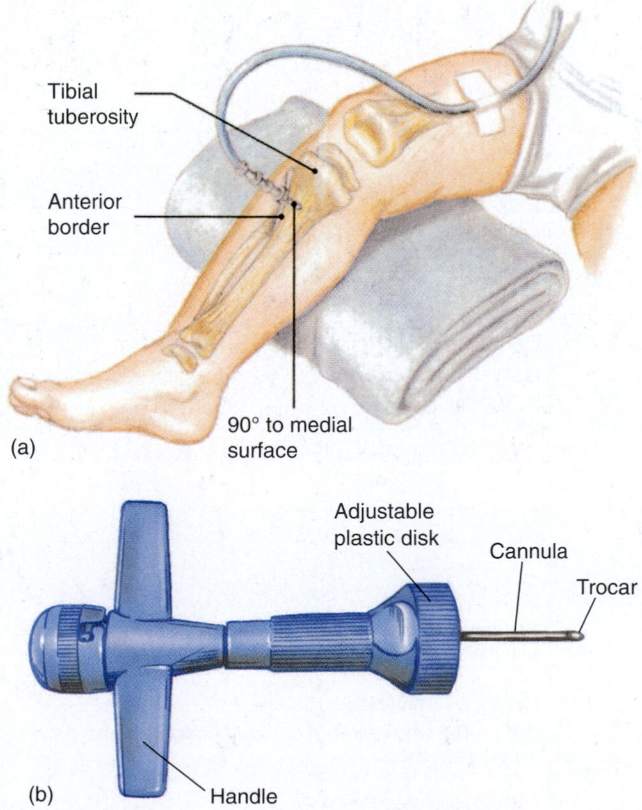

FIGURE 4-25 (a) Intraosseous administration in the pediatric patient. (b) An intraosseous needle.

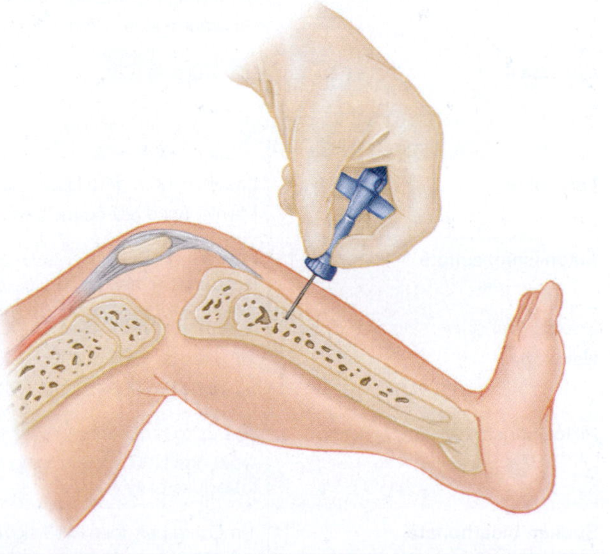

FIGURE 4-26 Correct needle placement for intraosseous administration. Note that the needle tip is in the marrow cavity.

Intravenous infusions in children should be closely monitored with frequent patient reassessment. Minidrip administration sets, flow limiters, or infusion pumps should be used routinely in pediatric cases.

Medications

Cardiopulmonary arrest in infants and children is almost always the result of a primary respiratory problem, such as drowning, choking, or smoke inhalation. The major aim in pediatric resuscitation is airway management and ventilation, as well as replacement of intravascular volume, if indicated. In certain cases, medications may be required. The objectives of medication therapy in pediatric patients include:

- Correction of hypoxemia
- Increased perfusion pressure during chest compressions
- Stimulation of spontaneous or more forceful cardiac contractions
- Acceleration of the heart rate
- Correction of metabolic acidosis
- Suppression of ventricular ectopy
- Maintenance of renal perfusion

The dosages of medications must be modified for the pediatric patient. Tables 4–10 and 4–11 illustrate recommended pediatric drug dosages in advanced cardiac life support.

CONTENT REVIEW

➤ Drugs Administered by Intraosseous Route
- Epinephrine
- Atropine
- Dopamine
- Lidocaine
- Sodium bicarbonate
- Dobutamine

Table 4-10 Drugs Used in Pediatric Advanced Life Support*

Drug	Dose	Remarks
Adenosine	0.1–0.2 mg/kg Maximum strength dose 12 mg	Monitor ECG Rapid IV/IO bolus
Amiodarone	5 mg/kg IV/IO; repeat up to 15 mg/kg. Maximum: 300 mg	Monitor ECG and blood pressure Adjust administration rate to urgency (give more slowly when perfusing rhythm present) Use caution when administering with other drugs that prolong the QT interval.
Atropine sulfate	0.02 mg/kg IV/IO 0.03 mg/kg ET† Repeat once if needed Minimum dose: 0.1 mg Maximum single dose: Child: 0.5 mg Adolescent: 1.0 mg	Higher doses may be used with organophosphate poisoning.
Calcium chloride (10%)	20 mg/kg per dose IV/IO (0.2 mL/kg)	Give slowly.
Epinephrine	0.01 mg/kg (0.1 mL/kg 1:10,000) IV/IO 0.1 mg/kg (0.1 mL/kg 1:1,000) ET† Maximum dose: 1 mg IV/IO; 10 mg ET†	May repeat every 3–5 minutes.
Glucose	0.5–1.0 g/kg IV/IO	$D_{10}W$: 5–10 mL/kg $D_{25}W$: 2–4 mL/kg $D_{50}W$: 1–2 mL/kg
Lidocaine	Loading: 1.0 mg/kg loading dose Maintenance: 20-50 mcg/kg per minute	
Magnesium sulfate	20–50 mg/kg IV/IO over 10–20 minutes; faster in *torsades de pointes*. Maximum dose: 2 g	
Naloxone	<5 years or <20 kg: 0.1 mg/kg IV/IO/ET* >5 years or >20 kg: 2 mg IV/IO/ET*	Use lower doses to reverse respiratory depression associated with therapeutic opioid use (1–15 mcg/kg).
Procainamide	15 mg/kg IV/IO over 30–60 minutes Adult dose: 20 mg/min IV up to a total dose of 17 mg/kg	Monitor ECG and blood pressure. Use caution when administering with other drugs that prolong the QT interval.
Sodium bicarbonate	1 mEq/kg per dose IV/IO slowly	After adequate ventilation.

*IV indicates intravenous route; IO, intraosseous route; ET, endotracheal route.

†Flush with 5 mL of normal saline and follow with five ventilations.

Table 4-11 Preparation of Infusions

Drug	Preparation*	Dose
Epinephrine	0.6 × body weight (kg) equals milligrams added to diluents† to make 100 mL	Then 1 mL/hr delivers 0.1 mcg/kg per minute; titrate to effect
Dopamine/dobutamine	0.6 × body weight (kg) equals milligrams added to diluents† to make 100 mL	Then 1 mL/hr delivers 0.3 mcg/kg per minute; titrate to effect

*Standard concentration can be used to provide more dilute or more concentrated drug solution, but then individual dose must be calculated for each patient and each infusion rate:

$$\text{Infusion Rate (mL/h)} = \frac{\text{Weight (kg)} \times \text{Dose (mcg/kg/min)} \times 60\ \text{min/hr}}{\text{Concentration (mcg/mL)}}$$

†Diluent may be 5 percent dextrose in water, 5 percent dextrose in half-normal, normal saline, or Ringer's lactate.

Electrical Therapy

You are less likely to use electrical therapy on pediatric patients than on adult patients, because ventricular fibrillation is much less common in children than adults. However, you should review and keep the following principles in mind for times when these emergencies arise:

- Administer an initial dosage of 2 to 4 joules per kilogram of body weight. (Keep in mind the estimated body weights in Table 4-5.)
- If this is unsuccessful, focus your attention on correcting hypoxia and acidosis.
- Transport to a pediatric critical care unit, if possible.

C-Spine Stabilization

Spinal injuries in children are not as common as in adults. However, because of a child's disproportionately larger and heavier head, the cervical spine (C-spine) is vulnerable to injury. Whenever an infant or child sustains a significant head injury, assume that a neck injury may also be present. Children can suffer a spinal cord injury with no noticeable damage to the vertebral column as seen on cervical spine X-rays, referred to as spinal cord injury without radiographic abnormality (SCIWORA). Thus, negative cervical spine X-rays do not necessarily ensure that a spinal cord injury does not exist. Because of this, children should remain stabilized until a spinal cord injury has been excluded by hospital personnel—typically through magnetic resonance imaging (MRI) and other imaging technologies. As previously noted, even a child secured in a car safety seat can suffer a neck injury if the head is propelled forward during a collision or sudden stop.

Always make sure that you use the appropriate-sized pediatric stabilization equipment. These supplies may include cervical collars, towel or blanket rolls, foam head blocks, commercial pediatric stabilization devices, vest-type or short wooden backboards, and long boards with the appropriate padding. For pediatric patients found in car seats, you can also use the seat for stabilization (Procedure 4-4). The Kendrick extrication device (KED) can be quickly modified to stabilize a pediatric patient. Because of the significant variations in the size of children, you must be creative in devising a plan for pediatric stabilization.

In securing the pediatric patient to the backboard, use appropriate amounts of padding to secure infants, toddlers, and preschoolers in a supine, neutral position. Never use sandbags when stabilizing a pediatric patient's head. If you must tip the board to manage vomiting, the weight of the sandbag may worsen the head injury. For steps in applying a pediatric stabilization system, see Procedure 4-5.

Whenever you stabilize a pediatric patient, remember that many children, especially those under age 5, will protest or fight restraint. Try to minimize the emotional stress by having a parent or caretaker stand near or touch the child. Often the child will stop struggling when secured totally in an stabilization device. Ideally, a rescuer or family member should remain with the child at all times to reassure and calm the child, if possible.

Transport Guidelines

In managing a pediatric patient, never delay transport to perform a procedure that can be done en route to the hospital. After deciding on necessary interventions—first BLS, then ALS—determine the appropriate receiving facility. In reaching your decision, consider three factors:

- Time of transport
- Specialized facilities
- Specialized personnel

If you live in an area with specialized prehospital crews, such as critical care crews and neonatal nurses, their availability should weigh in your decision as well. Consider whether the patient would benefit from transfer by one of these crews. If so, request support. If not, determine

Procedure 4-4 Stabilizing a Patient in a Child Safety Seat

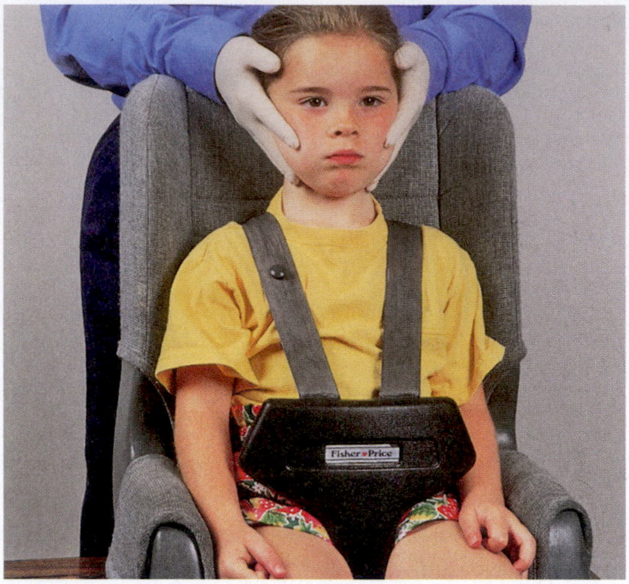

4-4a One paramedic stabilizes the car seat in an upright position and applies and maintains manual in-line stabilization to the child's head throughout the stabilization process.

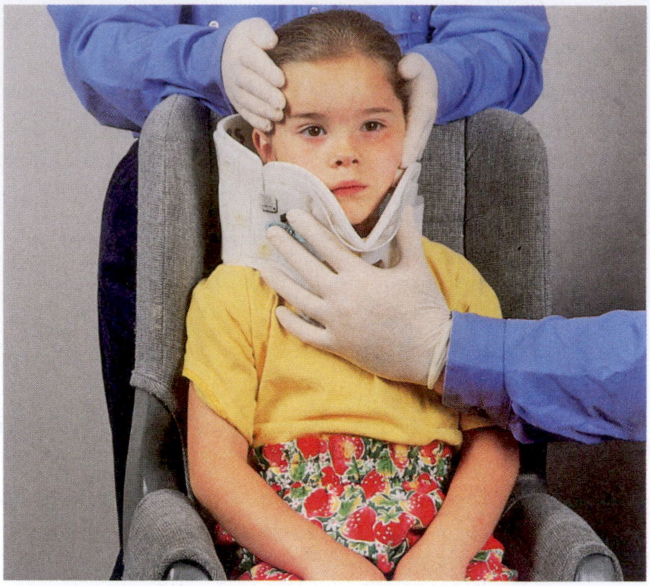

4-4b A second paramedic applies an appropriately sized cervical collar. If one is not available, improvise using a rolled hand towel.

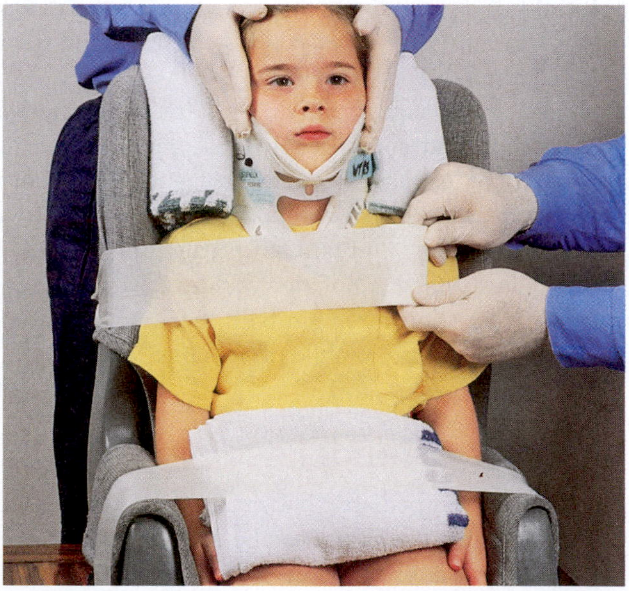

4-4c The second paramedic places a small blanket or towel on the child's lap, then uses straps or wide tape to secure the chest and pelvic areas to the seat.

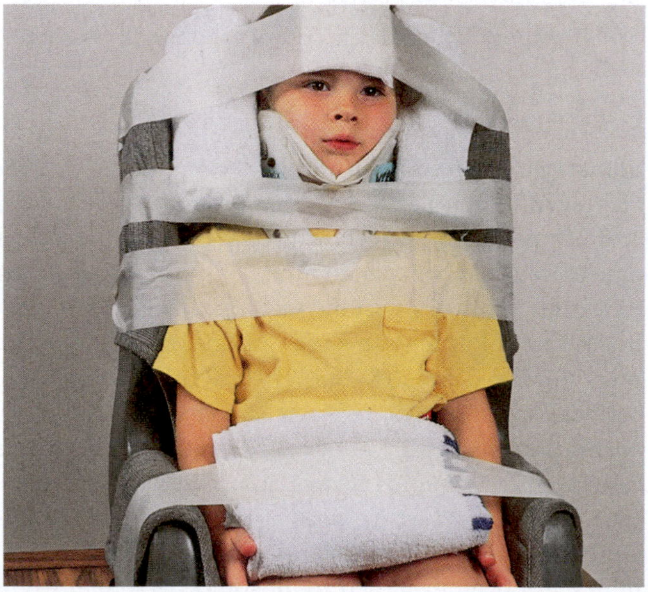

4-4d The second paramedic places towel rolls on both sides of the child's head to fill voids between the head and seat. The paramedic tapes the head into place, taping across the forehead and the collar, but avoiding taping over the chin, which would put pressure on the neck. The patient and seat can be carried to the ambulance and strapped to the stretcher, with the stretcher head raised.

Procedure 4-5 Applying a Pediatric Stabilization System

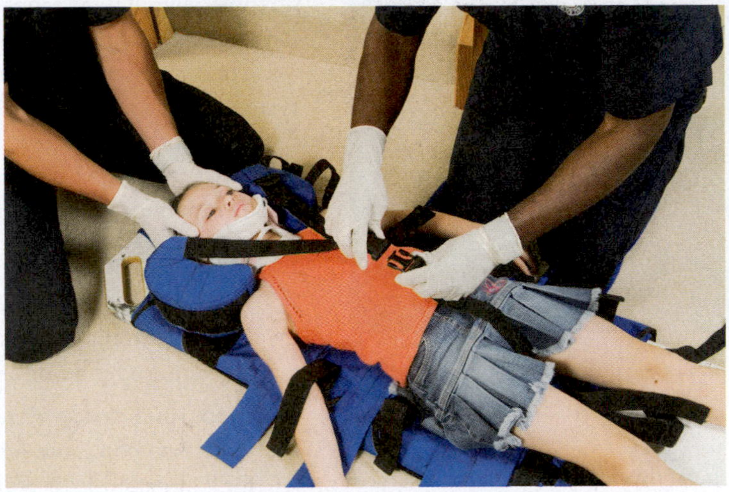

4-5a Position the patient on the stabilization system and adjust the color-coded straps to fit the child.

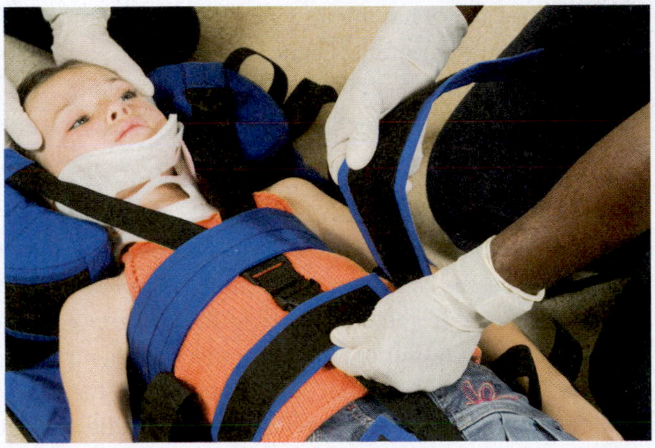

4-5b Attach the four-point safety system.

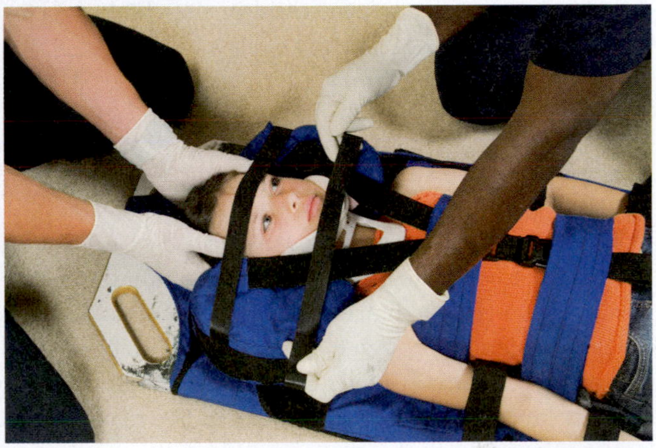

4-5c Fasten the adjustable head-support system.

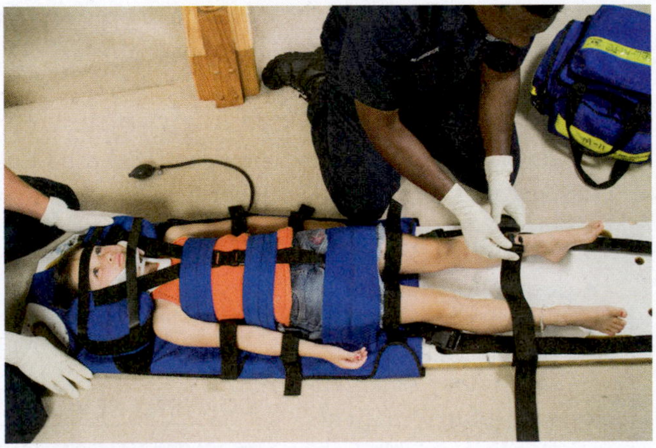

4-5d At this point, the patient is fully stabilized to the system.

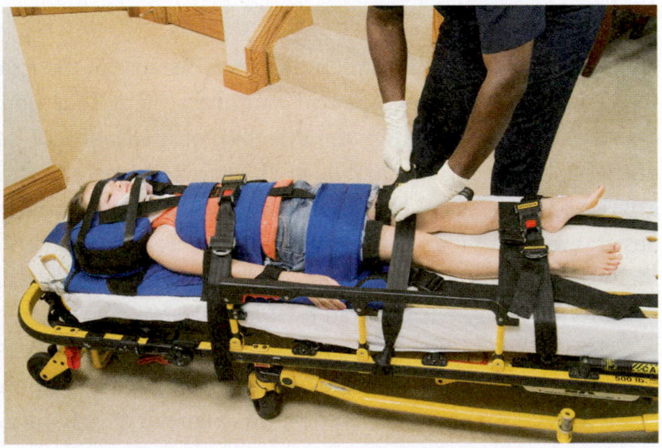

4-5e Move the stabilized patient onto the stretcher and fasten the loops at both ends to connect to the stretcher straps.

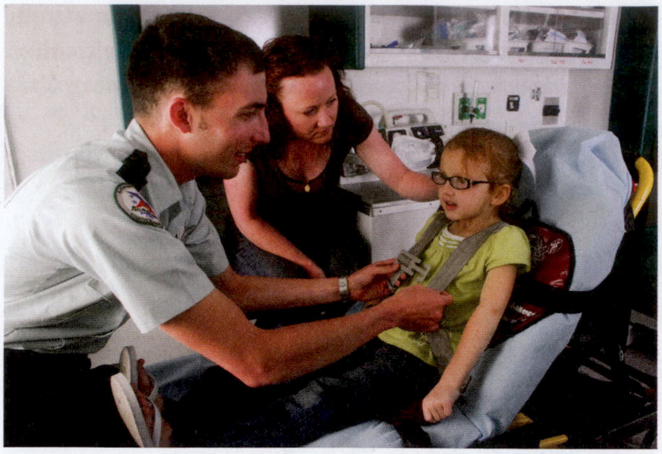

FIGURE 4-27 Emotional support of the infant or child continues during transport.

the closest definitive care facility for the infant or child placed in your care. Continue to reassure the child to reduce the fear involved in transition of care from the family to the hospital (Figure 4-27). Think of what you would do or say to calm your own child or the child of a close relative or friend.

Specific Medical Emergencies

As you already realize from your earlier training and experience, a variety of pediatric medical problems can activate the EMS system. Although the majority of childhood medical emergencies involve the respiratory system, other body systems can be involved as well. To help you recognize and treat pediatric medical emergencies, the following sections cover some of the specific conditions you may encounter.

Infections

Childhood is a time of frequent illnesses because of the relative immaturity of the pediatric immune system. Infectious diseases may be caused by the infection or infestation of the body by an infectious agent such as a virus, bacterium, fungus, or parasite. Most infections are minor and self-limiting. Several infections, however, can be life threatening. These include meningitis, pneumonia, and septicemia, a systemic infection (usually bacterial) in the bloodstream.

The impact of an infection on physiologic processes depends on the type of infectious agent and the extent of the infection. Signs and symptoms also vary, depending on the type of infection and the time since exposure. Any of the following conditions may indicate the presence of an infection: fever, chills, tachycardia, cough, sore throat, nasal congestion, malaise, tachypnea, cool or clammy skin, petechiae, respiratory distress, poor appetite, vomiting, diarrhea, dehydration, hypoperfusion (especially with septicemia), purpura (purple blotches resulting from hemorrhages into the skin that do not disappear under pressure), seizures, severe headache, irritability, stiff neck, or bulging fontanelle (in infants).

The management of infections depends on the body system or systems affected. Treatment of some of the most common and serious infections will be found in the sections that follow. As a general rule, you should adhere to these guidelines when treating an infectious illness:

- Take Standard Precautions because of the unknown cause of the infection.
- Become familiar with the common pediatric infections encountered in your area.
- If possible, try to determine which, if any, pediatric infections you have not been exposed to or vaccinated for. For example, if you did not have chickenpox (varicella) or measles (rubeola) as a child and were not vaccinated for them, then you should consider receiving vaccinations for these illnesses. If you encounter a child suspected of having an infectious disease to which you may be susceptible, consider allowing another rescuer to be the primary person to care for the child.

Respiratory Emergencies

Respiratory emergencies constitute the most common reason EMS is summoned to care for a pediatric patient. Respiratory illnesses can cause respiratory compromise because of their effect on the alveolar/capillary interface. Some illnesses are quite minor, causing only mild symptoms, but others can be rapidly fatal. Your approach to the child with a respiratory emergency will depend on the severity of respiratory compromise. If the child is alert and talking, then you can take a more relaxed approach. However, if the child appears ill and exhibits marked respiratory difficulty, then you must immediately intervene to prevent respiratory arrest and possible cardiopulmonary arrest.

Severity of Respiratory Compromise

The severity of respiratory compromise can be quickly classified into the following categories:

- Respiratory distress
- Respiratory failure
- Respiratory arrest

Respiratory emergencies in pediatric patients may progress quickly from respiratory distress to respiratory failure to respiratory arrest. You must learn to recognize the

CONTENT REVIEW

➤ Stages of Respiratory Compromise
- Respiratory distress
- Respiratory failure
- Respiratory arrest

phase your patient is in and take the appropriate interventions. Prompt recognition and treatment can literally mean the difference between life and death for an infant or child suffering from respiratory compromise.

RESPIRATORY DISTRESS The mildest form of respiratory impairment is classified as respiratory distress. The most noticeable finding is an increased work of breathing. One of the earliest indicators of respiratory distress is an increase in respiratory rate. Unfortunately, respiratory rate is one of the vital signs that is most often "estimated." As mentioned previously, it is essential to obtain an accurate respiratory rate in children. Ideally, the respiratory rate should be measured for an entire minute. If time does not allow it, or if the child is deteriorating, the respiratory rate should be measured for at least 30 seconds and multiplied by two to obtain the respiratory rate.

In addition to an increased work of breathing, the child in respiratory distress will initially have a slight decrease in the arterial carbon dioxide tension as the respiratory rate increases. However, as respiratory distress increases, the carbon dioxide tension will gradually increase.

The signs and symptoms of respiratory distress include:

- Normal mental status deteriorating to irritability or anxiety
- Tachypnea
- Retractions
- Nasal flaring (in infants)
- Poor muscle tone
- Tachycardia
- Head bobbing
- Grunting
- Cyanosis or hypoxia that improves with supplemental oxygen

If not corrected immediately, respiratory distress will lead to respiratory failure.

RESPIRATORY FAILURE Respiratory failure occurs when the respiratory system is not able to meet the demands of the body for oxygen intake and for carbon dioxide removal. It is characterized by inadequate ventilation and oxygenation. During respiratory failure, the carbon dioxide level begins to rise because the body is not able to remove carbon dioxide. This ultimately leads to respiratory acidosis.

The signs and symptoms of respiratory failure include:

- Irritability or anxiety deteriorating to lethargy
- Marked tachypnea, later deteriorating to bradypnea
- Marked retractions, later deteriorating to agonal respirations
- Poor muscle tone
- Marked tachycardia, later deteriorating to bradycardia
- Central cyanosis
- Hypoxia

Respiratory failure is a very ominous sign. If immediate intervention is not provided, the child will deteriorate to full respiratory arrest.

RESPIRATORY ARREST The end result of respiratory impairment, if untreated, is respiratory arrest. The cessation of breathing typically follows a period of bradypnea and agonal respirations.

Signs and symptoms of respiratory arrest include:

- Unresponsiveness deteriorating to coma
- Bradypnea deteriorating to apnea
- Absent chest wall motion
- Bradycardia deteriorating to asystole
- Profound cyanosis

Respiratory arrest will quickly deteriorate to full cardiopulmonary arrest if appropriate interventions are not made. The child's chances of survival markedly decrease when cardiopulmonary arrest occurs.

Management of Respiratory Compromise

The management of respiratory compromise should be based on the severity of the problem. The goals of management include increasing ventilation and increasing oxygenation. You should try to identify the signs and symptoms of respiratory distress early so that you can intervene before the child deteriorates.

Your initial attention should be directed at the airway. Is it patent? Is it maintainable with simple positioning? Is endotracheal intubation required?

After assessing the airway, ensure continued maintenance of the airway by positioning, placement of an airway adjunct (oropharyngeal or nasopharyngeal airway), or endotracheal intubation.

For children in respiratory distress or early respiratory failure, administer high-concentration oxygen. Some children will tolerate a nonrebreather mask. Others may not and may require that someone (perhaps a parent) hold blow-by oxygen for them to breathe. If the child fails to improve with supplemental oxygen administration, the patient should be treated more aggressively. Often it is necessary to separate the parents from the child so that you can provide the necessary care without interruption or distraction.

Pediatric patients with late respiratory failure or respiratory arrest require aggressive treatment. This includes:

- Establishment of an airway
- High-concentration, supplemental oxygen administration
- Mechanical ventilation with a BVM device attached to a reservoir delivering 100 percent oxygen

- Endotracheal intubation (or another acceptable airway) if mechanical ventilation does not rapidly improve the patient's condition
- Consideration of gastric decompression with an orogastric or nasogastric tube if abdominal distention is impeding ventilation
- Consideration of needle decompression of the chest if a tension pneumothorax is thought to be present
- Consideration of cricothyrotomy if complete airway obstruction is present and the airway cannot be obtained by any other method

In addition to the preceding treatments, you should obtain venous access. The child should be promptly transported to a facility staffed and equipped to handle critically ill children. While en route, continue to reassess the child. Signs of improvement include an improvement in skin color and temperature. As end-organ perfusion improves, the child will exhibit an increase in pulse rate, an increase in oxygen saturation, and an improvement in mental status. Provide emotional and psychological support to the parents and keep them abreast of the results of your care.

Specific Respiratory Emergencies

Respiratory problems typically arise from obstruction of a part of the respiratory tract or impairment of the mechanics of respiration. In the following discussion, we present the common pediatric respiratory emergencies based on the part of the airway they most affect.

Upper Airway Obstruction

Obstruction of the upper airway can be caused by many factors. As previously mentioned, upper airway obstruction may be partial or complete. It can be caused by inflamed or swollen tissues resulting from infection or by an aspirated foreign body. Appropriate care depends on prompt and immediate identification of the disorder and its severity. Whenever you find an infant, toddler, or young child in respiratory or cardiac arrest, assume complete upper airway obstruction until proven otherwise.

CROUP Croup, medically referred to as *laryngotracheobronchitis,* is a viral infection of the upper airway. It most commonly occurs in children six months to four years of age and is prevalent in the fall and winter. Croup causes an inflammation of the upper respiratory tract involving the subglottic region. The infection leads to edema beneath the glottis and larynx, thus narrowing the lumen of the airway. Severe cases of croup can lead to complete airway obstruction. Another form of croup, called *spasmodic croup,* occurs mostly in the middle of the night without any prior upper respiratory infection.

CONTENT REVIEW

➤ Common Causes of Upper Airway Obstructions
- Croup
- Epiglottitis
- Bacterial tracheitis
- Foreign body aspiration

Table 4-12 Symptoms of Croup and Epiglottitis

Croup	Epiglottitis
Slow onset	Rapid onset
Generally wants to sit up	Prefers to sit up
Barking cough	No barking cough
No drooling	Drooling; painful to swallow
Fever approximately 101°F–102°F (38.3°C–38.9°C)	Fever approximately 102°F–104°F (38.9°C–40.0°C)
	Occasional stridor

Assessment The history for croup is fairly classic. Often, the child will have a mild cold or other infection and be doing fairly well until evening. After dark, however, a harsh, barking, or brassy cough develops. The attack may subside in a few hours but can persist for several nights.

The physical exam will often reveal inspiratory stridor. There may be associated nasal flaring, tracheal tugging, or retraction. You should *never* examine the oropharynx. Often, in the prehospital setting, it is difficult to distinguish croup from epiglottitis (Table 4-12 and Figure 4-28). If epiglottitis is present, examination of the oropharynx may result in laryngospasm and complete airway obstruction. If the attack of croup is severe and progressive, the child may develop restlessness, tachycardia, and cyanosis. Although croup can result in complete airway obstruction and respiratory arrest, this is a rare event.

Management Management of croup consists of appropriate airway maintenance. Place the child in a position of comfort and administer cool mist air or oxygen by facemask or blow-by method. If the attack is severe, the physician may order the administration of racemic epinephrine or albuterol (if racemic epinephrine is not available). Recent studies have shown that standard epinephrine by nebulizer is just as effective as, and in some cases better than, racemic epinephrine in croup.[12] Steroids are recommended for moderate to severe croup because they appear to improve symptoms, shorten the course of the illness, and decrease hospitalizations.

In preparing the patient for transport, remember that the journey from the house to the ambulance will often allow the child to breathe cool air. Because cool air causes a decrease in subglottic edema, the child may be clinically improved by the time you reach the ambulance. If appropriate, keep the parent or caregiver with the infant or child. Do not agitate the patient, which could worsen the croup, by administering nonessential measures such as IVs or blood pressure readings.

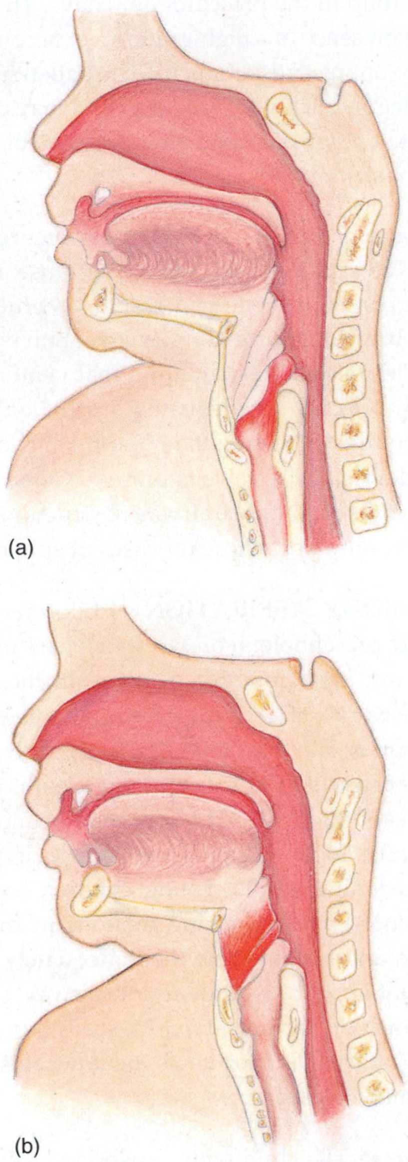

FIGURE 4-28 (a) Epiglottitis is characterized by inflammation of the epiglottis and supraglottic tissues. (b) Croup is characterized by subglottic edema.

EPIGLOTTITIS **Epiglottitis** is an acute infection and inflammation of the epiglottis and is potentially life threatening. (Recall that the epiglottis is a flap of cartilage that protects the airway during swallowing.) Epiglottitis, unlike croup, is caused by a bacterial infection, usually *Haemophilus influenzae* type B. As a result of the availability of *H. influenzae* vaccination, epiglottitis has become an uncommon occurrence. When it does occur, it tends to strike children three to seven years old.

Assessment Epiglottitis presents similarly to croup. Often, the child will go to bed feeling relatively well, usually with what parents or caregivers consider to be a mild infection of the respiratory tract. Later, the child awakens with a high temperature and a brassy cough. The progression of symptoms can be dramatic. There is often pain on swallowing, sore throat, high fever, shallow breathing, dyspnea, inspiratory stridor, and drooling (Figure 4-29).

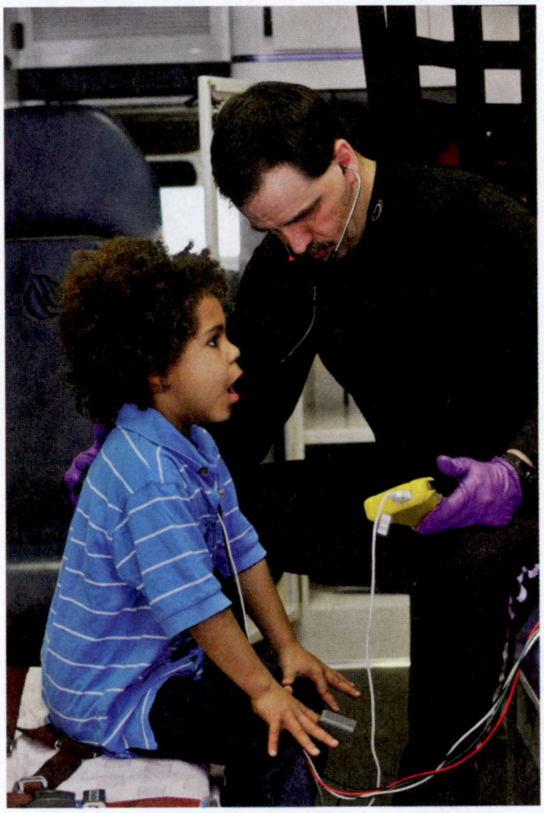

FIGURE 4-29 Posturing of the child with epiglottitis.

On physical examination, the child will appear acutely ill and agitated. *Never attempt to visualize the airway.* If the child is crying, the tip of the epiglottis can be seen posterior to the base of the tongue. In epiglottitis, the epiglottis is cherry red and swollen. As airway obstruction develops, the child will exhibit retractions, nasal flaring, and pulmonary hyperexpansion. As the epiglottis swells, he may not be able to swallow his saliva and will begin to drool. Often the child will want to remain seated. Patients will often assume the "tripod position" to help maximize their airway. If they lean backward or lie flat, the epiglottis can fall back and completely obstruct the airway.

Management Management of epiglottitis consists of appropriate airway maintenance and oxygen administration by facemask (Figure 4-30) or the blow-by technique. Ideally, the oxygen should be humidified to minimize drying of the epiglottis and airway. To reduce the child's anxiety, you might ask the parent or caregiver to administer the oxygen. If the airway becomes obstructed, two-rescuer ventilation with BVM is almost always effective. Make sure that all intubation equipment is available, including an appropriately sized endotracheal tube. Remember, however, that intubation is contraindicated unless complete obstruction has occurred.

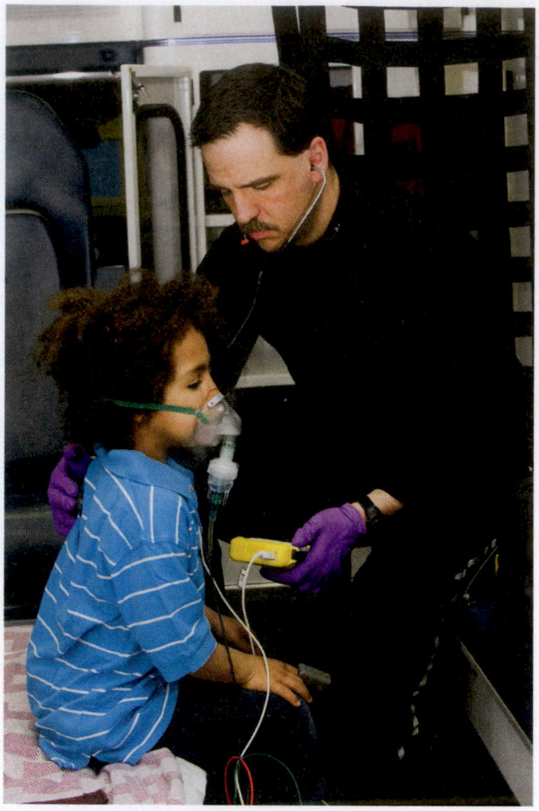

FIGURE 4-30 The child with epiglottitis should be administered humidified oxygen and transported in a comfortable position.

Also, do not intubate in settings with short transport times. If endotracheal intubation is required, it may be necessary to use a smaller endotracheal tube because of narrowing of the glottic opening. If you perform chest compression upon glottic visualization during intubation, a bubble at the tracheal opening may form. This may help to establish upper airway landmarks that are distorted by the disease. As a last resort, consider needle cricothyrotomy per medical direction.

Pediatric patients with epiglottitis require immediate transport. Handle the child gently, as stress could lead to total airway obstruction from spasms of the larynx and swelling tissues. Avoid IV sticks, do not take a blood pressure, and do not attempt to look into the mouth. During transport, reassure and comfort the child. Constantly monitor the child, and notify the hospital of any changes in status. Remember, if the patient is maintaining his airway, *do not put anything in the child's mouth*, including a thermometer. Always consider epiglottitis a critical condition.

BACTERIAL TRACHEITIS **Bacterial tracheitis** is a bacterial infection of the airway in the subglottic region. Although the condition is very uncommon, it is most likely to appear following episodes of viral croup. It afflicts mainly infants and toddlers one to five years of age.

Assessment In assessing this condition, parents or caregivers will typically report that the child has experienced an episode of croup in the preceding few days. They will also indicate the presence of a high-grade fever accompanied by coughing up of pus and/or mucus. The patient may exhibit a hoarse voice and, if able to talk, the child may complain of a sore throat. A physical examination may reveal inspiratory or expiratory stridor.

Management As with all respiratory emergencies, the child must be carefully monitored, because respiratory failure or arrest may be an end result. Carefully manage airway and breathing, providing oxygenation by facemask or blow-by technique. Keep in mind that ventilations may require high pressure to adequately ventilate the patient. This may require depressing the pop-off valve of the pediatric BVM device, if the valve is present. Consider intubation only in cases of complete airway obstruction. Transport guidelines are similar to those for cases of epiglottitis.

FOREIGN BODY ASPIRATION Children—especially toddlers and preschoolers, one to four years old—like to put objects into their mouths. As a result, these children are at increased risk of aspirating foreign bodies, especially when they run or fall. In fact, foreign body aspiration is the number-one cause of in-home accidental deaths in children under six years of age. In addition, many children choke on, or aspirate, food given to them by their parents or other well-meaning adults. Young children have not yet developed coordinated chewing motions in their mouth and pharynx and cannot chew food adequately. Common foods associated with aspiration and airway obstruction in children include hard candy, nuts, seeds, hot dogs, sausages, and grapes. Nonfood items include coins, balloons, and other small objects.

Assessment The child with a suspected aspirated foreign body may present in one of two ways. If the obstruction is complete, the child will have minimal or no air movement. If the obstruction is partial, the child may exhibit inspiratory stridor, a muffled or hoarse voice, drooling, pain in the throat, retractions, and cyanosis.

Management Whenever you suspect that a child has aspirated a foreign body, immediately assess the patient's respiratory efforts. If the obstruction is partial, make the child as comfortable as possible and administer humidified oxygen. If the child is old enough, place him in a sitting position. Do not attempt to look in the mouth. Intubation equipment should be readily available because complete airway obstruction can occur. Transport the child to a hospital, where the foreign body can be removed by hospital personnel in a controlled environment.

If the obstruction is complete, clear the airway with accepted basic life support techniques. Sweep visible obstructions with your gloved finger. Do not perform blind finger sweeps, because this can push a foreign body deeper into the airway. Following BLS foreign body removal procedures, attempt ventilation with a BVM. If unsuccessful, visualize the airway with a laryngoscope. If the foreign body is seen and readily accessible, try to remove it with Magill forceps. Intubate if possible. Continue BLS foreign body removal procedures. If the airway cannot be cleared by routine measures, consider needle cricothyrotomy per medical direction and only as a last resort. Transport following appropriate guidelines, avoiding further agitation of the child.

Lower Airway Distress

As already discussed, suspect lower airway distress when the following conditions exist: an absence of stridor, presence of wheezing during exhalation, and increased work of breathing. Common causes of lower airway distress include respiratory diseases such as asthma, bronchiolitis, and pneumonia. Although infrequent, you may also encounter cases of foreign body lower airway aspiration, especially in toddlers and preschoolers.

ASTHMA **Asthma** is a chronic inflammatory disorder of the lower respiratory tract. The disease affects more than 6 million Americans. It occurs before age 10 in approximately 50 percent of the cases, and before age 30 in another 33 percent of cases. The disease tends to run in families. It is also commonly associated with atopic conditions, such as eczema and allergies. Although deaths from other respiratory conditions have been declining steadily, asthmatic deaths have risen significantly in recent decades. Hospitalization of children for treatment of asthma has increased by more than 200 percent during the past 20 years. Because children can readily succumb to asthma, prompt prehospital recognition and treatment are essential.[13]

Pathophysiology Asthma is a chronic inflammatory disorder of the airways, characterized by bronchospasm and excessive mucus production. In susceptible children, this inflammation causes widespread, but variable, airflow obstruction. In addition to airflow obstruction, the airways become hyperresponsive.

Asthma may be induced by one of many different factors, commonly called *triggers*. The triggers vary from one child to the next. Common triggers include environmental allergens, cold air, exercise, foods, irritants, emotional stress, and certain medications.

CONTENT REVIEW

➤ Asthma Triggers
- Environmental allergens
- Cold air
- Exercise
- Foods
- Irritants
- Emotional stress
- Certain medications

Within minutes of exposure to the trigger, a two-phase reaction occurs. The first phase of the reaction is characterized by the release of chemical mediators such as histamine. These cause bronchoconstriction and bronchial edema that effectively decrease expiratory airflow, causing the classic "asthma attack." If treated early, asthma may respond to inhaled bronchodilators. If the attack is not aborted, or does not resolve spontaneously, a second phase may occur. The second phase is characterized by inflammation of the bronchioles as cells of the immune system invade the respiratory tract. This causes additional edema and further decreases expiratory airflow. The second phase is typically unresponsive to inhaled bronchodilators. Instead, anti-inflammatory agents, such as corticosteroids, are often required.

As the attack continues, and swelling of the mucous membranes lining the bronchioles worsens, there may be plugging of the bronchi by thick mucus. This further obstructs airflow. As a result, sputum production increases. In addition, the lungs become progressively hyperinflated, because airflow is more restricted in exhalation. This effectively reduces vital capacity and results in decreased gas exchange by the alveoli, resulting in hypoxemia. If allowed to progress untreated, hypoxemia will worsen, and unconsciousness and death may ensue.

Assessment Asthma can often be differentiated from other pediatric respiratory illnesses by the history. In many cases, there is a prior history of asthma or reactive airway disease. The child's medications may also be an indicator. Children with asthma often have an inhaler or a nebulized beta-agonist preparation.

On physical examination, the child is usually sitting up, leaning forward, and tachypneic. Often, there is an associated unproductive cough. Accessory respiratory muscle usage is usually evident. Wheezing may be heard. However, in a severe attack, the patient may not wheeze at all. This is an ominous finding. Some children will not wheeze, but will cough, often continuously. Generally there is associated tachycardia; this should be monitored, as virtually all medications used to treat asthma increase the heart rate. Pulse oximetry and capnography can help assess the severity of asthma and guide treatment.

Management The primary therapeutic goals in the asthmatic patient are to correct hypoxia, reverse bronchospasm, and decrease inflammation. First, it is imperative that you establish an airway. Next, administer supplemental, humidified oxygen as necessary to correct hypoxia. Initial pharmacological therapy is the administration of an inhaled beta agonist (Figure 4-31). All paramedic units should have the capability of administering nebulized bronchodilator medications such as albuterol, metaproterenol, or levalbuterol. Alternatively, a metered-dose inhaler (MDI) may be used. If the transport time is prolonged, the medical direction physician may also request administration of a steroid preparation.

Status Asthmaticus *Status asthmaticus* is defined as a severe, prolonged asthma attack that cannot be broken by

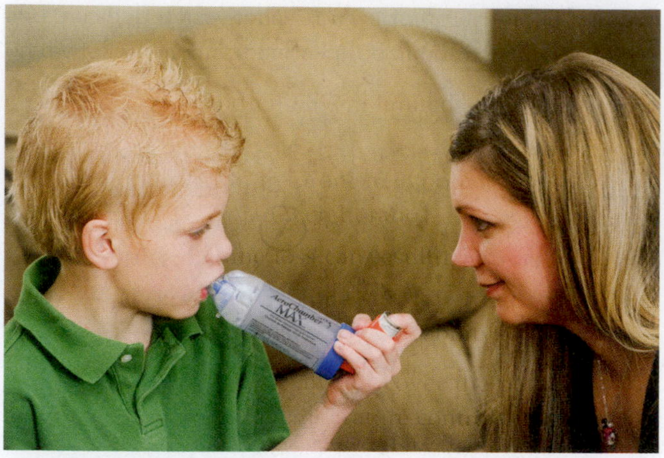

FIGURE 4-31 The young asthma patient may be making use of a prescribed inhaler to relieve symptoms.

aggressive pharmacological management. This is a serious medical emergency; prompt recognition, treatment, and transport are required. Often, the child suffering status asthmaticus will have a greatly distended chest from continued air trapping. Breath sounds, and often wheezing, may be absent. The patient is usually exhausted, severely acidotic, and often dehydrated. The management of status asthmaticus is basically the same as for asthma. However, you should recognize that respiratory arrest is imminent and remain prepared for endotracheal intubation. Transport should be immediate, with aggressive treatment continued en route.

BRONCHIOLITIS **Bronchiolitis** is a respiratory infection of the medium-sized airways—the bronchioles—that occurs in early childhood. It should not be confused with bronchitis, which is an infection of the larger bronchi. Bronchiolitis is caused by a viral infection, most commonly *respiratory syncytial virus* (RSV) that affects the lining of the bronchioles.

Bronchiolitis is characterized by prominent expiratory wheezing and clinically resembles asthma. It most commonly occurs in winter in children less than two years of age. Bronchiolitis often spreads quickly through day care and preschool facilities. Most children will develop lifelong immunity to RSV following infection. The exception is the very young infant who has an immature immune system.

Assessment A history is necessary to distinguish bronchiolitis from asthma. Often, with bronchiolitis, there is a family history of asthma or allergies, although neither is yet present in the child. In addition, a low-grade fever often exists. A major distinguishing factor is age. Asthma rarely occurs before the age of one year, whereas bronchiolitis is more frequent in this age group.

Your physical examination should be systematic. Pay particular attention to the presence of crackles or wheezes. In addition, note any evidence of infection or respiratory distress.

Management Prehospital management of suspected bronchiolitis is much the same as with asthma. Place the child in a semisitting position, if old enough, and administer humidified oxygen by mask or blow-by method. Ventilations should be supported as necessary. Equipment for intubation should be readily available. If respiratory distress is present, consider administration of a bronchodilator such as albuterol (Ventolin, Proventil) by small-volume nebulizer. The cardiac rhythm should be monitored constantly. Pulse oximetry, if available, should be used continuously. Remember that nasal suctioning in an infant can significantly improve respiratory distress.

PNEUMONIA Pneumonia is an infection of the lower airway and lungs. Either a bacterium or a virus may cause it. Pneumonia can occur at any age, but in pediatric patients, it most commonly appears in infants, toddlers, and preschoolers aged one to five years. Most cases of pneumonia in children are viral and self-limited. As children get older, they can contract bacterial pneumonias as adults do. A pneumonia vaccine is available for children and is highly effective. Pneumococcal conjugate vaccine (PCV13) is recommended for all children less than 5 years of age and for selected people 6 years of age and older that are at increased risk of pneumopcoccal disease. These include patients with an immune system problem or who are asplenic (lacking a spleen).

Assessment Persons with pneumonia often have a history of a respiratory infection, such as a severe cold or bronchitis. Signs and symptoms include a low-grade fever, decreased breath sounds, crackles, rhonchi, and pain in the chest area. Some children may present with increased respiratory rates, whereas others may initially present only with a tachycardia. Conduct a systematic assessment of a patient with suspected pneumonia, paying particular attention to evidence of respiratory distress.

Management Prehospital management of pneumonia is supportive. Place the patient in a position of comfort. Ensure a patent airway and administer supplemental oxygen via a nonrebreather device. If respiratory failure is present, support ventilations with a BVM device. If prolonged ventilation will be required, perform endotracheal intubation. Transport the patient in a position of comfort. Provide emotional and psychological support to the parents.

FOREIGN BODY LOWER AIRWAY OBSTRUCTION The same pediatric patients that are at risk from upper airway obstruction are at risk for lower airway obstruction. A foreign body can enter the lower airway if it is too small to lodge in the upper airway. The object is often food (nuts, seeds, candy), small toys, or parts of toys. The child will take a deep breath or will fall and accidentally aspirate the foreign body. The foreign body will fall into the lower airway until it reaches the airway area that is smaller than the foreign body. Depending on positioning, the foreign body can act as a one-way valve and either trap air in distal lung tissues or prevent aeration of distal lung tissues, causing a ventilation/perfusion mismatch.

Assessment The history often includes information about the child having a foreign body in the mouth and then the object suddenly disappears. The parents may be unsure whether the child swallowed it, aspirated it, or simply lost the object. If the object is fairly large and aspirated, then respiratory distress may be present. There is often considerable, often intractable, coughing. The child will be anxious and may have diminished breath sounds in the part of the chest affected by the foreign body. There may be crackles or rhonchi, usually unilateral. In some cases, there may be unilateral wheezing where some air is getting past the object. Unilateral wheezing should be considered to be due to an aspirated foreign body until proven otherwise.

Management The management of an aspirated foreign body is supportive. Place the child in a position of comfort and avoid agitation. Provide supplemental oxygen. Transport the child to a facility that has the capability of performing pediatric fiber-optic bronchoscopy. The bronchoscope can be used to visualize the airway and remove any foreign objects detected.

Shock (Hypoperfusion)

The second major cause of pediatric cardiopulmonary arrest—after respiratory impairment—is shock. Shock can most simply be defined as inadequate perfusion of the tissues with oxygen and other essential nutrients and inadequate removal of metabolic waste products. This ultimately results in tissue hypoxia and metabolic acidosis. Ultimately, if untreated, cellular death will occur.

When compared with the incidence of shock in adults, shock is an unusual occurrence in children because their blood vessels constrict so efficiently. However, when blood pressure does drop, it drops so far and so fast that the child may quickly develop cardiopulmonary arrest. A number of factors place infants and young children at risk of shock. As mentioned in the "Neonatology" chapter, newborns and neonates can develop shock as a result of loss of body heat. Other causes include dehydration (from vomiting and/or diarrhea), infection (particularly septicemia), trauma (especially from abdominal injuries), and blood loss. Less common causes of shock in infants and children include allergic reactions, poisoning, and cardiac events (rare).

CONTENT REVIEW

➤ Predisposing Factors of Pediatric Shock
- Hypothermia
- Dehydration (vomiting, diarrhea)
- Infection
- Trauma
- Blood loss
- Allergic reactions
- Poisoning
- Cardiac events (rare)

The definitive care of shock takes place in the emergency department of a hospital. Because shock is a life-threatening condition in pediatric patients, it is important to recognize early signs and symptoms—or even the possibility of shock in a situation when signs and symptoms have not yet developed. If you suspect a possibility of shock, provide oxygen to boost tissue perfusion and transport as quickly as possible. Also, keep the patient in a supine position and take steps to protect the child from hypothermia and agitation that might worsen the condition.

Severity of Shock

Shock is classified by degrees of severity as compensated, decompensated, and irreversible. The child responds to decreased perfusion by increasing heart rate and by increasing peripheral vascular resistance. The child has very little capacity to increase stroke volume. The key to early identification of shock is detecting the subtle signs that result from the body's various compensatory mechanisms.

COMPENSATED SHOCK Early shock is known as *compensated shock* because the body is able to compensate for decreased tissue perfusion through various physiologic mechanisms. In compensated shock, the patient exhibits a normal blood pressure. The signs and symptoms of compensated shock include:

- Irritability or anxiety
- Tachycardia
- Tachypnea
- Weak peripheral pulses, full central pulses
- Delayed capillary refill (more than 2 seconds in children less than 6 years of age)
- Cool, pale extremities
- Systolic blood pressure within normal limits
- Decreased urinary output

Compensated shock is generally reversible if appropriate treatment measures are instituted. Again, the key to a good outcome is prompt detection of the early signs and symptoms and initiation of therapy based on this. Management is directed at correcting the underlying problem. High-concentration oxygen should be administered and venous access obtained. If the patient is hypovolemic, then fluid replacement should be initiated. If the cause is cardiogenic, then medications should be administered to support cardiac output and increase peripheral vascular resistance. Sometimes definitive care of shock is surgical. However, in these cases, fluid therapy and oxygen administration will help buy time until the patient can be taken to surgery.

DECOMPENSATED SHOCK *Decompensated shock* develops when the body can no longer compensate for decreased tissue perfusion. The hallmark of decompensated shock is a fall in blood pressure (an ominous sign in children). This results in hypoperfusion and inadequate end-organ perfusion. It is important to remember that a child's compensatory mechanisms are quite efficient. Thus, when a child develops decompensated shock, a significant loss of fluid or a significant impairment of cardiac output has occurred. The signs and symptoms of decompensated shock (Figure 4-32) include:

- Lethargy or coma
- Marked tachycardia or bradycardia
- Absent peripheral pulses, weak central pulses
- Markedly delayed capillary refill
- Cool, pale, dusky, mottled extremities
- Hypotension
- Markedly decreased urinary output
- Absence of tears

Decompensated shock can become irreversible if aggressive treatment measures are not undertaken. In some cases, it may be irreversible despite the fact that aggressive treatment measures have been provided. Management is directed at treatment of the underlying cause. You should have a low threshold for initiating mechanical ventilation with a BVM device and 100 percent oxygen. Consider intubating the patient if mechanical ventilation will be prolonged.

IRREVERSIBLE SHOCK *Irreversible shock* occurs when treatment measures are inadequate or too late to prevent significant tissue damage and death. Sometimes, blood pressure and pulse can be restored. However, the patient later succumbs as a result of organ failure. The best treatment for irreversible shock is prevention.

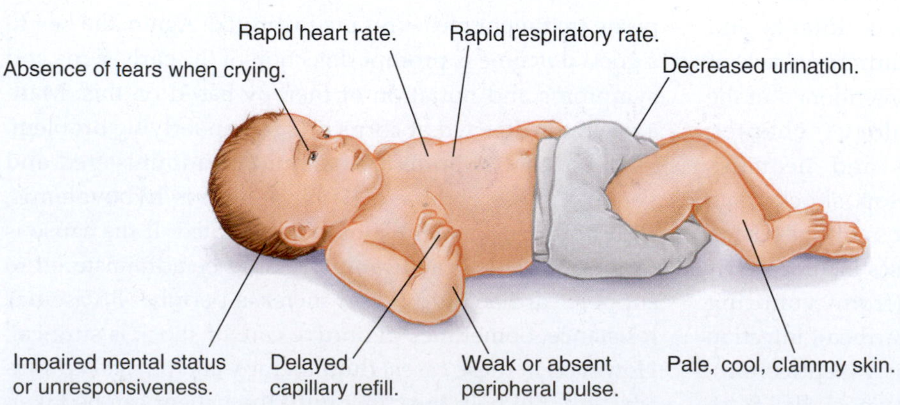

FIGURE 4-32 Signs and symptoms of shock (hypoperfusion) in a child.

Categories of Shock

Shock can be categorized in a number of ways. Shock can be categorized as *cardiogenic* (caused by impaired pumping power of the heart), *hypovolemic* (caused by decreased blood or water volume), *obstructive* (caused by an obstruction that interferes with the return of blood to the heart, such as a pulmonary embolism, cardiac tamponade, or tension pneumothorax), and *distributive* (caused by abnormal distribution and return of blood resulting from vasodilation, vasopermeability, or both, as in septic, anaphylactic, or neurogenic shock).

Often, shock is classified into two general categories: cardiogenic and noncardiogenic. As noted earlier, **cardiogenic shock** results from an inability of the heart to maintain an adequate cardiac output to the circulatory system and tissues. Cardiogenic shock in a pediatric patient is ominous and often fatal. **Noncardiogenic shock** includes types of shock that result from causes other than inadequate cardiac output. Causes may include hemorrhage, abdominal trauma, systemic bacterial infection, spinal cord injury, and others. In the following sections we first discuss types of noncardiogenic shock, then cardiogenic shock.

Noncardiogenic Shock

Noncardiogenic shock is more frequently encountered in prehospital pediatric care than cardiogenic shock. (Recall that children have a much lower incidence of cardiac problems than adults do.) The forms that you will most commonly assess and manage are hypovolemic and distributive shock. (See also the discussion of metabolic problems in children later in the chapter.)

HYPOVOLEMIC SHOCK **Hypovolemic shock** results from loss of intravascular fluids. In pediatric patients, the most common causes include severe dehydration from vomiting and/or diarrhea and blood loss, usually as a result of trauma. Trauma may include blood loss into a body cavity (particularly the abdomen) or frank external hemorrhage. Children are also at risk of fluid loss as a result of burns, the second leading cause of pediatric deaths in the United States.

Treatment of hypovolemic shock involves administration of supplemental oxygen and establishment of intravenous access. This should be followed by a 20 mL/kg bolus of lactated Ringer's or normal saline. Following the bolus, the child should be reassessed. If signs and symptoms of compensated shock still exist, then administer a second bolus. Some children may require 80 to 100 mL/kg of fluid, depending on the volume of fluid lost.

DISTRIBUTIVE SHOCK **Distributive shock** presents with a marked decrease in peripheral vascular resistance, usually owing to a loss of vasomotor tone. In pediatric patients, causes include sepsis from bacterial infection, anaphylactic reaction, and damage to the brain and/or spinal cord. Cardiac output and fluid volume are adequate.

Septic Shock This condition is caused by sepsis, an infection of the bloodstream by some pathogen, usually bacterial. Sepsis commonly occurs as a complication of an infection at some other site, such as pneumonia, meningitis, or a urinary tract infection. Meningitis is frequently associated with sepsis. The etiology can be varied, as can be the signs and symptoms.

The septic child is critically ill. Septic shock may develop when the pathogen causing the infection releases deadly toxins. These toxins cause peripheral vasodilation, leading to a drop in blood pressure and decreased tissue perfusion. Sepsis can be rapidly fatal if not promptly identified and treated.

Signs of sepsis include:

- Ill appearance
- Irritability or altered mental status
- Fever
- Vomiting and diarrhea
- Cyanosis, pallor, or mottled skin
- Nonspecific respiratory distress
- Poor feeding

Signs and symptoms of septic shock include:

- Very ill appearance
- Altered mental status
- Tachycardia
- Capillary refill time greater than 2 seconds
- Hyperventilation, leading to respiratory failure
- Cool and clammy skin
- Inability of child to recognize parents
- Acidosis (elevated lactate) and/or increasing CO_2 levels

Your goal in treating sepsis is to prevent the development of septic shock. Supplemental oxygen should be administered and intravenous access obtained. Administer a 20 mL/kg bolus of lactated Ringer's or normal saline. Consider initiating pressor therapy with epinephrine or dopamine. Begin at the designated starting dose and gradually increase the dose until the blood pressure improves or there is evidence of improved end-organ perfusion. Definitive treatment includes antibiotics and other therapy. Transport should be rapid, with care provided en route.

Anaphylactic Shock Anaphylactic shock results from exposure to an antigen to which the patient has been previously exposed. Milder cases may simply result in an allergic reaction. More severe reactions can impair tissue perfusion. This occurs primarily as a result of the release of histamine and other similar chemicals. Histamine causes peripheral vasodilation and leakage of fluid from the intravascular space into the interstitial space. Anaphylactic shock can be differentiated from a severe allergic reaction by the presence of signs and symptoms of impaired end-organ perfusion. These include:

- Tachycardia
- Tachypnea
- Wheezing
- Urticaria (hives)
- Anxiousness
- Edema
- Hypotension

Treatment of a severe allergic reaction includes administration of intramuscular epinephrine 1:1,000 and an antihistamine. Treatment of anaphylactic shock includes supplemental oxygen administration and intravenous access. If the patient is exhibiting decompensated shock, administer epinephrine 1:10,000 intravenously and diphenhydramine (Benadryl) intravenously. Patients not exhibiting hypotension may be given an initial dose of epinephrine intramuscularly. If this does not rapidly improve the situation, then an intravenous dose of epinephrine should be considered. Contact medical direction for additional assistance. EMS systems with long transport times may be asked to administer an initial dose of a corticosteroid such as methylprednisolone (Solu-Medrol).

Neurogenic Shock Neurogenic shock is due to sudden peripheral vasodilation resulting from interruption of nervous control of the peripheral vascular system. The most common cause is injury to the spinal cord. Cardiac output and intravascular fluid volume are usually adequate.

Treatment is directed at increasing peripheral vascular resistance. This is accomplished primarily through administration of a pressor agent such as dopamine. Care should also include stabilization of the injury and administration of supplemental oxygen (if the patient is hypoxic).

Cardiogenic Shock

Cardiogenic shock results from inadequate cardiac output. In children, cardiogenic shock usually results from a secondary cause such as near drowning or a toxic ingestion. Children, unlike adults, rarely have primary cardiac disease. The exceptions are congenital heart disease and cardiomyopathy.

Congenital heart disease is an abnormality or defect in the heart that is present at birth. Many congenital cardiac problems are detected at birth. However, some may not be detected until later in life. Cardiomyopathy causes a decrease in cardiac output owing to impairment of cardiac muscle contraction. Arrhythmias, although rare in children, can cause a decrease in cardiac output. Rapid arrhythmias may impair ventricular filling and thus cause a decrease in cardiac output. Likewise, slow arrhythmias may cause decreased cardiac output simply because of their slow rate.

In the following sections we discuss in more detail congenital heart disease, cardiomyopathy, and arrhythmias, which, as noted, are primary causes of pediatric cardiogenic shock. Remember, however, that cardiogenic shock in children most often results from secondary causes.

Congenital Heart Disease

Congenital heart disease is the primary cause of heart disease in children. As noted earlier, although most congenital heart problems are detected at birth, some problems may not be discovered until later in childhood. A common symptom of congenital heart disease is cyanosis. This occurs when blood going to the lungs for oxygenation mixes with blood bound for other parts of the body. This may result from holes in the internal walls of the heart or from abnormalities of the great vessels.

The child with congenital heart disease may develop respiratory distress, congestive heart failure, or a "cyanotic spell." *Cyanotic spells* occur when oxygen demand exceeds that provided by the blood. They begin as irritability, inconsolable crying or altered mental status, and progressive cyanosis in conjunction with severe dyspnea. In severe and prolonged cases, seizures, coma, or cardiac arrest may result. Noncyanotic problems associated with congenital heart disease include respiratory distress, tachycardia, decreased end-organ perfusion, drowsiness, fatigue, and pallor.

Treatment includes the standard primary assessment. Administer high-concentration oxygen. If necessary, provide ventilatory support. If the patient is having a cyanotic spell, place the child in the knee–chest position facing downward or, in an older child, have him squat. This will help increase the cardiac return. Apply the ECG monitor, and start an intravenous line at a keep-open rate. Transport immediately.

Cardiomyopathy

Cardiomyopathy is a disease or dysfunction of the cardiac muscle. Although fairly rare, cardiomyopathy can result from congenital heart disease or infection. A frequent cause of infectious cardiomyopathy is *Coxsackie* virus. Cardiomyopathy causes mechanical pump failure, which is usually biventricular. It often develops slowly and is not detectable until heart failure develops.

The signs and symptoms of cardiomyopathy include early fatigue, crackles, jugular venous distention, engorgement of the liver, and peripheral edema. Later, as the disease progresses, the signs and symptoms of shock can develop.

The prehospital treatment of cardiomyopathy is supportive. Supplemental oxygen should be administered via a nonrebreather mask. Fluids should be restricted. If possible, IV access should be obtained. Severe cases resulting in the development of severe dyspnea should be treated with furosemide and pressor agents (dobutamine, dopamine). The child should be transported to a facility capable of managing critically ill children. Most cases of cardiomyopathy are managed with medication. Definitive care in severe cases may include cardiac transplantation.

Arrhythmias

Arrhythmias in children are uncommon. When arrhythmias occur, bradyarrhythmias are the most common. Supraventricular tachyarrhythmias are uncommon and ventricular tachyarrhythmias are very uncommon. Arrhythmias can cause pump failure, ultimately leading to cardiogenic shock. Children have a very limited capacity to increase stroke volume. The primary mechanism through which they increase cardiac output is through changes in the heart rate. The treatment of arrhythmias is specific for the arrhythmia in question.

TACHYARRHYTHMIAS Tachyarrhythmias are arrhythmias in which the heart rate is greater than the estimated maximum normal heart rate for the child. These can result from primary cardiac disease or from secondary causes. Tachyarrhythmias from any cause are relatively uncommon in children.

Supraventricular Tachycardia True supraventricular tachycardia (SVT) is a narrow-complex tachycardia (QRS # 0.09 second) with a heart rate typically of 220 beats per minute or greater. SVT is usually caused by a problem in the cardiac conductive system. Rarely, it can be the result of a secondary cause, such as drug ingestion. It is occasionally seen in infants with no prior history. The cause is uncertain but may be due to immaturity of the cardiac conductive system. Rapid heart rates often do not allow time for adequate cardiac filling, eventually causing congestive heart failure and cardiogenic shock.

The signs and symptoms of supraventricular tachycardia include irritability, poor feeding, jugular venous distention, hepatomegaly (enlarged liver), and hypotension. The ECG will show a narrow-complex (supraventricular) tachycardia with a rate greater than 220 beats per minute. Children can often tolerate the rapid rate well.

Prehospital treatment of supraventricular tachycardia depends on the clinical findings. Children who are tolerating the heart rate (normal blood pressure) and are stable should receive supplemental oxygen (if they are hypoxic) and transport. Vagal maneuvers may be attempted unless the patient is unstable. In older children, carotid sinus massage or Valsalva maneuvers are safe. Adenosine should be considered if the child is stable. If the child is exhibiting signs of decompensation (hypotension, mental status change, poor skin color), then synchronized cardioversion should be attempted at an initial energy dose of 0.5 to 1.0 joules per kilogram of body weight. This can be increased to 2 joules per kilogram if the initial shock is unsuccessful. Consider amiodarone 5 mg/kg IO/IV or procainamide 15 mg/kg IO/IV for a patient with SVT unresponsive to vagal maneuvers and adenosine and/or electric cardioversion. These medications must be administered slowly with all monitors in place. The child should be transported to the appropriate facility.

Ventricular Tachycardia with a Pulse Ventricular tachycardia (wide-complex tachycardia) and ventricular fibrillation are exceedingly rare in children. They are occasionally seen following submersion/immersion injury or following a prolonged resuscitation attempt. Unlike adults, in whom ventricular tachyarrhythmias result from primary heart disease, ventricular tachyarrhythmias in children are almost always due to a secondary cause. The exception is structural, congenital heart disease.

The signs and symptoms of ventricular tachycardia with a pulse include poor feeding, irritability, and a rapid, wide-complex tachycardia. Children are unable to tolerate this arrhythmia for very long. They soon develop signs of shock.

The prehospital management of ventricular tachycardia with a pulse includes supplemental oxygen and intravenous access. Stable patients who are not hypotensive should be transported. Unstable patients (hypotension) should be treated aggressively. Initially, amiodarone, procainamide, or lidocaine should be administered. However, ventricular tachycardia due to structural heart disease often does not respond to antiarrhythmic drugs.

- ***Stable children with wide-complex tachycardia.*** Adenosine may be used to help distinguish supraventricular tachycardia from ventricular tachycardia (if the rhythm is regular and monomorphic). It may also convert supraventricular rhythms. Electrical cardioversion at 0.5 to 1.0 J/kg should be considered. This can be increased to 2 J/kg if needed. Pharmacological therapy should be considered (amiodarone or procainamide).
- ***Unstable children with wide-complex tachycardia.*** Electrical cardioversion at 0.5 to 1.0 J/kg should be considered. This can be increased to 2 J/kg if needed.

BRADYARRHYTHMIAS Bradyarrhythmias are the most common type of pediatric arrhythmia. They most frequently result from hypoxia. Although rare, they can also result from vagal stimulation from such causes as marked gastric distention.

The signs and symptoms of bradycardia include a slow (usually less than 60 beats per minute), narrow-complex rhythm. The child may be lethargic, or exhibiting early signs of congestive heart failure.

- ***Stable children with bradyarrhythmias.*** Stable children with bradyarrhythmias should receive supportive care that addresses ventilation and oxygenation. If the heart rate falls below 60 beats per minute they should be considered unstable.
- ***Unstable children with bradyarrhythmias.*** Likewise, unstable children (hypotension, altered mental status, signs of shock) should be ventilated with a BVM unit and 100 percent oxygen. If the heart rate does not increase readily, consider epinephrine IV or IO. Atropine may be used for suspected increased vagal tone of primary AV block. If pulseless arrest develops, perform chest compressions. If necessary, consider epinephrine or atropine down the endotracheal tube until intravenous or intraosseous access can be obtained. Transport rapidly with care provided en route.[10]

PULSELESS ARREST The absence of a cardiac rhythm is an ominous finding (Figure 4-33). Most cases are asystole. However, some cases may be a very fine ventricular fibrillation. If necessary, turn up the gain on the ECG to distinguish between the two.

Asystole Asystole is the absence of a rhythm and may be the initial rhythm seen in cardiopulmonary arrest. (Remember, children rarely develop ventricular fibrillation, which is often the precursor to arrest in adults.) Bradycardias can degenerate to asystole if appropriate intervention is not provided. The mortality rate associated with asystole in children is very high.

The child with asystole is pulseless and apneic. The cardiac rhythm is a straight line that should be confirmed in two leads. It is important to remember that pediatric cardiac arrest, unlike adult cardiac arrest, is often due to a respiratory cause. It is possible to have a return of a normal pulse in the pediatric patient following pulseless electrical activity (PEA) and/or asystole if the respiratory component of resuscitation has been addressed. However, CPR should be initiated, an IV or IO placed, and epinephrine administered every 3 to 5 minutes. The patient should receive an advanced airway and be ventilated with 100 percent oxygen. Chest compressions should be continued. Emergency resuscitative drugs (epinephrine) should be administered through the intraosseous or intravenous routes.[10]

Ventricular Fibrillation/Pulseless Ventricular Tachycardia Ventricular fibrillation and pulseless ventricular tachycardia are functionally the same rhythm. They are uncommon in children. Causes include electrocution and drug overdoses. The mortality rate is very high.

The child with ventricular fibrillation/pulseless ventricular tachycardia will be pulseless and apneic. The ECG will exhibit a wide-complex tachycardia or fibrillation. The

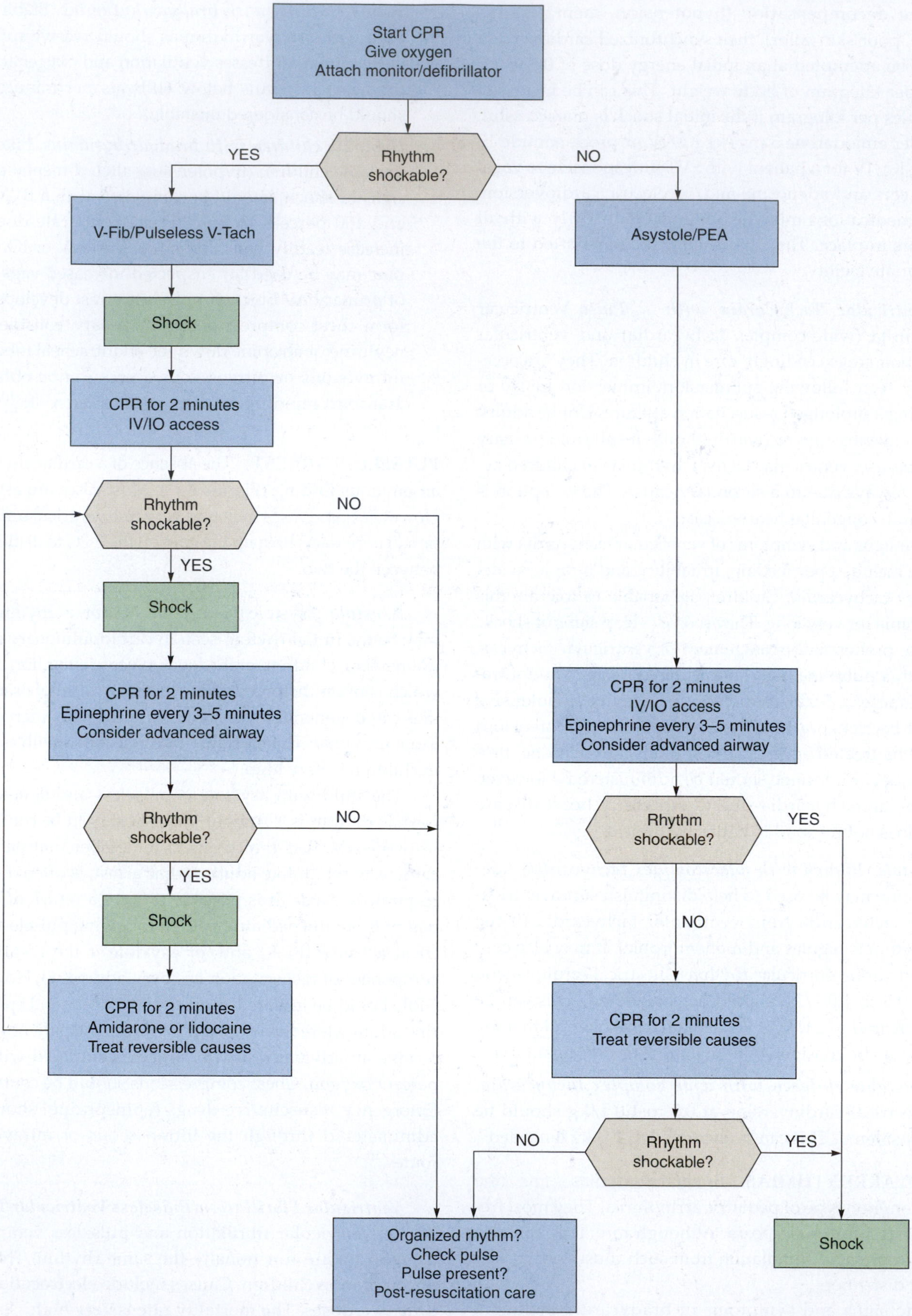

FIGURE 4-33 Pediatric cardiac arrest algorithm.

child should receive uninterrupted CPR for 2 minutes and IV/IO access obtained. After 2 minutes of CPR, the rhythm should be checked. If the patient is shockable, an initial shock of 2 J/kg should be provided and CPR resumed. Epinephrine should be administered every 3 to 5 minutes; an advanced airway should be placed and mechanical ventilation with 100 percent oxygen provided. If the patient remains in a shockable rhythm, the second and subsequent shocks should be at 4 J/kg. Amiodarone or lidocaine should be considered after the second unsuccessful shock. Transport as soon as possible.[10]

Pulseless Electrical Activity Pulseless electrical activity is the presence of a cardiac rhythm without an associated pulse. This is due to noncardiogenic causes such as hypoxia, pericardial tamponade, tension pneumothorax, trauma, acidosis, hypothermia, and hypoglycemia.

The patient with PEA is pulseless and apneic. Resuscitation should be directed toward correcting the underlying cause. Otherwise, treatment is the same as for asystole.[10]

Neurologic Emergencies

Neurologic emergencies in childhood are fairly uncommon. However, seizures can and do occur in children. In fact, they are a frequent reason for summoning EMS. In addition to seizures, meningitis tends to show up more often in children than in adults. Although your chances of encountering either of these two conditions are small, both are life threatening and should be promptly identified and treated.

Seizures

Seizures result from an abnormal discharge of neurons in the brain. Many people suffer seizures; it is a common reason for summoning EMS. People with chronic seizure disorders can often control their seizures with medications. A seizure can be an exceptionally scary event for both the parents and the child. This is especially true if the child has never had a seizure before.

Although the etiology for seizures is often unknown, several risk factors have been identified. They include:

- Fever
- Hypoxia
- Infections
- Idiopathic epilepsy (unknown origin)
- Electrolyte disturbances
- Head trauma
- Hypoglycemia
- Toxic ingestions or exposure
- Tumor
- CNS malformations

Seizures in pediatric patients may be either partial or generalized. (Recall that generalized seizures normally do not occur during the first month of life.) Simple partial seizures, sometimes called *focal motor seizures*, involve sudden jerking of a particular part of the body, such as an arm or a leg. Other characteristics include lip smacking, eye blinking, staring, confusion, and lethargy. There is usually no loss of consciousness. Generalized seizures involve sudden jerking of both sides of the body, followed by tenseness and relaxation of the body. In a generalized seizure, patients typically experience a loss of consciousness.

Keep in mind that children can have **status epilepticus**, a series of one or more generalized seizures, without any intervening periods of consciousness. Status epilepticus is a serious medical emergency because it involves a prolonged period of apnea, which in turn can cause hypoxia of vital brain tissues. The electrical discharges in the brain are harmful as well (see the chapter "Neurology").

Most of the pediatric seizures that you will probably encounter are febrile seizures. **Febrile seizures** are seizures that occur as a result of a sudden increase in body temperature. They occur most commonly between the ages of six months and six years. Often, the parents or caregivers will report the recent onset of fever or cold symptoms. The diagnosis of febrile seizure should not be made in the field. All pediatric patients suffering a seizure must be transported to the hospital so that other etiologies can be excluded.

ASSESSMENT The history is a major factor in determining seizure type. Febrile seizure should be suspected if the temperature is elevated. The history of a previous seizure may suggest idiopathic epilepsy or another CNS problem. However, there is also a tendency for recurrence of febrile seizures in children.

When confronted with a seizing child, determine whether there is a history of seizures or seizures with fever. Has the child had a recent illness? Also, determine how many seizures occurred during the incident. If the child is not seizing on your arrival, elicit a description of the seizure activity. Note the condition and position of the child when found. Question parents, caregivers, or bystanders about the possibility of head injury. A history of irritability or lethargy prior to the seizure may indicate CNS infection. If possible, find out whether the child suffers from diabetes or has recently complained of a headache or a stiff neck. Note any current medications, as well as possible ingestions.

The physical examination should be systematic. Pay particular attention to the adequacy of respirations, the level of consciousness, neurologic evaluation, and signs of injury. Also inspect the child for signs of dehydration. Dehydration may be evidenced by the absence of tears or, in an infant, by the presence of a sunken fontanelle.

MANAGEMENT Management of pediatric seizures is essentially the same as for seizing adults. Place patients on the floor or on the bed. Be sure to lay them on their side, away from the furniture. Do not restrain patients, but take steps to protect them from injury. Maintain the airway, but do not force anything, such as a bite stick, between the teeth. Administer supplemental oxygen if the patient is hypoxic. Then take and record all vital signs. If the patient is febrile, remove excess layers of clothing, while avoiding extreme cooling. If status epilepticus is present, institute the following steps:

- Start an IV of normal saline or lactated Ringer's and perform a glucometer evaluation.
- Administer diazepam or lorazepam as directed.
- Contact medical direction for additional dosing. Diazepam or lorazepam can be administered rectally if an IV cannot be established. Intranasal midazolam may also be considered.
- If the seizure appears to be caused by fever and a long transport time is anticipated, medical direction may request the administration of acetaminophen to lower the fever. Acetaminophen is supplied as an elixir or as suppositories. The dose should be 15 mg/kg body weight.

As mentioned previously, all pediatric patients should be transported. Reassure and support the parents or caregivers, as this is a very stressful and frightening situation for them.[14]

Meningitis

Meningitis is an infection of the meninges, the lining of the brain and spinal cord. Meningitis can result from both bacteria and viruses. Viral meningitis is frequently called *aseptic meningitis,* because an organism cannot be routinely cultured from cerebrospinal fluid (CSF). Aseptic meningitis is generally less severe than bacterial meningitis and is self-limiting. Bacterial meningitis most commonly results from *Streptococcus pneumoniae, Haemophilus influenzae,* and *Neisseria meningitides.* These infections can be rapidly fatal if they are not promptly recognized and treated appropriately.

ASSESSMENT Meningitis is more common in children than in adults. Findings in the history that may suggest meningitis include a child who has been ill for one day to several days, a recent ear or respiratory tract infection, high fever, lethargy or irritability, a severe headache, or a stiff neck. Infants generally do not develop a stiff neck. They will generally become lethargic and will not feed well. Some babies may simply develop a fever.

On physical examination, the child with meningitis will appear very ill. With an infant, the fontanelle may be bulging or full unless accompanied by dehydration. Extreme discomfort with movement, owing to irritability of the meninges, may be present (Figure 4-34).

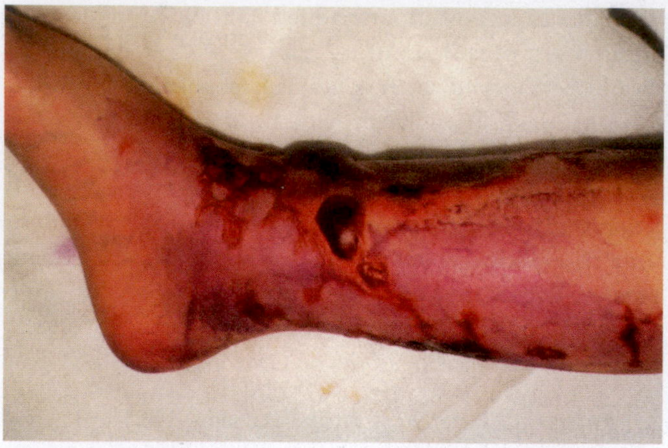

FIGURE 4-34 Petechial rash of meningococcal meningitis.
(Dr. Francois Bricaire/Science Source)

MANAGEMENT Prehospital care of the pediatric patient with meningitis is supportive. Complete the primary assessment rapidly and transport the child to the emergency department. If shock is present, treat the child with intravenous fluids (20 mL/kg) and oxygen.

Gastrointestinal Emergencies

Childhood gastrointestinal problems almost always present with nausea and vomiting as a chief complaint. As a child gets older, other gastrointestinal system emergencies, such as appendicitis, become more common.

Nausea and Vomiting

Nausea and vomiting are not diseases themselves, but are symptoms of other disease processes. Virtually any medical problem can cause these conditions in an infant or child. Common causes include fever, ear infections, and respiratory infections. In addition, many viruses and certain bacteria can infect the gastrointestinal system. These infections, collectively known as *gastroenteritis,* readily cause vomiting, diarrhea, or both.

The biggest risks associated with nausea and vomiting in children are dehydration and electrolyte abnormalities. Infants and toddlers can quickly become dehydrated from bouts of vomiting. If diarrhea or fever is also present, fluid loss is further accelerated, worsening the situation. Dehydration is more difficult to detect in infants and toddlers than in older children. (See Table 4-13 for a description of the signs and symptoms of dehydration.)

Treatment of pediatric nausea and vomiting is primarily supportive. If the child is dehydrated and unable to keep oral fluids down, intravenous fluid therapy may be indicated. Severe dehydration, as evidenced by prolonged capillary refill time, should be treated by 20 mL/kg fluid boluses of lactated Ringer's solution or 0.9 percent sodium chloride solution (normal saline).

Table 4-13 Signs and Symptoms of Dehydration

Signs/Symptoms	Mild	Moderate	Severe
Vital Signs			
Pulse	Normal	Increased	Markedly increased
Respirations	Normal	Increased	Tachypneic
Blood pressure	Normal	Normal	Hypotensive
Capillary refill	Normal	2–3 seconds	>2 seconds
Mental Status	Alert	Irritable	Lethargic
Skin	Normal	Dry and ashen	Dry, cool, mottled
Mucous Membranes	Dry	Very dry	Very dry/no tears

Diarrhea

Diarrhea is a common occurrence in childhood. Often, what parents call diarrhea is actually loose bowel movements. Generally, 10 or more stools per day is considered diarrhea. As with nausea and vomiting, the main concern associated with diarrhea is dehydration. Most diarrhea is caused by viral infections of the gastrointestinal system or arises secondary to infections elsewhere in the body. However, certain bacterial infections can cause significant, even life-threatening, diarrhea.

Treatment of the child suffering from diarrhea is primarily supportive. If dehydration is evident, administer fluids. Oral hydration works quite well. Severe dehydration should be treated with 20 mL/kg boluses of intravenous fluids (lactated Ringer's or normal saline).[15]

Metabolic Emergencies

Metabolic problems are uncommon in children. However, diabetes can occur in very young children. It is rarely diagnosed until the child comes to the hospital in diabetic ketoacidosis. Diabetic children can have great swings in their blood glucose levels owing to diet, growth, and physical activity. Because of this, hypoglycemia and hyperglycemia are possible. It is important to remember that very young children, unlike adults, can develop hypoglycemia without having diabetes. This can occur with severe illnesses such as meningitis, pneumonia, and severe dehydration. The following sections will present the prehospital treatment of pediatric hypoglycemia and hyperglycemia.

Hypoglycemia

Hypoglycemia is an abnormally low concentration of sugar (glucose) in the blood. It is a true medical emergency that must be treated immediately. Without treatment, low blood sugar may progress to unconsciousness and convulsions.

In the prehospital setting, hypoglycemia in pediatric patients usually occurs in newborn infants, children with type 1 diabetes, and children who accidently ingest oral diabetic medications used by parents and grandparents. Diabetic children increase their risk of hypoglycemia through overly strenuous exercise, too much insulin, and dehydration from illness. Nondiabetic children can develop hypoglycemia from physical activity, dietary changes, illness, and growth.

In known diabetics or hypoglycemics, preventive steps include:

- Taking extra snacks for extra activity
- Eating immediately after taking insulin if the blood sugar is less than 100 mg/dL
- Eating regular meals
- Regularly monitoring blood sugar
- Eating an extra snack of carbohydrate and protein if the blood sugar is less than 120 mg/dL at bedtime
- Replacing carbohydrates in the meal plan with things such as regular soda pop or regular popsicles on days when the child is sick

ASSESSMENT Suspect hypoglycemia when the patient exhibits the signs and symptoms listed in Table 4-14. Measure blood glucose with a glucometer and elicit a history of conditions known to cause hypoglycemia in infants and children. Treatment should be initiated whenever you have a high index of suspicion and/or blood sugar drops below 70 mg/dL (≤3.9 mmol/L).

MANAGEMENT As with all patients, continually monitor the ABCs. Be sure to find out whether parents or caregivers have given the patient any glucose tablets, gels,

Table 4-14 Signs and Symptoms of Hypoglycemia

Mild	Moderate	Severe
Hunger	Sweating	Decreased level of consciousness
Weakness	Tremors	Seizure
Tachypnea	Irritability	Tachycardia
Tachycardia	Vomiting	Hypoperfusion
Shakiness	Mood swings	
Yawning	Blurred vision	
Pale skin	Stomachache	
Dizziness	Headache	
	Dizziness	
	Slurred speech	

foods (cake icing, honey, maple syrup, sugar, raisins), or drinks (juice, regular soda pop, milk) to correct the situation. If so, find out what was given, how much was given, and when it was given. Administer a blood glucose test, if possible.

In the conscious, alert patient, administer oral fluids with sugar or oral glucose. (Amounts are age and/or weight specific, so check with medical direction.) If there is no response, or if the patient exhibits an altered mental status, transport immediately. Consult your medical direction physician on orders for the administration of dextrose or IM glucagon. Twenty-five percent dextrose solution ($D_{25}W$) can be prepared by diluting 50 percent dextrose solution 1:1 with sterile water or saline. A 10 percent dextrose solution ($D_{10}W$) will also work. It is easier to dose children with this concentration and it does not cause as much discomfort as intravenous administration. Repeat blood glucose tests within 10 to 15 minutes of infusion or the administration of glucose.[16]

In treating diabetic pediatric patients, remember that most children have been taught about their condition and can participate, in varying degrees, in their care. Most understand how glucometers work, for example, and can hand you a test strip (Figure 4-35). They may be sensitive to their condition, so avoid labeling any tests as "good" or "bad."

Hyperglycemia

Hyperglycemia is an abnormally high concentration of blood sugar. For patients with type 1 diabetes, hyperglycemia may lead to dehydration and **diabetic ketoacidosis**, a very serious medical emergency. Left untreated, the condition will deteriorate to coma. Hyperglycemia and diabetic ketoacidosis are the most common findings in new-onset diabetics.

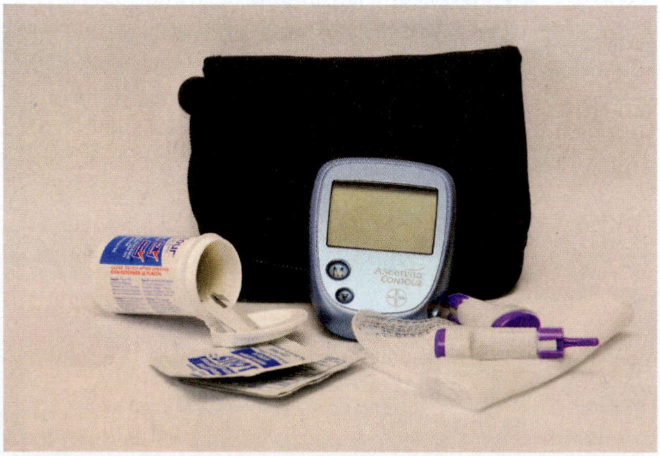

FIGURE 4-35 Many diabetic children have home glucometers to test their blood glucose levels. Older children know what the readings mean and will be curious about any glucose testing device that you may use.

In the prehospital setting, pediatric hyperglycemia is commonly associated with type 1 diabetes. Causes include:

- Eating too much food relative to injected insulin
- Missing an insulin injection
- Defective insulin pump, blockage of tubing, or disconnection of the insulin pump infusion set
- Illness or stress

Hyperglycemia can occur with other severe illnesses and not necessarily mean that the child is developing diabetes mellitus.

ASSESSMENT In cases of hyperglycemia, glucose is spilled into the urine, taking water with it through osmotic diuresis. This can result in a significant fluid loss with resultant dehydration.

Keep in mind that acidosis results from the accumulation of ketones, a byproduct of fat metabolism. A continual increase in the ketones eventually leads to metabolic acidosis, which produces the fruity breath odor commonly associated with hyperglycemia. For other signs and symptoms, see Table 4-15.

As with hypoglycemia, elicit a history to determine causes linked with hyperglycemia. If possible, confirm your suspicions with a blood glucose test. A blood sugar reading of greater than 200 mg/dL typically indicates hyperglycemia.

MANAGEMENT Carefully monitor the ABCs and vital signs. If you cannot confirm the presence of hyperglycemia with a blood glucose test, consider administering oral fluids with sugar or oral glucose in case the patient is hypoglycemic. If intravenous access is possible, consider initiating an IV of either normal saline or lactated Ringer's. Administer an IV bolus of 20 mL/kg, and repeat the bolus if the patient's vital signs do not change. Monitor the patient's mental status and be prepared to intubate if the respirations continue to decrease.

Remember, this is a potentially life-threatening situation. Consult with medical direction on all actions taken and transport immediately.

Table 4-15 Signs and Symptoms of Hyperglycemia

Early	Late	Ketoacidosis
Increased thirst Increased urination Weight loss	Weakness Abdominal pain Generalized aches Loss of appetite Nausea Vomiting Signs of dehydration, except increased urinary output Fruity breath odor Tachypnea Hyperventilation Tachycardia	Continued decreased level of consciousness progressing to coma Kussmaul's respirations (deep and slow) Signs of dehydration

Poisoning and Toxic Exposure

Accidental poisoning or toxic exposure is a common reason for summoning EMS. Pediatric patients account for the majority of poisonings treated by EMS. Most poisonings result from accidental ingestion of a toxic substance, usually by a young child. Toddlers and preschoolers like to taste things, especially colorful objects and substances that look like food or beverages. They also mimic their parents or caregivers, swallowing pills or drinking alcohol "just like Mommy and Daddy." Teenagers on antidepressants are also at risk of misusing or abusing their prescriptions, especially if given a one- or two-month supply of a medication.

Poisonings are the leading cause of preventable death in children under age five (Figure 4-36). Because of their immature respiratory and cardiovascular systems, even a single pill can poison or, in some cases, kill a child. Of all the substances ingested by young children, iron-containing supplements are the leading cause of poisonings, especially in toddlers and preschoolers.

The most dangerous rooms in a house in terms of poisons are the kitchen, where household cleaners are stored, and the bathroom, where many people keep their over-the-counter and prescription medications. Garages and utility rooms also contain toxic substances, made more attractive to children when they are poured into everyday containers such as coffee cans, soda bottles, or plastic cups. Living rooms may have poisonous plants and liquor bottles.

The best way to prevent pediatric poisonings is by helping the families in your communities learn how to "poison-proof" their homes. If your EMS system does not have information available on this topic, you can obtain guidelines from the U.S. Food and Drug Administration. Poisoning prevention should be a major goal of EMS prevention and community education programs.

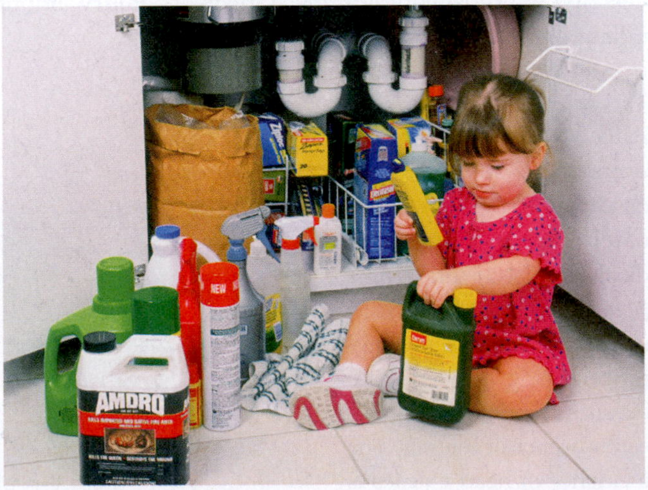

FIGURE 4-36 Poisonings are the leading cause of preventable death in children under age five.

Many EMS systems will dedicate a specific month out of the year to poisoning awareness and prevention.

Assessment

Assessment of a pediatric poisoning depends on the type of poison ingested or the extent to which a child was exposed to a toxic substance (Figure 4-37). Common substances involved in pediatric poisonings include:

- Alcohol, barbiturates, sedatives
- Amphetamines, cocaine, hallucinogens
- Anticholinergic agents (jimson weed, belladonna products)
- Aspirin, acetaminophen
- Lead
- Vitamins and iron-containing supplements
- Corrosives
- Digitalis and beta-blockers
- Hydrocarbons
- Narcotics
- Organic solvents (inhaled)
- Organophosphates (insecticides)

Poisoning can cause many different signs and symptoms, depending on the poison ingested, the route of exposure, and the time since exposure. Narcotics and some of the hydrocarbons can cause respiratory system depression. Digitalis, beta-blockers, calcium-channel blockers, and many antihypertensive agents can cause circulatory depression or collapse. Many agents can impair the central nervous system. These include alcohol, barbiturates, narcotics, and cocaine. Virtually any substance can affect thought and behavior. Common agents are the anticholinergics, alcohol, narcotics, hydrocarbons, and many others. Aspirin, corrosives, and hydrocarbons can irritate or destroy the gastrointestinal system. Acetaminophen can cause liver necrosis and, eventually, liver failure.

Management

Although scenarios vary, take these general steps in managing a pediatric poisoning patient:

Responsive Poisoning Patient

- Administer oxygen (if the patient is hypoxic).
- Contact medical direction and/or the poison control center.
- Consider the need for activated charcoal (rarely indicated).
- Transport. (Be sure to take any pills, substances, and containers to the hospital.)
- Monitor the patient continuously in case the child suddenly becomes unresponsive.

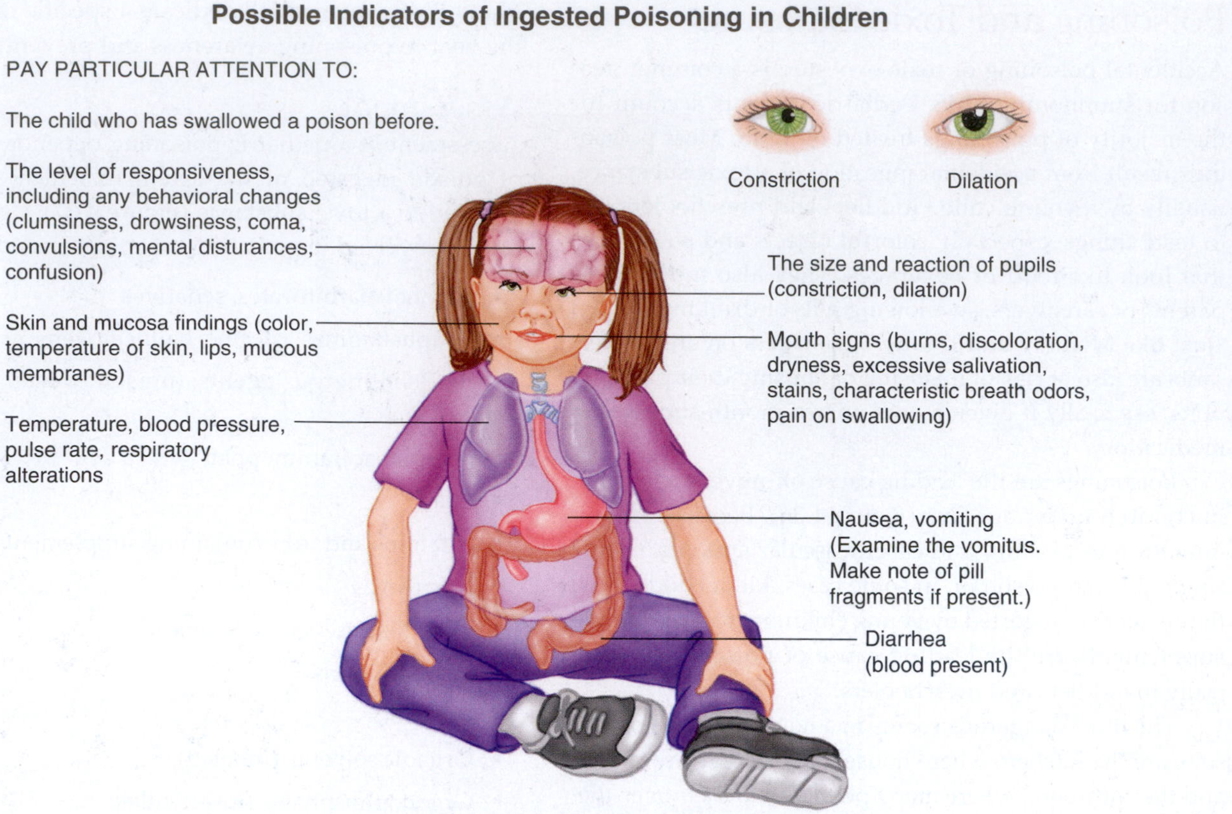

FIGURE 4-37 Possible indicators of ingested poisoning in children.

Unresponsive Poisoning Patient

- Ensure a patent airway. Apply suctioning, if necessary.
- Administer oxygen (if the patient is hypoxic).
- Be prepared to provide artificial ventilations if respiratory failure or cardiac arrest is present.
- Contact medical direction and/or the poison control center.
- Transport. (Be sure to take any pills, substances, and containers to the hospital.)
- Monitor the patient continuously, and rule out trauma as a cause of altered mental status.

For more on poisonings and toxic exposure, see the "Toxicology and Substance Abuse" chapter.

Trauma Emergencies

Trauma is the number-one cause of death in infants and children. Most pediatric injuries result from blunt trauma. As mentioned previously, children have thinner body walls that allow forces to be more readily transmitted to body contents, increasing the possibility of injury to internal tissues and organs. If you serve in an urban area, you can expect to see a higher incidence of penetrating trauma, mostly intentional and mostly from gunfire or knife wounds. Significant incidences of penetrating trauma are also seen outside cities—mostly unintentional, from hunting accidents and agricultural accidents.

Mechanisms of Injury

Although pediatric patients can be injured in the same way as adults, children tend to be more susceptible to certain types of injuries than adults are. The following categories describe the most common mechanisms of injury among infants and children.

Falls

Falls are the single most common cause of injury in children (Figure 4-38). Fortunately, serious injury or death from accidental falls is relatively uncommon, unless the fall is from a significant height. Falls from bicycles account for a significant number of injuries. The incidence of head injuries is declining, primarily because of bicycle safety helmets.

CONTENT REVIEW

➤ Most Common Pediatric Mechanisms of Injury
- Falls
- Motor vehicle collisions
- Car vs. pedestrian collisions
- Drownings
- Penetrating injuries
- Burns
- Physical abuse

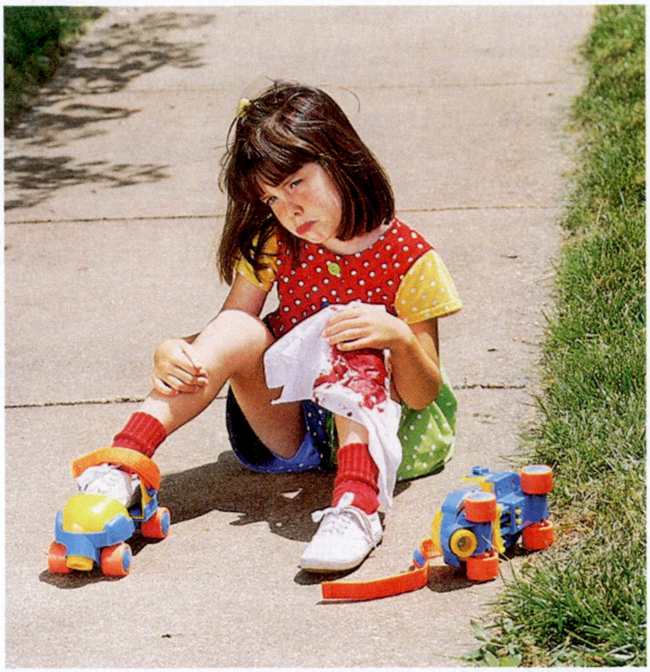

FIGURE 4-38 Falls are the most common cause of injury in young children.

Motor Vehicle Collisions

Approximately 25,000 American children die annually from trauma. Approximately one-third of these die from motor vehicle collisions, making motor vehicle collisions the leading cause of traumatic death in children. In addition, motor vehicle collisions are the leading cause of permanent brain injury and new-onset epilepsy. Improperly seated children are at increased risk of sustaining injury or death from automobile air bags when they deploy (Figure 4-39). This is an area in which EMS prevention strategies can make a difference. Public education programs on drunk driving, safe driving, air bags, and proper use of children's car seats can be a major focus of EMS personnel. Some states have given paramedics the ability to issue citations to persons who do not correctly buckle their children or place them in child safety seats.

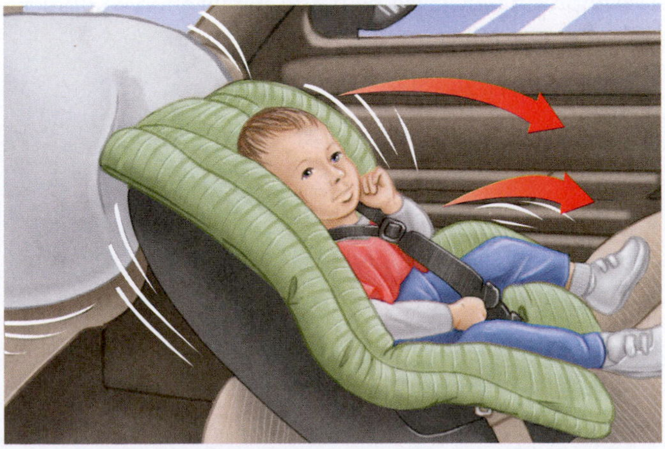

FIGURE 4-39 A deploying air bag can propel a child safety seat back into the vehicle's seat, seriously injuring the child secured in it.

Car-versus-Pedestrian Injuries

Car-versus-child pedestrian injuries are more common in cities where children play close to the street. Car-versus-pedestrian injuries are a particularly lethal form of trauma in children because children's short stature tends to push them down under the car. There are two phases of injury in car-versus-pedestrian collisions. The first group of injuries occurs when the auto contacts the child. Because of the energy present, the child may be propelled away from the car or pushed down underneath the car. It is at this point that the second group of injuries occurs, as the child contacts the ground or other objects. Head and spinal injuries often occur with the secondary impact. The best treatment for car-versus-child-pedestrian collisions is prevention. This, too, can be a major area of emphasis for prehospital prevention programs.

Submersion/Immersion Injuries

Among boys aged 1 to 4 years, drowning was the leading cause of death from unintentional injury in 2010 in the United States. Interestingly, the number of unintentional drowning deaths surpassed the number of motor vehicle traffic deaths in 2005, becoming the leading cause of death from unintentional injury in this age group. Drowning, as defined by the 2002 World Congress on Drowning, the American Red Cross, the World Health Organization, and other national and international authorities, is "the process of experiencing respiratory impairment as the result of submersion/immersion in a liquid medium." Drowning has three possible outcomes:

- No morbidity (no injury)
- Morbidity (injury)
- Mortality (death)

Older terms such as "near drowning" are no longer used. Drowning is considered to be a process, not an outcome. Thus, there can be "fatal" or "nonfatal" drownings. Many children who do not die from drowning suffer severe and irreversible brain injuries as a result of anoxia. Approximately 20 to 25 percent of near-drowning survivors exhibit severe neurologic deficits. The outcomes are better when the water is cold, because the body's protective mechanisms guard against brain injury.

Again, as with the other injury processes, the best treatment is prevention. EMS personnel, in conjunction with local building inspectors, can inspect pools for safety. A pool should be fenced off with a gate that closes automatically. Essential rescue equipment (pole, life preserver) should be immediately available and the local emergency number posted. The best time for drowning prevention programs is late spring and early summer. Encourage parents to enroll their children in water safety classes as early as possible.

Penetrating Injuries

Until 20 years ago, penetrating injuries in children were fairly uncommon. Since then, an increase in violent crime (although violent crime rates have both risen and fallen within that period) has resulted in an increasing number of children sustaining penetrating trauma. Stab wounds and firearm injuries account for approximately 10 to 15 percent of all pediatric trauma admissions. The risk of death increases with age. Children are usually innocent victims of crimes perpetrated against adults. However, children are sometimes the intended victims of gunfire and stabbings, as in the shootings that have taken place in schools.

It is important to remember that visual inspection of external injuries does not provide adequate evaluation of internal injuries. This is especially true with high-energy, high-velocity weapons that can cause massive internal injury with only minimal external trauma.

Paramedics can play a major role in preventing pediatric shootings. During public education and community service programs, it is prudent to talk about gun safety, including such measures as using trigger locks or locking weapons in places where children cannot reach them. You might emphasize the fact that children have an uncanny ability to find and gain access to weapons that adults think they have hidden and secured. As with many other pediatric emergencies, the best treatment is prevention.

Burns

Burn injuries are the leading cause of accidental death in the home for children under 14 years of age. Children can sustain both burn injuries and smoke inhalation in house fires. Unsupervised children with matches or cigarette lighters are responsible for many fires that result in pediatric injury.

Fire prevention programs are a major area of emphasis for fire departments. The importance of smoke detectors cannot be overemphasized. Citizens should be encouraged to change the batteries in their smoke detectors when the clock is moved backward or forward when daylight saving time changes. Many fire departments and EMS systems replace smoke detector batteries as a part of their fire prevention programs. Part of the fire prevention program should be specifically directed at children. It is especially important to teach children how to exit their houses in case fire erupts.

Physical Abuse

Unfortunately, children are at risk for physical abuse by adults and older children. Factors leading to child abuse are known to include social phenomena such as poverty, domestic disturbances, younger parents, substance abuse, and community violence. Paramedics are often the first members of the health care team to come into contact with the abused child. It is very important to not accuse the parents or confront a suspected abuser. Instead, document all pertinent findings, treatments, and interventions and report these to the proper authorities. (Child abuse is discussed in more detail later in this chapter.)

Special Considerations

As emphasized previously, children are not small adults. You should keep this in mind and modify treatment accordingly. Specific items to consider will be discussed next.

Airway Control

Special considerations are related to characteristics of the child's airway. These include the following:

- Maintain in-line stabilization in neutral instead of the sniffing position to prevent possible pinching of the trachea (Figure 4-40).
- Administer oxygen if the patient is hypoxic.
- Maintain a patent airway with suctioning and the jaw-thrust maneuver.
- Be prepared to assist ineffective respirations. Remember that airway pressures can be high in children and it may be necessary to depress the pop-off valve to ventilate the child adequately.
- Intubate the child when the airway cannot be maintained, while simultaneously maintaining cervical spine stabilization (Figure 4-41).
- A gastric tube should be placed following intubation to decompress the stomach.
- Needle cricothyrotomy is rarely indicated for traumatic upper airway obstruction.

Stabilization

Use appropriately sized pediatric stabilization equipment, including the following:

- Rigid cervical collar
- Towel or blanket roll
- Child safety seat
- Pediatric stabilization device
- Vest-type device (Kendrick extrication device)
- Short wooden backboard
- Straps and cravats
- Tape
- Padding

Keep infants, toddlers, and preschoolers supine with the cervical spine in a neutral in-line position by placing

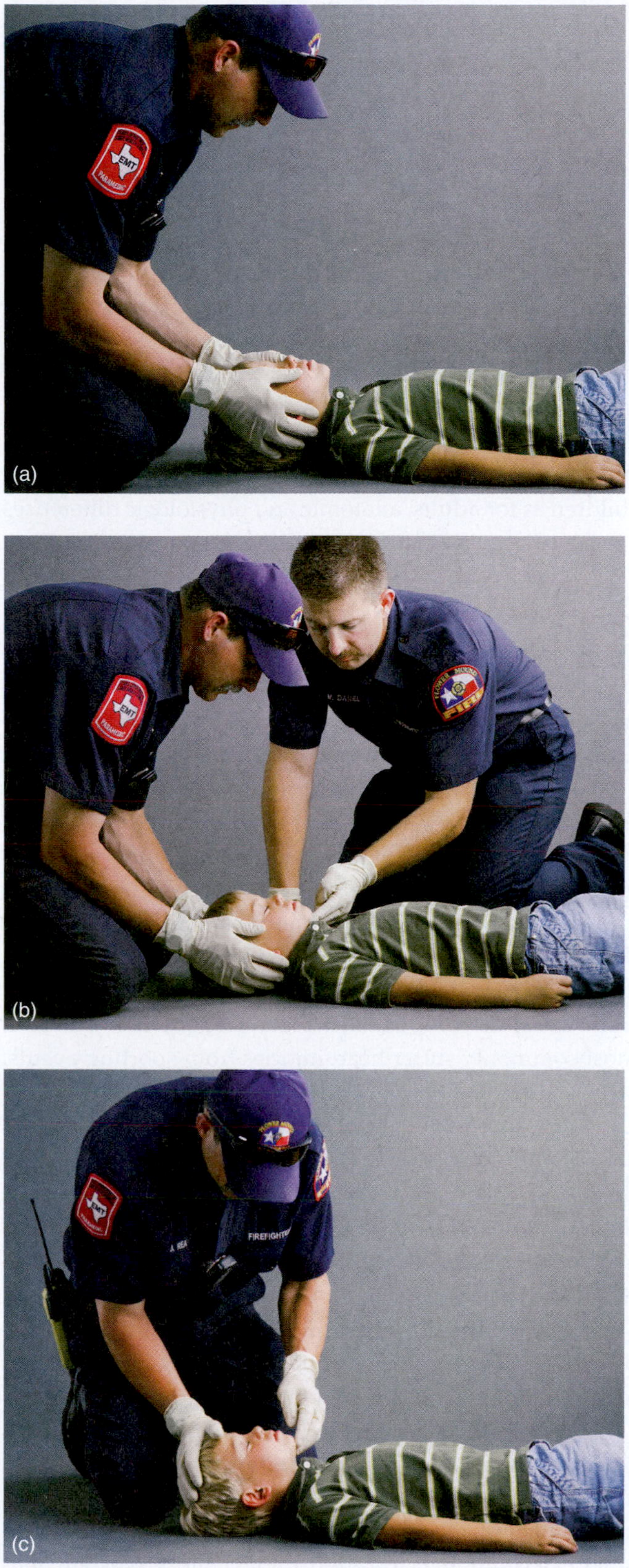

FIGURE 4-40 In the pediatric trauma patient, use the combination jaw-thrust/spine stabilization maneuver to open the airway. (a) Single paramedic kneels above child's head, holds head in neutral position while thrusting jaw forward with fingers. (b) Two paramedics working together; one holds head in neutral position while the other thrusts the jaw forward. (c) Single paramedic uses alternative technique to hold head in neutral position while thrusting jaw forward.

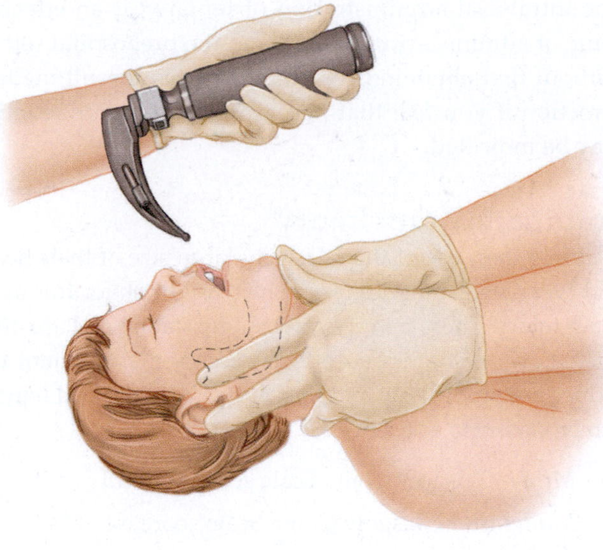

FIGURE 4-41 Simultaneous cervical spine stabilization and intubation in a pediatric patient.

padding from the shoulders to the hips. (Review the discussion of pediatric stabilization earlier in this chapter.)

Fluid Management

Management of the airway and breathing takes priority over management of circulation, because circulatory compromise is less common in children than in adults. When obtaining vascular access, remember the following:

- If possible, insert a large-bore intravenous catheter into a peripheral vein.
- Do not delay transport to gain venous access.
- Intraosseous access in children is an alternative when a peripheral IV cannot be obtained.
- Administer an initial fluid bolus of 20 mL/kg of lactated Ringer's solution or normal saline.
- Reassess the vital signs and give another bolus of 20 mL/kg if there is no improvement.
- If improvement does not occur after the second bolus, there is likely to be a significant blood loss that may require surgical intervention. Rapid transport is essential.

Pediatric Analgesia and Sedation

An often-overlooked aspect of prehospital pediatric care is pain control. Many pediatric injuries are painful and analgesics are indicated. These include burns, long-bone fractures, dislocations, and others. Unless there is a contraindication, pediatric patients should receive analgesics. Commonly used analgesics include morphine and fentanyl. Also, certain pediatric emergencies may benefit from sedation. These include such problems as penetrating eye injuries, prolonged rescue from entrapment in machinery, cardioversion, and other painful procedures.

The intranasal administration of fentanyl is an effective route of administering analgesia in the prehospital setting without first obtaining IV access. Always consult medical direction if you feel that pediatric analgesia or sedation may be indicated.

Traumatic Brain Injury

Children, because of the relatively large size of their heads and weak neck muscles, are at increased risk for traumatic brain injury. These injuries can be devastating and are often fatal. Early recognition and aggressive management can reduce both morbidity and mortality. Pediatric head injuries can be classified as follows:

- *Mild*—Glasgow Coma Scale score is 13–15
- *Moderate*—Glasgow Coma Scale score is 9–12
- *Severe*—Glasgow Coma Scale score is less than or equal to 8

Traumatic head injuries can cause intracranial bleeding or swelling. This ultimately results in an increase in intracranial pressure. The signs of increased intracranial pressure can be subtle. They include:

- Elevated blood pressure
- Bradycardia
- Rapid, deep respirations progressing to slow, deep respirations
- Bulging fontanelle in infants

Increased intracranial pressure will eventually lead to herniation of a portion of the brain through the foramen magnum. This is an ominous development that is often associated with irreversible injury. Signs and symptoms of herniation include:

- Asymmetrical pupils
- Decorticate posturing
- Decerebrate posturing

Specific management of traumatic head injuries in children is similar to that for adults. As a rule, follow these steps:

- Administer supplemental oxygen (if the patient is hypoxic).
- Provide ventilation. Consider intubation in children with a Glasgow Coma Scale score of less than or equal to 8 (severe head injury) and ventilate at a normal rate.
- Consider rapid sequence intubation (RSI) for children with a Glasgow Coma Scale score of less than or equal to 8 who have too much muscle tone to allow endotracheal intubation.

Consider hyperventilation only if there is a deterioration in the child's condition as evidenced by asymmetric pupils, active seizures, or neurologic posturing (indicating herniation). Children with traumatic head injuries do best at facilities that treat a great number of children and that have pediatric neurosurgeons on staff. Consider diverting to a pediatric trauma facility if a moderate or severe traumatic head injury is present.

Specific Injuries

As previously mentioned, more pediatric patients die of trauma than of any other cause. Statistics reveal that nearly 50 percent of these deaths occur within the first hour of injury. The quick arrival of EMS at the scene can literally mean the difference between life and death for a child. Although management of trauma is basically the same for children as for adults, anatomic and physiologic differences cause pediatric patients to have different patterns of injury.

Head, Face, and Neck

The majority of children who sustain multiple trauma will suffer associated head and/or neck injuries. As previously mentioned, the larger relative mass of the head and lack of neck muscle strength provide for increased momentum in acceleration–deceleration injuries and a greater stress on the cervical spine. The fulcrum of cervical mobility in the younger child is at the C-2–C-3 level. As a result, nearly 60 to 70 percent of pediatric fractures occur in C-1–C-2.[17]

Injuries to the head are the most common cause of death in pediatric trauma victims. School-age children tend to sustain head injuries from bicycle collisions, falls from trees, or car–pedestrian collisions. Older children most commonly suffer head injuries from sporting events. Head injuries in all age groups may result from abuse.

In treating head injuries, remember that diffuse injuries are common in children, whereas focal injuries are rare. Because the skull is softer and more compliant in children than in adults, brain injuries occur more readily in infants and young children. Because of open fontanelles and sutures, infants up to an average age of 16 months may be more tolerant to an increase in intracranial pressure and can have delayed signs. (Keep this fact in mind when taking the history of children in the one-month to two-year age range.)[18]

Children also frequently injure their faces. The most common facial injuries are lacerations secondary to falls. Young children are very clumsy when they first start walking. A fall onto a sharp object, such as the corner of a coffee table, can result in a laceration. Older children sustain dental injuries in falls from bicycles, skateboard accidents, fights, and sports activities.

Spinal injuries in children are not as common as in adults. However, as noted earlier, a child's proportionately larger and heavier head makes the cervical spine vulnerable to injury. Any time a child sustains a severe head injury, always assume that a neck injury may also be present.

Chest and Abdomen

Most injuries to the chest and abdomen result from blunt trauma. As noted earlier, infants and young children lack the rigid rib cages of adults. Therefore, they suffer fewer rib fractures and more intrathoracic injuries. Likewise, their relatively undeveloped abdominal musculature affords minimal protection to the viscera.

Because of the high mortality associated with blunt trauma, children with significant blunt abdominal or chest trauma should be transported immediately to a pediatric trauma center with appropriate care provided en route.

INJURIES TO THE CHEST Chest injuries are the second most common cause of pediatric trauma deaths. Because of the compliance of the chest wall, severe intrathoracic injury can be present without signs of external injury. Pneumothorax and hemothorax can occur in the pediatric patient, especially if the mechanism of injury was a motor vehicle collision.

Tension pneumothorax can also occur in children. Pediatric patients poorly tolerate the condition and a needle thoracostomy may be lifesaving. Tension pneumothorax presents with the following signs and symptoms:

- Diminished breath sounds over the affected lung
- Shift of the trachea to the opposite side
- Progressive decrease in ventilatory compliance

Keep in mind that children with cardiac tamponade may have no physical signs of tamponade other than hypotension. Also remember that flail chest is an uncommon injury in children. When chest injury is noted without a significant mechanism of injury, suspect child abuse.

INJURIES TO THE ABDOMEN Significant blunt trauma to the abdomen can result in injury to the spleen or liver. In fact, the spleen is the most commonly injured organ in children. Signs and symptoms of a splenic injury include tenderness in the left upper quadrant of the abdomen, abrasions on the abdomen, and hematoma of the abdominal wall. Symptoms of liver injury include right upper quadrant abdominal pain and/or right lower chest pain. Both splenic and hepatic injuries can cause life-threatening internal hemorrhage.

In treating blunt abdominal trauma, keep in mind the small size of the pediatric abdomen. Be certain to palpate only one quadrant at a time. In cases of both chest and abdominal trauma, treat for shock with positioning, fluids, and maintenance of body temperature.

Extremities

Extremity injuries in children are typically limited to fractures and lacerations. Children rarely sustain amputations and other serious extremity injuries. An exception includes farm children who may become entangled in agricultural equipment.

The most common injuries are fractures, usually resulting from falls (Figure 4-42). Because children have more flexible bones than adults, they tend to have incomplete fractures, such as **bend fractures**, **buckle fractures**, and **greenstick fractures**. In younger children, the bone growth plates have not yet closed. Some types of growth plate fractures can lead to permanent disability if not managed correctly. Whenever indicated, perform splinting to decrease pain and prevent further injury and/or blood loss.

Burns

Burns are the second leading cause of death in children. They are the leading cause of accidental death in the home for children under 14. Burns may be chemical, thermal, or electrical. The most common type of burn injury encountered by EMS personnel is scalding. Children can scald themselves by pulling hot liquids off tables or stoves. In cases of abuse, they can be scalded by immersion in hot water.

Estimation of the burn surface area is slightly different for children than for adults (Figure 4-43). In adults, the "rule of nines" assigns 9 percent of the body surface area (BSA) to each of 11 body regions: the entire head and neck; the anterior chest; the anterior abdomen; the

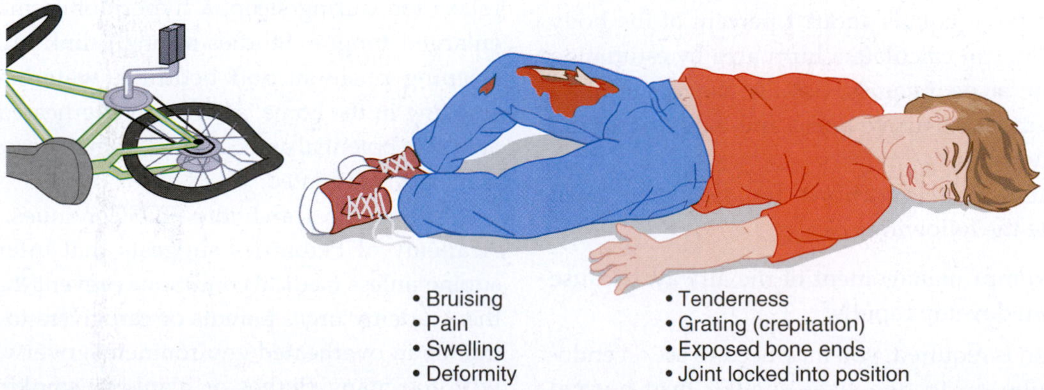

FIGURE 4-42 Signs and symptoms of a fracture in a child who has fallen off a bike.

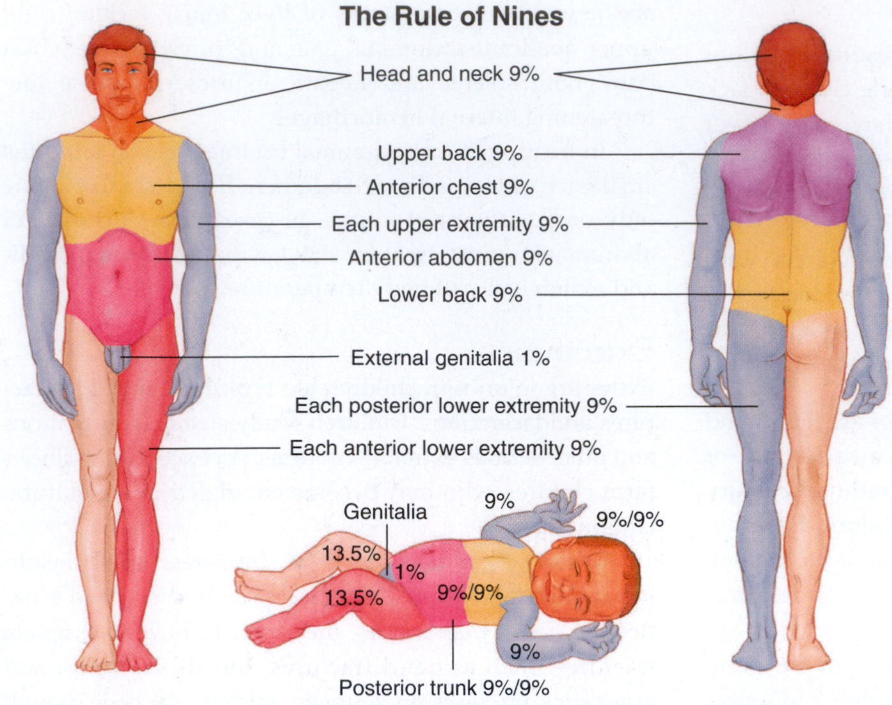

FIGURE 4-43 The rule of nines helps to estimate the extent of a burn in adults and children. Note the modifications for the child.

posterior chest; the lower back (posterior abdomen); the anterior surface of each lower extremity; the posterior surface of each lower extremity; and the entirety of each upper extremity. The remaining 1 percent is assigned to the genitalia.

In a child, the head accounts for a larger percentage of BSA, whereas the legs make up a smaller percentage. Thus, for children, the rule of nines is modified to take away 8 percent from the lower extremities (2 percent from the front and 2 percent from the back of each leg) plus the 1 percent assigned to the adult genitalia. This 9 percent that is taken from the lower part of the body is reassigned to the head. Therefore, whereas the adult's entire head and neck are counted as 9 percent, in the child the anterior head and neck count as 9 percent and the posterior head and neck count as another 9 percent.

You can also use the child's palm as a guide (the "rule of palm"). The palm equals about 1 percent of the body surface area. You can calculate a burn area by estimating how many palm areas it equals. Usually, the rule of nines works best for more extensive burns and the rule of palm for less extensive ones.

Management considerations for pediatric burn patients include the following:

- Provide prompt management of the airway, because swelling can develop rapidly.
- If intubation is required, you may need to use an endotracheal tube up to two sizes smaller than normal because of the swelling.
- Thermally burned children are very susceptible to hypothermia. Be sure to maintain body heat.
- When treating serious electrical burn patients, suspect musculoskeletal injuries and perform spinal stabilization.

Sudden Infant Death Syndrome

Sudden infant death syndrome (SIDS) is defined as the sudden death of an infant during the first year of life from an illness of unknown etiology. The incidence of SIDS in the United States is approximately 0.57 deaths per 1,000 births. SIDS is the leading cause of death between two weeks and one year of age. It is responsible for a significant number of deaths between one month and six months, with peak incidence occurring at two to four months.

SIDS occurs most frequently in the fall and winter months. It tends to be more common in boys than in girls. It is more prevalent in premature and low-birth-weight infants, in infants of young mothers, and in infants whose mothers did not receive prenatal care. Infants of mothers who used cocaine, methadone, or heroin during pregnancy are at greater risk. Occasionally, a mild upper respiratory infection will be reported prior to the death. SIDS is not caused by external suffocation from blankets or pillows, nor is it related to allergies to cow's milk or regurgitation and aspiration of stomach contents. It is not thought to be hereditary.

Current theories vary about the etiology of SIDS. Some authorities feel that it may result from an immature respiratory center in the brain that leads the child to simply stop breathing. Others think there may be an airway obstruction in the posterior pharynx as a result of pharyngeal relaxation during sleep, a hypermobile mandible, or an enlarged tongue. Studies strongly link SIDS to a prone sleeping position. Soft bedding, waterbed mattresses, smoking in the home, and/or an overheated environment are other potential associations. A small percentage of SIDS may be abuse related.

Although research into SIDS continues, the American Academy of Pediatrics suggests that infants be placed supine unless medical conditions prevent this. In addition, the Academy urges parents or caregivers to avoid placing infants in overheated environments, overwrapping them with too many clothes or blankets, smoking before and after pregnancy, and filling the crib with soft bedding.

Assessment

Infants suffering SIDS have similar physical findings. From an external standpoint, there is a normal state of nutrition and hydration. The skin may be mottled. There are often frothy, occasionally blood-tinged, fluids in and around the mouth and nostrils. Vomitus may be present. Occasionally, the infant may be in an unusual position as a result of muscle spasm or high activity at the time of death. Common findings noted at autopsy include intrathoracic petechiae (small hemorrhages) in 90 percent of cases. There is often associated pulmonary congestion and edema. Sometimes, stomach contents are found in the trachea. Microscopic examination of the trachea often reveals the presence of inflammatory changes.

Management

The immediate needs of the family with a SIDS baby are many. Unless the infant is obviously dead, undertake active and aggressive care of the infant to assure the family that everything possible is being done. A first responder or other personnel should be assigned to assist the parents and to explain the procedures. At all points, use the baby's name.

After arrival at the hospital, direct management toward the parents or caregivers, as nothing can be done for the child. Allow the family to see the dead child. Expect a normal grief reaction. Initially, there may be shock, disbelief, and denial. Other times, the parents or caregivers may express anger, rage, hostility, blame, or guilt. Often, there is a feeling of inadequacy as well as helplessness, confusion, and fear. The grief process is likely to last for years. SIDS has major long-term effects on family relations. It may also affect you, the on-scene paramedic. If so, do not be reluctant to seek counseling.

Apparent Life-Threatening Event

The term *apparent life-threatening event* (ALTE) is defined as a sudden event, often characterized by apnea or other abrupt changes in the child's behavior. Symptoms of an ALTE include one or more of the following:

- Apnea
- Change in color (cyanosis)
- Loss of muscle tone
- Coughing
- Gagging

These episodes may necessitate stimulation or resuscitation to arouse the child and reinitiate regular breathing. ALTE was once referred to as "near-miss SIDS." The true incidence is unknown. ALTE is often a result of another condition and is not an entity of its own. However, in some instances, the cause cannot be identified. Child abuse should be considered if other medical causes have been excluded. Home monitoring technology may be beneficial. From an EMS standpoint, the care provided should be based on your assessment and immediate life threats.[19,20]

Child Abuse and Neglect

A tragic truth is that some people cause physical and psychological harm to children, either through intentional abuse or through intentional or unintentional neglect. The estimated child mortality rate for child abuse and neglect is 18.4 per 100,000.

Abused children share several common characteristics. Often, the child is seen as "special" and different from others. Premature infants and twins stand a higher risk of abuse than other children. Many abused children are less than five years of age. Children with physical and mental handicaps, as well as those with other special needs, are at greater risk. So are uncommunicative (autistic) children. Boys are more often abused than girls. A child who is not what the parents wanted (e.g., the "wrong" gender) is at increased risk of abuse, too.

Perpetrators of Abuse or Neglect

A parent, a legal guardian, or a foster parent may instigate abuse or neglect. A person, an institution, or an agency or program entrusted with custody can carry it out. Abuse or neglect can also result from the actions of a caretaker, such as a babysitter or nanny.

The person who abuses or neglects a child can come from any geographic, religious, ethnic, racial, occupational, educational, or socioeconomic background. Despite their diversity, people who abuse children tend to share certain traits. The abuser is usually a parent or a full-time caregiver. When the mother spends the majority of the time with the child, she is the parent most frequently identified as the abuser. Most abusers were abused themselves as children.

Three conditions can alert you to the potential for abuse:

- A parent or adult who seems capable of abuse, especially one who exhibits evasive or hostile behavior
- A child in one of the high-risk categories noted in the preceding section
- The presence of a crisis, particularly financial stress, marital or relationship stress, or physical illness in a parent or child

Types of Abuse

Child abuse can take several forms, including:

- Psychological abuse
- Physical abuse

- Sexual abuse
- Neglect (either physical or emotional)

Abused children suffer every imaginable kind of mistreatment. They are battered with fists, belts, broom handles, hairbrushes, baseball bats, electric cords, and any other objects that can be used as weapons (Figure 4-44). They are locked in closets, denied food, or deprived of access to a toilet. They are intentionally burned or scalded with anything from hot water to cigarette butts to open flames (Figure 4-45). They are severely shaken, thrown into cribs, pushed down stairs, or shoved into walls. Some are shot, stabbed, or suffocated.

Sexual abuse ranges from adults exposing themselves to children to overt sexual acts to sexual torture. Sexual abuse can occur at any age, and the victims may be either male or female. Generally, the sexual abuser is someone the child knows and, perhaps, trusts. Stepchildren or adopted children face a greater risk for sexual abuse than biological children. Cases in which sexual abuse causes physical harm may get reported. Other cases, especially those with emotional and minor physical injury, may go undetected.

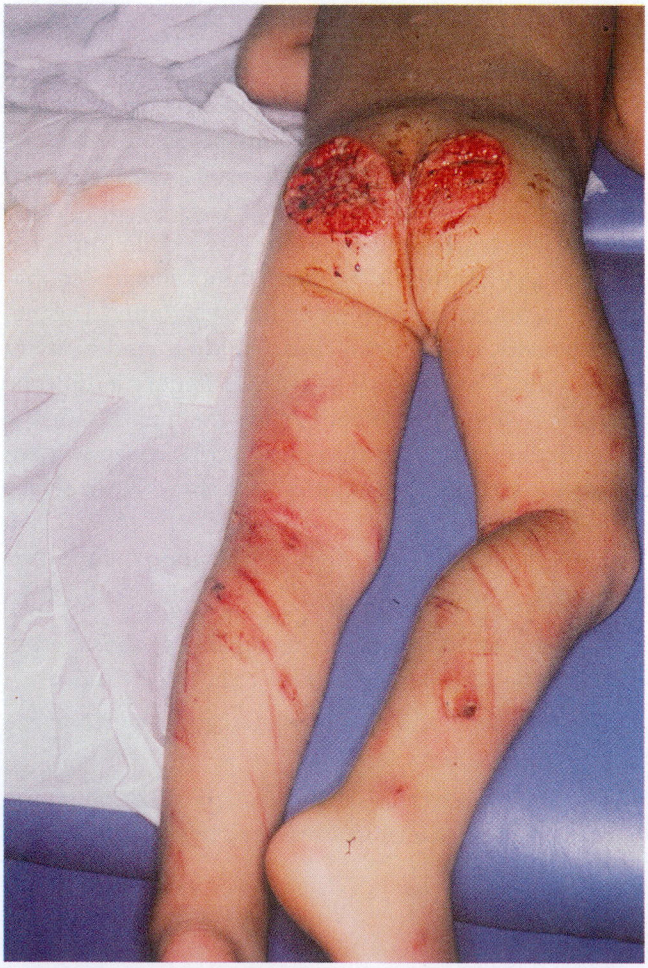

FIGURE 4-44 An abused child. Note the marks on the legs associated with beatings with an electric wire. The burns on the buttocks are from submersion in hot water.

(Courtesy of Scott and White Healthcare)

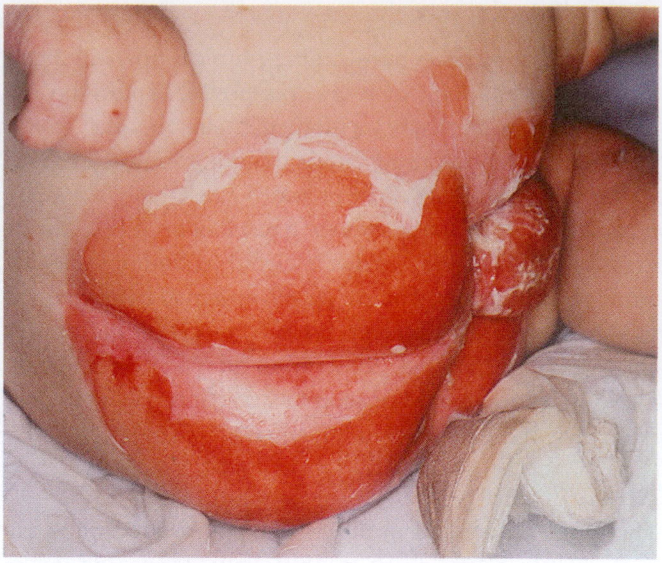

FIGURE 4-45 Burn injury from placing a child's buttocks in hot water as a punishment.

(Courtesy of Scott and White Healthcare)

Assessment of the Potentially Abused or Neglected Child

Signs of abuse or neglect can be startling. As a guide, the following findings should trigger a high index of suspicion:

- Any obvious or suspected fractures in a child under two years of age
- Multiple injuries in various stages of healing, especially burns and bruises (Figure 4-46)
- More injuries than usually seen in children of the same age or size
- Injuries scattered on many areas of the body

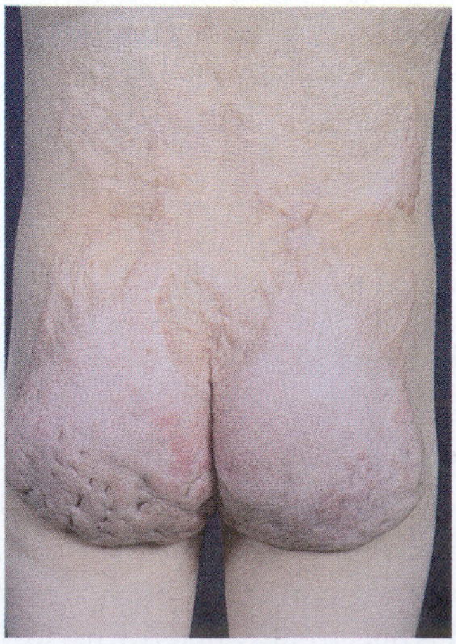

FIGURE 4-46 The effects of child abuse, both physical and mental, can last a lifetime.

(Courtesy of Scott and White Healthcare)

- Bruises or burns in patterns that suggest intentional infliction
- Increased intracranial pressure in an infant
- Suspected intraabdominal trauma in a young child
- Any injury that does not fit with the description of the cause given

Information in the medical history may also raise the index of suspicion. Examples include:

- A history that does not match the nature or severity of the injury
- Vague parental accounts or accounts that change during the interview
- Accusations that the child injured himself intentionally
- Delay in seeking help
- Child dressed inappropriately for the situation
- Revealing comments by bystanders, especially siblings

Suspect child neglect if you spot any of the following conditions:

- Extreme malnutrition
- Multiple insect bites
- Long-standing skin infections
- Extreme lack of cleanliness
- Verbal or social skills far below those you would expect for a child of similar age and background
- Lack of appropriate medical care

Management of the Potentially Abused or Neglected Child

In cases of child abuse or neglect, the goals of management include appropriate treatment of injuries, protection of the child from further abuse, and notification of proper authorities. You should obtain as much information as possible, in a nonjudgmental manner. Document all findings or statements in the patient report. Do not "cross-examine" the parents—this job belongs to the police or other authorities. Try to be supportive toward the parents, especially if it helps you to transport the child to the hospital. Remember: Never leave transport to the alleged abuser.

On arrival at the emergency department, report your suspicions to the appropriate personnel. Complete the patient report and all available documentation at this time, as delay may inhibit accurate recall of data.

Child abuse and neglect are particularly stressful aspects of emergency medical services. You must recognize and deal with your feelings, perhaps by seeking counseling.

Resources for Abuse and Neglect

You can contact your local child protection agency for additional information on child abuse. Consider taking a course in the recognition of child abuse and neglect. These are often offered by children's hospitals. The Internet has several sites that provide up-to-date information on child abuse.[21,22]

Infants and Children with Special Needs

For most of human history, infants and children with devastating congenital conditions or diseases either died or remained confined to a hospital. In recent decades, however, medical technology has lowered infant mortality rates and allowed a greater number of children with special needs to live at home. (See more about home care in the chapter "Acute Interventions for the Chronic Care Patient.") Some of these infants and children include:

- Premature babies
- Infants and children with lung disease, heart disease, or neurologic disorders
- Infants and children with chronic diseases, such as cystic fibrosis, asthma, childhood cancers, and cerebral palsy
- Infants and children with altered functions from birth, such as cerebral palsy, spina bifida, and other congenital birth defects

In caring for these children, family members receive education relative to the special equipment required by the infant or child. Even so, they may feel a great deal of apprehension when care moves from the hospital to the home. As a result, they may summon EMS at the first indication of trouble. This is especially true in the initial weeks following discharge.

Common Home Care Devices

Devices you might commonly find in the home include tracheostomy tubes, apnea monitors, home artificial ventilators, central intravenous lines, gastric feeding tubes, gastrostomy tubes, and shunts. In treating children with special needs, remember that the parents and caregivers are often very knowledgeable about their children and the devices that sustain their lives. Listen to them. They know their children better than anybody else.

Tracheostomy Tubes

Patients who are on prolonged home ventilators or who have chronic respiratory problems may have surgically placed tubes in the inferior trachea (Figure 4-47). A **tracheostomy** (trach) tube may be used as a temporary or a permanent device. Although various types of tubes are used, you might encounter some common complications. They include:

- Obstruction, usually by a mucus plug
- Site bleeding, either from the tube or around the tube
- An air leakage

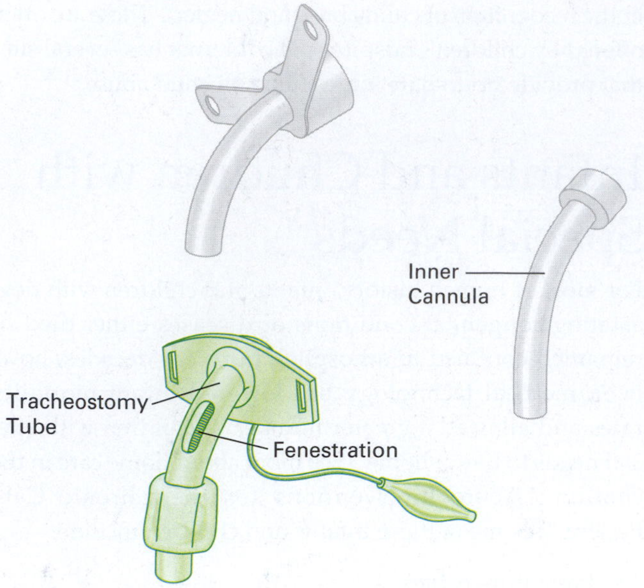

FIGURE 4-47 Tracheostomy tubes. Top: Plastic tube. Bottom: Metal tube with inner cannula.

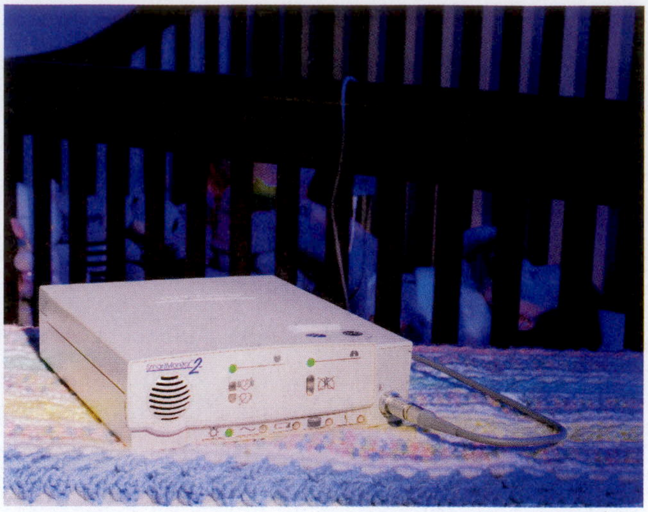

FIGURE 4-48 Home apnea monitor.

- A dislodged tube
- Infection—a condition that will worsen an already impaired breathing ability

Management steps for a patient with a tracheostomy include the following:

- Maintaining an open airway
- Suctioning the tube, as needed
- Allowing the patient to remain in a position of comfort, if possible
- Administering oxygen in cases of respiratory distress
- Assisting ventilations in cases of respiratory failure/arrest by:
  - Using the tracheostomy to ventilate
  - Intubating orally in the absence of an upper airway obstruction
  - Intubating via the **stoma** (surgical opening in the neck) if there is an upper airway obstruction
- Transporting the patient to the hospital

Apnea Monitors

Apnea monitors are used to alert parents or caregivers to the cessation of breathing in an infant, especially a premature infant. Some types of monitors signal changes in heart rate, such as bradycardia or tachycardia. They operate via pads attached to the baby's chest and connected to the monitor by wires. If the device does not detect a breath within a specific time frame or if the infant's heart rate is too slow or too fast, an alarm will sound (Figure 4-48).

When an apnea monitor is placed in a home, the parents are typically instructed on what to do if the alarm sounds (stimulate the child, provide artificial respirations, and so on). If these fail, EMS may be summoned. Also, nervous parents who have just brought a baby home on an apnea monitor may panic the first couple of times the alarm sounds and call 911. Be patient and kind while instructing them on what to do when the alarm sounds.

Home Artificial Ventilators

Various configurations exist for home ventilators. *Demand ventilators* sense the rate and quality of a patient's respiration as well as several other parameters, including pulse oximetry. They typically respond to preset limits. Other devices provide a constant PEEP (positive end-expiratory pressure) and a set oxygen concentration for the patient.

Two complications commonly result in EMS calls: (1) a device's mechanical failure and (2) shortages of energy during an electrical failure. Treatment typically includes:

- Maintaining an open airway
- Administering artificial ventilations via an appropriately sized BVM with oxygen
- Transporting the patient to a hospital until the home ventilator is working

Central Intravenous Lines

Children who require long-term IV therapy will often have central lines placed into the superior vena cava near the heart. If IV therapy is necessary for only several weeks, percutaneous intravenous catheter (PIC) lines may be placed in the arm and threaded into the superior vena cava. Otherwise, the lines are placed through subclavian venipuncture. **Central IV lines** are commonly used to administer intravenous nutrition, antibiotics, or chemotherapy for cancer.

Possible complications for central IV lines include:

- Cracked line
- Infection, either at the site or at more distal aspects of the line

- Loss of patency (e.g., clotting)
- Hemorrhage, which can be considerable
- Air embolism

Emergency medical care steps include control of any bleeding through direct pressure. If a large amount of air is in the line, try to withdraw it with a syringe. If this fails, clamp the line and transport. In cases of a cracked line, place a clamp between the crack and the patient. If the patient exhibits an altered mental status following the cracked line, position the child on the left side with head down. Transport the child to the hospital as quickly as possible.

Gastric Feeding Tubes and Gastrostomy Tubes

Children who are not capable of swallowing or eating receive nutrition through either a gastric feeding tube or a gastrostomy tube (Figure 4-49). (A gastric feeding tube is placed through the nostrils into the stomach. A gastrostomy tube is placed through the abdominal wall directly into the stomach.) These special devices are commonly used in disorders of the digestive system or in situations in which the developmental ability of the patient hinders feeding. Food consists of nutritious liquids.

Possible emergency complications include:

- Bleeding at the site
- Dislodged tube
- Respiratory distress, particularly if a tube feeding backs up into the esophagus and is aspirated into the trachea and lungs
- In the case of diabetics, altered mental status due to missed feedings

Emergency medical care involves supporting the ABCs, including possible suctioning and administration of supplemental oxygen. Patients should be transported to a definitive care facility, either in a sitting position or lying on the right side with the head elevated. The goal is to reduce the risk of aspiration, a serious condition.

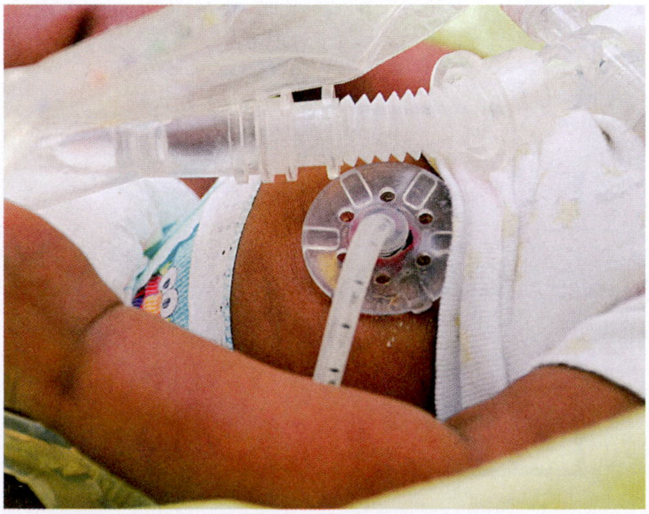

FIGURE 4-49 Infant with feeding tube.

Shunts

A **shunt** is a surgical connection that runs from the brain to the abdomen. It removes excess cerebrospinal fluid from the brain through drainage. A subcutaneous reservoir is usually palpable on one side of the patient's head. A pathologic rise in intracranial pressure, secondary to a blocked shunt, is a primary complication. Shunt failure may also result when the shunt's connections separate, usually because of a child's growth.

Cases of shunt failure present as altered mental status. The patient may exhibit drowsiness, respiratory distress, or the classic signs of pupil dysfunction or posturing. Be aware that an altered mental status may be caused by infection—a distinction to be made in a hospital setting.

Care steps involve maintenance of an open airway, administration of ventilations as needed, and immediate transport. Shunt failures require correction in the operating room, where the cerebrospinal fluid can be drained or, in rare cases, an infection identified and treated.

General Assessment and Management Practices

Remember that pediatric patients with special needs require the same assessment as other patients. Always evaluate the airway, breathing, and circulation. (Recall that in the primary assessment, "disability" refers to the patient's neurologic status, not to the child's special need.) If you discover life-threatening conditions in the primary assessment, begin appropriate interventions. Keep in mind that the child's special need is often an ongoing process. In most cases, you should concentrate on the acute problem.

During the assessment, ask pertinent questions of the patient, parent, or caregiver, such as "What unusual situation caused you to call for an ambulance?" As already mentioned, the parent or caregiver is usually very knowledgeable about the patient's condition.

In most cases, the physical examination is essentially the same as with other patients. It is important to explain everything that is being done, even if the patient does not seem to understand. Do not be distracted by the special equipment. Be aware of the help that the patient, parent, or caregiver may be able to provide in handling home care devices.

In managing patients with special needs, try to keep several thoughts in mind:

- Avoid using the term *disability* in reference to the child's special need. Instead, think of the patient's many abilities.
- Never assume that the patient cannot understand what you are saying.

- Involve the parents, caregivers, or the patient, if appropriate, in treatment. They manage the illness or congenital condition on a daily basis.
- Treat the patient with a special need with the same respect as any other patient.

Multiple-Casualty Incidents Involving Children

The criteria routinely used for triage of injured or ill patients at a multiple-casualty incident (MCI) are based on adult anatomic and physiologic data. However, as detailed earlier, children respond to injuries and illnesses somewhat differently because their anatomy and physiology are different. Recognizing this deficiency, noted pediatric emergency physician Lou Romig, MD, FAAP, FACEP, developed the JumpSTART™ system for pediatric triage.[20]

The *JumpSTART Pediatric MCI Triage Tool* is an objective tool developed specifically for the triage of children in the multicasualty/disaster setting. JumpSTART was developed in 1995 to parallel the structure of the START system—the adult MCI triage tool most commonly used in the United States and adopted in many countries around the world. JumpSTART's objectives are:

1. To optimize the primary triage of injured children in the MCI setting
2. To enhance the effectiveness of resource allocation for *all* MCI victims
3. To reduce the emotional burden on triage personnel who may have to make rapid life-or-death decisions about the injured

JumpSTART provides an objective framework that helps to ensure that injured children are triaged by responders using their heads instead of their hearts, thus reducing overtriage that might siphon resources from other patients who need them more. In addition, this system minimizes physical and emotional trauma to children from unnecessary painful procedures and separation from loved ones. Undertriage is addressed by recognizing the key differences between adult and pediatric physiology and using appropriate pediatric physiologic parameters at decision points.

JumpSTART was designed for use in disaster/multicasualty settings and not for daily EMS or hospital triage. The triage philosophies in the two settings are different and require different guidelines. JumpSTART is also intended for the triage of children with acute injuries and may not be appropriate for the primary triage of children with medical illnesses in a disaster setting.

Using the JumpSTART System

The entry category for the JumpSTART system is simple. That is, if the victim "appears to be a child," use the JumpSTART algorithm. If the victim appears to be a young adult or older, use the START system. (The START triage system is detailed in the chapter "Multiple Casualty Incidents and Incident Management.")

To use the JumpSTART system, follow this algorithm (see Figure 4-50):

1. ***Identify and direct all ambulatory patients to the designated minor (GREEN) area for secondary triage and***

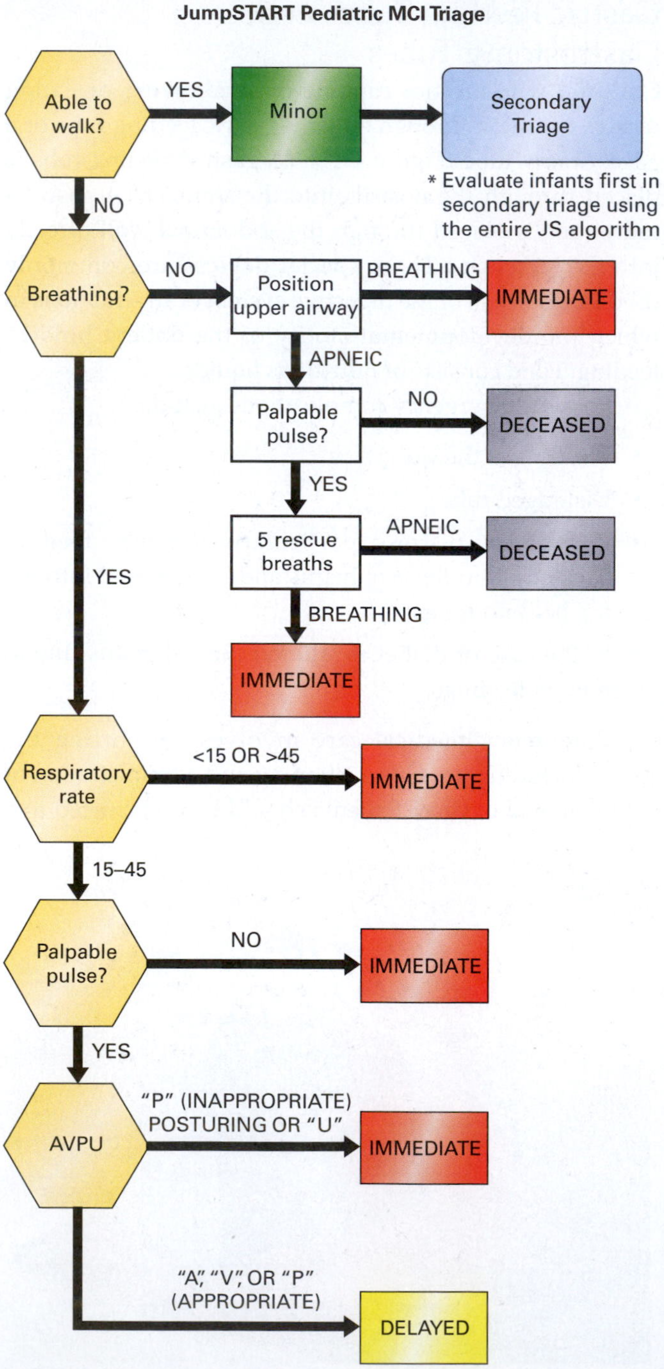

FIGURE 4-50 JumpSTART Pediatric MCI Triage Algorithm.

treatment. Begin assessment of nonambulatory patients as you come to them. Because children less than one year of age cannot walk, they should be carried to the minor (GREEN) area by other ambulatory victims and *must* be the first assessed by medical personnel in that area.

2. ***Assess breathing.*** If the child is breathing spontaneously, go on to the next step (assessing respiratory rate). If the child is apneic or with very irregular breathing, open the airway using standard positioning techniques. If positioning results in resumption of spontaneous respirations, tag the patient *immediate* (RED) and move on. If the child is not breathing after airway opening, check for peripheral pulse. If no pulse, tag the patient *deceased/nonsalvageable* (BLACK) and move on. If there is a peripheral pulse, give five mouth-to-barrier ventilations. If apnea persists, tag the patient *deceased/nonsalvageable* (BLACK) and move on. If breathing resumes after the "jumpstart" (ventilation attempt), tag the patient *immediate* (RED) and move on.
3. ***Assess respiratory rate.*** If the child's respiratory rate is 15 to 45 per minute, proceed to the next step (assess perfusion). If respiratory rate is 45 per minute or irregular, tag patient as *immediate* (RED) and move on.
4. ***Assess perfusion.*** If a peripheral pulse is palpable, proceed to the next step (assess mental status). If no peripheral pulse is present (in the least injured limb), tag the patient *immediate* (RED) and move on.
5. ***Assess mental status.*** Use the AVPU scale to assess mental status. If the patient is **a**lert, responsive to **ver**bal stimuli, or appropriately responsive to **p**ain, tag as *delayed* (YELLOW) and move on. If the patient is inappropriately responsive to **p**ain or is **u**nresponsive, tag as *immediate* (RED) and move on.

Modifications for Nonambulatory Children

All nonambulatory children must be immediately evaluated using the JumpSTART algorithm. Nonambulatory children include those who are too young to walk, children with a developmental delay, children with acute injuries that prevented them from walking *before* the incident, and children with chronic disabilities. If any are *immediate* (RED) criteria, tag as RED. If the child meets the *delayed* (YELLOW) criteria, further classify:

- *Delayed* (YELLOW) if significant external signs of injury are found (e.g., deep penetrating wounds, severe bleeding, severe burns, amputations, distended tender abdomen).
- *Minor* (GREEN) if no significant external injury.

Reassessing Dead/Nonsalvageable (Category BLACK) Victims

Unless clearly suffering from injuries incompatible with life, victims tagged in the *dead/nonsalvageable* (BLACK) category should be reassessed once critical interventions have been completed for *immediate* (RED) and *delayed* (YELLOW) patients. Care should be taken to preserve the dignity of the dead, at the same time being careful to not disturb any forensic evidence present.

Summary

Pediatric emergencies can be stressful for both you and the adults responsible for the child's wellbeing. Many of the pediatric emergencies for which you will be called will be the results of trauma, respiratory distress, ingestion of poisons, or febrile seizure activity. Keep in mind that pediatric medical emergencies are often caused by airway or breathing problems, so focus on these first.

With all pediatric calls, you must be on the lookout for signs and symptoms of child abuse or neglect and report them when found. Remember to never accuse or engage a family member or caregiver. Simply document your objective findings and relay the information to the receiving facility and to local law enforcement.

Keep in mind that the approach and management of pediatric emergencies must be modified for the age and size of the child. Certain skills generally considered routine, such as IV administration, become difficult in the pediatric patient because of size and other factors. As long as you remember that children are not "small adults" and approach them knowing that they have special considerations—both physical and emotional—that must be managed accordingly, you will be successful in assessing and appropriately treating your pediatric patient.

You Make the Call

Dispatch sends you to a residence in an affluent neighborhood. The call reports that "a child is hurt and bleeding." On arrival at the scene, the parents greet you and your crew with controlled anger. Apparently, the neighbors dialed 911 when they heard a child's loud cries coming from the house. The mother tells you that her 24-month-old son fell off the kitchen counter while trying to reach the cookie jar. "He's always climbing after something," she snaps. "I can't watch him 24 hours a day."

As you listen, the child remains strangely quiet. He avoids all eye contact and does not seek comfort from either his mother or father. You observe that a scalp laceration is bleeding profusely. You also observe a number of bruises and abrasions in various stages of healing on the patient's upper torso and arms.

1. What are your assessment priorities for this patient?
2. What interventions would you perform on scene and en route to the receiving hospital?
3. Describe possible transport considerations, including a potential refusal of transport by the angry parents.
4. What are the important factors in reporting this incident and documenting the call?

See Suggested Responses at the back of this book.

Review Questions

1. The ____________ was formed for the express purpose of improving the health of pediatric patients who suffer potentially life-threatening illnesses or injuries.
   a. APLS
   b. EMSC
   c. AHA
   d. PEPP
2. The term *neonate* describes infants from birth to what age?
   a. One week
   b. Two weeks
   c. One month
   d. Two months
3. Children in which age group should be examined in toe-to-head order?
   a. Infants, ages 1–5 months
   b. Infants, ages 6–12 months
   c. Preschoolers, ages 3–5 years
   d. School-age children, ages 6–12 years
4. Children in which age group worry about their physical image more than those in any other pediatric age group?
   a. Infants, ages 1–5 months
   b. Toddlers, ages 1–3 years
   c. School-age children, ages 6–12 years
   d. Adolescents, ages 13–18 years
5. The combination of increased oxygen requirements and decreased oxygen reserves makes infants and children especially susceptible to ____________
   a. trauma.
   b. hypoxia.
   c. epilepsy.
   d. diabetes.
6. Evaluation of breathing adequacy in the pediatric patient includes assessment of all of the following conditions *except* ____________
   a. breath sounds.
   b. heart rate.
   c. respiratory rate.
   d. respiratory effort.
7. Capillary refill time is considered reliable as a sign of perfusion primarily in children less than ____________ years of age.
   a. six
   b. seven
   c. eight
   d. nine
8. What finding in a distressed infant or child may indicate hypoxia and is an ominous sign of cardiac arrest?
   a. Retraction
   b. Bradycardia
   c. Tachycardia
   d. Head bobbing

9. Conditions that place a pediatric patient at risk of cardiopulmonary arrest include all of the following *except* ______________.
   a. respiratory rate greater than 40.
   b. delayed capillary refill.
   c. heart rate greater than 180 or less than 80 (under five years of age).
   d. heart rate greater than 180 or less than 60 (over five years of age).

10. Which of the following airways can be used with a 4-year-old pediatric patient?
    a. EOA
    b. PtL
    c. ETC
    d. LMA

11. Which of the following medications is *not* used in pediatric cardiac arrest?
    a. Epinephrine
    b. Atropine
    c. Lidocaine
    d. Oxygen

12. Which of the following is an example of a commonly used neuromuscular blocking agent that can be used in a pediatric RSI procedure?
    a. Fentanyl
    b. Etomidate
    c. Thiopental
    d. Succinylcholine

13. What should be the initial dosage of an isotonic crystaline solution for use in a 4-year-old hypovolemic shock patient?
    a. 10 mL/kg
    b. 20 mL/kg
    c. 25 mL bolus
    d. 30 mL bolus

14. What is the proper dose of amiodarone for a pediatric patient?
    a. 1.0 mg
    b. 0.5 mg/kg
    c. 2.5 mg
    d. 5.0 mg/kg

15. What is the initial setting for asynchronous cardioversion in a pediatric cardiac arrest patient displaying ventricular tachycardia?
    a. 2 joules per pound
    b. 4 joules per pound
    c. 2 joules per kilogram
    d. 4 joules per kilogram

16. The majority of childhood medical emergencies involve which body system?
    a. Nervous
    b. Endocrine
    c. Respiratory
    d. Cardiovascular

17. The mildest form of respiratory impairment is classified as respiratory ______________
    a. arrest.
    b. failure.
    c. distress.
    d. compromise.

18. Which stage of shock develops when the body can no longer compensate for decreased tissue perfusion and the patient enters cardiac arrest?
    a. Compensated
    b. Irreversible
    c. Anaphylactic
    d. Decompensated

19. What is the most common cause of pediatric bradyarrhythmias?
    a. Alkalosis
    b. Hypoxia
    c. Acidosis
    d. Hypothermia

20. What is the single most common cause of injury in children?
    a. Motor vehicle collisions
    b. Burns
    c. Falls
    d. Drownings

21. You are assessing a pediatric patient who has a rapid respiratory rate, absent alveolar breath sounds, a dropping pulse oximetry reading, and a spontaneous pulse of 102. What should you do next?
    a. Initiate positive pressure ventilation.
    b. Initiate an IV of normal saline or Ringer's lactate.
    c. Gather a SAMPLE history from the patient's parents.
    d. Apply oxygen via blow-by at 15 lpm.

22. During the management of a pediatric patient with a reactive airway disease and wheezing, you elect to provide a nebulized bronchodilator. Any of the following drugs could be used for this purpose in a pediatric patient *except* ______________
    a. levalbuterol.
    b. metaproterenol
    c. albuterol
    d. beclomethasone

See Answers to Review Questions at the end of this book.

References

1. Viner, R., C. Coffey, C. Mathers, et al. "50-year Mortality Trends in Children and Young People: A Study of 50 Low-Income, Middle-Income, and High-Income Countries." *Lancet* 377 (2011): 1162–1174.
2. Wood, D., E. J. Kalinowski, D. R. Miller, et al. "Pediatric Continuing Education for Emergency Medical Technicians. The National Council of State Emergency Medical Services Training Coordinators." *Prehosp Emerg Care* 20 (2004): 261–268.
3. U.S. Department of Health and Human Services. *Emergency Medical Services for Children*. (Available at http://bolivia.hrsa.gov/emsc/.)
4. Richard, J., M. H. Osmond, L. Nesbitt, and I. G. Stiell. "Management and Outcomes of Pediatric Patients Transported by Emergency Medical Services in a Canadian Prehospital System." *CJEM* 8 (2006): 6–12.
5. Diekmann, R. A., D. Brownstein, and M. Gausche-Hill. "The Pediatric Assessment Triangle: A Novel Approach for the Rapid Evaluation of Children." *Pediatr Emerg Care* 26 (2010): 312–315.
6. Corrales, A. Y. and M. Starr. "Assessment of the Unwell Child." *Aust Fam Physician* 39 (2010): 270–275.
7. Singh, S., W. D. Allen, Jr., S. T. Venkataraman, and M. S. Bhende. "Utility of a Novel Quantitative Handheld Microstream Capnometer during Transport of Critically Ill Children." *Am J Emerg Med* 24 (2006): 302–307.
8. Bhende, M. S. and W. D. Allen, Jr. "Evaluation of a Capno-Flo Resuscitator during Transport of Critically Ill Children." *Pediatr Emerg Care* 18 (2002): 414–416.
9. Moynihan, R. J., J. G. Brock-Utne, J. H. Archer, L. H. Feld, and T. R. Kreitzman. "The Effect of Cricoid Pressure on Preventing Gastric Insufflation in Infants and Children." *Anesthesiology* 78 (1993): 652–656.
10. de Caen, A. R., M. D. Berg, L. Chameides, et al. "Part 12: Pediatric Advanced Life Support: 2015 American Heart Association Guidelines for Cardiopulmonary Resuscitation and Emergency Cardiovascular Care." *Circulation* 132 (2015): S526–S542.
11. Ritter, S. C. and F. X. Guyette. "Prehospital Pediatric King LT-D Use: A Pilot Study." *Prehosp Emerg Care* 15 (2011): 401–404.
12. Bjornson, C., K. F. Russell, B. Vandermeer, et al. "Nebulized Epinephrine for Croup in Children." *Cochrane Database Syst Rev* 16 (2011): CD006649.
13. Stranges, E., C. T. Merrill, and C. A. Steiner. "Hospital Stays Related to Asthma, 2006 HCUP Statistical Brief # 58," August 2008.
14. Sharieff, G. Q. and P. L. Hendry. "Afebrile Pediatric Seizures." *Emerg Med Clin North Am* 29 (2011): 95–108.
15. Colletti, J. E., K. M. Brown, G. Q. Sharieff, et al. "The Management of Children with Gastroenteritis and Dehydration in the Emergency Department." *J Emerg Med* 38 (2010): 686–698.
16. Clarke, W., T. Jones, A. Rewers, et al. "Assessment and Management of Hypoglycemia in Children and Adolescents with Diabetes." *Pediatr Diabetes* 10 (Suppl) (2009): 134–145.
17. Klimo, P., Jr., M. L. Ware, N. Gupta, and D. Brockmeyer. "Cervical Spine Trauma in the Pediatric Patient." *Neurosurg Clin N Am* 18 (2007): 599–620.
18. Scaife, E. R. and K. D. Statler. "Traumatic Brain Injury: Preferred Methods and Targets for Resuscitation." *Curr Opin Pediatr* 22 (2010): 339–345.
19. Hall, K. L. and B. Zalman. "Evaluation and Management of Apparent Life-Threatening Events in Children." *Am Fam Physician* 15 (2005): 2301–2308.
20. Sanddal, T. L., T. Loyacono, and N. D. Sanddal. "Effect of JumpSTART Training on Immediate and Short-Term Pediatric Triage Performance." *Pediatr Emerg Care* 20 (2004): 749–753.
21. Child Abuse. Medline Plus/United States National Library of Medicine. (Available at http://www.nlm.nih.gov/medlineplus/childabuse.html.)
22. ChildAbuse.cofsm. (Available at http://www.childabuse.com/.)

Further Reading

American Academy of Pediatrics. *Pediatric Education for Prehospital Professionals*. 2nd ed. Sudbury, MA: Jones and Bartlett Publishers, 2006.

American Heart Association. *2015 American Heart Association Guidelines for CPR and ECC*. Dallas, TX: American Heart Association, 2015.

American Heart Association and American Academy of Pediatrics. *PALS Provider Manual*. Dallas, TX: American Heart Association, 2011.

Gausche-Hill, M., et al. *Pediatric Airway Management for the Prehospital Professional*. Sudbury, MA: Jones and Bartlett Publishers, 2004.

Markenson, D. S. *Pediatric Prehospital Care*. Upper Saddle River, NJ: Pearson/Prentice Hall, 2002.

Porter, R. S., et al. *The Merck Manual of Diagnosis and Therapy*. 19th ed. Whitehouse Station, NJ: Merck, Sharp, and Dohme, 2011.

Romig, L. E. The JumpSTART Pediatric MCI Triage Tool and Other Pediatric and Disaster Emergency Management Resources. (Available at http://www.jumpstarttriage.com/.)

Strange, G., et al. *Pediatric Emergency Medicine*. 3rd ed. New York: McGraw-Hill, 2009.

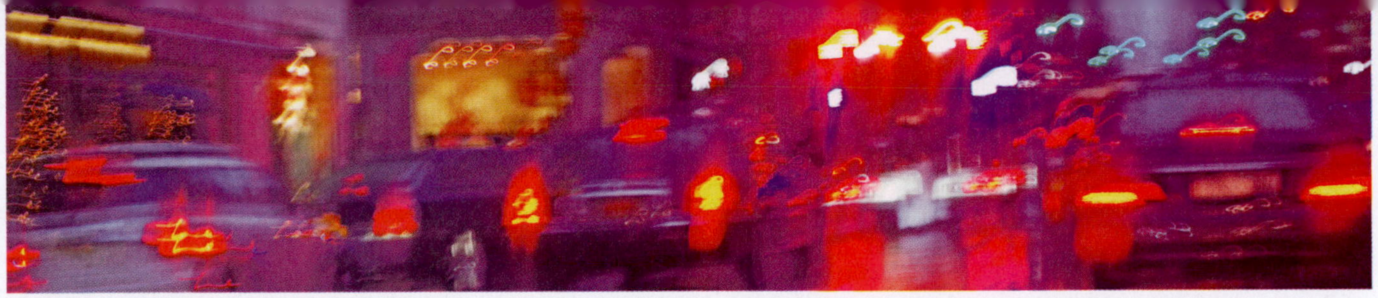

Chapter 5
Geriatrics

Bryan Bledsoe, DO, FACEP, FAAEM, EMT-P

STANDARD

Special Patient Populations (Geriatrics)

COMPETENCY

Integrates assessment findings with principles of epidemiology and pathophysiology and knowledge of psychosocial needs to formulate a field impression and implement a comprehensive treatment/disposition plan for patients with special needs.

Learning Objectives

Terminal Performance Objective: After reading this chapter, you should be able to integrate patient assessment findings, patient history, and knowledge of anatomy, physiology, pathophysiology, and basic and advanced life support interventions to recognize and manage emergencies in geriatric patients.

Enabling Objectives: To accomplish the terminal performance objective, you should be able to:

1. Define key terms introduced in this chapter.
2. Discuss the epidemiology and demographics of aging.
3. Explain the complex interactions between the effects of aging on the body systems and multiple disease processes in elderly patients.
4. Discuss the pathophysiology of aging on the major body systems of the elderly.
5. Identify how to adapt the scene size-up, primary assessment, patient history, secondary assessment, vital sign values, and use of monitoring technology to guide clinical reasoning in the elderly.
6. Identify and delineate between the common medical and traumatic emergencies in the elderly population, and how the paramedic should assess and manage these emergencies.
7. Identify common medications taken by the elderly population that can cause toxicological emergencies, and how these should be managed by the paramedic.
8. Describe special considerations in the elderly that necessitate maintaining a high index of suspicion for behavioral and psychiatric problems, including risk of suicide.
9. Given various geriatric scenarios, discuss how the paramedic should integrate assessment and management for these emergencies in the prehospital environment.

KEY TERMS

acute respiratory distress syndrome (ARDS) , p. 193
advance directive, p. 156
ageism, p. 154
Alzheimer's disease, p. 179
aneurysm, p. 176
ankylosing spondylitis, p. 185
anorexia nervosa, p. 163
anoxic hypoxemia, p. 169
aortic dissection, p. 176
aphasia, p. 180
assisted living, p. 155
autonomic dysfunction, p. 177
brain ischemia, p. 178
cataracts, p. 164
comorbidity, p. 160
congregate care, p. 155
delirium, p. 179
dementia, p. 179
dysphagia, p. 160
dysphoria, p. 192
elderly, p. 153
epistaxis, p. 177
fibrosis, p. 169
functional impairment, p. 159
geriatric abuse, p. 194
geriatrics, p. 154
gerontology, p. 154
glaucoma, p. 164
glomerulonephritis, p. 186
heatstroke, p. 186
hepatomegaly, p. 176
herpes zoster, p. 183
hiatal hernia, p. 170
hypertrophy, p. 169
hypochondriasis, p. 192
immune senescence, p. 171
incontinence, p. 162
intracerebral hemorrhage, p. 178
intractable, p. 179
kyphosis, p. 168
life-care community, p. 155
maceration, p. 184
Marfan syndrome, p. 170
melena, p. 182
Ménière's disease, p. 165
mesenteric ischemia or infarct, p. 182
nephrons, p. 171
nocturia, p. 176
old-old, p. 154
osteoarthritis, p. 184
osteoporosis, p. 171
Parkinson's disease, p. 180
personal-care home, p. 155
pill-rolling motion, p. 181
polycythemia, p. 179
polypharmacy, p. 160
pressure ulcer, p. 183
pruritus, p. 183
retinopathy, p. 182
senile dementia, p. 180
Shy-Drager syndrome, p. 181
sick sinus syndrome, p. 177
silent myocardial infarction, p. 175
spondylosis, p. 196
Stokes-Adams syndrome, p. 177
stroke, p. 178
subarachnoid hemorrhage, p. 178
substance abuse, p. 191
tinnitus, p. 165
transient ischemic attack (TIA) , p. 163
two-pillow orthopnea, p. 176
urosepsis, p. 186
Valsalva maneuver, p. 177
varicosities, p. 177
vertigo, p. 179

Case Study

"Turnpike Rescue, respond Priority One to 957 Homestead Road for a 79-year-old female with abdominal pain."

You've just arrived on duty when this call comes in to the station. "The day is starting early," you say to a coworker. Oh well, you think. It's a good chance to teach Andrew, the paramedic student intern assigned to your crew, about elderly patients. "Hey, Andy," you call out. "What are the causes of abdominal pain in an elderly patient?"

Andy tells you that the pain could be related to any number of bowel complaints—from obstruction to simple constipation. He also mentions problems such as ulcers, urinary infections, and even trauma. He ends with a quip: "Probably isn't related to too many beers and a taco, huh?"

You've just pulled up to the house, so you let Andy's remark slide for now. A man standing in the doorway calls out: "Come quickly—I think my mother may be dying."

You and your partner allow Andy to conduct a complete scene survey. You concur with his decision that the scene is safe at the present time and enter what appears to be a well-kept home.

"Does your mother live alone?" you ask. The son, who identifies himself as Michael, replies: "Yes, Mom lives alone. She's extremely independent. She drives everywhere, even at night. She does volunteer work and still likes to travel. This past summer, she took a cruise to the Bahamas all by herself." Michael then adds, "That's why I'm so worried. I stopped in to visit, and there was Mom still in bed, crying out in pain."

On entering the patient's bedroom, you see a well-nourished elderly woman, tossing and turning on her bed. "My stomach hurts so much," she sobs. Between cries of anguish, she manages to tell you that the pain woke her up early this morning. She has not gotten out of bed since. When you ask if she has fallen recently, she says "No."

You notice that Andy has instructed your partner to place the appropriate monitors. You nod in approval and ask him to begin the primary assessment. Meanwhile, you obtain a history from the son.

Michael explains that his mom, Mrs. Hildegaard, has been very healthy. She has hypertension, but is compliant with her medication of lisinopril and hydrochlorothiazide. When you ask about allergies, Michael mentions aspirin. He knows of no changes in his mother's diet and her appetite has been good. In fact, she and his brother Allen went out to dinner last night. Michael explains that Mrs. Hildegaard was clinically depressed after the death of her husband seven years ago, but "bounced back" after therapy. She has taken no antidepressants for more than five years.

After performing a primary assessment, Andy reports: "Airway is open and clear. Breathing is slightly fast at 22 per minute, but is interspersed with crying. Lungs are clear. Skin is cool, but dry. No overt bleeding. Pupils equal and reactive, with no neuro deficits noted." He then states the vital signs as BP 154/90 mmHg, pulse 110 and irregular, respirations 22 and nonlabored. SpO_2 is 97 percent on room air. On examination of the patient's abdomen, Andy found no evidence of guarding and no specific area of tenderness. Mrs. Hildegaard told him: "My stomach hurts all over, everywhere you touch."

Your partner has also established an IV line of normal saline and placed the patient on the cardiac monitor. The monitor shows atrial fibrillation with an average rate of 110 bpm.

The patient is packaged and transported to the emergency department. En route, you contact the receiving hospital.

In the ED, the attending physician orders blood work, a chest film, and an abdominal CT. Following an exploratory laparotomy, the physician admits Mrs. Hildegaard to the surgical intensive care unit. The diagnosis is an infarcted bowel. The patient's prognosis is poor.

Back at the station, you take time to address Andy's quip about the "beers and a taco." You say: "You probably know that as people age they often lose lifelong support systems, like a job or a spouse. But did you realize that the elderly sometimes turn to alcohol to relieve the pain, just like people our own age?"

You then offer some pointers for providing quality EMS care to the elderly. "The most important thing to remember about the elderly patient is that although many changes occur as a result of aging, you must avoid jumping to conclusions. Give proper attention to assessment and think about normal changes of aging versus changes as a result of disease. Provide prompt treatment because the elderly patient has less physiologic reserve than a younger patient. Once the elderly patient starts to deteriorate, the process is difficult to stop. Always remember that when complaints of abdominal pain are out of proportion to your exam, you should suspect a serious medical condition—in this case, bowel infarct."

As you walk away, you say: "So, Andy, do you want to talk about what went right with this call, and what we could have done better, while we restock the ambulance?"

"You bet," he replies.

Introduction

Aging—the gradual decline of biological functions—varies widely from one individual to another. Most people reach their biological peak in the years before age 30. For practical purposes, however, the aging process does not affect their daily lives until later years. Many of the decrements commonly ascribed to aging are caused by other factors, such as lifestyle, diet, behavior, or environment. The aging process becomes even more complicated if we remember that age-related changes in organ functions also occur at different rates. For example, a person's kidneys may decline rapidly with age while the heart remains strong, or vice versa.

As people age, they actually become less like one another, both physiologically and psychologically. Although some functional losses in old age are caused by normal age-related changes, many others result from abnormal changes, particularly disease. In assessing and treating older patients, it is important to distinguish, when possible, normal age-related changes from abnormal changes. The purpose of this chapter is to present some of the most common physiologic changes associated with aging and the implications of these changes to the quality of EMS care provided to the **elderly**, one of the fastest growing segments of our population.

Epidemiology and Demographics

The twentieth century—with its tremendous medical and technological advances—witnessed both a reduction in infant mortality rates and an increase in life expectancies. The cumulative effect was a population boom worldwide, with the greatest gains seen among people age 65 or older. During the 1900s, the population of the United States increased threefold, with the number of elderly increasing tenfold. Today, in the twenty-first century, the growing number of elderly patients presents a challenge to all health care services, including EMS, not only in terms of resources, but also in the enormous impact that aging has on our society.

Population Characteristics

America is getting older. Between 1960 and 1990, the number of elderly people in the United States nearly tripled. By late 2014, the total reached more than 45 million, with approximately 337,000 people aged 95 and older. As the twenty-first century opened, demographers talked about the "graying of America," a process in which the number of elderly people is pushing up the average age of the U.S. population as a whole. The percentage of elderly Americans is expected to increase by 19 percent by 2030. Reasons for this trend include the following:

- The mean survival rate of older persons is increasing.
- The birth rate is declining.
- There has been an absence of major wars and other catastrophes.
- Health care and standards of living have improved significantly since World War II.

In 2030, when the post–World War II baby boomers enter their 80s, more than 70 million people will be age 65 or older. By 2040, the elderly will represent roughly 20 percent of the population. In other words, one in five Americans will be aged 65 or older.

Not only will the elderly population increase in size, but its members also will live longer, which in turn will swell the number of the **old-old**. By 2040, the number of people aged 85 and older is expected to rise by 17 percent. Whether longer life spans mean longer years of active living or longer years of disease and disability is unknown (Figure 5-1).

Gerontology—the study of the effects of aging on humans—is a relatively new science. (The Gerontological Society of America was formed in 1945.) Gerontologists still do not fully understand the underlying causes of aging. However, most believe that some form of cellular damage or loss, particularly of nerve cells (neurons), is involved. The result is a general decline in the body's efficiency, such as a reduction in the size and function of most internal organs.

To treat age-related changes, physicians and other health care workers have increasingly specialized in the care of the elderly. This aspect of medicine, known as **geriatrics**, is essential in caring for our aging population.

The demographic changes will also affect your EMS career. Today, nearly 36 percent of all EMS calls involve the elderly. The percentage is expected to grow. Therefore, you will need to be familiar with the fundamental principles of geriatrics, especially those related to advanced prehospital care. You will also need to be aware of the social issues that can affect the health and mental well-being of the elderly patients that you will be treating.

Societal Issues

For a typical working person, the retirement years can be up to one-quarter of an average life span. The years include a series of transitions, such as reduced income, relocation, and loss of friends, family members, spouse, or partner.[1]

After years of working and/or raising a family, an elderly person must not only find new roles to fulfill but, in many cases, must also overcome the societal label of "old person." Many elderly people disprove **ageism**—and all the stereotypes it engenders—by living happy, productive, and active lives (Figure 5-2). Others, however, feel a sense of social isolation or uselessness. Physical and financial difficulties reinforce these feelings and help create an emotional context in which illnesses can occur. Therefore, successful medical treatment of elderly patients involves an understanding of the broader social situation in which they live.

Living Environments

The elderly live in both independent and dependent living environments. Many continue to live alone or with their partner well into their 80s or 90s. The "oldest" old are the most likely to live alone—and, in fact, nearly half of those age 85 and older live by themselves. The great majority of these people—an estimated 78 percent—are women. This is because married men tend to die before their wives, and widowed men tend to remarry more often than widowed women.

POVERTY AND LONELINESS Elderly persons living alone can be one of the most impoverished and vulnerable parts of society. Death of a partner reduces income sharply, especially for women whose savings are depleted by long illnesses and/or who relied on their husbands' retirement benefits. Such low incomes force the elderly to

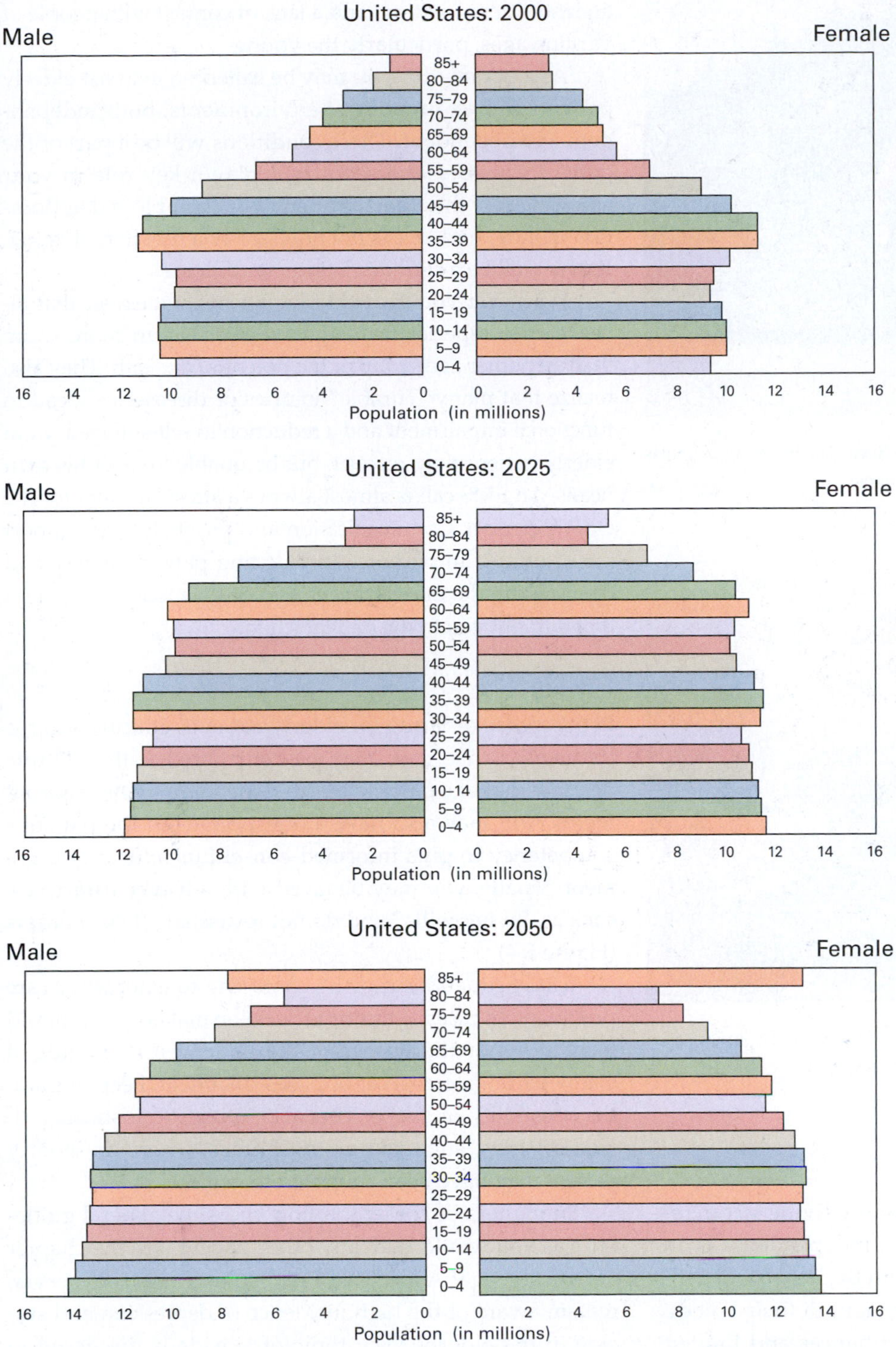

FIGURE 5-1 The elderly are rapidly becoming a large percentage of the population. These graphs represent predictions from the U.S. Census Bureau of future population distributions by age for the years 2025 and 2050.

choose among such basic necessities as food, shelter, or medicine.

In addition to poverty, many of the elderly who live alone, especially the old-old, have few or no living family members. Not surprisingly, more than 60 percent of those over age 75 report feelings of loneliness. Depression is also common, particularly among those who are both poor and alone.

Despite these difficulties, nearly 90 percent of the elderly who live alone choose to maintain their independence. Many fear any situation in which they would be treated as helpless human beings. Others do not want to burden family, friends, or even society with their problems. Some see their situation, including illness, as an inevitable part of aging and refuse to complain or ask for help. Keep this fact in mind whenever you question an elderly patient: The elderly often do not reveal problems beyond the chief complaint, either because they fear the loss of independence or because they consider the illnesses as "normal" for their age.

SOCIAL SUPPORT Of the elderly people who live alone and who cannot perform some everyday tasks, nearly 74 percent receive no form of assistance. To avoid the dangers of social isolation, doctors encourage the elderly to interact with other people. This helps them to build a network of social support, a factor critical to mental health and physical well-being (Figure 5-3). Interaction may be with family members, neighbors, or other elderly people at senior centers. Levels of interaction can be gauged by questions such as "Is there anyone you can call if you have trouble with your medications tonight?" "Can someone stay with you when you return from the hospital?"

Among the elderly who receive help, more than 43 percent rely on paid assistance. Another 54 percent use unpaid assistance, and 3 percent use both types of help. Elderly people who turn to dependent care arrangements may choose among a variety of options, including live-in nursing, **assisted living**, **life-care communities**, **congregate care**, or **personal-care homes**. Approximately 5 percent of the elderly live in nursing homes.

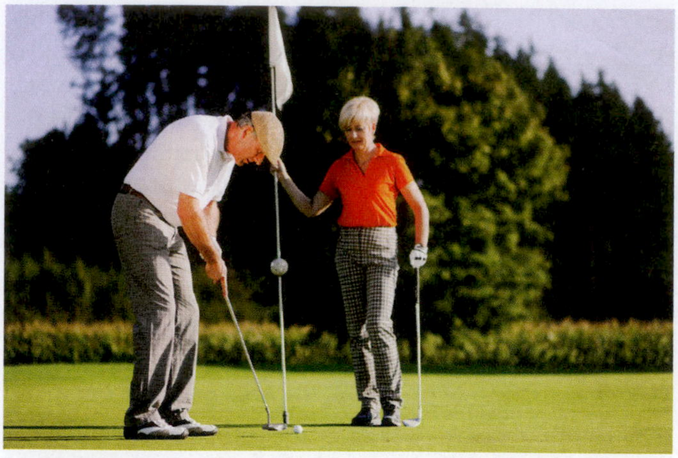

FIGURE 5-2 Many older adults live active lives, participating in sports and exercises popular among people of all ages.

(Kzenon/Fotolia)

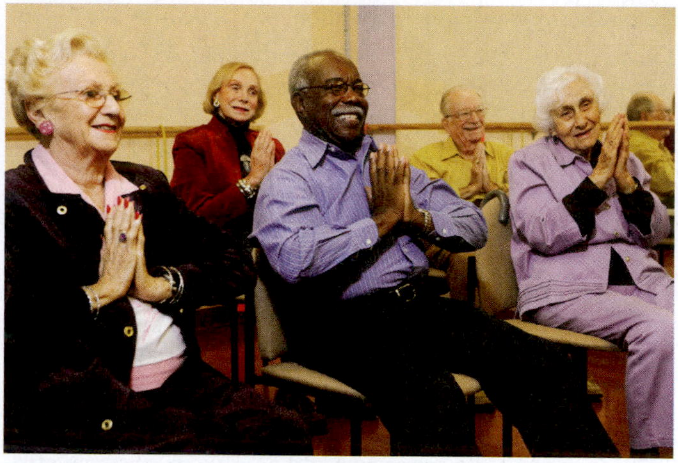

FIGURE 5-3 Many elderly people form social networks by joining a senior center or by taking part in volunteer programs.

(Monkey Business/Fotolia)

Both independent and dependent living arrangements have benefits and drawbacks. Independence is an important concept. Older persons with the desire and ability to do so should be allowed to remain in their homes. Keep in mind, however, that tight finances and limited mobility may prevent an independent elderly person from maintaining adequate nutrition and safety. As a result, elderly patients may be at increased risk of accidental hypothermia, carbon monoxide poisoning, or fires. They may also reduce their medications, or "half dose," to save money.

Many states have few or no restrictions on personal-care aides or others who provide assistance in the home. The elderly can be at risk for criminal activities. Living in an adult community or nursing home removes some of the concerns of self-care. Trade-offs include the loss, in varying degrees, of independence; exposure to illnesses found in an institutional setting; and a lack of contact with people of varying ages, particularly the young.

As a paramedic, you may be called on to assist elderly patients in any number of environments, both independent and dependent. These conditions will be a part of the patient's history and often will play a key role in your assessment of the elderly patient. For example, a deterioration in independence is not necessarily a function of aging. It may well be a sign of an untreated illness.

Whenever you treat elderly patients, remember that illness carries a special meaning for them. They are more aware than any other age group of the potential of death. They also realize that many "curable" injuries or diseases can lead to functional impairment and a reduction in self-sufficiency. An elderly patient may recover, but be unable to meet his own needs. An EMS call is almost always a stressful event for the elderly person. Communication and psychological support are of utmost importance in reducing patient anxiety and determining the underlying causes of the medical condition that brought you to the patient's home.

Ethics

In the course of caring for elderly patients, ethical concerns frequently arise. You may be confronted with multiple decision makers, particularly in dependent living environments. You may also have a question about the patient's competency to give informed consent or refusal of treatment. Finally, you may be faced with **advance directives**, such as "living wills" and do not resuscitate (DNR) orders (Figure 5-4).[2]

These situations may be confusing to emergency care providers. In cases of multiple decision makers, you should usually honor the wishes of the patient, if he is judged competent. If a caregiver opposes treatment, keep in mind the possibility of abuse. This also applies to institutionalized settings, such as nursing homes, where an elderly patient may have been subjected to neglect.

In matters of consent, follow the same general guidelines as you would with any other patient (see the chapter "Medical–Legal Aspects of Prehospital Care"). However, remain aware of the high incidence of depression and suicide in the elderly. (The topic of suicide is discussed in greater detail later in this chapter.) If you think a patient should be transported to the hospital, make every effort to get him there.

Whenever you are presented with advance directives, you should follow state laws and local EMS system protocols. Some states have standard legal forms for DNR orders to prevent confusion. Cases in which you receive an advance directive are truly life-and-death situations. If you have any doubt about what the directive says or its legality, begin treatment and contact medical direction. In all situations involving ethical decisions, document the reasons for your choice of action.

PREHOSPITAL DO NOT RESUSCITATE ORDER

ATTENDING PHYSICIAN

In completing this prehospital DNR form, please check part A if no intervention by prehospital personnel is indicated. Please check Part A and options from Part B if specific interventions by prehospital personnel are indicated. To give a valid prehospital DNR order, this form must be completed by the patient's attending physician and must be provided to prehospital personnel.

A) ____________ **Do Not Resuscitate (DNR):**
No Cardiopulmonary Resuscitation or Advanced Cardiac Life Support should be performed by prehospital personnel

B) ____________ **Modified Support:**
Prehospital personnel administer the following checked options:

____________ Oxygen administration
____________ Full airway support: intubation, airways, bag-valve-mask
____________ Venipuncture: IV crystalloids and/or blood draw
____________ External cardiac pacing
____________ Cardiopulmonary resuscitation
____________ Cardiac defibrillator
____________ Pneumatic anti-shock garment
____________ Ventilator
____________ ACLS meds
____________ Other interventions/medications (physician specify)
____

Prehospital personnel are informed that (print patient name)______________________________ should receive no resuscitation (DNR) or should receive Modified Support as indicated. This directive is medically appropriate and is further documented by a physician's order and a progress note on the patient's permanent medical record. Informed consent from the capacitated patient or the incapacitated patient's legitimate surrogate is documented on the patient's permanent medical record. The DNR order is in full force and effect as of the date indicated below.

____
Attending Physician's Signature

____
Print Attending Physician's Name

____
Attending Physician's Telephone

____
Date

____
____
____
Print Patient's Name and Location
(Home Address or Health Care Facility)

____
Expiration Date (6 Mos from Signature)

FIGURE 5-4 An example of a do not resuscitate order.

Financing and Resources for Health Care

Caring for an increasing number of elderly patients places a huge demand on traditional health care resources, including EMS. Currently, Social Security pays a significant portion of monthly bills, with medical support provided by various major publicly funded programs:

- ***Medicare.*** This program basically operates as a two-part complementary system. Part A covers in-hospital care; Part B provides medical insurance to cover physicians, outpatient care, therapy, and durable medical equipment. About 95 percent of all people over age 65 are enrolled in Part A; nearly all of them are also enrolled in Part B, which is voluntary. Under Medicare, people may enroll in health maintenance organizations (HMOs) that accept Medicare benefits. In 2006, the Medicare program was expanded to cover certain prescription drugs. This program, called Part D, made it easier for Medicare beneficiaries to receive needed prescription drugs.
- ***Medicaid.*** Under Medicaid, the federal and state governments share responsibility for providing health care to the aged poor, people who are blind, people with disabilities, and low-income families with dependent

children. Although Medicaid was created to help the poor, the high cost of medical care has brought large numbers of elderly people into the program. Today, Medicaid provides the largest share of public funding for long-term care. It contributes approximately 45 percent of the financing for nursing home services.

- ***Veterans Administration (VA).*** The Veterans Administration offers health care to veterans with disabilities or service-related problems. It operates more than 170 hospitals and more than 100 nursing homes. Services may be provided free or on a sliding scale.
- ***Local government.*** In many communities, publicly funded hospitals and clinics provide care for those unable to find health care. In many instances, persons less than 65 years of age and those who do not have legal resident status are not eligible for Medicare or Medicaid. In these instances, health care needs are met by public hospitals and clinics typically funded through taxes.

With the number of younger taxpaying workers shrinking, publicly funded medical programs face an uncertain future. A growing number of private insurers have started offering policies for long-term care during a person's older years. These policies, however, may be too expensive for many of the elderly, and younger people may not be willing to purchase them when they are young and premiums are low. Many experts worry that the booming elderly population projected for the 2030s and 2040s may have to rely increasingly on private savings, retirement plans, and state assistance in whatever form it exists.

Hospital Alternatives

One of the biggest health care debates of the early twenty-first century centers around the question of preventing death at all costs. A significant amount of health care dollars is spent during a person's last month of life, much of which is spent during the final ten days. Governmental and independent agencies have advised that it might be better to spend money on preventing disease rather than preventing death.

In an effort to bring down the cost of acute medical care, hospitals have shifted patient care increasingly to the home. The emphasis on home care, with appropriate medical and nursing assistance, has become a recognized medical practice (see the chapter "Acute Interventions for the Chronic Care Patient.") This development has gone hand in hand with the hospice movement, which allows terminally ill patients to live the remainder of their lives outside a hospital. Both trends have a deep impact on EMS personnel, who will be called on to provide more complicated care for more patients, particularly the elderly, in an out-of-hospital setting.

Prevention and Self-Help

In treating the elderly, remember that the best intervention is prevention (Table 5-1). The goal of any health care service, including EMS, should be to help keep people from becoming sick or injured in the first place. As previously mentioned,

Table 5-1 Prevention Strategies for the Older Person

Issues	Strategies
Lifestyle	
Exercise	Weight-bearing and cardiovascular exercise (walking) for 20–30 minutes at least three times a week
Nutrition	Varies, but generally low fat, adequate fiber (complex carbohydrates), reduced sugar (simple carbohydrates), moderate protein; adequate calcium, especially for women*
Alcohol/tobacco	Moderate alcohol, if any; abstinence from tobacco
Sleep	Generally 7–8 hours a night
Accidents	
	Maintain good physical condition; add safety features to home (handrails, nonskid surfaces, lights, etc.); modify potentially dangerous driving practices (driving at night with impaired night vision, traveling in hazardous weather, etc.)
Medical Health	
Disease/illness	Routine screening for hearing, vision, blood pressure, hemoglobin, cholesterol, etc.; regular physical examinations; immunizations (tetanus booster, influenza vaccine, once-in-a-lifetime pneumococcal vaccine)
Pharmacologic	Regular review of prescription and over-the-counter medications, focusing on potential interactions and side effects
Dental	Regular dental checkups and good oral hygiene (important for nutrition and general well-being)
Mental/emotional	Observe for evidence of depression, disrupted sleep patterns, psychosocial stress; ensure effective support networks and availability of psychotherapy; compliance with prescribed antidepressants

*Vitamin supplements may be required, but should be taken only after other medications are reviewed and in correct dosages. Excessive doses of vitamin A or D, for example, can be toxic.

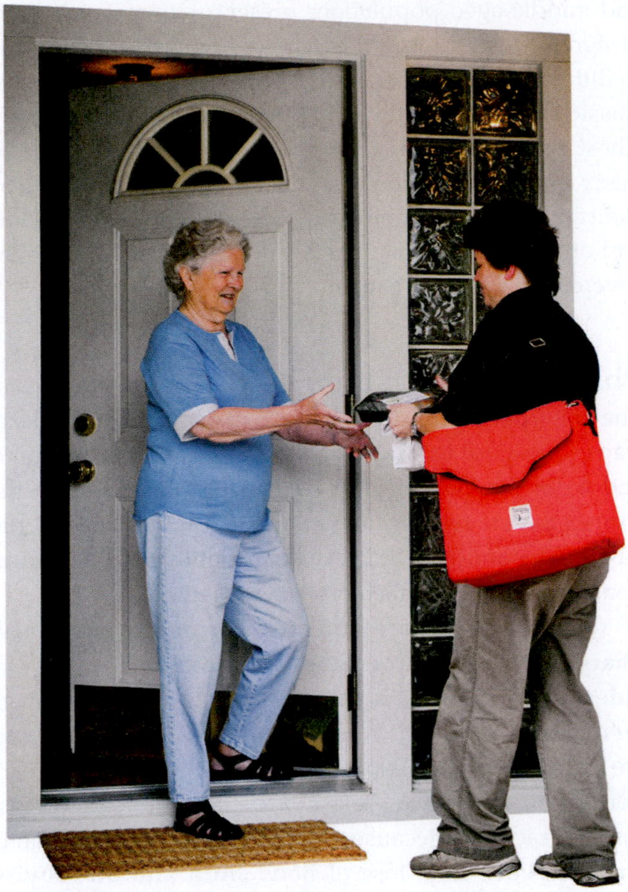

FIGURE 5-5 Meals on Wheels helps ensure that elderly people receive adequate nutrition by providing from one to three meals a day.

disease and disability in later life are often linked to unhealthy or unsafe behavior. As a paramedic, you can reduce morbidity among the elderly by taking part in community education programs and by cooperating with agencies or organizations that support the elderly. Some possible resources are described in the following sections.

SENIOR CENTERS Many communities have senior centers, which provide a social atmosphere for education, recreation, and entertainment. These centers also support health care endeavors such as flu shots, blood pressure monitoring, and transport to clinics. Meals on Wheels, a program that provides from one to three meals a day, may be part of a senior volunteer organization (Figure 5-5).

RELIGIOUS ORGANIZATIONS Religious organizations commonly serve as a resource for the elderly. Some provide services, including dependent living environments, for their members. Others keep in touch with governmental agencies, provide food or clothing for the aged poor, and offer volunteer programs in which the elderly can make useful contributions, thus reducing their sense of isolation.

NATIONAL AND STATE ASSOCIATIONS A number of associations serve as clearinghouses for information to aid the elderly. Some of these groups include AARP, the Alzheimer's Association, and the Association for Senior Citizens. These organizations provide significant advocacy for retired persons. They often have local chapters within a county or region and usually maintain web pages where elderly patients can access information from their homes. AARP is one of the largest, most visible, and most politically connected nonprofit organizations in the world today advocating for the elderly.

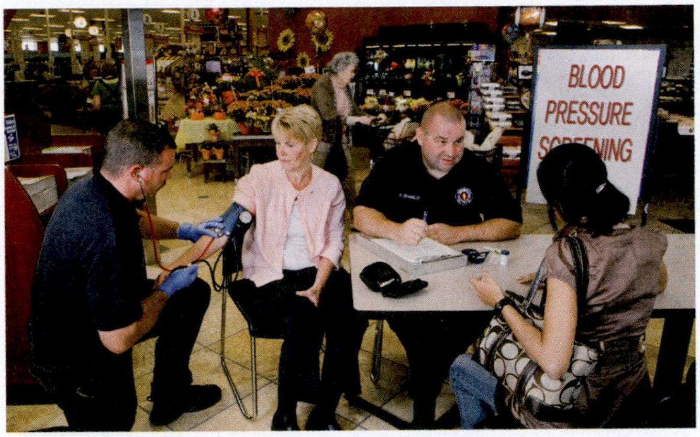

FIGURE 5-6 In some communities, paramedics offer free medical screening programs, such as blood pressure checks, to the elderly

GOVERNMENTAL AGENCIES A wide range of services can be found through governmental agencies, such as the Department of Health and Human Services. Many areas maintain an office for the aging, which refers the elderly to a wide range of community programs, including nutrition centers, senior citizen law projects, home-care services, senior citizen discount programs, and transportation services.

Familiarize yourself with agencies and organizations in your area that work with the elderly. They can be found through use of the Internet, the Department of Health, or special pages in the telephone book, usually at the front or in the Yellow Pages under the heading "Senior Citizens." You can either pass this information on to elderly patients, as needed, or work with one of these groups to initiate programs such as free blood pressure checks (Figure 5-6). You might also start a prevention program that helps the elderly to safeguard their environment against fires, theft, carbon monoxide poisoning, or extremes in temperature.

General Pathophysiology, Assessment, and Management

In treating elderly patients, it is important to recall several facts. First, medical disorders in the elderly often present as **functional impairment** and should be treated as an early warning of a possibly undetected medical problem.

Second, signs and symptoms do not necessarily point to the underlying cause of the problem or illness. For example, whereas confusion often indicates a brain disease in younger patients, this may not be the case in an elderly patient. The confused patient may be suffering from a wide range of disorders, including drug toxicity, malnutrition, or accidental hypothermia.

A thorough evaluation must always be done to detect possible causes of an impairment. If identified early, an environmental- or disease-generated impairment can often be reversed. Your success depends on a knowledge of age-related changes and the implications of these changes for patient assessment and management.

Pathophysiology of the Elderly Patient

As mentioned, patients become less like one another as they enter their elderly years. Even so, certain generalizations can be made about age-related changes and the disease process in the elderly.

Multiple-System Failure

There is no escaping the fact that the body becomes less efficient with age, increasing the likelihood of malfunction. The body is susceptible to all the disorders of young people, but its maintenance, defense, and repair processes are weaker. As a result, the elderly often suffer from more than one illness or disease at a time. On average, six medical disorders may coexist in an elderly person—and perhaps even more in the old-old. Neither the patient nor the patient's doctor may be aware of all these problems. Furthermore, disease in one organ system may result in the deterioration of other systems, compounding existing acute and/or chronic conditions.

Because of concomitant diseases (**comorbidity**) in the elderly, complaints may not be specific to any one disorder. Common complaints of the elderly include fatigue and weakness, dizziness/vertigo/syncope, falls, headaches, insomnia, **dysphagia**, loss of appetite, inability to void, and constipation/diarrhea.

CONTENT REVIEW

➤ Common Complaints in the Elderly
- Fatigue/weakness
- Dizziness/vertigo/syncope
- Falls
- Headaches
- Insomnia
- Dysphagia
- Loss of appetite
- Inability to void
- Constipation/diarrhea

Elderly patients often accept medical problems as a part of aging and fail to monitor changes in their condition. In some cases, such as a silent myocardial infarction, pain may be diminished or absent. In others, an important complaint, such as constipation, may seem trivial.

Although many medical problems in the young and middle-aged populations present with a standard set of signs and symptoms, the changes involved in aging lead to different presentations. In pneumonia, for example, the classic symptom of fever is often absent in the elderly. Chest pain and a cough are also less common. Finally, many cases of pneumonia among the elderly are caused by aspiration, not infection. The presentation of pneumonia and other diseases commonly found in the elderly will be covered later in this chapter.

Pharmacology in the Elderly

The existence of multiple chronic diseases in the elderly leads to the use of multiple medications. Persons age 65 and older use one-third of all prescription drugs in the United States, taking an average of 4.5 medications per day. This does not include over-the-counter (OTC) medications, vitamin supplements, or herbal remedies.

If medications are not correctly monitored, **polypharmacy** can lead to a number of problems among the elderly. In general, a person's sensitivity to drugs increases with age. When compared with younger patients, the elderly experience more adverse drug reactions, more drug–drug interactions, and more drug–disease interactions. Because of age-related pharmacokinetic changes, such as a loss of body fluid and atrophy of organs, drugs concentrate more readily in the plasma and tissues of elderly patients. As a result, drug dosages often must be adjusted to prevent toxicity.[3] (The problem of toxicity is discussed in more detail later in this chapter.)

In taking a medical history of an elderly patient, remember to ask questions to determine whether a patient is taking a prescribed medication as directed. Noncompliance with drug therapy—usually underadherence—is common among the elderly. Up to 40 percent do not take medications as prescribed. Of these individuals, 35 percent experience some type of medical problem. Factors that can decrease compliance in the elderly include:

- Limited income
- Memory loss owing to decreased or diseased neural activity
- Limited mobility
- Sensory impairment (cannot hear/read/understand directions)
- Multiple or complicated drug therapies
- Fear of toxicity
- Childproof containers (especially with arthritic patients)
- Duration of drug therapy (the longer the therapy, the less likely a patient will stick with it)

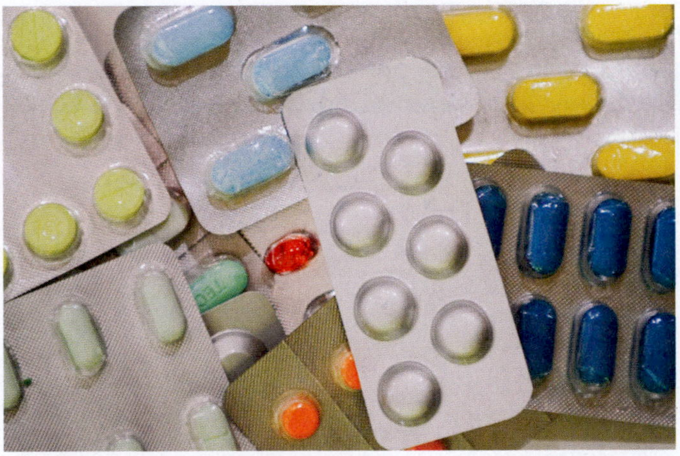

FIGURE 5-7 "Childproof" pill vials are sometimes "elder-proof" as well. Blister-pack packaging makes it easier for elderly patients, especially those suffering from arthritis, to take their medicines, thus furthering compliance.

Factors that can increase compliance among the elderly include:

- Good patient–physician communication
- Belief that a disease or illness is serious
- Drug calendars or reminder cards
- Compliance counseling
- Blister-pack or other easy-to-open packaging (Figure 5-7)
- Multiple-compartment pillboxes
- Transportation services to pharmacy
- Clear, simple directions written in large type
- Ability to read

Problems with Mobility and Falls

Regular exercise and a good diet are two of the most effective preventive measures for ensuring mobility among the elderly. However, not all elderly people take these measures. They may suffer from severe medical problems, such as crippling arthritis. They may fear for their personal safety, either from accidental injury or intentional injury, such as robbery. Certain medications also may increase their lethargy. Whatever the cause, a lack of mobility can have detrimental physical and emotional effects. Some of these include:

- Poor nutrition
- Difficulty with elimination
- Poor skin integrity
- A greater predisposition for falls
- Loss of independence and/or confidence
- Depression from "feeling old"
- Isolation and lack of a social network

Falls present an especially serious problem for the elderly. Fall-related injuries represent the leading cause of accidental death among the elderly and the seventh highest cause of death overall. Only children and young adults have a higher incidence of falls. However, unlike the elderly, children and young adults rarely die from fall-related injuries.

Falls may be either intrinsic (related to the patient) or extrinsic (related to the environment). Intrinsic factors include a history of repeated falls, dizziness, a sense of weakness, impaired vision, an altered gait, CNS problems, decreased mental status, or use of certain medications. Extrinsic factors include environmental hazards such as slippery floors, a lack of handrails, or loose throw rugs (Table 5-2).

Table 5-2 Making a Home Safe for the Elderly

Hazard	Intervention	Reason
Torn or slippery rugs	Repair or replace.	To prevent tripping or slipping
Chair without armrests	Install armrests.	To provide leverage in getting out of chair
Chair with low back	Replace with chair with high backs.	To support neck; to prevent falling backward for patients who must rock to get out of a chair
Chair with wheels	Replace with chair with sturdy legs.	To prevent chair from sliding when patient is getting into or out of it
Obstructing furniture	Move items so clutter is minimized and pathways are clear.	To help those with poor mobility and poor peripheral vision
Slippery bathtub	Install skid-resistant strips or mat.	To provide more stable footing
Dim lighting	Provide adequate lighting in all areas, perhaps with automatic timers.	To improve ability to see, especially in darkened rooms and at night
High cabinet shelves	Place frequently used items on lower shelves or in easy-to-reach places.	To eliminate unnecessary reaching or climbing
Missing handrails on stairways	Install handrail.	To allow elder to grab onto railing for support
High steps on stairways	Rebuild for a rise of less than 6 inches between steps or install a ramp.	To reduce the risk of tripping, falling, or overexertion (especially for cardiac or pulmonary patients)

Table 5-3 Age-Related Sensory Changes and Implications for Communication

Sensory Change	Result	Communication Strategy
Clouding and thickening of lens in eye	Cataracts; poor vision, especially peripheral vision	Position yourself in front of patient where you can be seen; put hand on arm of blind patient to let patient know where you are; locate a patient's glasses, if necessary.
Shrinkage of structure in ear	Decreased hearing, especially ability to hear high-frequency sounds; diminished sense of balance	Speak clearly; check hearing aids as necessary; write notes if necessary; allow the patient to put on the stethoscope, while you speak into it like a microphone.
Deterioration of teeth and gums	Patient needs dentures, but they may inflict pain on sensitive gums, so patient doesn't always wear them	If patient's speech is unintelligible, ask patient to put in dentures, if possible.
Lowered sensitivity to pain and altered sense of taste and smell	Patient underestimates the severity of the problem or is unable to provide a complete pertinent history	Probe for significant symptoms, asking questions aimed at functional impairment.

In assessing an elderly patient who has fallen, remember that a fall can result from any of multiple causes. An overmedicated patient, for example, may trip over a throw rug. A fall may also be a presenting sign of an acute illness, such as a myocardial infarction, or a sign that a chronic illness has worsened. Bear in mind the possibility of physical abuse, especially if the injury does not match the story.

Communication Difficulties

Most elderly patients suffer from some form of age-related sensory changes. Normal physiologic changes may include impaired vision or blindness, impaired or loss of hearing, an altered sense of taste or smell, and/or a lower sensitivity to pain (touch). Any of these conditions can affect your ability to communicate with the patient. Table 5-3 lists some communication strategies you can use with elderly patients. (A discussion on the implications of sensory impairment on patient assessment appears later in this chapter.)

Problems with Continence and Elimination

The elderly often find it embarrassing to talk about problems with continence and elimination. They may feel stigmatized, isolated, and/or helpless. When confronted with these problems, *do not* make a big deal out of them. Respect the patient's dignity and assure the person that, in many cases, the problem is treatable.

INCONTINENCE The problem of **incontinence** can affect nearly any age group, but is most commonly associated with the elderly. Incontinence may be either urinary or fecal. An estimated 15 percent of the elderly who live at home experience some form of urinary incontinence. Nearly 30 percent of the hospitalized elderly and 50 percent of those living in nursing homes suffer from the same condition. Although fecal, or bowel, incontinence is less common, it seriously impairs activity and may lead to dependent care. Between 16 and 60 percent of the institutionalized elderly have some kind of fecal incontinence.

Incontinence can lead to a variety of conditions, such as rashes, skin infections, skin breakdown (ulcers), urinary tract infections, sepsis, and falls or fractures. The condition can also take a high emotional toll on both the patient and the caregiver. Management of incontinence costs billions of dollars each year.

In general, effective continence requires several physical conditions. These include:

- An anatomically correct GI/GU tract
- Competent sphincter mechanism
- Adequate cognition and mobility

Although incontinence is not necessarily caused by aging, several factors predispose older patients to this condition. As mentioned, the elderly tend to have several medical disorders, each of which may require drug therapy. These disorders and/or the drugs used to treat them may compromise the integrity of either the urinary or bowel tracts. In addition, bladder capacity, urinary flow rate, and the ability to postpone voiding appear to decline with age. Certain diseases, such as diabetes and autonomic neuropathy, may also cause sphincter dysfunction. Diarrhea or lack of physical sensation may produce bowel incontinence as well.

Management of incontinence depends on the cause, which cannot be easily diagnosed in the field. Some cases of incontinence can be managed surgically. In most cases, however, patients use some type of absorptive devices, such as leakproof underwear or panty liners. Indwelling catheters are less common and may cause infections when used, particularly if not properly managed. Of critical importance is respect for the patient's modesty and dignity.

ELIMINATION Difficulty with elimination can be a sign of a serious underlying condition (Table 5-4). It can also lead to other complications. Straining to eliminate may have serious effects on the cerebral, coronary, and peripheral arterial circulations. In elderly people with cerebrovascular disease or impaired baroreceptor reflexes, efforts to force a bowel movement can lead to a **transient ischemic attack (TIA)** or syncope. In the case of prolonged constipation, the elderly may experience colonic ulceration, intestinal obstruction, and urinary retention.

In assessing a patient with difficulty eliminating, remember to inquire about his medications. Any of the following drugs can cause constipation:

- Opioids
- Anticholinergics (e.g., antidepressants, antihistamines, muscle relaxants, antiparkinsonian drugs)
- Cation-containing agents (e.g., antacids, calcium supplements, iron supplements)
- Neurally active agents (e.g., opiates, anticonvulsants)
- Diuretics

Assessment Considerations

As with all patients, be sure to take Standard Precautions when assessing an elderly patient. Because of the increased risk of tuberculosis in patients who are in nursing homes, consider wearing a HEPA or N-95 respirator. Remain alert to the environment, particularly the temperature of the surroundings and evidence of prescription medications.

In general, assessment of the elderly patient follows the same basic approach used with any patient. However, you need to keep in mind several factors that will improve the quality of your evaluation and make subsequent treatment more successful.

General Health Assessment

As already mentioned, you need to set a context for illness when assessing an elderly patient. When performing a general health assessment, take into account the patient's living situation, level of activity, network of social support, level of independence, medication history (both prescription and nonprescription), and sleep patterns.

CONTENT REVIEW

➤ Factors in Forming a General Assessment
- Living situation
- Level of activity
- Network of social support
- Level of independence
- Medication history
- Sleep patterns

Pay particular attention to the patient's nutrition. Elderly patients often have a decreased sense of smell and taste, which decreases their pleasure in eating. They also may be less aware of internal cues of hunger and thirst. Although caloric requirements generally decrease with age, an elderly patient can still suffer from malnutrition. Conditions that may complicate or discourage eating among the elderly include:

- Breathing or respiratory problems
- Abdominal pain
- Nausea/vomiting, sometimes a drug-induced condition as with antibiotics or aspirin
- Poor dental care
- Medical problems, such as hyperthyroidism, hypercalcemia, and chronic infections (e.g., cancer or tuberculosis)
- Medications (e.g., digoxin, vitamin A, fluoxetine)
- Alcohol or drug abuse
- Psychological disorders, including depression and **anorexia nervosa**
- Poverty
- Problems with shopping or cooking

As with any person, nutrition greatly affects a patient's overall health. For the reasons just cited, patients may suffer from a number of by-products of malnutrition, including vitamin deficiencies, dehydration, and hypoglycemia. Also remember that when a malnourished elderly person is fed, the food may produce other side effects, including electrolyte abnormalities, hyperglycemia, aspiration pneumonia, and a significant drop in blood pressure.

Table 5-4 Possible Causes of Elimination Problems

Difficulty in Urination	Difficulty with Bowel Movements
Enlargement of the prostate in men	Diverticular disease
Urinary tract infection	Constipation*
Acute or chronic renal failure	Colorectal cancer

*Constipation may be related to dietary, medical, or surgical conditions. It could also be the result of a malignancy, intestinal obstruction, or hypothyroidism. Treat constipation as a serious medical problem.

Pathophysiology and Assessment

Assessment of the elderly reflects the pathophysiology of this age group. As already mentioned, the chief complaint of the elderly patient may seem trivial or vague at first. Also, the patient may fail to report important symptoms. Therefore, you should try to distinguish the patient's chief complaint from the patient's primary problem. A patient may report nausea, which

CONTENT REVIEW

➤ By-Products of Malnutrition
- Vitamin deficiencies
- Dehydration
- Hypoglycemia

Cultural Considerations

How Well Are They Living? Unfortunately, many elderly persons are economically disadvantaged. In fact many, especially elderly women, live at or below the poverty line. The reasons for this are many. Most important, these persons are likely to live on a fixed income—from retirement pensions and/or Social Security benefits. Although this income remains fixed, the cost of living continues to increase. Thus, some elderly persons must make decisions as to what they can and cannot afford. Some will forgo certain medications. Others will try to live with reduced heating or cooling to save energy costs. Unfortunately, others will forgo food to maintain their independence.

When called to assess geriatric patients, try to get an idea about how well they are living. Is the house unusually hot or cold? Are they forgoing certain medications that they consider to be too expensive? Is the house safe and clean? Are they eating well? Are they able and motivated to prepare meals for themselves? Most important, do family members or friends periodically check in on them? If you have any concerns, you should notify the proper authorities or the hospital staff so that social services can provide an evaluation to ensure that these persons can live safely in their present setting.

is the chief complaint. The primary problem, however, may be the rectal bleeding that the patient neglected to mention.

The presence of multiple diseases also complicates the assessment process. The presence of chronic problems may make it more difficult to assess an acute problem. It is easy to confuse symptoms from a chronic illness with those of an acute condition. When confronted with an elderly patient who has chest pain, for example, it is difficult to determine whether the presence of frequent premature ventricular contractions is acute or chronic. If you lack access to the patient's medical record, you should treat the patient on a "threat-to-life" basis.

Other complications stem from age-related changes in an elderly patient's response to illness and injury. Pain may be diminished, causing both you and the patient to underestimate the severity of the primary problem. In addition, the temperature-regulating mechanism may be altered or depressed. This can result in the absence of fever, or a minimal fever, even in the face of a severe infection. Alterations in the temperature-regulating mechanism, coupled with changes in the sweat glands, also makes the elderly more prone to environmental thermal problems.

Because of the complexity of factors that can affect assessment, you must probe for significant symptoms and, ultimately, the primary problem. Patience, respect, and kindness will elicit the answers needed for a pertinent medical history.

History

You should be prepared to spend more time obtaining histories from elderly patients. You may need to split the interview into sessions. For example, you might need to allow patients time to rest if they become fatigued during the interview, or you might take a break to talk with caregivers.

When gathering the history, keep in mind the complications that arise from multiple diseases and multiple medications. Medications can be an especially important indicator of the patient's diseases. Therefore, you should find the patient's medications and take them to the hospital with the patient. Try to determine which of the medications, including OTC medications, are currently being taken. In cases of multiple medications, there is an increased incidence of medication errors, drug interactions, and noncompliance.

COMMUNICATION CHALLENGES As previously mentioned, communication may be more difficult when dealing with the aged. **Cataracts** (Figure 5-8) and **glaucoma** can diminish sight. Cataracts cause clouding of the lens, leading to impairments in vision (Figure 5-9). Blindness, often resulting from diabetes and stroke, is more common in the elderly. The level of anxiety increases when a patient is unable to see his surroundings clearly. As a result, you should talk calmly to patients with visual impairments. Yelling does not help. Instead, position yourself so the patient can see (if he is not totally blind) or touch you.

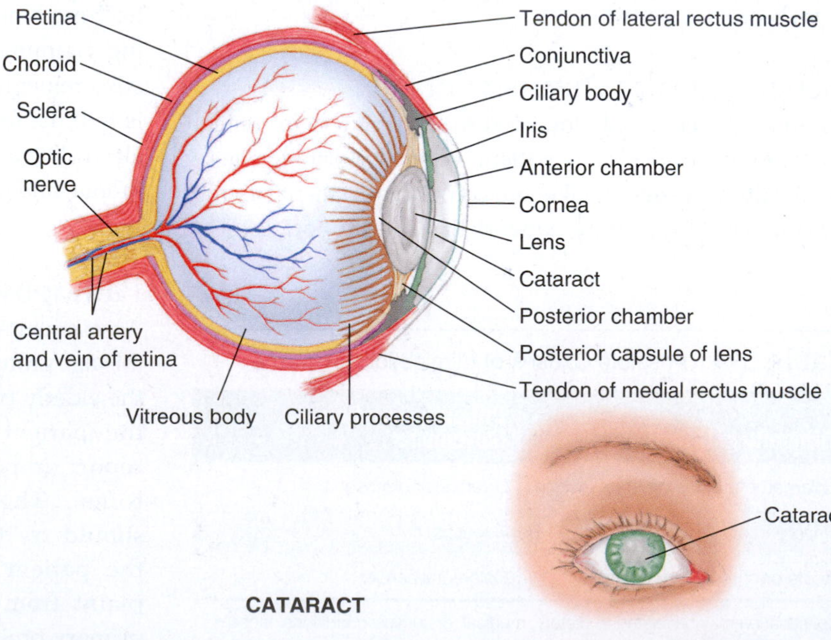

FIGURE 5-8 Cataracts, which cloud the lens, can diminish eyesight in the elderly.

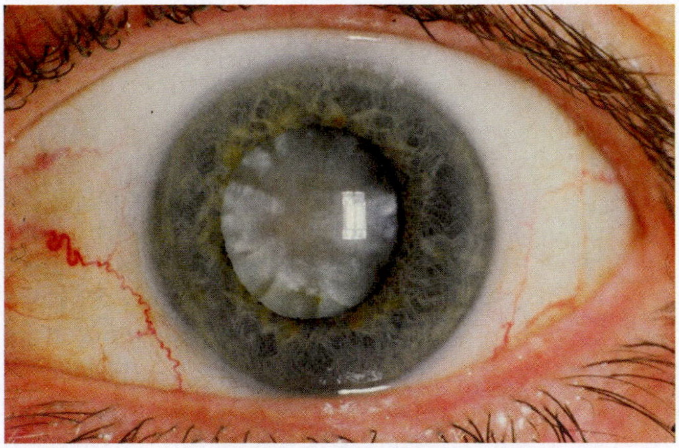

FIGURE 5-9 A clearly visible mature cataract.
(National Eye Institute, National Institutes of Health)

Age also affects hearing. Overall hearing decreases and patients may suffer from auditory disorders such as **tinnitus** or **Ménière's disease**. Diminished hearing or deafness can make it virtually impossible to obtain a history. In such cases, try to determine the history from a friend or family member. *Do not* shout at the patient. This will not help if the patient is deaf, and it may distort sounds and make it difficult for the patient who still has some hearing to understand you. Write notes if necessary. If the patient can lip-read, speak slowly and directly toward the patient. Whenever possible, verify the history with a reliable source. Also, because loss of hearing may result from other causes (such as a buildup of earwax), confirm whether deafness is a preexisting condition.

Patients may also have trouble with speech. They find it difficult to retrieve words. They will often speak slowly and exhibit changes in voice quality, which may be a normal age-related change. If a patient has forgotten to put in dentures, politely ask him to do so.

To improve your skill at communicating with the elderly, keep these techniques in mind:

- Always introduce yourself.
- Speak slowly, distinctly, and respectfully.
- Speak to the patient first, rather than to family members, caregivers, or bystanders.
- Speak face to face, at eye level with eye contact (Figure 5-10).
- Locate the patient's hearing aid or eyeglasses, if needed (Figure 5-11).
- Allow the patient to put on the stethoscope, while you speak into it like a microphone.
- Turn on the room lights.
- Display verbal and nonverbal signs of concern and empathy.
- Remain polite at all times.
- Preserve the patient's dignity.
- Do not be afraid to rephrase a question or ask the patient again if you could not understand or hear the patient.
- Always explain what you are doing and why.
- Use your power of observation to recognize anxiety—tempo of speech, eye contact, tone of voice—during the telling of the history.

ALTERED MENTAL STATUS AND CONFUSION Remember that age sometimes diminishes mental status. The patient can be confused and unable to remember details. In addition, the noise of radios, ECG equipment, and strange voices may add to the confusion. Both senility and organic brain syndrome may manifest themselves similarly. Common symptoms include:

- Delirium
- Confusion

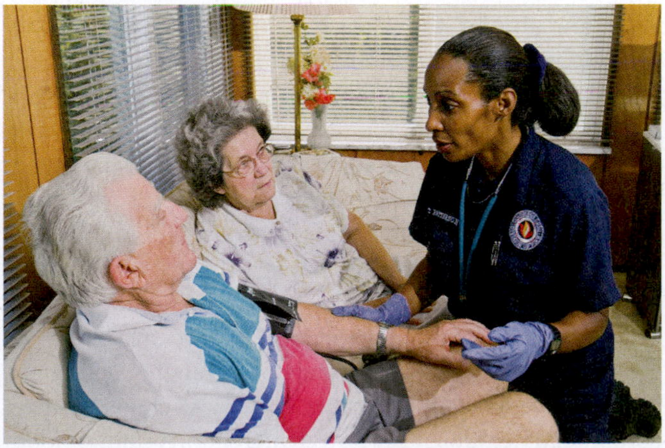

FIGURE 5-10 If possible, talk *to* the elderly patient rather than talking about the patient to others.

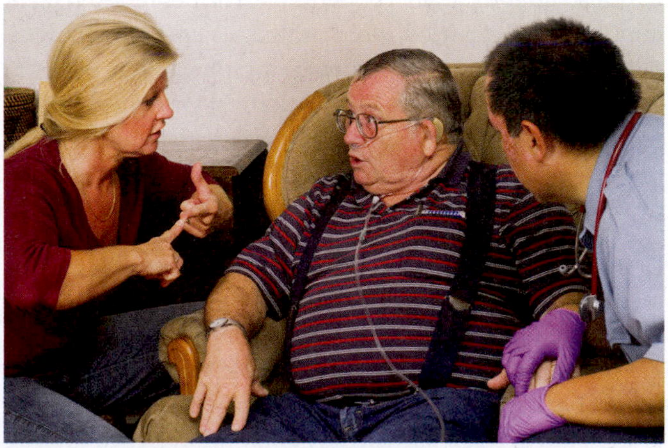

FIGURE 5-11 Make sure the elderly patient is wearing his eyeglasses and hearing aids, if required.

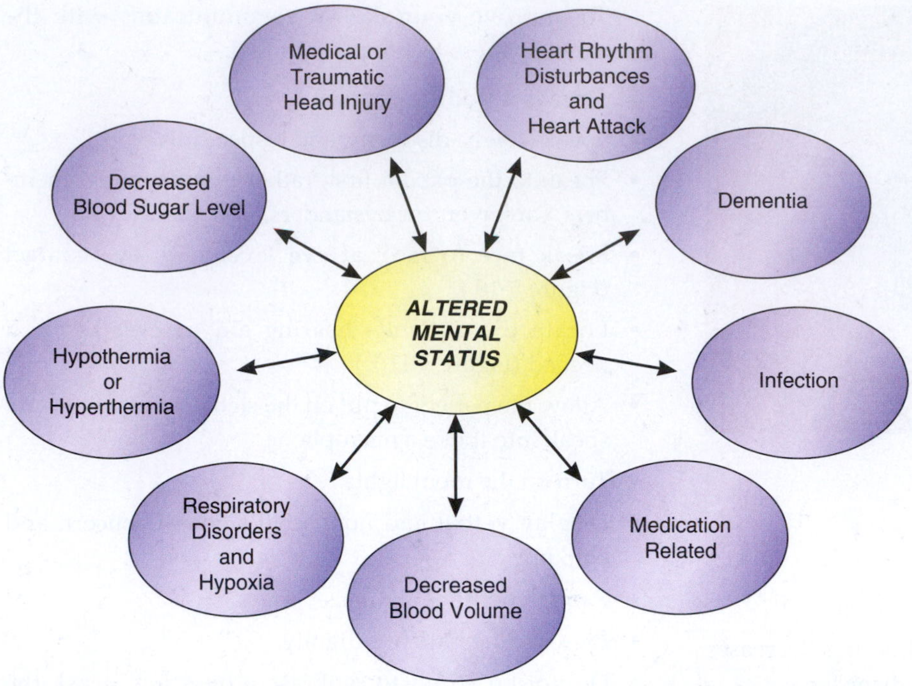

FIGURE 5-12 *Do not* assume that an altered mental status is a normal age-related change. A number of serious underlying problems may be responsible for changes in consciousness.

- Distractibility
- Restlessness
- Excitability
- Hostility

When confronted with a confused patient, try to determine whether the patient's mental status represents a significant change from normal. *Do not* assume that a confused, disoriented patient is "just senile," thus failing to assess for a serious underlying problem (Figure 5-12). Alcoholism, for example, is more common in the elderly than was once recognized. It can further complicate taking the history.

Another complication results from depression, which can be mistaken for many other disorders. It can often mimic senility and organic brain syndrome. Depression may also inhibit patient cooperation. The depressed patient may be malnourished, dehydrated, overdosed, contemplating suicide, or simply imagining physical ailments to gain attention. If you suspect depression, question the patient regarding drug ingestion or suicidal ideation. It is important to remember that suicide is a common cause of death among the elderly in the United States.

CONCLUDING THE HISTORY After obtaining the history, and if time allows, try to verify the patient's history with a credible source. This will often be less offensive to the patient if done out of his presence. While at the scene, it is important to observe the surroundings for indications of the patient's self-sufficiency. Look for evidence of drug or alcohol ingestion and for MedicAlert tags, Vial of Life, or similar medical identification items. It is also important to spot signs of abuse or neglect, particularly in dependent living arrangements.

Physical Examination

Certain considerations must be kept in mind when examining the elderly patient. Remember that some patients may be easily fatigued and unable to tolerate a long examination. Also, because of the problems with temperature regulation, the patient may be wearing several layers of clothing, which can make examination difficult. Be sure to explain all actions clearly before initiating the examination, especially to patients with impaired vision. Be aware that the patient may minimize or deny symptoms because of a fear of becoming institutionalized or a loss of self-sufficiency.

Try to distinguish signs of chronic disease from an acute problem. Peripheral pulses may be difficult to evaluate, because of peripheral vascular disease and arthritis. The elderly may also have nonpathologic crackles (rales) on lung auscultation. In addition, the elderly often exhibit an increase in mouth breathing and a loss of skin elasticity, which may be easily confused with dehydration. Dependent edema may be caused by inactivity, not congestive heart failure. Only experience and practice will allow you to distinguish acute from chronic physical findings.

Management Considerations

Elderly patients can present a unique challenge in terms of assessment and management. You will need to tailor your management plan to fit a patient's illness, injury, and overall general health. Because of the potential for rapid deterioration among the elderly, you must quickly spot conditions requiring rapid transport.

As with any other patient, your first concern is the primary assessment. Remain alert at all times for changes in an elderly patient's neurologic status, vital signs, and general cardiac status. (Management of specific disorders and the administration of medications to the elderly are covered in other sections of this chapter.)

In general, remember that transport to a hospital is often more stressful for the elderly than to any other age group, except for the very young. Avoid lights and sirens in all but the most serious cases, such as when you suspect a pulmonary embolism or bowel infarction. A calm, smooth transport helps to reduce patient anxiety—and the resulting strain that anxiety places on an elderly patient's heart.

Provide emotional support at every phase of the call. Nearly any serious illness or injury in the elderly can provoke a sense of impending doom. Death is a very real possibility to this age group. To help reduce patient fears, keep these guidelines in mind:

- Encourage patients to express their feelings.
- *Do not* trivialize their fears.
- Acknowledge nonverbal messages.
- Avoid questions that are judgmental.
- Confirm what the patient says.
- Recall all you have learned about communicating with the elderly, thus avoiding communication breakdowns.
- Assure patients that you understand that they are adults on an equal footing with their care providers, including you.

System Pathophysiology in the Elderly

Although aging begins at the cellular level, it eventually affects virtually every system in the body (Figure 5-13). Age-related changes in the structure and function of organs increase the probability of disease, modify the threshold at which signs and symptoms appear, and affect assessment

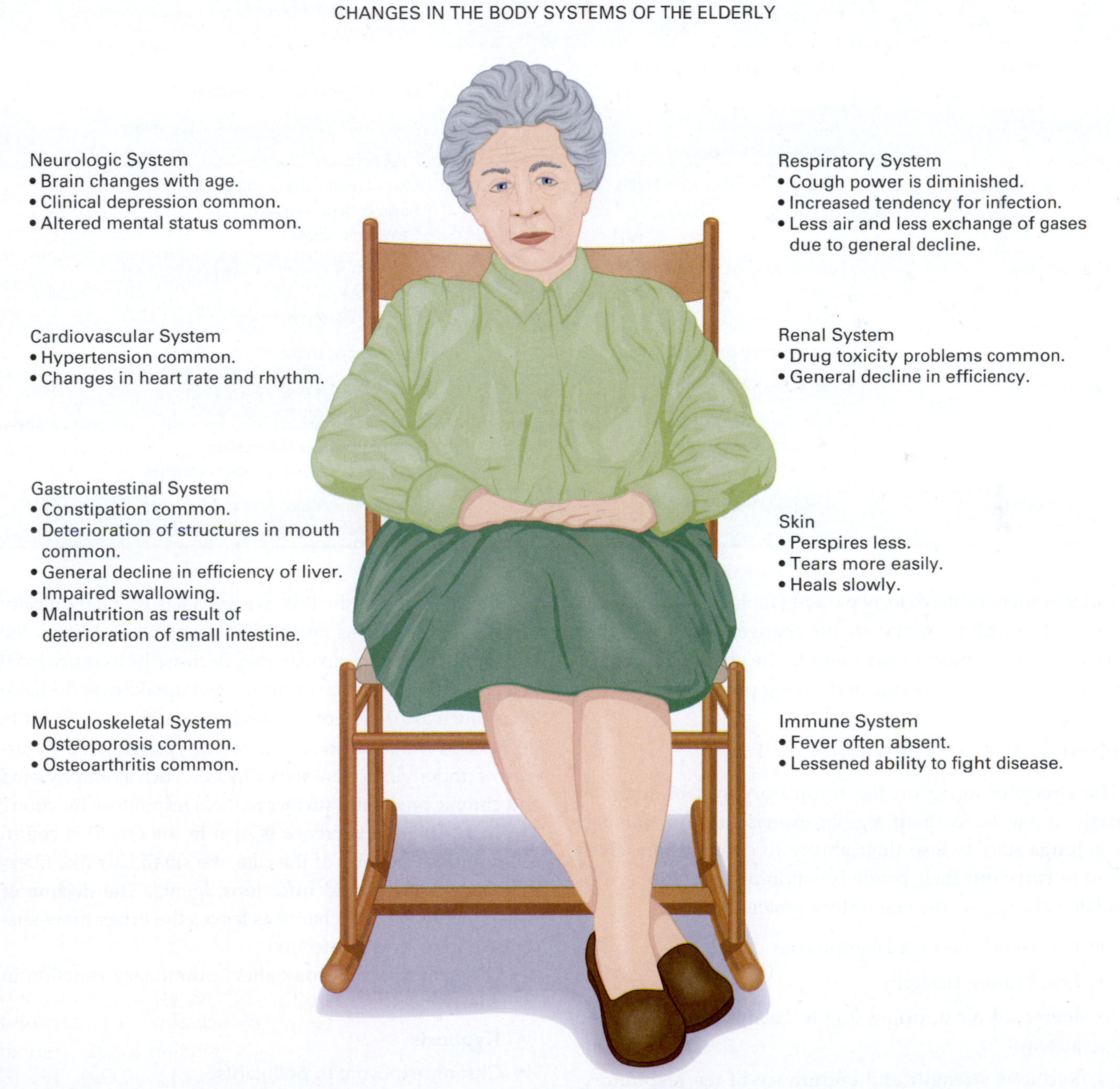

FIGURE 5-13 Some changes in the body systems of the elderly.

Table 5-5 Common Age-Related Systemic Changes

Body System	Changes with Age	Clinical Importance
Respiratory	Loss of strength and coordination in respiratory muscles Cough and gag reflex reduced	Increased likelihood of respiratory failure
Cardiovascular	Loss of elasticity and hardening of arteries Changes in heart rate, rhythm, efficiency	Hypertension common Greater likelihood of strokes, heart attacks Great likelihood of bleeding from minor trauma
Neurologic	Brain tissue shrinks Loss of memory Clinical depression common Altered mental status common Impaired balance	Delay in appearance of symptoms with head injury Difficulty in patient assessment Increased likelihood of falls
Endocrine	Lowered estrogen production (women) Decline in insulin sensitivity Increase in insulin resistance	Increased likelihood of fractures (bone loss) and heart disease Diabetes mellitus common with greater possibility of hyperglycemia
Gastrointestinal	Diminished digestive functions	Constipation common Greater likelihood of malnutrition
Thermoregulatory	Reduced sweating Decreased shivering	Environmental emergencies more common
Integumentary (skin)	Thins and becomes more fragile	More subject to tears and sores Bruising more common Heals more slowly
Musculoskeletal	Loss of bone strength (osteoporosis) Loss of joint flexibility and strength (osteoarthritis)	Greater likelihood of fractures Slower healing Increased likelihood of falls
Renal	Loss of kidney size and function	Increased problems with drug toxicity
Genitourinary	Loss of bladder function	Increased urination/incontinence Increased urinary tract infection
Immune	Diminished immune response	More susceptible to infections Impaired immune response to vaccines
Hematologic	Decrease in blood volume and/or RBCs	Slower recuperation from illness/injury Greater risk of trauma-related complications

and treatment of the elderly patient (Table 5-5). You should be familiar with normal systemic changes related to aging so that you can more easily identify the abnormal changes that may point to a serious underlying problem.

Respiratory System

The effects of aging on the respiratory system begin as early as age 30. Without regular exercise and/or training, the lungs start to lose their ability to defend themselves and to carry out their prime function of ventilation. Age-related changes in the respiratory system include:

- Decreased chest wall compliance
- Loss of lung elasticity
- Increased air trapping due to collapse of the smaller airways
- Reduced strength and endurance of the respiratory muscles

Functionally, by the time we reach age 65, vital capacity may be reduced by as much as 50 percent. In addition, the maximum breathing capacity may decrease by as much as 60 percent, whereas the maximum oxygen uptake may decrease by as much as 70 percent. These changes ultimately result in decreased ventilation and progressive hypoxemia. Any presence of underlying pulmonary diseases, such as emphysema and chronic bronchitis, further reduces respiratory function.

In addition, a decrease is seen in the effective cough reflex and the activity of the cilia, the small hair-like fibers that trap particles and infectious agents. The decline of these two defense mechanisms leaves the lungs more susceptible to recurring infection.

Other factors that may affect pulmonary function in the elderly include:

- **Kyphosis**
- Chronic exposure to pollutants
- Long-term cigarette smoking

The management of respiratory distress in elderly patients is essentially the same as for all age groups. Position the patient for adequate breathing, usually upright or sitting. Teach breathing patterns that assist in exhalation, such as pursed-lip breathing. (Tell patients to pretend they are blowing out a candle with each exhalation.) Use bronchodilators as needed, and provide supplemental oxygen to correct hypoxia.

At all times, remain attentive for possible complications, such as **anoxic hypoxemia**. Monitor ventilations closely because an elderly patient can become easily fatigued from any increase in the work of breathing. Remember that many elderly patients with respiratory disease have underlying cardiac disease. With this in mind, drugs such as beta agonists should be used with extreme caution. Monitor cardiovascular status and administer IV fluids judiciously. *Do not* overload fluids. When infusing fluids, frequently reassess lung sounds to check for the pressure of pulmonary edema.

Cardiovascular System

A number of variables unrelated to aging influence cardiovascular function. They include diet, smoking and alcohol use, education, socioeconomic status, and even personality traits. Of particular importance is the level of physical activity. Even though maximum exercise capacity and maximum oxygen consumption decline with age, a well-trained elderly person can match—or even exceed—the aerobic capacity of an unconditioned younger person.

This said, the cardiovascular system still experiences age-related deterioration, in varying degrees. The wall of the left ventricle may thicken and enlarge (**hypertrophy**), often by as much as 25 percent. This is even more pronounced if there is associated hypertension. In addition, **fibrosis** develops in the heart and peripheral vascular system, resulting in hypertension, arteriosclerosis, and decreased cardiac function.

The aorta also becomes stiff and lengthens. This results from deposits of calcium and changes in the connective tissue. These changes predispose the aorta to partial tearing, resulting in dissection (thoracic) or aneurysm (abdominal).

As a person ages, the pattern of ventricular filling changes. Less blood enters the left ventricle during early diastole when the mitral valve is open. Therefore, filling and stretch (preload) depend on atrial contraction. Loss of the atrial kick (as will occur with atrial fibrillation) is not well tolerated in the elderly.

Over time, the conductive system of the heart degenerates, often causing arrhythmias and varying degrees of heart block. Ultimately, the stroke volume declines and the heart rate slows, leading to decreased cardiac output. Because of this, the heart's ability to respond to stress diminishes. In such situations, expect exercise intolerance—that is, an inability of the heart to meet an exercising muscle's need for oxygen.

To adequately manage complaints related to the cardiovascular system, ask the patient to stop all activity. This reduces the myocardial oxygen demand. *Do not* walk a patient with a cardiovascular complaint to your ambulance. Take the following basic steps per local protocols:

- Administer oxygen if the patient is hypoxic.
- Start an IV for medication administration. Medications will vary with the complaint, but may include:
  - Antianginal agents
  - Aspirin
  - Diuretics
  - Antiarrhythmics
- Inquire about age-related dosages.
- Monitor vital signs and rhythm.
- Acquire a 12-lead ECG.
- Remain calm, professional, and empathetic. A heart attack is one of the most fear-inducing situations for the elderly.

Nervous System

Unlike cells in other organ systems, nerve cells in the central nervous system cannot significantly reproduce. The brain can lose as much as 45 percent of its cells in certain areas of the cortex. Overall, people experience an average 10 percent reduction in brain weight from age 20 to age 90. Keep in mind that reductions in brain weight and ventricular size are not well correlated with intelligence, and elderly people may still be capable of highly creative and productive thought. Once again, *do not* assume that an elderly person possesses less cognitive skill than a younger person. Slight changes that may be expected include:

- Difficulty with recent memory
- Psychomotor slowing
- Forgetfulness
- Decreased reaction times

Although brain size may not have clinical implications in terms of intelligence, it does have implications for trauma. A reduction in brain size allows mass effects (bleeding, tumors) to become larger before they become clinically significant. Thus, following a blow to the head, a subdural hematoma may take longer to manifest when compared with one in a younger person. In cases of altered mental status or seizure, maintain a suspicion of trauma, especially when an accident has been reported.

Whenever you assess an elderly patient for mental status, determine a baseline. Presume your patient to have been mentally sharp unless proven otherwise. (Talk with partners, caregivers, family members, and so on.) Focus on the patient's perceptions, thinking processes, and communication. In questioning an elderly patient, provide an environment with minimal distractions. As already mentioned, ask clear and unhurried questions.

In forming a patient plan, observe for weakness, chronic fatigue, changes in sleep patterns, and syncope or near syncope. If you suspect a stroke, assign the patient a priority status. (Additional material on strokes appears later in this chapter.) Consider blood pressure control per local protocol, but remember that perfusion of the brain tissue depends on an adequate blood pressure. In most cases, *do not* plan to reduce the blood pressure in stroke because raising the blood pressure is the body's response to increase cerebral blood flow to ensure brain perfusion. Consider the causes of changes in mental status, keeping in mind the possibility of trauma. Apply oxygen if the patient is hypoxic, monitor ventilations with capnography (if available), and continually reassess the patient.

Endocrine System

Early diagnosis of disorders in the endocrine system offers some of the greatest opportunities to prevent disabilities through appropriate hormonal therapy and/or lifestyle changes. Diabetes mellitus, for example, is extremely common among the elderly. However, normalization of glucose levels through diet, exercise, and/or drug therapy can reduce some of the devastating vascular and neurologic complications.

Thyroid disorders are "clinical masqueraders," especially in the elderly. Common signs and symptoms may be absent or diminished. When signs and symptoms are present, they may be attributed to aging or tied to other diseases, such as cardiovascular, GI, or neuromuscular disorders. However, it has been shown that thyroid disorders, especially hypothyroidism and thyroid nodules, increase with age. (For more on thyroid disorders, see the section "Metabolic and Endocrine Disorders" later in this chapter.)

With the exception of glucose disorders, most endocrine disorders cannot be easily determined in the field. Many endocrine emergencies will present as altered mental status, especially with insulin-related diseases. Monitor for cardiovascular effects of endocrine changes such as aortic aneurysm in a patient with **Marfan syndrome**, a disorder resulting in abnormal growth of distal tissues and a dilation of the root of the aorta. Also remain alert to blood pressure swings in thyroid disorders such as hyperthyroidism and hypothyroidism.

Gastrointestinal System

Age affects the gastrointestinal system in various ways. The volume of saliva may decrease by as much as 33 percent, leading to complaints of dry mouth, nutritional deficiencies, and a predisposition to choking. Gastric secretions may decrease to as little as 20 percent of the quantity present in younger people. Esophageal and intestinal motility also decrease, making swallowing more difficult and delaying digestive processes. The production of hydrochloric acid also declines, further disrupting digestion and, in some adults, contributing to nutritional anemia. Gums atrophy and the number of taste buds decreases, reducing even further the desire to eat.

Other conditions may also develop. **Hiatal hernias** are not age related per se, but can have serious consequences for the elderly. They may incarcerate or strangulate the contents of the hernia (esophagus, stomach), or, in the most severe cases, result in massive GI hemorrhage. Diminished liver function, which is associated with aging, can delay or impede detoxification. A common drug toxicity problem for EMS personnel is the use of various medications (e.g., amiodarone) for ventricular arrhythmias. (See the section "Toxicologic Emergencies" later in this chapter.) Diminished liver function can also reduce the production of clotting proteins, which in turn leads to bleeding abnormalities.

Complications in the gastrointestinal system can be life threatening. Use shock protocols as necessary, and remember that not all fluid loss occurs outside the body.

Thermoregulatory System

The elderly and infants are highly susceptible to variations in environmental temperatures. This occurs in the elderly because of altered or impaired thermoregulatory mechanisms. Aging seems to reduce the effectiveness of sweating in cooling the body. Older persons tend to sweat at higher core temperatures and have less sweat output per gland than younger people. As people age, they also experience deterioration of the autonomic nervous system, including a decrease in shivering and a lower resting peripheral blood flow. In addition, the elderly may have a diminished perception of the cold. Drugs and disease can further affect an elderly patient's response to temperature extremes, resulting in hyperthermia or accidental hypothermia.

Environmental emergencies are common causes of EMS calls, especially among the elderly living alone or in poverty. For more on these emergencies, see the discussion of heatstroke, hypothermia, and hyperthermia later in this chapter.

Integumentary System

As people age, the skin loses collagen, a connective tissue that gives elasticity and support to the skin. Without this support, the skin is subject to a greater number of injuries from bumping or tearing. The lack of support also makes it more difficult to start an IV, because the veins tend to "roll away." Furthermore, the assessment of tenting skin becomes an inaccurate indicator of fluid status in the elderly. Without elasticity, the skin often will remain tented regardless of water balance.

As the skin thins, cells reproduce more slowly. In the elderly, injury to skin is often more severe than in younger patients and healing time is increased. As a rule, the elderly are at a higher risk of secondary infection, skin tumors, drug-induced eruptions, and fungal or viral infections. Decades of exposure to the sun also makes the elderly vulnerable to melanoma and other sun-related carcinomas (e.g., basal cell carcinoma, squamous cell carcinoma).

Musculoskeletal System

An aging person may lose as much as 2 to 3 inches of height from narrowing of the intervertebral disks and osteoporosis. Much of the height loss is caused by vertebral fractures.[4] **Osteoporosis** is the loss of mineral from the bone, resulting in softening of the bones. This is especially evident in the vertebral bodies, thus causing a change in posture. The posture of the aged individual often reveals an increase in the curvature of the thoracic spine, commonly called kyphosis, and slight flexion of the knee and hip joints. The demineralization of bone makes the patient much more susceptible to hip and other fractures. Some fractures may even occur from simple actions such as sneezing.

In addition to skeletal changes, a decrease in skeletal muscle weight commonly occurs with age, especially with sedentary individuals. To compensate, elderly women develop a narrow, short gait, whereas older men develop a wide gait. These changes make the elderly more susceptible to falls and, consequently, a possible loss of independence.

Because of the changes in the musculoskeletal system, simple trauma in the elderly can lead to complex injuries. In treating musculoskeletal disorders, supply supplemental oxygen (if the patient is hypoxic), initiate an IV line, and consider pain control. Many extremity injuries should be splinted as found because of changes in the bone and joint structure of the elderly. To determine the cause of any injury, be sure to look beyond the obvious. Keep in mind the possibility of underlying medical conditions, drug complications, abuse or neglect, and ingestion of alcohol or drugs.

Renal System

Aging affects the renal system through a reduction in the number of functioning **nephrons**, which may be decreased by 30 to 40 percent. Renal blood flow may also be reduced by up to 45 percent, increasing the waste products in the blood and upsetting the fluid and electrolyte balance. Because the kidneys are responsible for the production of erythropoietin (which stimulates the production of red blood cells in the bone marrow) and renin (which stimulates vasoconstriction), a decrease in renal function may result in anemia or hypertension in the older patient.

Prehospital treatment of complaints involving the renal and urinary systems is directed toward adequate oxygenation, fluid status, monitoring output, and pain control. Pay attention to the airway because nausea and vomiting are complications of pain secondary to renal obstruction. Monitor vital signs to detect changes in blood pressure and pulse.

Genitourinary System

As people age, they experience a progressive loss of bladder sensation and tone. The bladder does not empty completely and, consequently, the patient may sense a frequent need to urinate. This urge increases the risk of falls, especially during the middle of the night when lighting is dim or the patient is sleepy. Furthermore, the lack of emptying increases the likelihood of urinary tract infection and perhaps sepsis. In the male, the prostate often becomes enlarged (benign prostatic hypertrophy), causing difficulty in urination or urinary retention. As already mentioned, the elderly also commonly develop, in varying degrees, problems with incontinence.

Treatment for a complaint in the genitourinary system is described in the preceding section on the renal system and in the earlier discussion of incontinence.

Immune System

As a person ages, the function of T cells declines, making them less able to notify the immune system of invasion by antigens. A diminished immune response, sometimes called **immune senescence**, increases the susceptibility of the elderly to infections. It also increases the duration and severity of an infection.

Barring contraindications, the elderly should receive vaccinations suggested by the health department. However, keep in mind that aging impairs the immune response to vaccines. The best prevention is adequate nutrition, infection control measures (e.g., washing hands), and exercise. Recognition and treatment of diseases such as diabetes mellitus, heart failure, thyroid disease, and occult malignancy also reduce the risk and severity of infections. As a paramedic, you should treat alterations in immune status as life threats and seek to prevent exposure of patients to infectious agents. Take necessary precautions so that you do not transmit an illness—even a mild cold—to an elderly patient.

Hematologic System

The hematologic system is affected by a failure of the renal system to stimulate the production of red blood cells (RBCs). Changing coagulation factors and vessel damage increase the chance of thromboembolic events in the elderly. Nutritional abnormalities may also produce abnormal RBCs. Because the elderly have less body water, blood volume is decreased. This makes it difficult for an elderly patient to recuperate from an illness or injury. Intervention must be started early to make a lasting difference.

In addition to providing supplemental oxygen if the patient is hypoxic, you should prepare for increases in bleeding time. Monitor the elderly patient closely because deterioration is difficult to stop.

Common Medical Problems in the Elderly

In general, the elderly suffer from the same kinds of medical emergencies as younger patients. However, illnesses may be more severe, complications more likely, and classic signs and symptoms absent or altered. In addition, the elderly are more likely to react adversely to stress and deteriorate much more quickly than young or middle-aged adults. The following are some of the medical disorders that you may encounter.

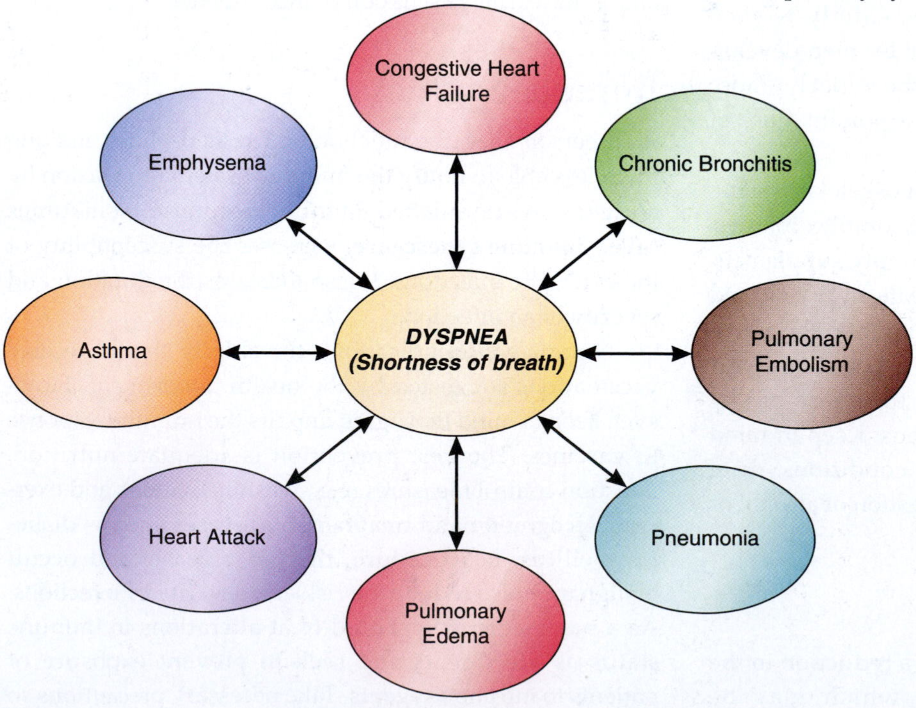

FIGURE 5-14 Dyspnea can be caused by a number of respiratory and cardiac problems in the elderly.

Pulmonary/Respiratory Disorders

Respiratory emergencies are some of the most common reasons elderly persons summon EMS or seek emergency care. Most elderly patients with a respiratory disorder present with a chief complaint of dyspnea. However, coughing, congestion, and wheezing are also common chief complaints.

Many factors can trigger respiratory distress among the elderly (Figure 5-14). Descriptions of the most common ones follow.

Pneumonia

Pneumonia is an infection of the lung. It is usually caused by a bacterium or virus. However, aspiration pneumonia may also develop as a result of difficulty swallowing.

Pneumonia is a serious disease for the elderly. It is the seventh-leading cause of death in people age 65 and older. Its incidence increases with age at a rate of 10 percent for each decade beyond age 20. It is found in up to 60 percent of the autopsies performed on the elderly. Reasons the elderly develop pneumonia more frequently than younger patients include:

- Decreased immune response
- Reduced pulmonary function
- Increased colonization of the pharynx by Gram-negative bacteria
- Abnormal or ineffective cough reflex
- Decreased effectiveness of mucociliary cells of the upper respiratory system (Figure 5-15)

The elderly who are at greatest risk for contracting pneumonia include frail adults and those with chronic, multiple diseases or compromised immunity. Institutionalized patients in hospitals or nursing homes are especially vulnerable because of increased exposure to microorganisms and limited mobility. A patient in an institutional setting is up to 50 times more likely to contract pneumonia than an elderly patient receiving home care.

Common signs and symptoms of pneumonia include increasing dyspnea, congestion, fever, chills, tachypnea, sputum production, and altered mental status. Occasionally, abdominal pain may be the only symptom. Because of thermoregulatory changes, a fever may be absent in an elderly patient.

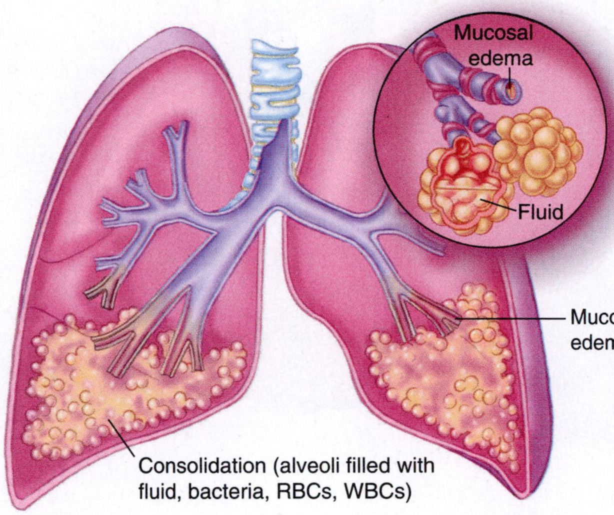

FIGURE 5-15 Pneumonia is an infection of the lung or lungs usually caused by bacteria. It is a common cause of death in the elderly.

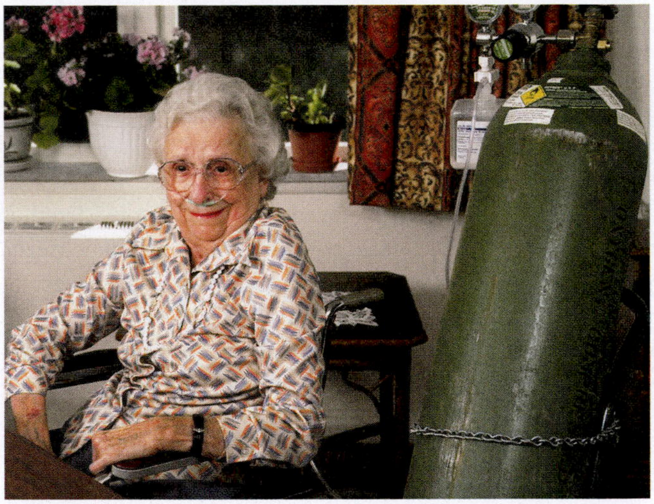

FIGURE 5-16 The COPD patient may use a nasal cannula with an oxygen unit.

Prevention strategies include immunization with the current pneumonia and influenza vaccines. Efforts should also be taken to reduce exposure to infectious patients and to promote patient mobility.

In treating an elderly patient with pneumonia, manage all life threats. Maintain adequate oxygenation. Transport the patient to the hospital for diagnosis, keeping in mind that patients with respiratory disease often have other underlying problems.

Chronic Obstructive Pulmonary Disease

Chronic obstructive pulmonary disease (COPD) is really a collection of diseases, characterized by chronic airflow obstruction with reversible and/or irreversible components. Although each COPD has its own distinct features, elderly patients commonly have two or more types at the same time. COPD usually refers to some combination of emphysema, chronic bronchitis, and, to a lesser degree, asthma. Pneumonia, as well as other respiratory disorders, can further complicate chronic obstructive pulmonary disease in the elderly.

In the United States, chronic obstructive pulmonary disease is the third leading cause of death. Its prevalence has been increasing during the past 20 years. Several factors combine to produce the damage of COPD:

- Cigarette smoking, a contributing factor in up to 80 percent of all cases of COPD
- Existence of a childhood respiratory disease
- Exposure to environmental pollutants
- Genetic predisposition

The physiology of COPD varies, but may include inflammation of the air passages with increased mucus production or actual destruction of the alveoli. The outcome is decreased airflow in the alveoli, resulting in reduced oxygen exchange. Usual signs and symptoms include:

- Accessory muscle use
- Cough
- Dyspnea
- Exercise intolerance
- Increased sputum production
- Pleuritic chest pain
- Pursed-lip breathing
- Tachypnea
- Tripod positioning
- Wheezing

COPD is progressive and debilitating (Figure 5-16). The patient can often keep the signs and symptoms under control until the body is stressed. When the condition becomes disabling, it is called *exacerbation of COPD*. This condition can lead rapidly to patient death because the accompanying hypoxia and hypercapnia alter the acid–base balance and deprive the tissues of the oxygen needed for efficient energy production.

The most effective prevention involves elimination of tobacco products and reduced exposure to cigarette smoke (in nonsmokers). Recent legislation has sought to keep public places smoke free and to discourage cigarette smoking in the young. Once the disease is present, patients are taught to identify stresses that exacerbate the condition. Appropriate self-care includes exercise, avoidance of infections, appropriate use of drugs, and, when necessary, calling EMS.

When confronted with an elderly patient with COPD, treatment is essentially the same as for all age groups. Supply supplemental oxygen to correct hypoxia and possibly drug therapy, usually for reducing dyspnea.

Pulmonary Embolism

Pulmonary embolism (PE) should always be considered as a possible cause of respiratory distress in the elderly. Although statistics for the elderly are unavailable, approximately 650,000 cases occur annually in the United States alone. Of this number, a pulmonary embolism is the primary cause of death in 100,000 people and a contributing factor in another 100,000 deaths. Nearly 11 percent of PE deaths take place in the first hour and 38 percent in the second hour after occurrence.

Blood clots are the most frequent cause of pulmonary embolism. However, the condition may also be caused by fat, air, bone marrow, tumor cells, or foreign bodies. Risk factors for developing pulmonary embolism include:

- Atrial fibrillation
- Deep venous thrombosis
- Fractures of the pelvis, hip, or leg
- Major surgery
- Malignancy (tumors)
- Obesity
- Paralysis
- Presence of a venous catheter
- Prolonged immobility, common among the elderly
- Trauma to the leg vessels
- Use of hormones (estrogen and progestin) in women

Pulmonary emboli usually originate in the deep veins of the thigh and calf. The condition should be suspected in any patient with the acute onset of dyspnea. Often, it is accompanied by pleuritic chest pain and right heart failure. If the pulmonary embolus is massive, you can often expect severe dyspnea, cardiac arrhythmias, and, ultimately, cardiovascular collapse (Figure 5-17).

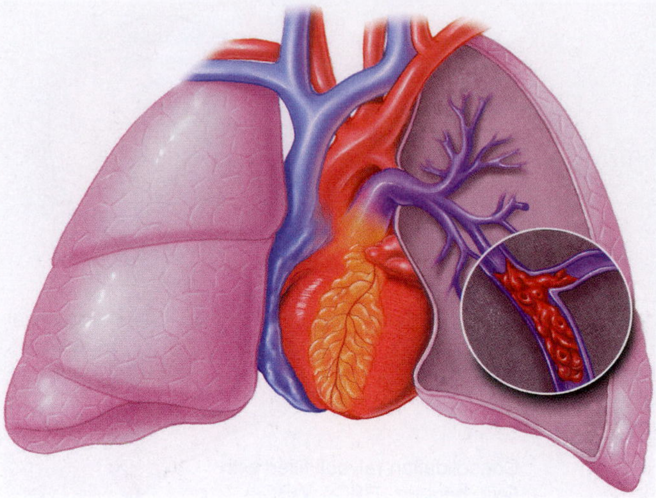

FIGURE 5-17 A pulmonary embolism is a blood clot lodged in a pulmonary artery, thus interrupting blood flow and adversely affecting the oxygenation of hemoglobin.

Definitive diagnosis of a pulmonary embolism takes place in a hospital setting. The goals of field treatment are to manage and minimize complications of the condition. General treatment considerations include delivery of supplemental oxygen via mask to maintain a SpO_2 >95 percent. Establishing an IV for possible administration of medications is appropriate, but vigorous fluid therapy should be avoided, if possible.

Prehospital pharmacological therapy for pulmonary embolism is limited. On advice from medical direction, you may administer small doses of morphine sulfate to reduce patient anxiety. After confirming the absence of GI bleeding, medical direction may also prescribe anticoagulants to prevent clot formation and/or to speed clot dissolution. If the administration of a vasopressor is indicated by low blood pressure, then dopamine or a similar vasopressor may be prescribed. In such cases, remember to titrate the vasopressor to a desirable blood pressure.

The risk of death from pulmonary embolism is greatest in the first few hours. As a result, rapid transport is essential. Position the patient in an upright position and avoid lifting the patient by the legs or knees, which may dislodge thrombi in the lower extremities. During transport, continue to monitor changes in skin color, pulse oximetry, and breathing rate and rhythm. Your field assessment and interventions can save the patient's life and guide the hospital physician in a direction that will result in an accurate diagnosis and rapid treatment.

Pulmonary Edema

Pulmonary edema is an effusion or escape of serous fluids into the alveoli and interstitial tissues of the lungs. Acute pulmonary edema can develop rapidly in the elderly. Although most commonly associated with acute myocardial infarction and congestive heart failure (acute on chronic congestive heart failure), it can also result from pulmonary infections, inhaled toxins, narcotic overdose, pulmonary embolism, and decreased atmospheric pressure.

Pulmonary edema causes severe dyspnea associated with congestion. Other signs and symptoms include rapid labored breathing, cough with blood-stained sputum, cyanosis, and cold extremities. Physical examination usually reveals the presence of moist crackles and accessory muscle use. Severe cases will exhibit rhonchi.

Treatment is directed toward altering the cause of the condition. The existence of pulmonary edema can be life threatening and is often the symptom of a fatal cardiovascular disease.

Lung Cancer

North America has the highest incidence of lung cancer in the world. The incidence increases with age, with about 65 percent of all lung cancer deaths occurring among people age 65 and older. The leading cause of lung cancer is cigarette smoking.

Often, progressive dyspnea will be the first presentation of a cancerous lesion. Hemoptysis (bloody sputum), chronic cough, and weight loss are also common symptoms.

Treatment of lung cancer occurs in a hospital setting. However, you may be called to assist with the follow-up home care or, in terminal stages, in a hospice situation. (See the chapter on "Acute Interventions for the Chronic Care Patient" for more information on this subject.)

Cardiovascular Disorders

The leading cause of death in the elderly is cardiovascular disease. Assessment and treatment of cardiovascular disease in the elderly patient is often complicated by non–age-related factors and disease processes in other organ systems. In conducting your history, determine the patient's level of cardiovascular fitness, changes in exercise tolerance, recent diet history, use of medications, and use of cigarettes and/or alcohol. Ask questions about breathing difficulty, especially at night, and evidence of palpitations, flutter, or skipped beats.

In performing the physical exam, look for hypertension and orthostatic hypotension (a decrease in blood pressure and an increase in heart rate when rising from a seated or supine position). Watch for dehydration or dependent edema. When taking an elderly patient's blood pressure, consider checking both arms. Routinely determine pulses in all the extremities. In auscultating the patient, remember that a bruit or noise in the neck, abdomen, or groin indicates a high probability of carotid, aortorenal, or peripheral vascular disease. Keep in mind, too, that heart sounds are generally softer in the elderly, probably because of a thickening of lung tissue between the heart and chest wall.

In evaluating the problem, recall the cardiovascular disorders commonly found in elderly patients. They include angina pectoris, myocardial infarction, heart failure, arrhythmias, aortic dissection, aneurysm, hypertension, and syncope.

Angina Pectoris

The likelihood of developing angina increases dramatically with age. This is especially true of women, who are protected by estrogen until after menopause. Angina is usually triggered by physical activity, especially after a meal, and by exposure to very cold weather. Attacks vary in frequency, from several a day to occasional episodes separated by weeks or months.

Angina pectoris literally means "pain in the chest." However, the pain of angina is actually felt in only about 10 to 20 percent of elderly patients. The changes in sensory nerves, combined with the myocardial changes of aging, make dyspnea a more likely symptom of angina than pain.

Angina develops when narrowing of coronary vessels as a result of plaque or vasospasm leads to an inability to meet the oxygen demands of the heart muscle. The heart muscle usually responds by sending out pain signals, which represent a buildup of lactic acid. In an elderly patient, exercise intolerance is a key symptom of angina. In obtaining a history, you should ask the patient about sudden changes in routine. In addition, inquire about any increased stresses on the heart, such as anemia, infection, arrhythmias, and thyroid changes.

General prevention strategies in the elderly are similar to those in young patients. Blood pressure control combined with diet, exercise, and smoking modifications reduces the risk in all groups.

Myocardial Infarction

A myocardial infarction (MI) involves actual death of muscle tissue owing to a partial or complete occlusion of one or more of the coronary arteries. The greatest number of patients hospitalized for acute myocardial infarction are older than 65. The elderly patient with myocardial infarction is less likely to present with classic symptoms, such as chest pain, than a younger counterpart. Atypical presentations that may be seen in the elderly include:

- Absence of pain
- Confusion/dizziness
- Dyspnea—common in patients over age 85
- Exercise intolerance
- Fatigue/weakness
- Neck, dental, and/or epigastric pain
- Syncope

The mortality rate associated with myocardial infarction and/or resulting complications doubles after age 70. Unlike younger patients, the elderly are more likely to suffer a **silent myocardial infarction**. They also tend to have larger myocardial infarctions. The majority of deaths that occur in the first few hours following a myocardial infarction are caused by arrhythmias.

A myocardial infarction is most commonly triggered by some form of physical exertion or a preexisting heart disease. Because of the high mortality associated with myocardial infarctions in the elderly, early detection and emergency management are critical.

Heart Failure

Heart failure takes place when cardiac output cannot meet the body's metabolic demands. The incidence rises exponentially after age 60. The condition is widespread among the elderly and is the most common diagnosis in hospitalized patients over age 65. The causes of heart failure fall into one of four categories: impairment to flow, inadequate cardiac filling, volume overload, and myocardial failure.

Typical age-related factors, such as prolonged myocardial contractions, make the elderly vulnerable to heart failure. Other factors that place them at risk include:

- Anemia
- Arrhythmias (e.g., atrial fibrillation)
- Hypoxia
- Infection
- Ischemia
- Noncompliance with drug therapy
- Thermoregulatory disorders (hypothermia/hyperthermia)
- Use of nonsteroidal anti-inflammatory drugs (excluding low-dose aspirin)

Signs and symptoms of heart failure vary. In most patients, regardless of age, some form of edema exists. However, edema in the elderly can indicate a range of problems, including musculoskeletal injury. Assessment findings specific to the elderly include:

- Fatigue (left failure)
- **Two-pillow orthopnea** (needing two pillows to breathe easily)
- Dyspnea on exertion
- Paroxysmal nocturnal dyspnea
- Dry, hacking cough progressing to productive cough
- Dependent edema (right failure)
- **Nocturia** (excessive urination at night)
- Anorexia, **hepatomegaly** (enlarged liver), ascites

Nonpharmacological management of heart failure includes modifications in diet (e.g., less fat and cholesterol), exercise, and reduction in weight, if necessary. Pharmacological management may include treatment with diuretics, vasodilators, antihypertensive agents, or inotropic agents. Check to see whether the patient is already on any of these medications and if the patient is compliant with scheduled doses.

Arrhythmias

Many cardiac arrhythmias develop with age. Atrial fibrillation is the most common arrhythmia encountered and can be a predictor of long-term mortality in elderly patients.[5]

Arrhythmias occur primarily as a result of degeneration of the patient's conductive system. Anything that decreases myocardial blood flow can produce an arrhythmia. They may also be caused by electrolyte abnormalities.

CONTENT REVIEW

➤ Possible Pacemaker Complications
- Electrode dislodgment
- Failed battery
- Fibrosis around the catheter site
- Lead fracture

To complicate matters further, the elderly do not tolerate extremes in heart rate as well as a younger person would. For example, a heart rate of 140 in an older patient may cause syncope, whereas a younger patient can often tolerate a heart rate greater than 180. In addition, arrhythmias can lead to falls from cerebral hypoperfusion. They can also result in congestive heart failure (CHF) or a transient ischemic attack.

Treatment considerations depend on the type of arrhythmia. Patients may already have a pacemaker in place. In such cases, keep in mind that pacemakers have a low but significant rate of complications such as a failed battery, fibrosis around the catheter site, lead fracture, or electrode dislodgment. In a number of situations, drug therapy may be indicated. Whenever you discover an arrhythmia, remember that an abnormal or disordered heart rhythm may be the only clinical finding in an elderly patient suffering acute myocardial infarction.

Aortic Dissection/Aneurysms

Aortic dissection is a degeneration of the wall of the aorta, either in the thoracic or abdominal cavity. It can result in an **aneurysm** or in a rupture of the vessel. Generally speaking, dissections are more common in the thoracic aorta, whereas aneurysms are more common in the abdominal aorta—although both can occur in either location.

Approximately 80 percent of thoracic aneurysms are the result of atherosclerosis combined with hypertension. The remaining cases occur secondary to other factors, including blunt trauma to the chest. Patients with dissections will often present with tearing chest pain radiating through to the back or, if rupture occurs, cardiac arrest. Marfan syndrome is a connective system disorder resulting in abnormal growth of distal tissues and a dilation of the root of the aorta. It can cause aortic aneurysm and dissection; these should be considered in elderly patients with this condition.

The distal portion of the aorta is the most common site for abdominal aneurysms. Approximately 1 in 250 people over age 50 die from a ruptured abdominal aneurysm. The aneurysm may appear as a pulsatile mass in a patient with a normal girth, but lack of an identifiable mass does not eliminate this condition. Patients may present with tearing abdominal pain or unexplained low back pain. Pulses in the legs are diminished or absent and the lower extremities feel cold to the touch. The patient may experience sensory abnormalities such as numbness, tingling, or pain in the legs. The patient may fall when attempting to stand.

Treatment of an aneurysm depends on its size, location, and the severity of the condition. In the case of thoracic aortic dissection, continuous IV infusion and/or administration of drug therapy to lower the arterial pressure and to diminish the velocity of left ventricle contraction may be indicated. Rapid transport is essential, especially for the older patient who most commonly requires care and observation in an intensive care unit.

Hypertension

Hypertension appears to be a product of industrial society. In developed nations, such as the United States, the systolic and diastolic pressures have a tendency to rise until age 60. Systolic pressure may continue to rise after that time, but diastolic pressure stabilizes. Because this rise in blood pressure is not seen in less developed nations, experts believe that hypertension is not a normal age-related change.

Today, more than 50 percent of Americans over age 65 have clinically diagnosed hypertension, which is defined as blood pressure greater than 140/90 mmHg. Prolonged elevated blood pressure will eventually damage the heart, brain, or kidneys. As a result of hypertension, elderly patients are at greater risk for heart failure, stroke, blindness, renal failure, coronary heart disease, and peripheral vascular disease. In men with blood pressure greater than 160/95 mmHg, the risk of mortality nearly doubles.

Hypertension increases with atherosclerosis, which is more common with the elderly than other age groups. Other contributing factors include obesity and diabetes. The condition can be prevented or controlled through diet (sodium reduction), exercise, cessation of smoking, and compliance with medications.

Hypertension is often a silent disease that produces no clinically obvious signs or symptoms. It may be associated with nonspecific complaints such as headache, tinnitus, **epistaxis**, slow tremors, or nausea and vomiting. An acute onset of high blood pressure without any kidney involvement is often a telltale indicator of thyroid disease.

Treatment of hypertension for those between 60 and 80 years of age has been shown to increase their life span, whereas treatment of those above 80 years of age has not shown to increase life span. The management of hypertension depends on its severity and the existence of other conditions. For example, hypertension is often treated with angiotensin-converting enzyme (ACE) inhibitors or angiotensin II receptor blockers. Other medications, such as beta-blockers (medications that are contraindicated in patients with chronic obstructive lung disease, asthma, or heart block greater than first degree) and calcium-channel blockers can be effective. Diuretics, another common drug used in treating hypertension, should be prescribed with care for patients on digitalis. Keep in mind that centrally acting agents are more likely to produce negative side effects in the elderly. Unlike younger patients, the elderly may experience depression, forgetfulness, sleep problems, or vivid dreams and/or hallucinations.

CONTENT REVIEW

➤ Hypertension Prevention Strategies
- Modified diet (low sodium)
- Exercise
- Smoking cessation
- Compliance with medications

Syncope

Syncope is a common presenting complaint among the elderly. The condition results when blood flow to the brain is temporarily interrupted or decreased. It is most often caused by problems with either the nervous system or the cardiovascular system. In general, syncope has a higher incidence of death in elderly patients than in younger individuals.[6] The following are some of the common presentations that you may encounter:

- ***Vasodepressor syncope.*** Vasodepressor syncope is commonly termed "fainting." It may occur following emotional distress; pain; prolonged bed rest; mild blood loss; prolonged standing in warm, crowded rooms; anemia; or fever.
- ***Orthostatic syncope.*** Orthostatic syncope occurs when a person rises from a seated or supine position. There are several possible causes. First, the person may have a disproportion between blood volume and vascular capacity. That is, there is a pooling of blood in the legs, reducing blood flow to the brain. Causes of this include hypovolemia, venous **varicosities**, prolonged bed rest, and **autonomic dysfunction**. Many drugs, especially blood pressure medicines, can cause drug-induced orthostatic syncope due to the effects of the medications on the capacitance vessels.
- ***Vasovagal syncope.*** Vasovagal syncope occurs as a result of a **Valsalva maneuver**, which happens during defecation, coughing, or similar maneuvers. This effectively slows the heart rate and cardiac output, thus decreasing blood flow to the brain.
- ***Cardiac syncope.*** Cardiac syncope results from transient reduction in cerebral blood flow due to a sudden decrease in cardiac output. It can result from several mechanisms. Syncope can be the primary symptom of silent myocardial infarction. In addition, many arrhythmias can cause syncope. Arrhythmias that have been shown to cause syncope include bradycardias, **Stokes-Adams syndrome**, Brugada syndrome, heart block, tachyarrhythmia, and **sick sinus syndrome**.

- *Seizures.* Syncope may result from a seizure disorder or prolonged syncope may cause seizure activity. Syncope due to seizures tends to occur without warning. It is associated with muscular jerking or convulsions, incontinence, and tongue biting. Postictal confusion may follow.
- *Transient ischemic attacks.* Transient ischemic attacks occur more frequently in the elderly and they may cause syncope.

Neurologic Disorders

Elderly patients are at risk for several neurologic emergencies. Often, the exact cause is not initially known and may require probing at the hospital.

Many of the neurologic disorders that you will encounter in the field will exhibit an alteration in mental status. You may discover a range of underlying causes from stroke to degenerative brain disease. Some of the most common causes of altered mental status include:

- Cerebrovascular disease (stroke or transient ischemic attack)
- Fluid and electrolyte abnormalities (dehydration)
- Infection
- Lack of nutrients (hypoglycemia)
- Medication-related problems (drug interactions, drug underdose, and drug overdose)
- Myocardial infarction
- Seizures
- Structural changes (dementia, subdural hematoma)
- Temperature changes (hypothermia, hyperthermia)

As mentioned, it is often impossible to distinguish in the field the cause of an altered mental status. Even so, you should carry out a thorough assessment. Administer supplemental oxygen if the patient is hypoxic. As soon as practical, obtain a blood glucose level to exclude hypoglycemia as a possible cause. Overall, the approach to the elderly patient with altered mental status is the same as that for any other patient presenting with similar symptoms.

Cerebrovascular Disease (Stroke/TIAs)

Stroke is the fourth-leading cause of death in the United States. Annually, about 795,000 people suffer strokes and about 130,000 die. Incidence of stroke and the likelihood of dying from a stroke increase with age. Occlusive stroke is statistically more common in the elderly and relatively uncommon in younger individuals. Older patients are at higher risk of stroke because of atherosclerosis, hypertension, immobility, limb paralysis, congestive heart failure, and atrial fibrillation. Transient ischemic attacks are also more common in older patients. More than one-third of patients suffering TIAs will develop a major, permanent stroke. As previously mentioned, TIAs are a frequent cause of syncope in the elderly.

Strokes usually fall into one of two major categories. **Brain ischemia**—injury to brain tissue caused by an inadequate supply of oxygen and nutrients—accounts for about 80 percent of all strokes. Brain hemorrhage, the second major category, may be either **subarachnoid hemorrhage** or **intracerebral hemorrhage**. These different patterns of bleeding have different presentations, causes, and treatments. However, together they account for a high percentage of all stroke deaths (Figure 5-18).

Because of the various kinds of strokes, signs and symptoms can present in many ways: altered mental status, coma, paralysis, slurred speech, a change in mood, and seizures. Stroke should be highly suspect in any elderly patient with a sudden change in mental status.

Whenever you suspect a stroke, it is essential that you complete the Los Angeles Prehospital Stroke Screen or Cincinnati Prehospital Stroke Scale for later comparison in the emergency department. Fibrinolytic agents administered to a patient suffering an occlusive (ischemic) stroke can decrease the severity of damage if administered within 4.5 hours of onset. Rapid transport is essential for avoiding brain damage or limiting its extent. In the case of stroke, "time is brain tissue."

By far, the most preferred treatment is prevention of strokes in the first place. Strategies include:

- Cessation of recreational drugs
- Cessation of smoking
- Control of hypertension

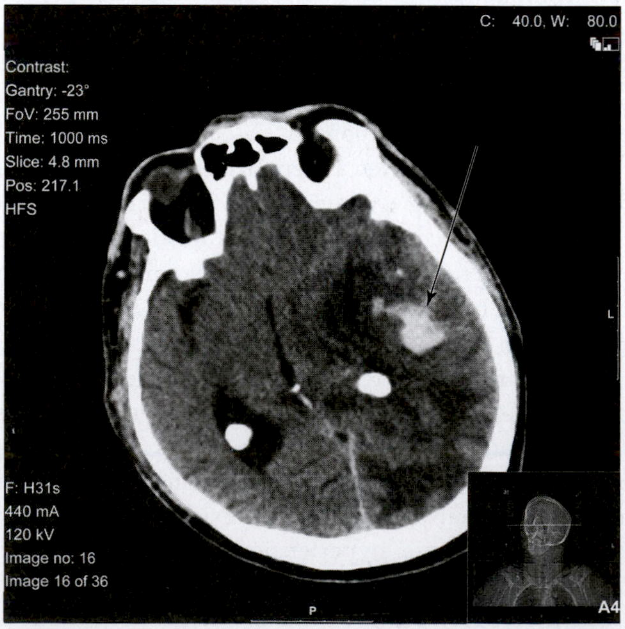

FIGURE 5-18 Large intracerebral hemorrhage with resultant midline shift.

(© Dr. Bryan E. Bledsoe)

- Good eating habits
- Moderate use of alcohol
- Regular exercise
- Treatment of blood disorders, such as anemia and **polycythemia** (excess of red blood cells)
- Treatment of cardiac disorders, including arrhythmias and coronary artery disease

Seizures

Seizures can be easily mistaken for strokes in the elderly. In addition, a first-time seizure may occur as a result of damage from a previous stroke. Not all seizures experienced by the elderly are of the major motor type. Some are more subtle. Many causes of seizure activity in the elderly have been identified. Common causes include:

- Alcohol withdrawal
- Hypoglycemia
- Mass lesion (tumor or bleed)
- Recent or past head trauma
- Seizure disorder (epilepsy)
- Stroke
- Syncope

Often the cause of the seizure cannot be determined in the field. Examination of the patient's home medications may give an indication as to whether the patient has a seizure disorder. Common antiseizure medications include:

- Carbamazepine (Tegretol)
- Ethosuximide (Zarontin)
- Gabapentin (Neurontin)
- Lacosamide (Vimpat)
- Lamotrigine (Lamictal)
- Levetiracetam (Keppra)
- Phenobarbital (Luminal)
- Phenytoin (Dilantin)
- Valproic acid (Depakote)

Because the cause of a seizure cannot always be determined, treat the condition as a life-threatening emergency and transport as quickly as possible to eliminate the possibility of stroke. If the patient has fallen during a seizure, check for evidence of trauma and treat accordingly.

Dizziness/Vertigo

Dizziness is a frightening experience and a frequent complaint of the elderly. The complaint of dizziness may actually mean that the patient has suffered syncope, presyncope, light-headedness, or true **vertigo**. Vertigo is a specific sensation of motion perceived by the patient as spinning or whirling. Many patients will report that they feel as though they are spinning. Vertigo is often accompanied by sweating, pallor, nausea, and vomiting. Ménière's disease can cause severe, **intractable** vertigo. It is often, however, associated with a constant "roaring" sound in the ears, as well as ear "pressure."

Vertigo results from so many factors that it is often hard, even for the physician, to determine the actual cause. Any factor that impairs visual input, inner-ear function, peripheral sensory input, or the central nervous system can cause dizziness. In addition, alcohol and many prescription drugs can cause dizziness. So can hypoglycemia in its early stages. It is virtually impossible to distinguish dizziness, syncope, and presyncope in the prehospital setting.

Delirium, Dementia, and Alzheimer's Disease

Approximately 15 percent of all Americans over age 65 have some degree of dementia or delirium. **Dementia** is a chronic global cognitive impairment, often progressive or irreversible. The best known form of dementia is **Alzheimer's disease**, a condition that affects 5.5 million Americans. **Delirium** is a global mental impairment of sudden onset and self-limited duration. (For differences between dementia and delirium, see Table 5-6.)

DELIRIUM Many conditions can cause delirium. The cause may be either organic brain disease or disorders that occur elsewhere in the body. Delirium in the elderly is a serious condition. According to some estimates, about 18 percent of hospitalized elderly patients with delirium die. Possible etiologies or causes include:

- Subdural hematoma
- Tumors and other mass lesions
- Drug-induced changes or alcohol intoxication
- CNS infections

Table 5-6 Distinguishing Dementia and Delirium*

Dementia	Delirium
Chronic, slowly progressive development	Rapid in onset, fluctuating course
Irreversible disorder	May be reversed, especially if treated early
Greatly impairs memory	Greatly impairs attention
Global cognitive deficits	Focal cognitive deficits
Most commonly caused by Alzheimer's disease	Most commonly caused by systemic disease, drug toxicity, or metabolic changes
Does not require immediate treatment	Requires immediate treatment

*These are general characteristics that apply to most, but not all, cases.

- Electrolyte abnormalities
- Heart failure
- Fever
- Metabolic disorders, including hypoglycemia
- Chronic endocrine abnormalities, including hypothyroidism and hyperthyroidism
- Postconcussion syndrome

The presentation of delirium varies greatly and can change rapidly during assessment. Common signs and symptoms include the acute onset of anxiety, an inability to focus, disordered thinking, irritability, inappropriate behavior, fearfulness, excessive energy, or psychotic behavior such as hallucinations or paranoia. Aphasia or other speech disorders and/or prominent slurring of speech may be present. Normal patterns of eating and sleeping are almost always disrupted.

In distinguishing between delirium and dementia, err on the side of delirium. The condition is often caused by life-threatening, but reversible, conditions. Causes of delirium, such as infections, drug toxicity, and electrolyte imbalances, generally have a good prognosis if identified quickly and managed promptly.

DEMENTIA Dementia is more prevalent in the elderly than delirium. More than 50 percent of all nursing home patients have some form of dementia. It is usually caused by an underlying neurologic disease. This mental deterioration is often called organic brain syndrome, **senile dementia**, or senility. It is important to find out whether an alteration in mental status is acute or chronic. Causes of dementia include:

- Small strokes
- Atherosclerosis
- Age-related neurologic changes
- Neurologic diseases
- Certain hereditary diseases (e.g., Huntington's disease)
- Alzheimer's disease

Signs and symptoms of dementia include progressive disorientation, shortened attention span, **aphasia** or nonsense talking, and hallucinations. Dementia often hampers treatment through the patient's inability to communicate, and it can exhaust caregivers. In moderate to severe cases, you will need to rely on the caregiver for information. (Remain alert to signs of abuse or neglect, which occurs in a disproportionate number of elderly suffering from dementia.)

ALZHEIMER'S DISEASE Alzheimer's disease, a particular type of dementia, is a chronic degenerative disorder that attacks the brain and results in impaired memory, thinking, and behavior.[7] It accounts for more than half of all forms of dementia in the elderly (Figure 5-19).

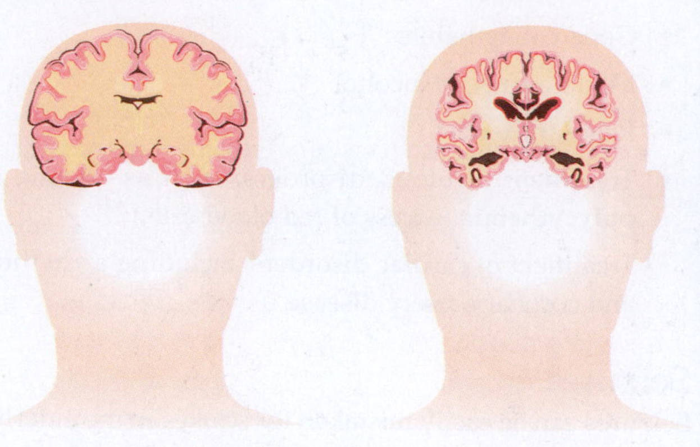

FIGURE 5-19 Illustration of normal human brain (left) and the brain of an Alzheimer's patient (right). Note the pronounced atrophy and ventricular enlargement.

Alzheimer's disease generally occurs in stages, each with different signs and symptoms. These stages are:

- ***Early stage.*** Characterized by loss of recent memory, inability to learn new material, mood swings, and personality changes. Patients may believe someone is plotting against them when they lose items or forget things. Aggression or hostility is common. Poor judgment is evident.
- ***Intermediate stage.*** Characterized by a complete inability to learn new material; wandering, particularly at night; increased falls; and loss of ability for self-care, including bathing and use of the toilet.
- ***Terminal stage.*** Characterized by an inability to walk and regression to infant stage, including the loss of bowel and bladder function. Eventually the patient loses the ability to eat and swallow.

Families caring for an Alzheimer's patient at home also present signs of stress. Remember to treat both the Alzheimer's patient and the family and/or caregivers with respect and compassion. Evaluate the needs of the family and make an appropriate report at your facility. Support groups are available to assist families.

Parkinson's Disease

Parkinson's disease is a degenerative disorder characterized by changes in muscle response, including tremors, loss of facial expression, and gait disturbances. It mainly appears in people over age 50 and peaks at age 70. The disease affects about 1 million Americans, with 50,000 new cases diagnosed each year. It is the fourth most common neurodegenerative disease among the elderly.

The cause of primary Parkinson's disease remains unknown.[8] However, it affects the basal ganglia in the

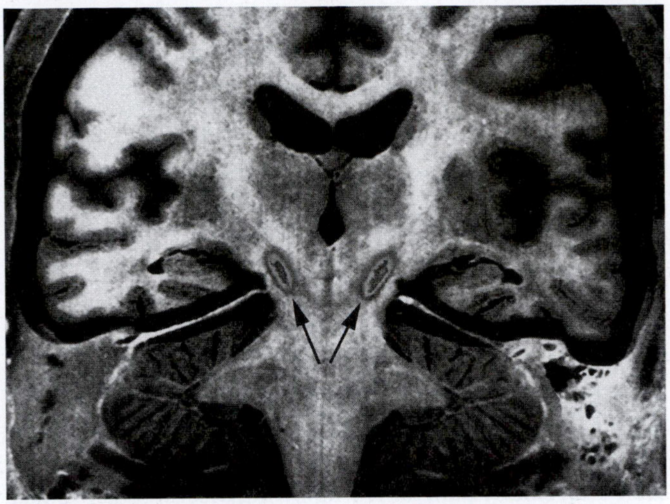

FIGURE 5-20 Degenerative disease of the extrapyramidal system (substantia nigra, arrows) in a 50-year-old man with Parkinson's disease.

(SPL/Science Source)

brain, an area that deciphers messages going to muscles (Figure 5-20). Secondary Parkinson's disease is distinguished from primary Parkinson's disease by having a known cause. Some of the most common causes include:

- Viral encephalitis
- Atherosclerosis of cerebral vessels
- Reaction to certain drugs or toxins, such as antipsychotics or carbon monoxide
- Metabolic disorders, such as anoxia
- Tumors
- Head trauma
- Degenerative disorders, such as **Shy-Drager syndrome**

It is impossible in a field setting to distinguish primary and secondary Parkinson's disease. The most common initial sign of a Parkinson's disorder is a resting tremor combined with a **pill-rolling motion**. As the disease progresses, muscles become more rigid and movements become slower and/or more jerky. In some cases, patients may find their movements halted while carrying out some routine task. Their feet may feel "frozen to the ground." Gait becomes shuffled with short steps and unexpected bursts of speed, often to avoid falling. Kyphotic deformity is a hallmark of the disease.

Patients with Parkinson's disease commonly develop mask-like faces devoid of all expression. They speak in slow, monotone voices. Difficulties in communication, coupled with a loss of mobility, often lead to anxiety and depression.

There is no known cure for Parkinson's disease, with the exception of drug-induced secondary Parkinson's disorders. Exercise may help maintain physical activity or teach the patient adaptive strategies. In calls involving a Parkinson's patient, observe for the conditions that involved the EMS system, such as a fall or the inability to move. Manage treatable conditions and transport as needed.

Metabolic and Endocrine Disorders

As previously mentioned, the endocrine system undergoes a number of age-related changes that affect hormone levels. The most common endocrine disorders include diabetes mellitus and problems related to the thyroid gland. Of the two, you will more often treat diabetic-related emergencies, particularly hypoglycemia.

Diabetes Mellitus

An estimated 20 percent of older adults have diabetes mellitus, primarily type II diabetes. Almost 40 percent have some type of glucose intolerance. The elderly develop these disorders for these reasons:

- Poor diet
- Decreased physical activity
- Loss of lean body mass
- Impaired insulin production
- Resistance by body cells to the actions of insulin

Diagnosis of type 2 diabetes usually occurs during routine screening in a physical exam. In some cases, urine tests may register negative because of an increased renal glucose threshold in the elderly. The condition may present, in its early stages, with vague constitutional symptoms such as fatigue or weakness. If allowed to progress, diabetes can result in neuropathy and visual impairment. These manifestations often lead to more aggressive blood testing, which in most cases will reveal elevated glucose levels.

The treatment of diabetes involves diet, exercise, the use of sulfonylurea agents, and/or insulin. Many diabetics use self-monitoring devices to test glucose levels. Unfortunately, the cost of these devices and the accompanying test strips sometimes discourages the elderly from using them. Elderly patients on insulin also risk hypoglycemia, especially if they accidentally take too much insulin or do not eat enough food following injection. The lack of good nutrition can be particularly troublesome to elderly diabetics. They often find it difficult to prepare meals, fail to enjoy food because of altered taste perceptions, have trouble chewing food, or are unable to purchase adequate and/or the correct food because of limited income.

Management of diabetic and hypoglycemic emergencies for the elderly is generally the same as for any other patient. *Do not* rule out alcohol as a complicating factor, especially in cases of hypoglycemia. In addition, remember that diabetes places the elderly at increased risk of other complications, including atherosclerosis, delayed healing, **retinopathy**, blindness, altered renal function, and severe peripheral vascular disease, leading to foot ulcers and even amputations.

Thyroid Disorders

With normal aging, the thyroid gland undergoes moderate atrophy and changes in hormone production. An estimated 2 to 5 percent of people over age 65 experience hypothyroidism, a condition resulting from inadequate levels of thyroid hormones. It affects women in greater numbers than men, and the prevalence rises with age.

Less than 33 percent of the elderly who have hypothyroidism present with typical signs and symptoms of hypothyroidism. When they do, their complaints are often attributed to aging. Common nonspecific complaints in the elderly include mental confusion, anorexia, falls, incontinence, and decreased mobility. Some patients also experience an increase in muscle or joint pain. Treatment involves thyroid hormone replacement.

Hyperthyroidism is less common among the elderly but may result from medication errors such as an overdose of thyroid hormone replacement. The typical symptom of heat intolerance is often present. Otherwise, hyperthyroidism presents atypically in the elderly. Common nonspecific features or complaints include atrial fibrillation, failure to thrive (weight loss and apathy combined), abdominal distress, diarrhea, exhaustion, and depression.

The diagnosis and treatment of thyroid disorders does not take place in the field. Elderly patients with known thyroid problems should be encouraged to go to the hospital for medical evaluation.

Gastrointestinal Disorders

Gastrointestinal emergencies are common among the elderly. The most frequent emergency is gastrointestinal bleeding. However, older people will also describe a variety of other gastrointestinal complaints: nausea, poor appetite, diarrhea, and constipation, to name a few. Remember that, like other presenting complaints, these conditions may be symptomatic of more serious diseases. Bowel problems, for example, may point to cancer of the colon or other abdominal organs.

Regardless of the complaint, remember that prompt management of a GI emergency is essential for young and old alike. For the elderly, there is a significant risk of hemorrhage and shock. There is a tendency to take GI patients less seriously than those suffering moderate or severe external hemorrhage. This is a serious mistake. Patients with gastrointestinal complaints, especially the elderly, should be managed aggressively. Keep in mind that older patients are far more intolerant of hypotension and anoxia than younger patients are. Treatment should include:

- Airway management
- Support of breathing and circulation
- Supplemental oxygen therapy if the patient is hypoxic
- IV fluid replacement with a crystalloid solution
- Rapid transport

Some of the most critical GI problems that you may encounter in the field will involve internal hemorrhage and bowel obstruction. You may also be called on to treat **mesenteric ischemia or infarct**, a serious and life-threatening condition in an elderly patient. The following descriptions will help you to recognize each of these gastrointestinal disorders.

GI Hemorrhage

Gastrointestinal bleeding falls into two general categories: upper GI bleed and lower GI bleed.

UPPER GI BLEED This form of gastrointestinal bleeding includes:

- ***Peptic ulcer disease:*** injury to the mucous lining of the upper part of the gastrointestinal tract due to stomach acids, digestive enzymes, and other agents, such as anti-inflammatory drugs
- ***Gastritis:*** an inflammation of the lining of the stomach
- ***Esophageal varices:*** an abnormal dilation of veins in the lower esophagus; a common complication of cirrhosis of the liver
- ***Mallory-Weiss tear:*** a tear in the lower esophagus that is often caused by severe and prolonged retching

LOWER GI BLEED Conditions categorized as lower gastrointestinal bleeding include:

- ***Diverticulosis:*** the presence of small pouches on the colon that tend to develop with age; causes 70 percent of life-threatening lower GI bleeds
- ***Tumors:*** tumors of the colon can cause bleeding when the tumor erodes into blood vessels within the intestine or surrounding organs
- ***Ischemic colitis:*** an inflammation of the colon resulting from impaired or decreased blood supply
- ***Arteriovenous malformations:*** an abnormal link between an artery and a vein

Signs of significant gastrointestinal blood loss include the presence of "coffee-grounds" emesis; black, tarlike stools (**melena**); obvious blood in the emesis or stool; orthostatic hypotension; pulse greater than 100 (unless the patient is on beta-blockers); and confusion. Gastrointestinal

CONTENT REVIEW

- ➤ Signs and Symptoms of Bowel Obstruction
  - Diffuse abdominal pain
  - Bloating
  - Nausea
  - Vomiting
  - Distended abdomen
  - Hypoactive/absent bowel sounds

bleeding in the elderly may result in such complications as a recent increase in angina symptoms, congestive heart failure, weakness, or dyspnea.

Bowel Obstruction

Bowel obstruction in the elderly typically involves the small bowel. Causes include tumors, prior abdominal surgery, use of certain medications, and occasionally the presence of vertebral compression fractures. The patient will typically complain of diffuse abdominal pain, bloating, nausea, and vomiting. The abdomen may feel distended when palpated. Bowel sounds may be hypoactive or absent, or hyperactive and "tinkling." If the obstruction has been present for a prolonged period of time, the patient may have fever, weakness, shock, and various electrolyte disturbances.

Mesenteric Ischemia/Infarct

Vessels arising from the superior or inferior mesenteric arteries generally serve the bowel. An infarct occurs when a portion of the bowel does not receive enough blood to survive. Certain age-related changes make the elderly more vulnerable to this condition. First, as a person ages, changes in the heart (such as atrial fibrillation) or the vessels (atherosclerosis) predispose the patient to a clot lodging in one of the branches serving the bowel. Second, changes in the bowel itself can promote swelling that effectively cuts off blood flow.

The primary symptom of a bowel infarct is pain out of proportion to the physical exam. Signs include:

- Bloody diarrhea, but usually not a massive hemorrhage
- Some tachycardia, although there may be a vagal effect masking the sign
- Abdominal distention

The patient is at great risk for shock because the dead bowel attracts interstitial and intravascular fluids, thus removing them from use. Necrotic products are released to the peritoneal cavity, leading to a massive infection. The prognosis is poor due, in part, to decreased physiologic reserves on the part of the older patient.

Skin Disorders

Younger and older adults experience common skin disorders at about the same rates. However, age-related changes in the immune system make the elderly more prone to certain chronic skin diseases and infections. They are also more likely to develop **pressure ulcers** (bedsores) than any other age group.

Skin Diseases

Elderly patients commonly complain about **pruritus**, or itching. This condition can be caused by dermatitis (eczema) or environmental conditions, especially during winter (i.e., from hot dry air in the home and cold windy air outside). Keep in mind that generalized itching can also be a sign of systemic diseases, particularly liver and renal disorders. When itching is strong and unrelenting, suspect an underlying disease and encourage the patient to seek medical evaluation.

Slower healing and compromised tissue perfusion in the elderly make them more susceptible to bacterial infection of wounds, appearing as cellulitis, impetigo, and, in the case of immunocompromised adults, staphylococcal scalded skin. The elderly also experience a higher incidence of fungal infections, partly because of decreases in the cutaneous immunologic response. In addition, they suffer higher rates of **herpes zoster** (shingles), which peaks between ages 50 and 70. Although these skin disorders also occur in the young, their duration and severity increases markedly with age.

In treating skin disorders, remember that many conditions may be drug induced. Beta-blockers, for example, can worsen psoriasis, which occurs in about 3 percent of elderly patients. Question patients about their medications, keeping in mind that certain prescription drugs (e.g., penicillins and sulfonamides) and some OTC drugs can cause skin eruptions. Also ask about topical home remedies, such as alcohol or soaps that may cause or worsen the disorder. Find out whether the patient is compliant with prescribed topical treatments. Finally, remember that some drugs and topical medications commonly used to treat skin disorders in the young can worsen or cause other problems for the elderly. Antihistamines and corticosteroids are two to three times more likely to provoke adverse reactions in the elderly than in younger adults.

Pressure Ulcers (Decubitus Ulcers)

Most pressure ulcers occur in people over age 70. As many as 20 percent of patients enter the hospital with a pressure ulcer or develop one while hospitalized. The highest incidence occurs in nursing homes, where up to 25 percent of patients may develop this condition.[9]

Pressure ulcers typically develop from the waist down, usually over bony prominences, in bedridden patients. However, they can occur anywhere on the body and with the patient in any position. Pressure ulcers usually result from tissue hypoxia and affect the skin, subcutaneous tissues, and muscle (Figure 5-21). Factors that can increase the risk of this condition include:

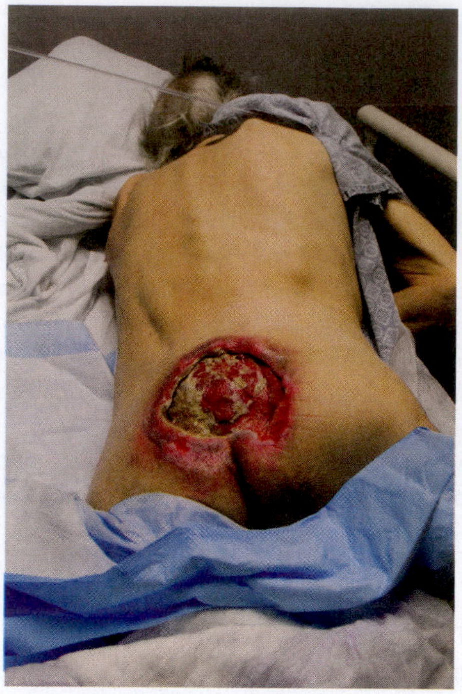

FIGURE 5-21 Multiple decubitus ulcers ("bedsores" or "pressure sores"). These often become infected, leading to the patient's death. They can be prevented with good nursing care.

(Robert A. Penne-Casanova/Science Source)

- External compression of tissues (i.e., pressure)
- Altered sensory perception
- **Maceration**, caused by excessive moisture
- Decreased activity
- Decreased mobility
- Poor nutrition
- Friction or shear

To reduce the development of pressure ulcers or to alleviate their condition, you can take these steps:

- Assist the patient in changing position frequently, especially during extended transport, to reduce the length of time pressure is placed on any one point.
- Use a pull sheet to move the patient, reducing the likelihood of friction.
- Reduce the possibility of shearing by padding areas of skin prior to movement.
- Unless a life-threatening condition is present, take time to clean and dry areas of excessive moisture, such as urinary or fecal incontinence and excessive perspiration.
- Clean ulcers with normal saline solution and cover with hydrocolloid or hydrogel dressings, if available. With severe ulcers, pack with loosely woven gauze moistened with normal saline.

Musculoskeletal Disorders

The skeleton, as you know, is a metabolically active organ. Its metabolic processes are influenced by a number of factors, including age, diet, exercise, and hormone levels. The musculoskeletal system is also subject to disease. In fact, musculoskeletal diseases are the leading cause of functional impairment in the elderly. Although usually not fatal, musculoskeletal disorders often produce chronic disability, which in turn creates a context for illness. Two of the most widespread musculoskeletal disorders are osteoarthritis and osteoporosis.

Osteoarthritis

Osteoarthritis is the leading cause of disability among people age 65 and older. Many experts think the condition may not be one disease but several with similar presentations. Although wear and tear, as well as age-related changes such as loss of muscle mass, predispose the elderly to osteoarthritis, other factors may play a role as well. Presumed contributing causes include:

- Obesity
- Primary disorders of the joint, such as inflammatory arthritis
- Trauma
- Congenital abnormalities, such as hip dysplasia

Osteoarthritis in the elderly presents initially as joint pain, worsened by exercise and improved by rest. As the disease progresses, pain may be accompanied by diminished mobility, joint deformity, and crepitus or grating sensations. Late signs include tenderness on palpation or during passive motion.

The most effective treatment involves management before the disability develops or worsens. Prevention strategies include stretching exercises and activities that strengthen stress-absorbing ligaments (Figure 5-22). Immobilization, even for short periods, can accelerate the condition. Drug therapy is usually aimed at lessening pain and/or inflammation. Surgery (i.e., total joint replacement) is usually the last resort after more conservative methods have failed.

Osteoporosis

Osteoporosis affects an estimated 20 million Americans and is largely responsible for fractures of the hip, wrist, and vertebral bones following a fall or other injury. Risk factors include:

- ***Age.*** Peak bone mass for men and women occurs in their third and fourth decades of life and declines at varying rates thereafter. Decreased bone density generally becomes a treatment consideration at about age 50.
- ***Gender.*** The decline of estrogen production places women at a higher risk of developing osteoporosis

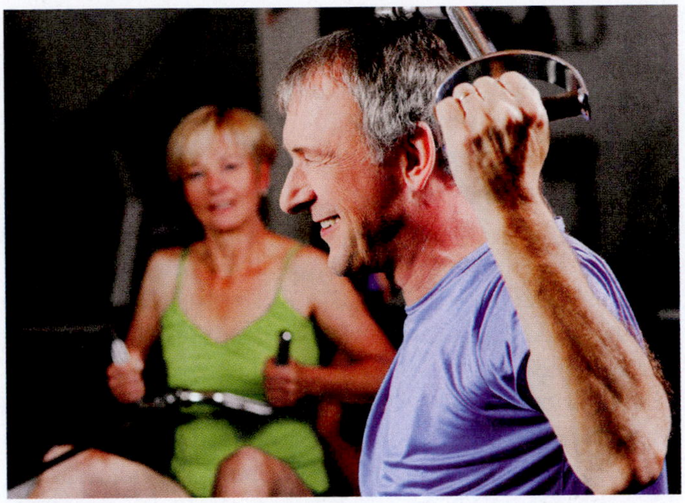

FIGURE 5-22 Regular stretching and weight-bearing exercises help prevent the development of osteoarthritis.

(Kzenon/Fotolia)

than men. Women are more than twice as likely to have brittle bones, especially if they experience early menopause (before age 45) and do not take estrogen replacement therapy.

- ***Race.*** Whites and Asians are more likely to develop osteoporosis than African Americans and Latinos, who have higher bone mass at skeletal peak.
- ***Body weight.*** Thin people, or people with low body weight, are at greater risk of osteoporosis than obese people. Increased skeletal weight is thought to promote bone density. However, weight-bearing exercise can have the same effect.
- ***Family history.*** Genetic factors (i.e., peak bone mass attainment) and a family history of fractures may predispose a person to osteoporosis.
- ***Miscellaneous.*** Late menarche, nulliparity, and use of caffeine, alcohol, and cigarettes are all thought to be important determinants of bone mass.

Unless a bone density test is conducted, persons with osteoporosis are usually asymptomatic until a fracture occurs. The precipitating event can be as slight as turning over in bed, carrying a package, or even a forceful sneeze (Figure 5-23). Management includes prevention of fractures through exercise and drug therapy, such as the administration of calcium, vitamin D, estrogen, and other medications or minerals. Once the condition occurs, pain management also becomes a consideration.

Ankylosing Spondylitis

Ankylosing spondylitis (AS) is a form of inflammatory arthritis that primarily affects the spine. It is estimated that approximately 500,000 people in the United States have the disease. AS primarily causes inflammation of the joints

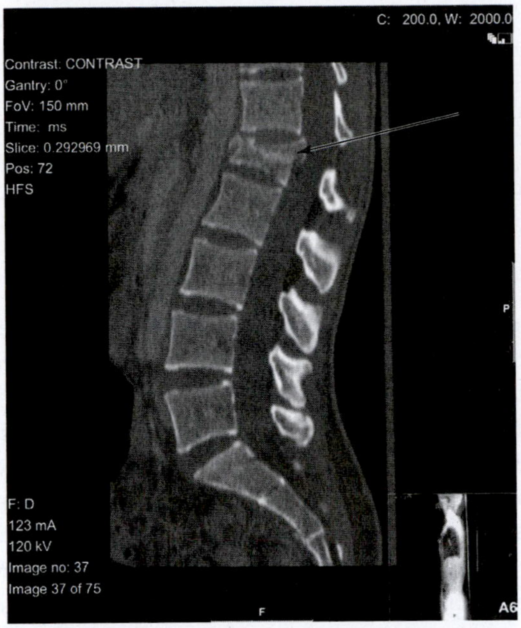

FIGURE 5-23 Sagittal CT image of a traumatic L1 compression fracture with retropulsion of bone fragments into the spinal canal.

(© Dr. Bryan E. Bledsoe)

between the vertebrae of the spine and the sacroiliac joints in the pelvis (Figure 5-24). It can also cause inflammation and pain in other parts of the body. As the condition worsens and the inflammation persists, new bone forms as a part

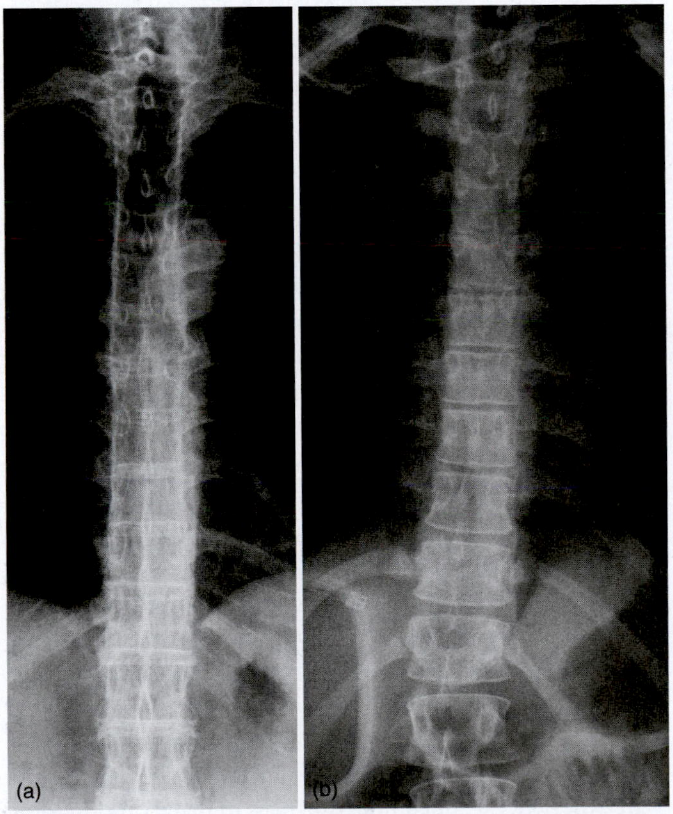

FIGURE 5-24 Typical "bamboo spine" as seen in ankylosing spondylitis (a) compared with a normal spine (b).

(Spondylitis Association of America)

of the healing process. The bone may grow from the edge of the vertebra across the disk space between two vertebrae, resulting in a bony bridge; this may occur throughout the spine so that the spine becomes stiff and inflexible—effectively fusing the spine. On spinal X-rays, this phenomenon is referred to as "bamboo spine." This fusion can also affect the rib cage, restricting lung capacity and function.

As the disease progresses, the spine becomes fused into a single unit incapable of flexion, extension, or lateral movement. Usually the fusion progresses with the spine assuming a flexed position and the patient is forced to walk bent over.

EMS providers called to care for a victim of AS must remember that the patient's spine is inflexible and cannot be moved. Furthermore, the fused spine can be extremely fragile and subject to fracture, with resultant spinal cord injury. Numerous EMS techniques must be modified to accommodate patients with AS. These include airway management techniques, splinting techniques, and transport considerations. Because most AS patients have spinal flexion, it is important to adequately pad underneath the patient's head, neck, and upper back with pillow or pillows.[10] Likewise, airway management techniques must be applied without extending the neck. Airway devices that do not require visualization (e.g., extraglottic airways) should be considered instead of endotracheal intubation, with cricothyrotomy used as a last resort.

Although patients with AS are not common, improper EMS care of them can be devastating. Learn to identify the signs and symptoms of AS and be careful to protect the patient's spine accordingly.

Renal Disorders

The most common renal diseases in the elderly include renal failure, **glomerulonephritis**, and renal blood clots. These problems may be traced to two age-related factors: (1) loss in kidney size and (2) changes in the walls of the renal arteries and in the arterioles serving the glomeruli. In general, a person's kidney loses approximately one-third of its weight between the ages of 30 and 80. Most of this loss occurs in the tissues that filter blood. When filtering tissue is gone, blood is shunted from the precapillary side directly to venules on the postcapillary side, thus bypassing any tissue still capable of filtering. The result is a reduction in kidney efficiency. This condition is complicated by changes in renal arteries, which promote the development of renal emboli and thrombi.

With renal changes, elderly patients are more likely to accumulate toxins and medications within the bloodstream. Occasionally, this will be obvious to the patient because he will experience a substantial decrease in urine output. More often, however, the elderly are prone to a type of renal failure in which urine output remains normal to high while the kidney remains ineffective in clearing wastes.

Processes that precipitate acute renal failure include hypotension, heart failure, major surgery, sepsis, angiographic procedures (the dye is nephrotoxic), and use of nephrotoxic antibiotics (e.g., gentamicin, tobramycin). Ongoing hypertension also figures in the development of chronic renal failure.

Urinary Disorders

Urinary tract infections (UTIs) affect as much as 10 percent of the elderly population each year. Younger women generally suffer more UTIs than young men, but in the elderly the distribution is almost even. Most of these infections result from bacteria and easily lead to **urosepsis** owing to reduced immune system function among the elderly.

A number of factors contribute to the high rate of UTIs among the elderly:

- Atrophic vaginitis (in women)
- Bladder outlet obstruction from benign prostatic hyperplasia (in men)
- Dementia, with resulting poor hygiene
- Diabetes
- Immobilization
- Stroke
- Upper urinary tract stone
- Use of indwelling bladder catheters

Signs or symptoms of a UTI range from cloudy, foul-smelling urine to the typical complaints of bladder pain and frequent urination. Urosepsis presents as an acute process, including fever, chills, abdominal discomfort, and other signs of septic shock. The septicemia generally begins within 24 to 72 hours after catheterization or cystoscopy.

Treatment of urosepsis commonly includes placement of a large-bore IV catheter for administration of fluids and parenteral antibiotics. Diagnosis of urosepsis is based on history and other physical findings. Prompt transport is critical. The prognosis for elderly patients with urosepsis is poor, with a mortality rate of approximately 30 percent. Maintenance of fluid balance, as well as adequate blood pressure, is essential.

Environmental Emergencies

As previously mentioned, environmental extremes represent a great health risk for the elderly. Nearly 50 percent of all **heatstroke** deaths in the United States occur among people over age 50. The elderly are just as susceptible to low temperatures, suffering numerous winter deaths annually, primarily from hypothermia and "winter risks" such as pneumonia and influenza. As you may already know from your EMT experience, thermoregulatory emergencies represent some of the most common EMS calls involving the elderly.

Hypothermia

A number of factors predispose the elderly to hypothermia:

- Accidental exposure to cold
- AV shunts, which increase heat loss
- Chronic illness
- CNS disorders, including head trauma, stroke, tumors, or subdural hematomas
- Drugs that interfere with heat production, including alcohol, antidepressants, and tranquilizers
- Endocrine disorders, including hypoglycemia and diabetes (patients with diabetes are six times as likely to develop hypothermia as other patients)
- Forced inactivity as a result of arthritis, dementia, falls, paralysis, or Parkinson's disease
- Inflammatory dermatitis
- Low or fixed income, which discourages the use of home heating
- Malnutrition or starvation

Signs and symptoms of hypothermia can be slow to develop. Many times, elderly patients with hypothermia lose their sensitivity to cold and fail to complain. As a result, hypothermia may be missed. Nonspecific complaints may suggest a metabolic disorder or stroke. Hypothermic patients may exhibit slow speech, confusion, and sleepiness. In the early stages, patients will exhibit hypertension and an increased heart rate. As hypothermia progresses, however, blood pressure drops and the heart rate slows, sometimes to a barely detectable level.

Remember that the elderly patient with hypothermia often does not shiver. Check the abdomen and back to see if the skin is cool to the touch. Expect subcutaneous tissues to be firm. If your unit has a low-temperature thermometer, check the patient's core temperature. (Regular thermometers often do not "shake down" far enough for an accurate reading.)

As with other medical disorders, prevention is the preferred treatment. However, once elderly patients develop hypothermia, they become progressively impaired. Treat even mild cases of hypothermia, or suspected hypothermia, as a medical emergency. Focus on the rewarming techniques used with other patients and rapid transport. Maintain reassessment to ensure that the hypothermia does not complicate existing medical problems or heretofore untreated disorders. Death most commonly results from cardiac arrest or ventricular fibrillation.

Hyperthermia (Heatstroke)

Age-related changes in sweat glands and increased incidence of heart disease place the elderly at risk of heat stress. They may develop heat cramps, heat exhaustion, or heatstroke. Although the first two disorders rarely result in death, heatstroke is a serious medical emergency. Risk factors for severe hyperthermia include:

- Alcoholism
- Altered sensory output, which would normally warn a person of overheating
- Commonly prescribed medications that inhibit sweating such as antihistamines and tricyclic antidepressants
- Concomitant medical disorders
- Decreased functioning of the thermoregulatory center
- Inadequate liquid intake
- Low or fixed income, which may result in a lack of air conditioning or adequate ventilation
- Use of diuretics, which increase fluid loss

Like hypothermia, early heatstroke may present with nonspecific signs and symptoms, such as nausea, lightheadedness, dizziness, or headache. High temperature is the most reliable indicator, but consider even a slight temperature elevation as symptomatic if coupled with an absence of sweating and neurologic impairment. Severe hypotension also exists in many critical patients.

Prevention strategies include adequate fluid intake, reduced activity, shelter in an air-conditioned environment, and use of light clothing. If hyperthermia develops, however, rapid treatment and transport are necessary.

Toxicologic Emergencies

As previously mentioned, aging alters pharmacokinetics and pharmacodynamics in the elderly. Functional changes in the kidneys, liver, and gastrointestinal system slow the absorption and elimination of many medications. In addition, the various compensatory mechanisms that help buffer against medication side effects are less effective in the elderly than in younger patients.

A significant number of all hospital admissions are a result of drug-related illnesses. Many of these result in drug-related deaths in people over age 60. Accidental overdoses may occur more frequently in the aged as a result of confusion, vision impairment, self-selection of medications, forgetfulness, and concurrent drug use. Intentional drug overdose also occurs in attempts at self-destruction. Another complicating factor is the abuse of alcohol among the elderly.

The paramedic must be familiar with the range of side effects that can be caused by the polypharmacy of medications taken by geriatric patients. The usage of multiple doctors and polypharmacy in the aging patient increase the chances of receiving multiple medications for the same medical conditions. This problem is further compounded as a result of the usage of both trade and generic medication names.

In assessing the geriatric patient, always take these steps:

- Obtain a full list of medications currently taken by the patient.
- Elicit any medications that are newly prescribed. (Some side effects appear within a few days of taking a new medication.)
- Obtain a good past medical history. Find out if your patient has a history of renal or hepatic depression.
- Know your medications, their routes of elimination, and their potential side effects.
- If possible, always take all medications to the hospital along with the patient.

A knowledge of pharmacology is important in all patients; however, it is critical in recognizing potential toxicologic emergencies in the geriatric patient. Some of the drugs or substances that have been identified as commonly causing toxicity in the elderly are described in the following sections.

Beta-Blockers

Beta-blockers are widely used to treat hypertension, angina pectoris, and cardiac arrhythmias. Commonly prescribed beta-blockers include propranolol hydrochloride (Inderal), nadolol, atenolol, sotalol, timolol, esmolol, metoprolol, penbutolol, and labetalol.

Although fairly well tolerated in younger adults, elderly patients tend to be more susceptible to the side effects of these agents. In particular, central nervous system side effects—depression, lethargy, and sleep disorders—are more common in the elderly.

Because geriatric patients often have preexisting cardiovascular problems that can cause decreased cardiac function and output, beta-blockers will limit the heart's ability to respond to postural changes, causing orthostatic hypotension. Beta-blockers also limit the heart's ability to increase contractile force and cardiac output whenever a sympathetic response is necessary in situations such as exercise or hypovolemia. This can be detrimental to the trauma patient who is hemorrhaging and cannot mount the sympathetic response necessary to maintain perfusion of vital organs. Also remember that all beta-blockers can worsen heart failure in patients with poor left ventricular function. Beta-blockers decrease intraocular pressure and are often used to treat glaucoma in the elderly. Remember, even beta-blocker eyedrops can cause systemic effects.

Treatment of beta-blocker overdose includes general supportive measures, the removal of gastric contents, cardiorespiratory support, fluids, and administration of nonadrenergic inotropic agents, such as glucagon, for hypotension. Excessive bradycardia can be treated with atropine.

Antihypertensives/Diuretics

Diuretics act on the kidneys to increase urine flow and the excretion of water and sodium. They are used primarily in the treatment of hypertension and congestive heart failure.

This group of medications includes hydrochlorothiazide (HCTZ), furosemide, bumetanide, and torsemide. Of these drugs, furosemide is the most widely used diuretic in the elderly. The elimination half-life of furosemide is markedly prolonged in the patient with acute pulmonary edema and renal and hepatic failure. As a result, the geriatric patient is at risk for a drug buildup.

Because the elderly may be sensitive to adult dosages, a smaller dose is often prescribed and the patient usually takes a daily potassium supplement. Excessive urination caused by the drug may put the elderly at risk for postural hypotension, circulatory collapse, potassium depletion, and renal function impairment.

Angiotensin-Converting Enzyme Inhibitors

Angiotensin-converting enzyme (ACE) inhibitors are a relatively recent addition to the group of medications used in the treatment of hypertension and congestive heart failure. They are used either as a first-line treatment or when other, more established, drugs are contraindicated, are poorly tolerated, or fail to produce the desired effect. Specific examples of ACE inhibitors include captopril, enalapril, lisinopril, fosinopril, benazepril, quinapril, and ramipril.

For the treatment of congestive heart failure, ACE inhibitors reduce renin–angiotensin-mediated vasoconstriction, which reduces the pressure against which the heart has to pump (afterload). Geriatric patients generally respond well to treatment with ACE inhibitors. However, these drugs can cause chronic hypotension in patients with severe heart failure if they are also taking high-dose loop diuretics. ACE inhibitors can also cause plasma volume reduction and hypotension with prolonged vomiting and diarrhea, especially in the elderly. Some hemodialysis patients can experience anaphylactic reactions if treated with ACE inhibitors.

Other side effects of ACE inhibitors include dizziness or light-headedness upon standing; presence of a rash; muscle cramps; swelling of the hands, face, or eyes; cough (especially in women); headache; stomach upset; and fatigue. Captopril, in particular, can cause a loss of taste.

Digitalis (Digoxin, Lanoxin)

Digoxin is the most widely used cardiac glycoside for the management of congestive heart failure, atrial fibrillation, atrial flutter, paroxysmal atrial tachycardia, and cardiogenic shock. The drug is unique in that it has a positive inotropic effect, but a negative chronotropic effect. In congestive heart failure, digoxin increases the strength of myocardial contractions (positive inotropic effect) with a resulting increase in cardiac output. Digoxin also slows conduction and increases the refractory period in cardiac conducting tissue, resulting in a reduced ventricular rate (negative chronotropic effect). This allows the ventricle to adequately fill with blood, also improving cardiac output.

In the patient with moderate to severe heart failure, digitalis is often combined with ACE inhibitors and diuretics. Remember that digoxin has a low therapeutic index. As a result, the dose must be adjusted for each patient.

Digoxin serum levels should be monitored carefully during therapy. The drug is excreted in the urine, with 50 to 70 percent of the dose as unchanged drug. The half-life ranges from 32 to 48 hours in patients with normal renal function. Because the elderly have a reduced volume of distribution for digoxin and may have impaired renal or hepatic function, the dose should be reduced and individualized to minimize the risk of toxicity. Digitalis-induced appetite loss is also a danger in frail elderly patients.

The most common adverse drug effect that occurs in elderly patients is digoxin toxicity. The primary reason is that digoxin has a low margin of safety and a narrow therapeutic index. The amount of the drug needed to produce beneficial or therapeutic effects is close to the toxic amount.

Digoxin toxicity in the elderly can result from accidental or intentional ingestion. For the renal-impaired elderly patient, any change in kidney function usually warrants an alteration in the dosing of digoxin. Failure to adjust the dose can lead to toxicity. Diuretics, which are often given to patients with congestive heart failure, cause the loss of large amounts of potassium in the urine. If potassium is not adequately replenished in the patient taking digoxin, toxicity will develop. Therefore, elderly patients on digoxin should be taking a daily potassium supplement such as potassium chloride (Micro-K, K-Tabs, Slow-K).

Signs and symptoms of digoxin toxicity include visual disturbances, fatigue, weakness, nausea, loss of appetite, abdominal discomfort, dizziness, abnormal dreams, headache, and vomiting. Patients who are taking digoxin for the first time are instructed to call their physician if any of these symptoms occur.

Low potassium (hypokalemia) is also common with chronic digoxin toxicity due to concurrent diuretic therapy. Arrhythmias commonly associated with digoxin toxicity include sinoatrial (SA) exit block, SA arrest, second- or third-degree AV block, atrial fibrillation with a slow ventricular response, accelerated AV junctional rhythms, patterns of premature ventricular contractions (bigeminy and trigeminy), ventricular tachycardia, and atrial tachycardia with AV block.

Management of digoxin toxicity includes gastric lavage with activated charcoal, correction of confirmed hypokalemia with K^+ supplements, treatment of bradycardias with atropine or pacing, and treatment of rapid ventricular rhythms with an antiarrhythmic. A digoxin-specific FAB fragment antibodies treatment (Digibind), an antidote for digoxin toxicity, is used in the treatment of potentially life-threatening situations.

Anticoagulants

The use of anticoagulant medications by the elderly is common. Low-dose aspirin is commonly used as an antiplatelet inhibitor for the prophylaxis of cardiovascular and cerebrovascular disease. A commonly encountered anticoagulant is warfarin (Coumadin). It is used to prevent blood clots from forming or enlarging. It is commonly used in patients with atrial fibrillation, those who have prosthetic (artificial) heart valves, and in selected patients following cardiac events (STEMI). It is also used to prevent pulmonary emboli and deep venous thrombosis.

Warfarin can be difficult to dose and requires routine monitoring of the patient's prothrombin time (PT) or the derivative value called the International Normalized Ratio (INR). The goal is to keep the INR within a target range—not too high or the patient will bleed, or too low where it is ineffective. Warfarin toxicity can be reversed with vitamin K if required.

Several newer anticoagulants are available. These include dabigatran (Pradaxa), rivaroxaban (Xarelto), and apixaban (Eliquis). These medications are effective and do not require PT or INR monitoring. However, there is no reversal agent. Patients on anticoagulants (besides aspirin) are at an increased risk for hemorrhage following trauma—especially head trauma.

Antipsychotics/Antidepressants

Psychotropic medications comprise a variety of agents that affect mood, behavior, and other aspects of mental function. The elderly often experience a high incidence of psychiatric disorders and may take any number of medications, including antidepressants, antianxiety agents, sedative-hypnotic agents, and antipsychotics.

Depression is the most common mental disorder in the elderly. Drug therapy may be prescribed to help resolve the feelings of sadness or hopelessness that result from the death of a spouse, divorce, declining health, and/or loss of independence. Commonly prescribed antidepressants include serotonin reuptake inhibitors (SSRIs) such as fluoxetine (Prozac) and bupropion (Wellbutrin). Tricyclic antidepressants (amitriptyline [Elavil] and imipramine [Tofranil]) are less popular. Monoamine oxidase inhibitors (isocarboxazid [Marplan] and phenelzine [Nardil]) are rarely used.

Antidepressant use in the elderly may result in side effects such as sedation, lethargy, and muscle weakness. Some antidepressants tend to produce anticholinergic effects, including dry mouth, constipation, urinary retention, and confusion. Newly prescribed tricyclic antidepressants can also cause orthostatic hypotension, which can be compounded if the geriatric patient is taking diuretics or other antihypertensive medications. Side effects such as sedation and confusion may also impair the patient's cognitive abilities and possibly endanger the elderly patient who lives alone.

Elderly patients with a history of bipolar disorder may be treated with lithium carbonate. This drug stabilizes the mood swings associated with bipolar disorder. Because lithium cannot be degraded by the body into an inactive form, the kidneys are the sole routes of elimination for this drug. If renal function is impaired, the drug may quickly accumulate to toxic levels, causing lithium toxicity. Symptoms include a metallic taste in the mouth, hand tremors, nausea, muscle weakness, and fatigue. As the levels of toxicity increase, blurred vision, lack of coordination, coma, and even death may occur.

Antipsychotic medications produce a number of minor side effects such as sedation and anticholinergic effects. Extrapyramidal side effects can also occur, including restlessness and involuntary muscle movements, particularly in the face, jaw, and extremities. Examples of these medications include chlorpromazine (Thorazine), thioridazine (Mellaril), chlorprothixene (Taractan), thiothixene (Navane), and haloperidol (Haldol).

Sedative-hypnotic drugs are prescribed to relax the patient, allay anxiety, and promote sleep. Antianxiety medications, chemically similar to the sedative-hypnotics, are intended to decrease anxiety without producing sedation. These drugs are helpful in geriatric patients who suffer from insomnia and feelings of fear or apprehension.

Benzodiazepines are the most commonly prescribed sedative-hypnotic and anxiolytic drugs. These medications can produce drowsiness, sluggishness, and addiction if used over a long period of time. Examples of benzodiazepines include flurazepam (Dalmane), temazepam (Restoril), and triazolam (Halcion). Specific antianxiety agents include diazepam (Valium), lorazepam (Ativan), and chlordiazepoxide (Librium).

Field treatment for overdoses of these medications are aimed primarily at the ABCs, with special emphasis on airway management.

Medications for Parkinson's Disease

Parkinson's disease is a common disorder of the elderly and is caused by a breakdown of dopamine-secreting neurons located in the basal ganglia. This leads to an imbalance in other neurotransmitters, which eventually results in the parkinsonian motor symptoms of rigidity, bradykinesia, resting tremor, and postural instability. Drug treatment is aimed at restoring the balance of neurotransmitters in the basal ganglia. The most commonly prescribed medications include carbidopa/levadopa (Sinemet), bromocriptine (Parlodel), benztropine mesylate (Cogentin), and amantadine (Symmetrel).

Toxicity of these drugs commonly presents as dyskinesia (the inability to execute voluntary movements) and psychological disturbances such as visual hallucinations and nightmares. When these medications are first taken, orthostatic hypotension may also occur.

Tolcapone (Tasmar) is a Parkinson's drug that is given in combination with Sinemet. It potentiates the effects of Sinemet and can cause liver failure. Toxicity in a patient on Tasmar will present as acute jaundice.

The goal of field management is aimed at decreasing the patient's anxiety and providing a supportive environment. Remember that patients with gross involuntary motor movements are at risk for aspiration and choking. Continued assessment of this patient is necessary.

Antiseizure Medications

Seizure disorders are not uncommon in elderly patients. In most cases, the cause of seizures is related to a previous central nervous system injury such as stroke or trauma, tumor, or degenerative brain disease. The selection of a specific antiseizure medication depends on the type of seizure present in the patient.

The most common side effect of antiseizure medications is sedation. Other side effects include GI distress, headache, dizziness, lack of coordination, and dermatologic reactions (rashes). Recommended treatment involves airway management and supportive therapy.

Analgesics and Anti-Inflammatory Agents

Treatment of pain and inflammation for chronic conditions such as rheumatoid arthritis and osteoarthritis includes narcotics and nonnarcotic analgesics and corticosteroids. The narcotic analgesics used to reduce pain in the elderly include codeine, meperidine (Demerol), morphine, hydrocodone (Vicodin), oxycodone (Percodan, Percocet), and hydromorphone (Dilaudid). Remember that these agents alter pain perception, rather than eliminating the condition. As they wear off, pain reappears, encouraging a patient to increase the frequency of dosage.

Adverse side effects of these drugs include sedation, mood changes, nausea, vomiting, and constipation. Orthostatic hypotension and respiratory depression may also occur. Over long periods of time, patients may develop drug tolerance and physical dependence on narcotic agents.

The nonsteroidal anti-inflammatory drugs (NSAIDs) and acetaminophen (Tylenol) are prescribed for mild to moderate pain. They are also the principal therapeutic agents for osteoarthritis and other inflammatory musculoskeletal considerations. The most common side effect of these agents is gastric irritation. Higher doses can cause renal and hepatic toxicity. Acetaminophen is particularly toxic to the liver when taken in high doses. Confusion and hearing problems (ringing or buzzing in the ears) and gastrointestinal hemorrhaging may occur with aspirin use.

Corticosteroids

Corticosteroids are powerful anti-inflammatory agents used to treat rheumatoid arthritis and other inflammatory conditions. Side effects from these agents include hypertension, peptic ulcer, aggravation of diabetes mellitus, glaucoma, increased risk of infection, and suppression of normally produced corticosteroids. Commonly prescribed corticosteroids include cortisone (Cortone), hydrocortisone (Hydrocortone), and prednisone (Deltasone).

Substance Abuse

Substance abuse is a widespread problem in the United States. It affects nearly all age groups, including the elderly. Many Americans over age 60 are addicted to substances. That number is expected to rise as the baby boomer generation swells to the size of the elderly population.

In general, the factors that contribute to substance abuse among the elderly are different from those of younger people. They include:

- Age-related changes
- Loneliness
- Loss of employment
- Loss of spouse or partner
- Malnutrition
- Moving from a long-loved house to an apartment
- Multiple prescriptions

Like people in other age groups, the elderly may intentionally abuse substances to escape pain or life itself. Other times, particularly in the case of prescription drugs, the abuse is accidental. Substance abuse in the elderly may involve drugs, alcohol, or both drugs and alcohol.

Drug Abuse

As previously mentioned, people age 65 and older have more illnesses, consume more drugs, and are more sensitive to adverse drug reactions than younger adults. The sheer number of medications taken by the elderly makes them vulnerable to drug abuse. Of the 1.5 billion prescriptions written each year in the United States, more than one-third go to the elderly. People age 65 and older fill an average of 13 prescriptions per year. The elderly also use a disproportionate percentage of OTC drugs.

Polypharmacy, coupled with impaired vision and/or memory, increases the likelihood of complications. The elderly might experience drug–drug interactions, drug–disease interactions, and drug–food interactions.

The elderly who become physically and/or psychologically dependent on drugs (or alcohol) are more likely to hide their dependence and less likely to seek help than other age groups. Common signs and symptoms of drug abuse include:

- Decreased vision/hearing
- Drowsiness
- Falling
- Memory changes
- Mood changes
- Orthostatic hypotension
- Poor dexterity
- Restlessness
- Weight loss

In cases of suspected drug abuse, carefully document your findings. Collect medications for identification at the hospital, where the patient can be evaluated and, if necessary, referred for substance abuse treatment.

Alcohol Abuse

In a national survey, nearly 50 percent of the elderly reported abstinence from alcohol. However, the same survey found that 15 percent of the men and 12 percent of the women interviewed regularly drank in excess of the one-drink-a-day limit suggested by the National Institute on Alcohol Abuse and Alcoholism. Those percentages are expected to rise with the aging of the baby boomer generation, which has generally used alcohol more frequently than their predecessors.

The use or abuse of alcohol places the elderly at high risk of toxicity. Physiologic changes, such as organ dysfunction, makes older adults more susceptible to the effects of alcohol. Consumption of even moderate amounts of alcohol can interfere with drug therapy, often leading to dangerous consequences. Severe stress and a history of heavy and/or regular drinking predisposes a person to alcohol dependence or abuse in later life.

Unless a patient is openly intoxicated, discovery of alcohol abuse depends on a thorough history. Signs and symptoms of alcohol abuse in the elderly may be very subtle or confused with other conditions. Remember that even small amounts of alcohol can cause intoxication in an older person. If possible, question family, friends, or caregivers about the patient's drinking patterns. Pertinent findings include:

- Anorexia
- Confusion
- History of falls
- Insomnia
- Mood swings, denial, and hostility (especially when questioned about drinking)
- Nausea
- Visible anxiety

Treatment follows many of the same steps as for any other patient with a pattern of abusive drinking. (See the chapter "Toxicology and Substance Abuse.") *Do not* judge the patient. Evaluate the need for fluid therapy, and keep in mind the possibility of withdrawal. Transport the patient to the hospital for evaluation and referral for treatment. Ideally, these patients will seek support from community organizations such as Alcoholics Anonymous (AA). Many communities have AA groups specifically for senior citizens.

Behavioral/Psychological Disorders

When behavioral or psychological problems develop later in life, they are often dismissed as normal age-related changes. This attitude denies an elderly person the opportunity to correct a treatable condition and/or overlooks an underlying physical disorder. Studies have shown that the elderly retain their basic personalities and their adaptive cognitive abilities. In other words, intellectual decline and/or regressive behavior are not normal age-related changes. Unless an organic brain disorder is involved, alterations in behavior should be considered symptomatic of a possible psychological problem.

It is important to keep in mind the emotionally stressful situations facing many elderly people: isolation, loneliness, loss of self-dependence, loss of strength, fear of the future, and more. The elderly also face a higher incidence of secondary depression as a result of neuroleptic medications such as Haldol and Thorazine. Some of the common classifications of psychological disorders related to age include:

- Affective disorders (depression)
- Dissociative disorders (paranoid schizophrenia)
- Organic brain syndrome
- Personality disorders (dependent personality)

As with other people, the emotional well-being of the elderly affects their overall physical health. Therefore, it is important that you note evidence of altered behavior in any elderly patient you assess and examine. Common signs and symptoms of a psychological disorder include lapses in memory, cognitive difficulty, changes in sleep patterns, fear of death, changes in sexual interest, thoughts of suicide, or withdrawal from society.

In general, management of psychological disorders in the elderly is the same as that for other age groups. Two of the most common emotional disturbances that you may encounter in the elderly are depression and suicide.

Depression

Up to 15 percent of the noninstitutionalized elderly experience depression. Within institutions, that figure rises to about 30 percent. The incidence of depression among the elderly has risen in the early twenty-first century as the baby boomers—with their larger population numbers and more prevalent depression at an earlier age—enter their 60s and 70s.

Some of the general signs and symptoms noted previously may indicate depression. Ask the patient about feelings of sadness or despair. Determine whether he has suffered episodes of crying. Inquire about past psychological treatment and current stressful events, particularly the death of a loved one. Keep in mind that sensory changes, especially deafness and blindness, may make the patient vulnerable to depression. Serious acute diseases can have the same effect. If the patient recognizes the depression, ask about the duration and any prior bouts. Find out whether the patient has been given any medications to treat the depression. If so, check compliance.

Some depressed patients may exhibit **hypochondriasis** (hypochondria). If this condition is a side effect of the depression, the patient will still show some degree of emotional pain and/or **dysphoria**. Although you may not be able to identify hypochondria in the field, remember that the condition is an illness and requires treatment by trained medical personnel.

In general, depressed patients should receive supportive care. Encourage them to talk, delicately raising questions about suicidal thoughts. The seriously depressed patient should be transported to the hospital. Treatment of depression usually entails psychotherapy and/or antidepressants.

Suicide

The highest suicide rates in the United States are among people over age 65, especially men. The elderly account for 20 percent of all suicides, but represent only 12 percent of the total population. Someone over age 65 commits suicide about every 90 minutes. Suicide is the third-leading cause of death among the elderly, following falls and car accidents.

Depression is the leading cause of suicide among the elderly. As a group, the elderly are less likely to seek help than the young. They are also less likely to express their anger or sorrow, turning their feelings inward instead. Other stressors that put the elderly at risk of suicide include:

- Bereavement
- Chronic illness
- Family history of suicide
- Family issues
- Financial problems
- Isolation and loneliness
- Living in a youth-oriented society
- Low serotonin levels (serotonin declines with age)
- Physical impairment
- Substance abuse
- Unrelieved pain

Suicidal behavior is related to stress. As a paramedic, you should try to evaluate the stress from an elderly patient's point of view, keeping the preceding factors in mind. In cases of a seriously depressed patient, elicit behavior patterns from family, friends, or caregivers. Warning signs may include:

- Loss of interest in activities that were once enjoyable
- Curtailing social interaction, grooming, and self-care
- Breaking from medical or exercise regimens
- Grieving a personal loss ("I don't want to live without him/her")
- Feeling useless ("nobody would miss me")
- Putting affairs in order, giving away things, finalizing a will
- Stockpiling medications or other lethal means of self-destruction, including firearms

Be particularly alert to suicide among the acutely ill. With more patients being returned home to care for themselves, there is a higher incidence of suicide among the terminally ill, especially cancer victims. A lack of postacute hospital care can be interpreted as a lack of caring in general.

Prevention of suicide among the elderly involves intervention by all levels of society, from family to EMS to hospital workers. It is important to dispel the common myths about aging and age-related diseases. Recognition of warning signs and involvement of appropriate individuals and agencies is critical.

Your first priorities in the management of a suicidal elderly patient are to protect yourself and then to protect the patient from self-harm. To do this, you must gain access to the patient. This may require breaking into a house or room, particularly if the patient is unconscious or can be readily seen. Remember to summon law enforcement personnel as necessary. *Do not* rule out firearm use among the elderly.

If you reach the patient, emergency care has the highest priority secondary to crew safety. Conduct a brief interview with the patient, if possible, to determine the need for further action. *Do not* leave the suicidal patient alone. Administer medications with caution, keeping in mind polypharmacy and drug interactions in the elderly. (Consult with medical direction.) *All* suicidal elderly patients should be transported to the hospital.

Trauma in the Elderly Patient

Older patients who sustain moderate to severe injuries are more likely to die than their younger counterparts. Postinjury disability is also more common in the elderly than in the young.

Contributing Factors

A number of factors contribute to the high incidence and severity of trauma among the elderly. Slower reflexes, arthritis, and diminished eyesight and hearing predispose the elderly to accidents, especially falls. The elderly, because of their physical state and vulnerability, are also at high risk from trauma caused by criminal assault. Purse snatching, armed robbery, and assault occur all too frequently in the elderly population, especially among those living in urban areas. Fall and trauma prevention programs can be effective in reducing elderly trauma—especially falls.[11]

Age-related factors that place the elderly at risk of severe injury and complications include:

- ***Osteoporosis and muscle weakness***—increased likelihood of fractures
- ***Reduced cardiac reserve***—decreased ability to compensate for blood loss
- ***Decreased respiratory function***—increased likelihood of **acute respiratory distress syndrome (ARDS)**
- ***Impaired renal function***—decreased ability to adapt to fluid shifts
- ***Decreased elasticity in the peripheral blood vessels***—greater susceptibility to tearing
- ***Use of anticoagulant medications***—renders patient more susceptible to hemorrhage.

General Assessment

As with any other trauma patient, determine the mechanism of injury. Leading causes of trauma in the elderly include falls, motor vehicle crashes, burns, assault or abuse, and underlying medical problems such as syncope.

In assessing elderly trauma patients, remember that blood pressure readings may be deceptive. Older patients typically have higher blood pressures than younger patients. Although a blood pressure of 110/70 mmHg may be normal for a 30-year-old, it could represent a low blood pressure, and possibly shock, for an older patient. Elderly trauma patients also may not exhibit an elevated pulse, a common early sign of hypoperfusion. This may be because of a chronic heart disease or the use of medications to treat hypertension or a myocardial infarction. Fractures may also be obscured or concealed because of a diminished sense of pain among the elderly. One of the best indicators of shock in the elderly is an altered mental status or changes in consciousness during assessment. Elderly trauma patients who exhibit confusion or agitation are candidates for rapid transport.

Observing for Abuse/Neglect

Make sure you observe the scene for signs of abuse and neglect. Abuse of the elderly is as big a problem in our society as child abuse and neglect. **Geriatric abuse** is defined as a syndrome in which an elderly person has received serious physical or psychological injury from family members or other caregivers. Abuse of the elderly knows no socioeconomic bounds. It often occurs when an older person is no longer able to be totally independent, and the family members have difficulty upholding their commitment to care for the patient. It can also occur in nursing homes and other health care facilities. The profile for the potential geriatric abuser may often show a great deal of life stress. In many cases, there is sleep deprivation, marital discord, financial problems, and work-related problems. As the abuser's life falls into further disarray, and as the patient further deteriorates, abuse may be the outcome.

Signs and symptoms of geriatric abuse and neglect are often obvious. Unexplained trauma is usually the primary presentation. The average abused patient is older than 80 and has multiple medical problems, such as cancer, congestive heart failure, heart disease, and incontinence. Senile dementia is often present. In these cases, it can be hard to determine whether the dementia is chronic or acute, especially if there is an increased likelihood of head trauma from abuse.[12]

Whenever you suspect geriatric abuse, obtain a complete patient and family history. Pay particular attention to inconsistencies. *Do not* confront the family. Instead, report your suspicions to the emergency department and the appropriate governmental authority. Many states have very strong laws protecting the elderly from abuse or neglect. In fact, many states consider it a criminal offense *not* to report suspected geriatric abuse. These states also offer legal immunity to those who report geriatric abuse, as long as the report is made in good faith.

General Management

The priorities of care for the elderly trauma patient are similar to those for any trauma patient. However, you must keep in mind age-related systemic changes and the presence of chronic diseases. This is especially true of the cardiovascular, respiratory, and renal systems.

Cardiovascular Considerations

Recent or past myocardial infarctions may contribute to the risk of arrhythmia or congestive heart failure in the trauma patient. In addition, there may be a decreased response of the heart, in adjusting heart rate and stroke volume, to hypovolemia. An elderly trauma patient may require higher than usual arterial pressures for perfusion of vital organs, owing to increased peripheral vascular resistance and hypertension. Care must be taken in intravenous fluid administration because of decreased myocardial reserves. Hypotension, hypovolemia, and hypervolemia are poorly tolerated in the elderly patient.

Respiratory Considerations

In managing the airway and ventilation in an elderly trauma patient, you must consider the physical changes that may affect treatment. Check for dentures and determine whether they should be removed. Keep in mind that age-related changes can decrease chest wall movement and vital capacity. Age also reduces the tolerance of all organs for anoxia. Remember, too, that chronic obstructive pulmonary disease is widespread among the elderly.

Make necessary adjustments in treatment to provide adequate oxygenation and appropriate CO_2 removal. Monitor with oximetry and capnography.

Renal Considerations

The decreased ability of the kidneys to maintain a normal acid–base balance and to compensate for fluid changes can further complicate the management of the elderly trauma patient. Any preexisting renal disease can decrease the kidney's ability to compensate. The decrease in renal function, along with a decreased cardiac reserve, places the elderly injured patient at risk for fluid overload and pulmonary edema. Remember, too, that renal changes allow toxins and medications to accumulate more readily in the elderly.

Transport Considerations

You may have to modify the positioning, stabilization, and packaging of the elderly trauma patient before transport. Be attentive to physical deformities such as arthritis, spinal abnormalities, or frozen limbs that may cause pain or require special care (Figure 5-25). Recall the frailty of an elderly person's skin and avoid creating skin tears or pressure sores. Keep in mind that trauma places an elderly person at increased risk of hypothermia. Ensure that the patient is kept warm at all times.

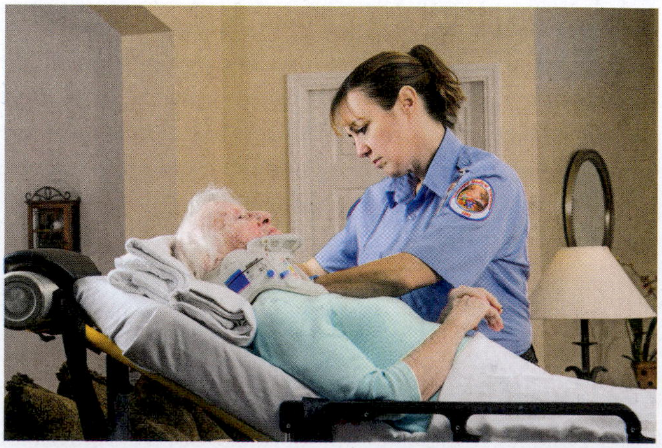

FIGURE 5-25 Use padding to ensure that the elderly patient is comfortable.

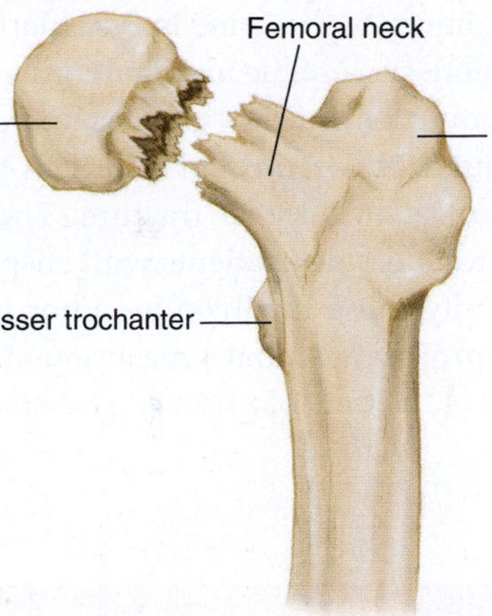

FIGURE 5-26 Subcapital femoral neck fracture. Patients with a displaced femoral neck fracture present with groin pain and a shortened externally rotated leg.

Specific Injuries

The elderly can be subject to a variety of injuries, just like any other age group. The three most common categories of injuries among the elderly are orthopedic injuries, burns, and injuries of the head and spine.

Orthopedic Injuries

As previously mentioned, the elderly suffer the greatest mortality and greatest incidence of disability from falls. Some falls in the elderly result in at least one fractured bone (Figure 5-26). The most common fall-related fracture is a fracture of the hip or pelvis. Osteoporosis and general frailty contribute to this. The older patient who has fallen should be assumed to have a hip fracture until proven otherwise. Signs and symptoms of a hip fracture include tenderness over the affected joint and shortening and external rotation of the leg. The patient is unable to bear weight on the affected leg. Patients who live alone may not be able to get to a phone to summon help. Because of this, they may remain on the floor for a prolonged period of time. This can lead to hypothermia, hyperthermia, and/or dehydration.

Falls also result in a variety of other stress fractures in the elderly, including fractures of the proximal humerus, distal radius, proximal tibia, and thoracic and lumbar bodies. Falls may also lead to soft-tissue injuries and hot-water burns if the incident occurred in a tub or hot shower.

CONTENT REVIEW

➤ Common Fractures among the Elderly
- Hip or pelvis fractures
- Proximal humerus
- Distal radius
- Proximal tibia
- Thoracic and lumbar bodies

In treating orthopedic injuries, remember to ask questions aimed at detecting an underlying medical condition. Ask whether the patient recalls "blacking out." Remain alert for evidence of potential cardiac emergencies. Package and transport the patient according to the general guidelines mentioned earlier.

Burns

People aged 60 and older are more likely to suffer death from burns than any other age group except neonates and infants. Several factors help explain the high mortality rate among elderly burn victims:

- Reaction time slows as people age, so the elderly often stay in contact with thermal sources longer than their younger counterparts.
- Preexisting diseases place the elderly being treated for burns at risk of medical complications, particularly pulmonary and cardiac problems.
- Age-related skin changes (thinning) result in deeper burns and slower healing time.
- Immunologic and metabolic changes increase the risk of infection.
- Reductions in physiologic function and the reduced reserve of several organ systems make the elderly more vulnerable to major systemic stress.

Management of elderly burn patients follows the same general procedures as other patients. However, remember that the elderly are at increased risk of shock. Administration of fluids is important to prevent renal tubular damage. Assess hydration in the initial hours after a burn injury by blood pressure, pulse, and urine output (at least 1 to 2 mL/kg per hour).

In the case of the elderly, complications from a burn may manifest themselves in the days and weeks following the incident. For serious burns to heal, the body may use up to 20,000 calories a day. Elderly patients, with altered metabolism and complications such as diabetes, may not be able to meet this demand, increasing the chances for infection and systemic failure. Part of your job may be to prepare the family for such a delayed response and to provide necessary psychological support.

Head and Spinal Injuries

As a group, the elderly experience more head injuries, even from relatively minor trauma, than their younger counterparts. Elderly patients with a seemingly less severe head injury often have increased mortality and decreased functional outcomes compared with non-elderly patients. A major factor is the difference in proportion between the brain and the skull. As mentioned earlier, the brain decreases in size and weight with age. The skull, however, remains constant in size, allowing the brain more room to move, thus increasing the likelihood of brain injury. Because of this, signs of brain injury may develop more slowly in the elderly, sometimes over days and weeks. In fact, the patient may often have forgotten the offending injury.

The cervical spine is also more susceptible to injury due to osteoporosis and spondylosis. **Spondylosis** is a degeneration of the vertebral body. The elderly often have a significant degree of this disease. In addition, arthritic changes can gradually compress the nerve rootlets or spinal cord. Thus, injury to the spine in the elderly makes the patient much more susceptible to spinal cord injury. In fact, sudden neck movement, even without fracture, may cause spinal cord injury. This can occur with less than normal pain, owing to the absence of fracture. Therefore, it is important to provide older patients with suspected spinal injuries, especially those involved in motor vehicle collisions, with appropriate spinal precautions (based upon local protocols) at the time of primary assessment.

Summary

Providing EMS in the twenty-first century means treating a growing elderly population. The "graying of America" has resulted in a greater number of people aged 65 and older, many of whom are in home settings. When treating elderly patients, keep in mind the anatomic, physiologic, and emotional changes that occur with age. However, never jump to conclusions based solely on age. Weigh normal age-related changes against abnormal changes—that is, those resulting from a medical condition or trauma. Recall that elderly patients are much more susceptible to medication side effects and toxicity than younger patients. They also are more susceptible to trauma and environmental stressors. Abuse of the elderly occurs; you should bear this in mind whenever injuries do not match the history. Any suspected abuse or neglect of an elderly patient should be reported to the emergency department and/or the appropriate governmental authorities.

Just as in pediatric calls, the call for an elderly patient can present with a variety of scenarios that are unique to the population or related to the normal physiology. Maintaining a current knowledge and understanding of these two unique populations will help you make quicker, more accurate assessments and treatment plans.

You Make the Call

Just after 3 A.M., a call comes in to the station to assist an elderly man who has fallen. His wife requests lifting assistance because she has a disability. She reports: "I have arthritis and cannot possibly help him back into bed."

You arrive at a small, one-family home just off a major thoroughfare. A small, severely arthritic woman in a wheelchair greets you: "He's inside. The nerve of him. He won't even answer me—just makes fun of me by repeating everything I say and slurring his words. I'll bet he's been drinking and didn't want me to know. As if I couldn't tell by his behavior! We've been married for 47 years, and he still takes care of me. But not tonight!"

The home is clean and well cared for—not a speck of dust or a single cobweb to be seen. The woman's husband is lying on his side on the carpeted floor next to the bed. He is awake, drooling, and repeating words in a thick speech.

During the primary assessment, the patient is at V on the AVPU scale. Pupils are deviated left. You ensure that all spinal precautions are taken. Then you check hand grasp; the left is strong, the right absent. The airway is open, but needs suctioning of saliva. Respirations are present and unlabored. You note strong, but irregular, distal pulses.

You apply oxygen to correct mild hypoxia and determine that the patient, Mr. Jones, is a high priority due to the field diagnosis of a stroke. His airway will need close management and definitive treatment.

1. What general impression do you have of this patient?
2. Do you suspect that this is an acute or chronic problem? Explain.
3. During the primary assessment, the patient is at V on the AVPU scale. Pupils are deviated left. You ensure that all spinal precautions are taken. Then you check hand grasp; the left is strong, the right absent. The airway is open, but needs suctioning of saliva. Respirations are present and unlabored. You note strong, but irregular, distal pulses.
4. You apply oxygen to correct mild hypoxia and determine that the patient, Mr. Jones, is a high priority due to the field diagnosis of a stroke. His airway will need close management and definitive treatment.
5. Aside from the patient's presentation and response to your interventions, what other information should be included in your hospital report?
6. What support do you provide for Mrs. Jones?

See Suggested Responses at the back of this book.

Review Questions

1. What term is used to describe discrimination against aged or elderly people by an individual?
   a. Ageism
   b. Polypharmacy
   c. Congregate
   d. Comorbidity
2. Where is the most common fall injury in elderly patients?
   a. Hip or pelvis
   b. Radius or ulna
   c. Femur or tibia
   d. Wrist or hand
3. Multiple drug therapy in which there is a concurrent use of a number of drugs is termed ______________
   a. multipharmacy.
   b. polypharmacy.
   c. hyperpharmacy.
   d. comorbidity.
4. What trauma mechanism is the leading cause of accidental death among the elderly?
   a. Burn
   b. Fall-related
   c. Abuse-related
   d. Vehicle collision
5. By-products of malnutrition may include all of the following *except* ______________
   a. vitamin deficiencies
   b. dehydration
   c. hypoglycemia
   d. hyperthermia
6. A pathophysiologic change may cause a reduction in brain size, leaving room for increased bleeding following a blow to the head, making the elderly more prone to what type of brain injury that is typically underdiagnosed?
   a. Hypoxic brain injury
   b. Brain infection
   c. Epidural hematoma
   d. Subdural hematoma
7. You are on scene with an elderly patient who is complaining of dyspnea. The patient has had this problem for the past 4 days, and states that he has "chills" and a low-grade fever. He uses a home nebulizer for his COPD, but he says this is not helping any. Breath sounds are slightly diminished, with absent breath sounds in the lower right lobe, which also displays increased tactile fremitus. What would be your field impression at this time?
   a. Exacerbation of COPD
   b. Pneumothorax
   c. Pneumonia
   d. Congestive heart failure
8. Which pathophysiology underlies the leading cause of death in the elderly population?
   a. Renal diseases
   b. Respiratory diseases
   c. Cardiovascular diseases
   d. Neurologic diseases

9. Which of the following is a common manifestation related to myocardial infarction in a patient who is over 85 years of age?
   a. Anoxia
   b. Dyspnea
   c. Vomiting
   d. Diaphoresis

10. Toxicity in a patient on tolcapone (Tasmar) will present as acute ________
    a. hypoxia.
    b. jaundice.
    c. anxiety.
    d. anemia.

See Answers to Review Questions at the end of this book.

References

1. Administration on Aging, Department of Health and Human Services. *Aging into the 21st Century*. (Available at http://www.aoa.gov/AoARoot/Aging_Statistics/future_growth/aging21/program.aspx.)
2. Grudzen, C. R., J. R. Hoffman, W. J. Koenig, et al. "The LA Story: What Happened after a New Policy Allowing Paramedics to Forgo Resuscitation Attempts in Prehospital Cardiac Arrest." *Resuscitation* 81 (2010): 685–690.
3. Byrd, L. "More Drugs Equal More Problems: Polypharmacy in Elders—More Problems than Benefits?" *Geriatr Nurs* 31 (2010): 389–390.
4. Xu, W., S. Parera, D. Medich, et al. "Height Loss, Vertebral Fractures, and the Misclassification of Osteoporosis." *Bone* 48 (2011): 301–311.
5. Testa, G., F. Cacciatore, D. Della-Morte, et al. "Role of Permanent Atrial Fibrillation (AF) on Long-Term Mortality in Community-Dwelling Elderly People with and without Chronic Heart Failure (CHF)." *Arch Gerontol Geriatr* 54 (2011): 121–126.
6. Kessler, C., J. M. Tristano, and R. DeLorenzo. "The Emergency Department Approach to Syncope: Evidence-Based Guidelines and Prediction Rules." *Emerg Med Clin N Am* 28 (2010): 487–500.
7. Querfurth, H. W. and F. M. LaFeria. "Alzheimer's Disease." *N Engl J Med* 362 (2010): 329–344.
8. Lees, A. "The Bare Essentials: Parkinson's Disease." *Pract Neurol* 10 (2010): 240–246.
9. Naccarato, M. K. and T. Kelechi. "Pressure Ulcer Prevention in the Emergency Department." *Adv Emerg Nurs J* 33 (2011): 155–162.
10. Carnell, J., J. Fahimi, and C. P. Wills. "Cervical Spine Fracture in Ankylosing Spondylitis." *West J Emerg Med* 10 (2009): 267.
11. Weiss, S. J., R. Chong, M. Ong, A. A. Ernst, and M. Balash. "Emergency Medical Services Screening of Elderly Falls in the Home." *Prehosp Emerg Care* 7 (2003): 79–84.
12. Rinker, A. G., Jr. "Recognition and Perception of Elder Abuse by Prehospital and Hospital-Based Care Providers." *Arch Gerontol Geriatr* 48 (2009): 110–115.

Further Reading

Abrams, W. B., et al., eds. *The Merck Manual of Geriatrics*. 3rd ed. Whitehouse Station, NJ: Merck Research Laboratories, 2000.

American Geriatrics Society, National Council of State EMS Coordinators. *Geriatric Education for Emergency Medical Services*. 2nd ed. Burlington, MA: Jones and Bartlett Learning, 2016.

Bledsoe, B. and D. Clayden. *Prehospital Emergency Pharmacology*. 7th ed. Upper Saddle River, NJ: Pearson/Prentice Hall, 2012.

"Drug Therapy in the Elderly," in Beers, M. H., et al., eds. *The Merck Manual of Diagnosis and Therapy*. 19th ed. Whitehouse Station, NJ: Merck Research Laboratories, 2011.

"Geriatric Trauma" and "Abuse in the Elderly and Impaired," in Tintinalli, J. E., et al., eds. *Emergency Medicine: A Comprehensive Study Guide*. 7th ed. New York: McGraw-Hill, 2013.

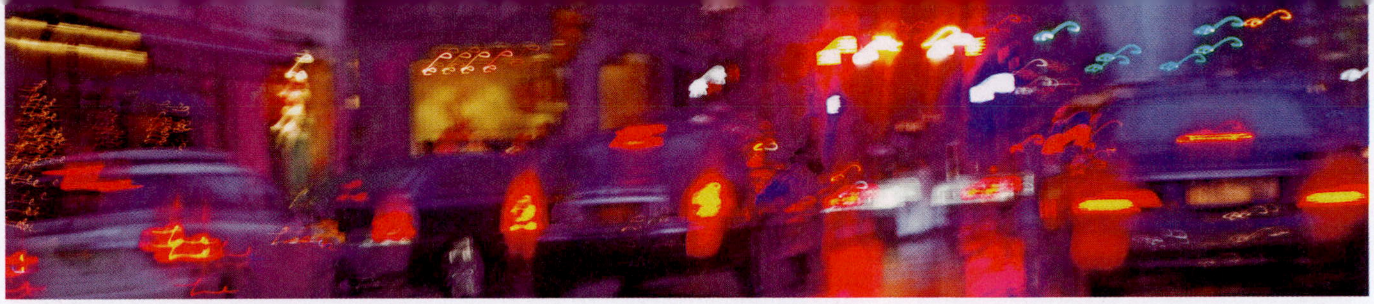

Chapter 6

Abuse, Neglect, and Assault

Bryan Bledsoe, DO, FACEP, FAAEM, EMT-P

STANDARD

Special Patient Populations (Patients with Special Needs)

COMPETENCY

Integrates assessment findings with principles of epidemiology and pathophysiology and knowledge of psychosocial needs to formulate a field impression and implement a comprehensive treatment/disposition plan for patients with special needs.

Learning Objectives

Terminal Performance Objective: After reading this chapter, you should be able to integrate patient assessment findings, patient history, and knowledge of therapeutic communication and medical/legal considerations to recognize and manage patients suffering from abuse, neglect, and assault.

Enabling Objectives: To accomplish the terminal performance objective, you should be able to:

1. Define key terms introduced in this chapter.
2. Describe the epidemiology and demographics of abuse, assault, neglect, and hate crimes.
3. Describe the characteristics of abusers and abused and neglected patients, including partner abuse, elder abuse, child abuse, and hate crimes.
4. Identify patterns of injuries and behavior suspicious for abuse, neglect, assault, and hate crimes.
5. Recognize the effects of date rape drugs.
6. Discuss how to report and document relevant observations and information regarding suspected abuse, assault, neglect, and hate crimes.
7. Identify the paramedic's role in the suspicion, identification, and assessment of patients involved in some form of human trafficking.
8. Given various scenarios, discuss how the paramedic should integrate assessment and management for emergencies related to abuse, neglect, assault, and hate crimes.

KEY TERMS

bias-motivated crime, p. 211
chain of evidence, p. 210
child abuse, p. 204
domestic elder abuse, p. 203
hate crime, p. 211
human trafficking, p. 209
institutional elder abuse, p. 203
partner abuse, p. 201
rape, p. 207
sexual assault, p. 207

Case Study

You are awakened during the middle of the night to respond to an unknown emergency. You arrive to find a police officer on the scene with a 36-year-old woman who was found at the side of the road, partially clothed. She is crying and nearly incoherent. You learn from scattered comments and from remarks by the police officer that a male assailant abducted the patient at gunpoint and sexually assaulted her. He then threw the patient from a moving vehicle and fled the scene. A passing motorist spotted the woman curled up along the roadside and used a cell phone to summon police.

Because you have a female partner, you decide that she might be a more appropriate choice than you to maintain contact with this patient. As you return to the ambulance to retrieve equipment, your partner begins the primary assessment. She looks for immediate life threats, while exhibiting a compassionate and consoling attitude just as any EMS professional should do. During the secondary assessment, she uses a blanket to protect the patient's privacy. All clothing removed during the assessment is placed in a paper bag and given to the police officer as evidence.

Because of the mechanism of injury, you and your partner decide to apply spinal immobilization. You find extensive abrasions when you logroll the patient, but do not detect any life-threatening injuries. Because your partner has noted blood around the patient's perineum, she places a dressing over the patient's genitals.

Vital signs are good, so you begin transport to a hospital designated as a rape crisis center. En route, you notify the receiving hospital so the staff can prepare for your arrival. The staff readies a private room for the patient and summons a social worker, a nurse with specialized training as a sexual assault nurse examiner (SANE), and a detective.

After you transfer the patient, you complete your patient report, giving special attention to the narrative. Both you and your partner realize that you might be called to testify in court sometime in the future.

Introduction

Because of underreporting, it is difficult to provide accurate statistics on the incidence of abuse and assault in the United States today. That makes available figures even more overwhelming in their seriousness. To grasp the magnitude of the problem, consider these facts:

- Nearly three million children suffer abuse each year and almost five children a day die as a result of child abuse.[1]
- Between 2 and 4 million women each year are battered by their partners or spouses.
- Elder abuse occurs at an incidence of 700,000 to 1.1 million elderly people annually.[2]

Abuse and assaults transcend gender, race, age, and socioeconomic status. The effects are serious and long-lasting. Victims may die as a result of their injuries or have long-term health care problems. No victim ever forgets his or her pain. Even after the physical wounds have healed, the emotional injuries never fade completely.

Unfortunately, the pattern of abuse and assault forms a cycle that is difficult to break. Parents who harm each other are more likely to abuse their children. Children who suffer abuse have a greater likelihood of becoming abusers themselves. At some point in their lives, they may abuse their dates, their partners, their children, their elders, or others.

The EMS system is involved with many cases of abuse. Although law enforcement is not always present, you have a responsibility to identify victims of abuse and initiate some kind of action. In many areas, laws require health care personnel to report actual or suspected incidences of abuse. Early detection is critical to breaking the cycle of abuse through social services support and alterations in behavior.

Partner Abuse

The potential for **partner abuse** has existed for as long as couples have interacted. It results when a man or woman subjects a domestic partner to some form of physical or psychological violence. The victim may be a husband or wife, someone who shares a residence, or simply a boyfriend or girlfriend.

The most widespread and best known form of abuse involves the abuse of women by men. However, battery is not limited to women. Men can be—and are—abused by women. They suffer the same feelings of guilt, humiliation, and loss of control. A battered man feels trapped, just like a battered woman, but is often even less likely to report the abuse, out of either a sense of shame, a lack of resources for support, or both.

Battery also affects same-sex couples. Abusive relationships between men or between women follow the same patterns and the same conditioning as those seen in heterosexual relationships. What can be said of women battered by men can generally be said of most battery situations, regardless of the gender of the victim or the abuser.

Reasons for Not Reporting Abuse

Victims of partner abuse hesitate or fail to report the problem for a number of reasons. Fear is one of the biggest obstacles to taking action. Most battered partners fear reprisals, either to themselves or to their children. They also fear being humiliated for their powerlessness or inability to stop the violence, especially if the battered partner is a male.

Reporting abuse is usually the last resort. Many partners hope that the abusive behavior will simply just end. This hope is fueled when the abuser promises to change—a common reaction after a violent episode. The abused partner may also be in denial, claiming that the situation is less serious than it is or rationalizing that the violence was somehow justified. Some abused women, for example, believe that they are the cause of the abusive behavior or that the abuse is part of the marriage and should be endured to preserve the family.

Finally, many victims of abuse lack the knowledge or financial means to seek help. They may not know where to turn or whom to trust. They may also lack the money to seek counseling, intervention, or a safe place to live. A partner who lacks job training and/or who must support dependent children may find the prospect of starting life anew more frightening than the abuse. Unfortunately, an abusive situation rarely ceases without some kind of separation or intervention. Escalation of violence is common, with injuries becoming more severe. Over time, abuse becomes more frequent, often occurring without provocation, and more inclusive. If children were not initially involved, they may become victims as the episodes escalate. All too often, victims of abuse are eventually killed by their abuser.

CONTENT REVIEW

- Reasons for Not Reporting Abuse
  - Fear of reprisal
  - Fear of humiliation
  - Denial
  - Lack of knowledge
  - Lack of financial resources

Identification of Partner Abuse

Partner abuse can fall into several categories. The most obvious form is physical abuse, which involves the application of force in ways too numerous to list here. In addition to direct personal injury, physical abuse may exacerbate existing medical conditions, such as hypertension, diabetes, or asthma. These conditions can also be affected by verbal abuse, which consists of words chosen to control or harm a person. Verbal abuse may leave no physical mark, but it damages a person's self-esteem and can lead to depression, substance abuse, or other self-destructive behavior.

Sexual abuse, which is a form of physical abuse, can also occur between partners. It involves forced sexual contact and includes marital or date rape. (For more on sexual abuse and assault, see material later in this chapter.)

In identifying an abusive family situation, keep in mind the 10 generic risk factors identified in *Domestic Violence: Cracking the Code of Silence*, a source often cited.[3] These 10 factors, based on research on battered women, are as follows:

1. Male is unemployed.
2. Male uses illegal drugs at least once a year.
3. Partners have different religious backgrounds.
4. Family income is below the poverty level.
5. Partners are unmarried.
6. Either partner is violent toward children at home.
7. Male did not graduate from high school.
8. Male is unemployed or has a blue-collar job.
9. Male is between 18 and 30 years old.
10. Male saw his father hit his mother.

Characteristics of Partner Abusers

As already indicated, partner abuse occurs in all demographic groups. However, abuse is more common in lower socioeconomic levels in which wage earners have trouble paying bills, holding down jobs, or keeping pace with technological changes that make their job skills outdated or obsolete.

A history of family violence makes a person more likely to repeat the pattern as an adult. Typically, the abuser does not like being out of control but at the same time feels powerless to change. The situation is made worse if both parties do not know how to back down from a conflict. Lacking any alternative, one or both of the partners may

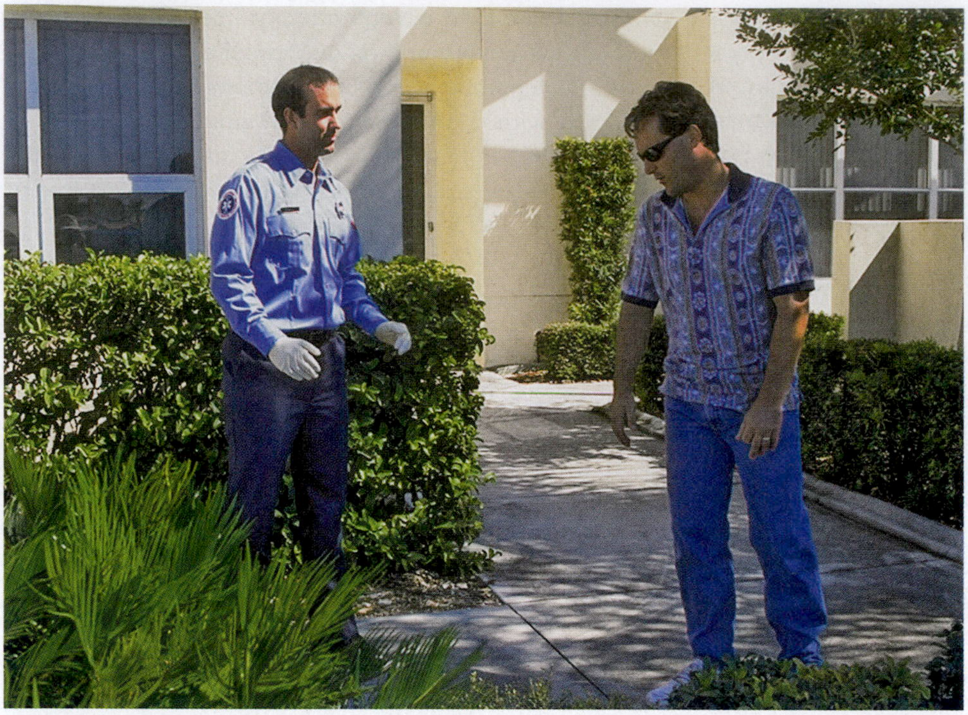

FIGURE 6-1 When called to the scene of domestic violence, you may encounter hostility from the person responsible for the abuse. Remain calm when you speak to the person and do not enter his personal space. Remain alert to changes in emotional status, and be prepared to summon law enforcement officials as necessary.

turn to physical and/or verbal violence (Figure 6-1). In some cases, abusers will think they are demonstrating discipline rather than violent behavior.

Abusers usually exhibit overly aggressive personalities—an outgrowth of low self-esteem. They often feel insecure and jealous, flying into sudden and unpredictable rages. Use of alcohol or drugs increases the likelihood that the abuser will lose control and may not even clearly remember his or her actions.

In the aftermath of an abusive incident, the abuser often feels a sense of remorse and shame. The person may seek to relieve his or her guilt by promising to change or even seeking help. For a time, the abuser may appear charming or loving, convincing an abused partner to think that perhaps the pattern has finally been broken. All too often, however, the cycle of violence repeats itself in just a few days, weeks, or months.[4]

Characteristics of Abused Partners

It may be difficult to identify an abused partner. As mentioned, the primary risk factor for abuse is a history of violence between parents, a factor that will not be immediately known to you or other EMS providers. However, studies have revealed that abused partners share certain common characteristics. They include:

- ***Pregnancy:*** Many women suffer some form of battery during pregnancy.
- ***Substance abuse:*** Abused partners often seek the numbing effect of alcohol and/or drugs.
- ***Emotional disorders:*** Abused partners frequently exhibit depression, evasiveness, anxiety, or suicidal behavior.

As mentioned earlier, the victim may seek to protect the attacker, either by delaying care and/or by providing alternative explanations for injuries. Remain alert to subtle signs that the patient is being less than honest. Many victims, for example, avoid eye contact, exhibit nervous behavior, and/or watch the abuser, if present (Figure 6-2). The victim may also provide verbal clues, saying such things as "We've been having some problems lately" or "I always seem to be causing some kind of trouble."

Approaching the Abused Patient

In assessing the abused patient, direct questioning usually works best. Convey an awareness that the person's partner may have caused the harm or created conditions that led to the injury and/or the emotional trauma. Once the subject of abuse has been introduced, exhibit a willingness to discuss it. Remember to avoid both judgmental questions

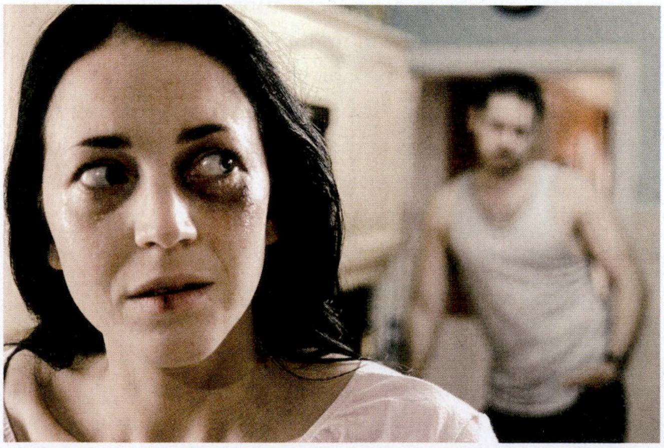

FIGURE 6-2 A domestic abuse situation is among the most dangerous of situations an EMS crew can encounter. The abuser is often aggressive, but it is not uncommon to have the abused person become aggressive as well. Alcohol and drugs of abuse are often confounding factors in these situations.

(Ian Thraves/Alamy Images)

such as "Why don't you leave?" or judgmental statements such as "How awful!"

Throughout the assessment, listen carefully to the patient. Indicate your attention by saying, "I hear what you are telling me." Often victims of abuse feel a sense of relief when someone else knows about the situation. This can be the first step toward seeking help.

Keep in mind that in cases of partner abuse, the abuser may be reported and taken into custody by the police. However, the person may soon be released on his own recognizance, sometimes within a matter of hours. The patient may already know this and be reluctant to take any action. If the patient does not know this, it is your duty to inform the patient of this possibility and to provide information about available protection programs.

Elder Abuse

As noted in the chapter "Geratrics," elder abuse is a widespread medical and social problem caused by many factors, including:

- Increased life expectancies
- Increased dependency on others, as a result of longevity
- Decreased productivity in later years
- Physical and mental impairments, especially among the old-old
- Limited resources for long-term care of the elderly
- Economic factors, such as strained family finances
- Stress on middle-aged caretakers responsible for two generations—children and parents

The problem of elder abuse is expected to grow along with the size of the elderly population, which will increase dramatically within the next 20 to 30 years as baby boomers turn 65 and older. It is your responsibility to be aware of this situation and to remain alert to signs of elder abuse (Figure 6-3).

Identification of Elder Abuse

The two basic types of elder abuse are domestic and institutional. **Domestic elder abuse** takes place when an elder is being cared for in a home-based setting, usually by relatives. **Institutional elder abuse** occurs when an elder is being cared for by a person with a legal or contractual responsibility to provide care, such as paid caregivers, nursing home staff, or other professionals. Both types of abuse can be either acts of commission (acts of physical, sexual, or emotional violence) or acts of omission (neglect).[5]

In some cases, signs of elder abuse are subtle, such as theft of the victim's belongings or loss of freedom. Other signs, such as wounds, untreated decubitus ulcers, or poor hygiene, are more obvious. For additional information on the signs of elder abuse, see the "Geriatrics" chapter.

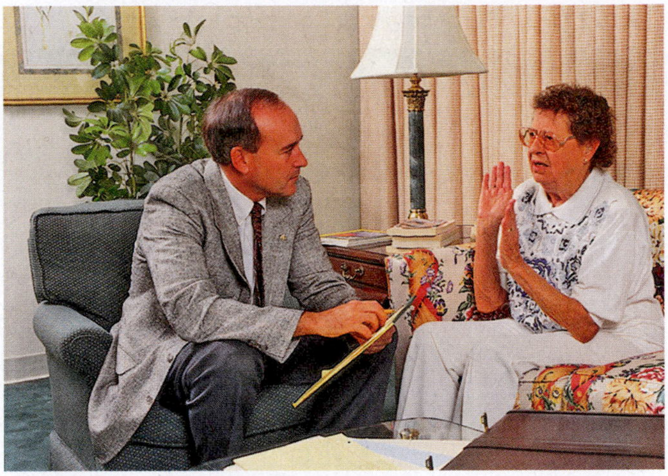

FIGURE 6-3 You are obligated to report suspected elder abuse to the appropriate authorities. In the case of institutional elder abuse, your actions may result in an investigation by an outside agency who will question the patient more closely.

Theories about Domestic Elder Abuse

There are four main theories about causes of domestic elder abuse. Commonly, caregivers feel stressed and overburdened. They are ill equipped to provide care or simply lack the knowledge to do the job correctly. Another cause of elder abuse is the patients' physical and/or mental impairment. Elders in poor health are more likely to be abused than elders in good health. This situation results, in part, from their inability to report the abuse. Yet another cause of elder abuse is family history, or the cycle of violence mentioned earlier. Finally, elder abuse increases proportionately with the personal problems of the caregivers. Abusers of the elderly tend to have more difficulties, either financial or emotional, than nonabusers.

Characteristics of Abused Elders

Like partner abuse, elder abuse cuts across all demographic groups. As a result, it is difficult to outline an accurate profile of the abused elder. The most common cases involve elderly women abused by their sons. However, this pattern is skewed by the fact that women live longer than men. Elder abuse most frequently occurs among people who are dependent on others for their care, especially among those elders who are mentally or physically challenged. In such cases, elders may be repeatedly abused by relatives who believe the elder will not or cannot ask for help.

In cases of neglect, abused elders most commonly live alone. They may be mentally competent, but fear asking for help because relatives have complained about providing care or have threatened to place them in a nursing home. Like abused partners, they may be reluctant to give information about their abusers for fear of retaliation.

Table 6-1 Perpetrators of Domestic Elder Abuse

Group	Percentage
Adult children	32.5
Grandchildren	4.2
Spouse	14.4
Sibling	2.5
Other relatives	12.5
Friend/neighbor	6.5
All others	18.2
Unknown	8.2

Characteristics of Elder Abusers

It is also difficult to profile the people who are most likely to abuse elders. According to the National Aging Resource Center on Elder Abuse, the percentages in Table 6-1 reflect the reported perpetrators of elder abuse in domestic settings. As you can see, the most typical abusers are adult children who are either overstressed by care of the elder or who were abused themselves.

As with partner abusers, several characteristics in common are found in abusers of the elderly. Often, the perpetrators exhibit alcoholic behavior, drug addiction, or some mental impairment. The abuser may also be dependent on the income or assistance of the elder, a situation that can cause resentment, anger, and, in some cases, violence.

For more on the management of elder abuse, see the "Geriatrics" chapter.

Child Abuse

As pointed out in the chapters "Neonatology" and "Pediatrics," child abuse is one of the most difficult circumstances that you will face as a paramedic. **Child abuse** may range from physical or emotional impairment to neglect of a child's most basic needs (Figure 6-4). It can occur from infancy to age 18 and can be inflicted by any number of caregivers: parents, foster parents, stepparents, babysitters, siblings, stepsiblings, or other relatives or friends charged with a child's care.

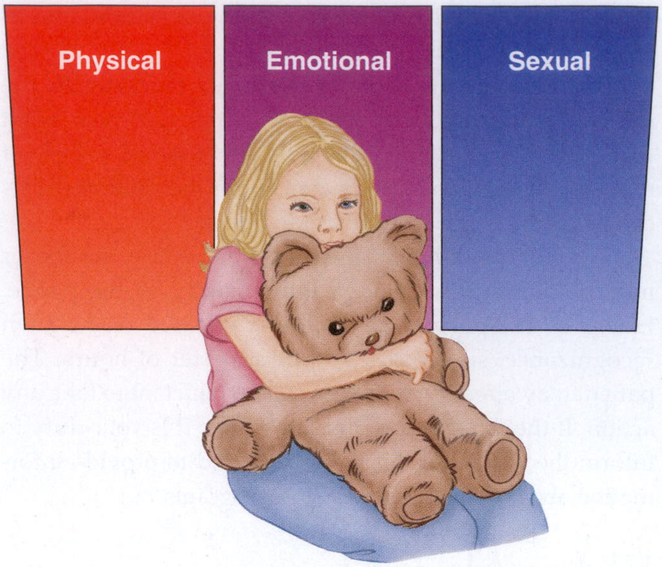

FIGURE 6-4 Child abuse comes in many forms. Be alert and report any concerns you may have regarding abuse or neglect.

Although you may be familiar with some of the following information from your training or from other chapters in this book, it bears repeating. The damage done to a child can last a lifetime and, as stressed earlier, can perpetuate a cycle of violence in generations to come.

Characteristics of Child Abusers

As with other types of abusers, you cannot relate child abuse to social class, income, or education. However, certain patterns do emerge, most notably a history of abuse within their own families. Most child abusers were physically or emotionally abused as children. They often would prefer to use other forms of discipline, but under stress they regress to their earliest and most familiar patterns. Once they resort to physical discipline, the punishments become more severe and more frequent.

In cases of reported physical abuse, perpetrators tend to be men. However, the statistics for men and women even out when neglect is taken into account. As indicated earlier, potential child abusers can include a wide variety of caregivers. In most cases, however, one or both parents are the most likely abusers. Frequent behavioral traits include:

- Use or abuse of drugs and/or alcohol
- Immaturity and preoccupation with self
- Lack of obvious feeling for the child, rarely looking at or touching the child
- Apparent lack of concern about the child's injury, treatment, or prognosis
- Open criticism of the child, with little indication of guilt or remorse for involvement in the child's condition
- Little identification with the child's pain, whether it is physical or emotional

Any one of these signs should raise suspicion in your mind of possible child abuse. The infant or child will provide other clues, even before you begin your physical examination.

Characteristics of Abused Children

A child's behavior is one of the most important indicators of abuse. Some behavior is age related. For example, abused children under age six usually appear excessively passive, whereas abused children over age six seem aggressive. Other behavioral clues include:

- Crying, often hopelessly, during treatment—or not crying at all
- Avoiding the parents or showing little concern for their absence
- Unusual wariness or fear of physical contact
- Apprehension and/or constant alertness for danger
- Being prone to sudden behavioral changes
- Absence of nearly all emotions
- Neediness, constantly requesting favors, food, or things

In general, use your instincts and knowledge of age-appropriate behavior (see the "Neonatology" and "Pediatrics" chapters) to guide your first impression of the child. If the child's behavior is atypical, maintain an index of suspicion throughout your assessment.[6]

Cultural Considerations

Medicinal Practices of the Hmong. Some cultural folk medicine practices can be easily mistaken for child abuse. An Asian population, referred to as the Hmong or "Hill People," is among the oldest populations in Asia. Many Hmong were recruited by the Central Intelligence Agency and were allied with the United States in the secret war in Laos that was fought contemporaneously with the war in Vietnam. When these countries fell, more than 100,000 Hmong were killed by the Communist insurgents. Numerous Hmong families immigrated to the United States—usually with the help of various church groups—and settled primarily in southern California and the Midwest.

In the Hmong folk medicine belief system, coining, cupping, and pinching are common practices. With coining, a utensil with a rounded edge (such as a coin or spoon) is used to rub the skin until bruising appears. This procedure leaves an oval ecchymotic area with an irregular border. Cupping treatment creates a vacuum effect that is thought to draw out pain. It is done by burning cotton in a small jar and placing the jar over the affected area after the flame is out. The sign of this is a round ecchymotic area. Pinching is commonly used to alleviate headaches. It is performed by pinching the skin until bruising appears. The result is a narrow bruise, often found between the eyes. As noted, all these folk remedies result in bruising. It is also common to puncture and bleed these ecchymotic areas in an effort to release toxins thought to cause the illness. The puncture usually is done with a sewing needle.

Soon after their settlement in the United States, numerous Hmong children were referred to child protection authorities for investigation of suspected child abuse—usually by well-meaning health care professionals. Some of the bruising secondary to coining, cupping, or pinching seemed symptomatic of child abuse to those unfamiliar with Hmong culture. However, following investigation, it was learned that these were loving actions designed to make the child or adult well.

In areas where Hmong are present, cultural diversity education programs are available to provide information on the folk medicine and cultural practices of this interesting group of people.[7]

Identification of the Abused Child

CONTENT REVIEW

- ➤ Conditions Commonly Mistaken for Abuse
  - Car seat burns
  - Staphylococcal scalded skin syndrome
  - Chickenpox (cigarette burns)
  - Hematologic disorders that cause easy bruising

As you know, children very commonly get injured, and not all injured children are abused. If a child volunteers the story of his injury without hesitation and if it matches the story told by the parent and the symptoms of injury, child abuse is very unlikely. However, if the behavior of a caregiver and/or child has raised an index of suspicion, you may face a challenge in distinguishing between an intentional injury and an authentic accident. Conditions commonly mistaken for abuse are car seat burns, staphylococcal scalded skin syndrome, chickenpox (which may look like cigarette burns), and hematologic disorders that can cause bruising. In assessing a child, look for common patterns of physical abuse, evidence of emotional abuse, and/or environmental clues of neglect.

Physical Examination

In most cases, signs of physical mistreatment of a child should be the easiest type of abuse for you to recognize. Soft tissue injuries are the most common indicators, especially multiple bruises in different places of the body, in different stages of healing, and with distinctive shapes (Table 6-2). Other common warning signs include defensive wounds on the hands and forearms and symmetrical injuries such as bites or burns. Any of these conditions carries a high index of suspicion of abuse.

Table 6-2 Determining the Age of a Bruise by Its Color

Color of Bruise	Age of Bruise
Red (swollen, tender)	0–2 days
Blue, purple	2–5 days
Green	5–7 days
Yellow	7–10 days
Brown	10–14 days
No further evidence of bruising	2–4 weeks

From Portable Guides to Investigating Child Abuse, *Office of Juvenile Justice and Delinquency Prevention, Office of Justice Programs, U.S. Department of Justice.* https://www.ncjrs.gov/html/ojjdp/portable_guides/abuse/bruises.html *(accessed May 30, 2012)*

BURNS AND SCALDS Some injuries often have distinctive patterns that indicate the implement or source used to injure the child. The burns tend to be in certain common locations: the soles of the feet, palms of the hands, back, or buttocks. They may or may not be found in conjunction with other injuries.

Because children have thinner skin than adults (other than elders), they also tend to scald more easily. The temperature of hot water in most residences is about 140°F, which can scald an adult in only about 5 seconds. (Bathwater for children should be kept below 120°F.) When children accidentally get into water that is too hot, you can expect to see "splash" burns—marks created by spattering water as children try to escape. Intentional scalding, however, is characterized by the conspicuous lack of splash burns. Such "dipping injuries" are a common form of child abuse.

FRACTURES Fractures constitute the second most common form of child abuse. Sites of fractures include the skull, nose, facial structures, and upper extremities (Figure 6-5). Twisting and jerking fractures result from grabbing a child by an extremity, and neck injuries occur from shaking a child. Because children have soft, pliable ribs, they rarely experience accidental fractures to this region. As a result, you should maintain a high index of suspicion of abuse whenever you encounter a child with fractured ribs.

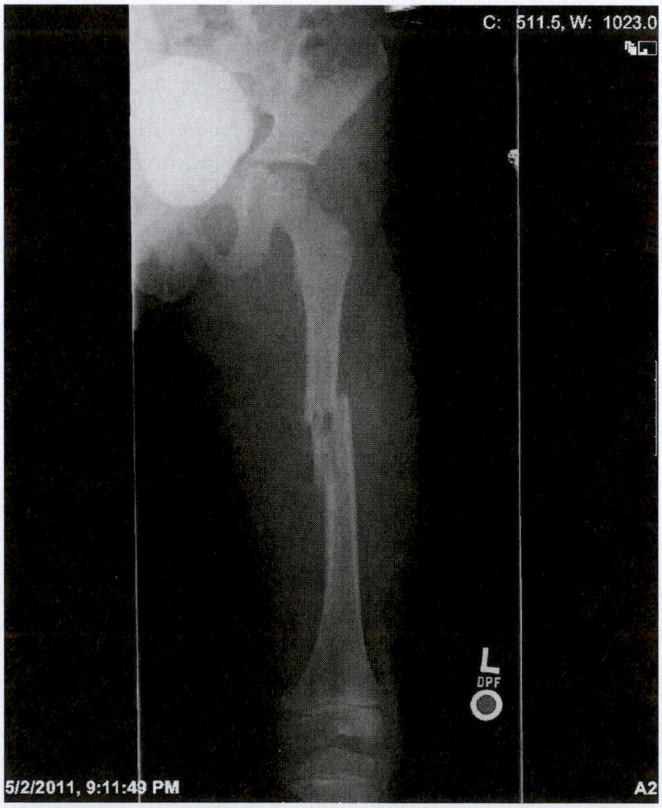

FIGURE 6-5 Evidence of child abuse—X-ray of a femur fracture in a six-year-old girl.

(© Dr. Bryan E. Bledsoe)

HEAD INJURIES Over time, injuries from abuse tend to progress from the extremities and trunk to the head. Head injuries commonly found in abused children include scalp wounds, skull fractures, subdural hematomas, and repeated contusions.

Injuries to the head claim the largest number of lives among abused children. They also account for most of the long-term disability associated with child abuse.

SHAKEN BABY SYNDROME Shaken baby syndrome frequently occurs when a parent or caregiver becomes frustrated with a crying infant and all other attempts to quiet the baby have failed. It happens when a person picks up the infant and shakes the baby vigorously. The movement can cause permanent brain damage, such as subdural hematomas or diffuse swelling. It may also result in injuries to the neck and spine or retinal hemorrhages, which, in turn, can lead to blindness. If the infant is shaken hard enough or repeatedly, the baby may die from the injuries.

ABDOMINAL INJURIES Although abdominal injuries represent a small proportion of the injuries suffered by abused children, they are usually very serious. Blunt force can result in trauma to the liver, spleen, or mesentery. You should look for pain, swelling, and vomiting, as well as hemodynamic compromise from these injuries.

Maternal Drug Abuse

Drug abuse by the mother during pregnancy is a subtle, but devastating, form of child abuse. Certain drugs, particularly cocaine and alcohol, are associated with long-term problems for the fetus. Fetal alcohol syndrome (FAS) can occur following repeated exposure to alcohol during the first trimester of pregnancy. In addition, maternal use of cocaine can result in a specific pattern. Children of mothers addicted to cocaine, most commonly "crack cocaine," are a particular problem. Premature birth and numerous complications are often seen in cocaine babies or "crack babies" (Figure 6-6).

Signs of Neglect

Some forms of child abuse are less obvious than physical injuries. Abuse may result from neglect. Caregivers simply do not provide children with adequate food, clothing, shelter, or medical care.

As a paramedic, you may be in a unique position to observe and report neglect. Unlike many other health care or public safety workers, EMS personnel get an opportunity to see the child's home environment for themselves. Unhealthy or unclean conditions are clear evidence of a caregiver's inability to provide for a child's safety or well-being.

In examining a child, keep in mind the following common signs of neglect:

- Malnutrition (neglected children are often underweight, sometimes by up to 30 percent)
- Severe diaper rash

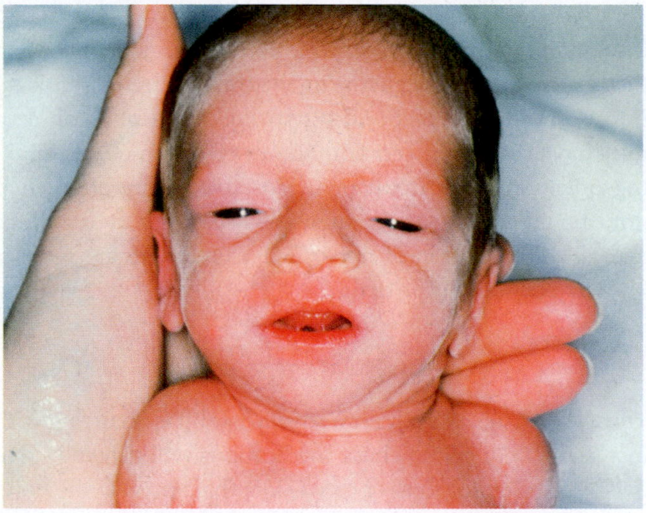

FIGURE 6-6 Face of a premature cocaine baby. The mother of this child was a cocaine addict. Developmental abnormalities are common. The infant may develop acute cocaine withdrawal signs and symptoms.
(*© Stevie Grand/Science Source*)

- Diarrhea and/or dehydration
- Hair loss
- Untreated medical conditions
- Inappropriate, dirty, torn clothing or lack of clothing
- Tired and listless attitudes
- Near constant demands for physical contact or attention

Signs of Emotional Abuse

Emotional abuse is often the hardest form of abuse to identify. It may take any one of the following six forms:

1. Parents or caregivers simply ignore the child, showing indifference to the child's needs and failing to provide any stimulation.
2. Parents or caregivers reject, humiliate, or criticize the child.
3. The child may be isolated and deprived of normal human contact or nurturing.
4. A child may be terrorized or bullied through verbal assaults and threats, creating feelings of fear and anxiety.
5. A parent or caregiver may encourage destructive or antisocial behavior.
6. The child may be overpressured by unrealistic expectations of success.

Recording and Reporting Child Abuse

As with all other forms of abuse, you have a responsibility to report suspected cases of child abuse. In some instances, you might have a chance to provide early intervention. An abusive adult may actively seek help or may send out signals for help. For example, a potential abuser may make several calls within a 24-hour period. The person may also summon help for inconsequential symptoms or demonstrate an inability to handle an impeding crisis. These are warning signs and should be duly noted.

When confronted with an actual case of child abuse, try to conduct the examination with another colleague present. You must keep your personal reactions to yourself and record only your objective observations. Assumptions must not be included in your report. The final document should be objective, legible, and written with the knowledge that it may be used in a future court or child custody case. At all times, put the child's interest first, treating him with the utmost kindness and gentleness. (For more on your EMS and legal responsibilities, see material later in this chapter.)

Sexual Assault

Anyone can be a victim of sexual violence. Statistics from the National Victims Center and the U.S. Department of Justice reveal that males and females of all backgrounds, from infancy to old age, have reported crimes involving forced or unwanted sexual contact. According to the Bureau of Justice Statistics, more than 260,000 rapes and nearly 100,000 sexual assaults are reported each year. However, these figures reflect only a small percentage of cases, with an estimated 63 to 74 percent of all incidents going unreported.[8]

Although the legal definitions vary from state to state, courts generally interpret **sexual assault** as unwanted sexual contact, whether it is genital, oral, rectal, or manual. **Rape** is usually defined as penile penetration of the genitalia or rectum (however slight) without the consent of the victim. Both forms of sexual violence are prosecuted as crimes, with rape constituting a felony offense. As a result, your actions at the scene and the report that you file will, in all likelihood, affect the outcome of a trial.

Characteristics of Victims of Sexual Assault/Rape

It is difficult to profile a victim of sexual assault or rape because of the variety of victims. However, statistics reveal certain patterns. The group most likely to be victimized is adolescent females younger than age 18. Nearly two-thirds of all rapes and sexual assaults take place between the hours of 6 P.M. and 6 A.M. at the victim's home or at the home of a friend, relative, or acquaintance. A woman is raped, on average, every 2 minutes in the United States; a woman is four times as likely to be raped by someone she knows than by a stranger.

Particularly alarming is the number of children who suffer some form of sexual abuse. According to the Department of Justice, one in two rape victims is under age 18; one in six is under age 12. Other government figures show that approximately one-third of all juvenile victims of sexual abuse are children younger than six years of age. Typically, contact involves a male assailant and a female victim, but not always. The contact can range from exposure to fondling to penetration. Although sexual abuse can occur in families of all descriptions, children raised in families in which there is domestic violence are eight times more likely to be sexually molested within that family.

Sexual assault and rape carry serious consequences. Victims may be physically injured, or even killed, during the assault. They commonly suffer internal injuries, particularly if multiple assailants are involved in the attack. Rape can result in infections, sexually transmitted diseases, and unwanted pregnancies. The psychological damage is deep and long lasting. Shame, anger, and a lack of trust can persist for years—or even for a lifetime.

Children, in particular, find it difficult to speak about molestation. It is likely that they know the person and fear reprisal or, in some instances, even seek to protect the individual. In many cases, the assailants physically explore the child without intercourse or force the child to touch or fondle them. Victims, especially very young children, may be confused about the situation or, lacking physical evidence of abuse, fear that nobody will believe them. Symptoms of sexual abuse, regardless of its form, may include:

- Nightmares
- Restlessness
- Withdrawal tendencies
- Hostility
- Phobias related to the offender
- Regressive behavior, such as bed wetting
- Truancy
- Promiscuity, in older children and teens
- Drug and alcohol abuse

Characteristics of Sexual Assailants

Like the victims of sexual assaults, the assailants can come from almost any background. However, the violent victimizers of children are substantially more likely than the victimizers of adults to have been physically or sexually abused as children. Many assailants, particularly adolescents and abusive adults, think domination is part of any relationship. Such thinking can lead to date rape or marital rape. In a significant percentage of all cases, the assailants are under the influence of alcohol or drugs. Nearly 30 percent of all rapists use weapons, underscoring the fact that sexual assaults are violent crimes.

In cases of date rape, the assailant may have drugged the unknowing victim with one of the drugs described in the next section. The victim may exhibit extreme intoxication without a corresponding strong smell of alcohol or may have drug-induced amnesia (a common effect), making questioning difficult or impossible. More often than not, the alleged assailant in such cases lives on a college campus, the location of most EMS calls involving what is known as a "date rape drug."

Date Rape Drugs

The use of drugs to facilitate a sexual assault is occurring with increasing frequency.[9] These medications will generally render a person unresponsive or weaken the person to the point of being unable to resist an attacker. Some of these medications cause amnesia, thus eliminating or distorting the victim's recall of the assault. Because these drugs have become more commonplace in society, it is important for EMS personnel to be aware of these agents and their effects. Date rape drugs have a rapid onset of action with a varying duration of effect. Drugs that have been associated with rape, which are also known as *predator drugs*, include the following:

- ***Rohypnol.*** Rohypnol is a potent benzodiazepine that produces a sedative effect, amnesia, muscle relaxation, and slowing of the psychomotor response. It is widely prescribed outside the United States as a sleeping pill. It is colorless, odorless, and tasteless and can be dissolved in a drink without being detected. Rohypnol can be potentiated by the concomitant effects of alcohol. Street names for rohypnol include *Roofies, Rope, Ruffies, R2, Ruffles, Roche, Forget-Pill,* and *Mexican Valium.*
- ***GHB.*** Gamma-hydroxybutyrate, commonly called GHB, is an odorless, colorless liquid depressant with anesthetic-type qualities. It is also used as an amino acid supplement by body builders. The drug causes relaxation, tranquility, sensuality, and loss of inhibitions. Street names for GHB include *Liquid Ecstasy, Liquid X, Scoop, Easy Lay,* and *Grievous Bodily Harm.*
- ***Ketamine.*** Ketamine is a potent anesthetic agent. Widely used in veterinary practice, ketamine is also used in human anesthesia. It is chemically similar to the hallucinogenic LSD. It causes hallucinations, amnesia, and dissociation. Street names for ketamine include *K, Special K, Vitamin K, Jet,* and *Super Acid.*
- ***MDMA.*** 3,4-Methylenedioxymethamphetamine (MDMA) is most commonly known as *Ecstasy.* It is known to cause psychological difficulties including confusion, depression, sleep problems, drug craving, severe anxiety, and paranoia (both during and sometimes weeks after taking the drug). It can also cause physical symptoms such as muscle tension, involuntary teeth clenching, nausea, blurred vision,

rapid eye movement, faintness, and chills or sweating. Street names for MDMA, in addition to *Ecstasy*, include *Beans, Adam, XTC, Roll, E,* and *M.*

Persons attending parties and other events should be cautious with regard to predator drugs. It is best not to drink from a punch bowl or a bottle that is being passed around. Notice the behavior of others at the party. If a person seems more intoxicated than the amount of alcohol consumed would warrant, then consider the possibility of predator drugs. If a rape victim thinks she has been drugged, a drug screen should be requested on arrival at the emergency department. EMS personnel should note any suspicions or observations that may point to the use of a predator drug.

EMS Responsibilities

Your response to a call involving a sexual assault is similar in many ways to your response to any abusive situation. In both instances, your primary responsibility is safety—both your own and that of the patient. You should never enter a scene if your safety is compromised, and you should leave the scene as soon as you feel unsafe.

You can expect victims of assault or abuse to feel unsafe as a result of the violence they have suffered. One of your primary responsibilities is to provide a safe environment for an already traumatized patient. Sometimes you can provide safety merely by your official presence. Other times, you may have to move the patient to the ambulance, where you can lock the doors, or move to a different location entirely. In still other instances, you may have to summon additional personnel. (For more on crime scene management, see the chapter "Crime Scene Awareness.")

You are also responsible for providing proper psychosocial care for the victims of abuse and assault. Privacy is a major consideration. In many cases, a paramedic of the same sex as the victim should maintain contact with the victim (Figure 6-7). Although you may need to expose the victim during assessment, you should cover the patient and remove him or her from public view as soon as possible.

When talking with the patient, use open-ended questions to reestablish a sense of control. You might say, for example, "Would you like to sit on a seat or ride on the stretcher?" Or you might ask, "Is there someone you would like us to call?" As mentioned in earlier sections, remain nonjudgmental throughout treatment, avoiding subjective comments about both the patient and the assailant. In a reassuring voice, encourage the patient to report the rape, explaining the importance of preserving evidence.

Medical treatment of victims of abuse and assault is essentially the same as with other patients. However, you should always remember the origins of the patient's injuries and provide appropriate emotional support. Keep in mind that the patient has been harmed by another human being, in many cases a person that the patient knows intimately.

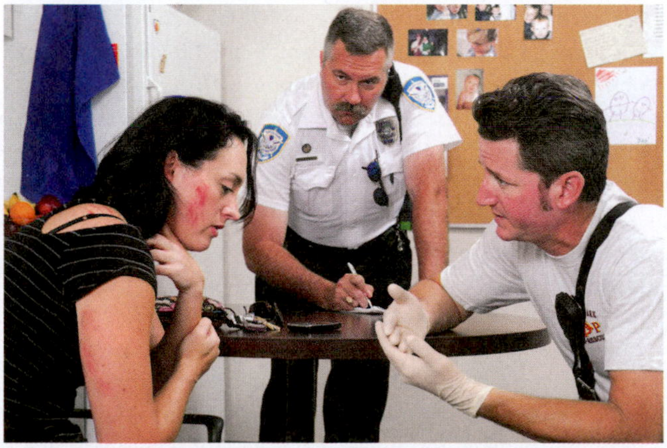

FIGURE 6-7 The paramedic should maintain contact with the victim of abuse or rape, staying with the patient during any interview by police and accompanying the patient to the hospital.

Human Trafficking

Human trafficking is defined as the trade of humans, or the illegal movement of people, usually for forced labor or commercial sexual exploitation (Figure 6-8). It is, in essence, a form of modern slavery where people profit from the control and exploitation of others. There are various forms of human trafficking, including sex trafficking, labor trafficking, forced marriages, and similar abuses (such as the extraction of organs and/or tissues to sell). In most cases, traffickers use violence, threats, deception, debt bondage, and similar manipulative tactics to force vulnerable people into engaging in commercial sex or to provide labor services against their will (often domestic or manual labor). Traffickers place people into forced labor and sex trafficking by exploiting their vulnerabilities such as their legal status within the country, inability to speak English,

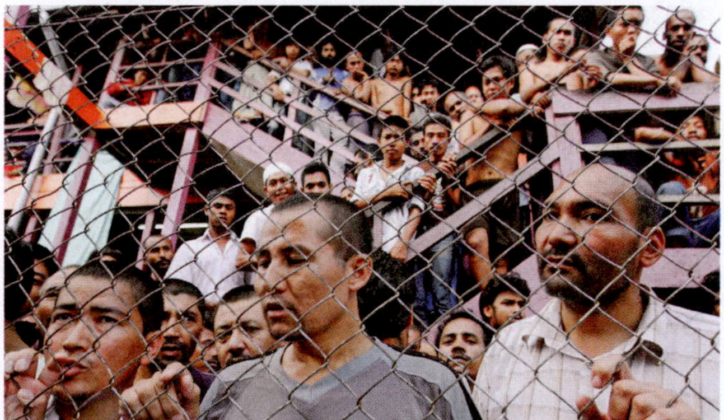

FIGURE 6-8 Human trafficking takes place in the United States and around the world. In this photo, detainees in Malaysia have been accused of forced labor of Myanmar migrants.

(©Mark Baker/Associated Press)

poverty, and cultural influences. Traffickers are often of the same national, ethnic or cultural backgrounds as those who are being exported. The underlying motive is almost always a profit.

Human trafficking is defined legally as "the recruitment, transport, transfer, harboring or receipt of a person by such means as threat or use of force or other forms of coercion, of abduction, of fraud or deception for the purpose of exploitation." In the United States, human trafficking can be generally divided into three vulnerable populations, including:

- Children under 18 years of age induced into commercial sex
- Adults over age 18 who are induced into commercial sex through force, fraud, or coercion
- Children and adults induced to perform labor or services through force, fraud, or coercion

EMS personnel are uniquely positioned to identify the signs and symptoms of human trafficking. Recognition is the first step in identifying victims and can actually save a life. The following questions identify common indicators of human trafficking:

- Does the person appear disconnected from family, friends, community organizations, or houses of worship?
- Has a child stopped attending school?
- Has the person had a sudden or dramatic change in behavior?
- Is a juvenile engaged in commercial sex acts?
- Is the person disoriented or confused, or showing signs of mental or physical abuse?
- Does the person have bruises in various stages of healing?
- Is the person fearful, timid, or submissive?
- Does the person show signs of having been denied food, water, sleep, or medical care?
- Is the person often in the company of someone to whom he or she defers? Or someone who seems to be in control of the situation, e.g., where they go or who they talk to?
- Does the person appear to be coached on what to say?
- Is the person living in unsuitable conditions?
- Does the person lack personal possessions and appear not to have a stable living situation?
- Does the person have freedom of movement? Can the person freely leave where he or she lives? Are there unreasonable security measures?

Not all the indicators included in the above list are present in every human trafficking situation, and the presence or absence of any of the indicators is not necessarily proof of human trafficking.

If you believe you have identified someone who is or may presently be in a human trafficking situation, alert law enforcement immediately. It may be unsafe to attempt to rescue a human trafficking victim yourself. You have no way to know how the trafficker may react and retaliate against the victim and you. If, however, you

Legal Considerations

As noted throughout this chapter, abuse and assault constitute crimes. Although the nature and extent to which an assault is considered a crime often depends on local laws, you have a responsibility to report suspected cases to the appropriate law enforcement officials. Because the assailants may be detained only a short time, you also have an obligation to find out about the victim and witness protection programs available in your area.

Specialized resources include both private and state or federally funded programs. Make a point of learning about hospital units for the victims of sexual assault, public and private shelters for battered persons, and state agencies responsible for youths and their families. Also acquaint yourself with nurses trained as sexual assault nurse examiners (SANEs). They have completed programs allowing them to perform the physical exam for sexual assaults. They have detailed information on the protection of evidence, something that you must keep in mind throughout the call.

As you have read, your actions can affect the prosecution of a crime. Clothing should be removed from a patient only when necessary for assessment and treatment. All items should then be turned over to the proper authorities.

In the case of rape, patients should not urinate, defecate, douche, bathe, eat, drink, or smoke. Some jurisdictions have specific rules for evidence protection, such as using paper bags to collect evidence or placing bags over the patient's hands to preserve trace evidence. Remember that any evidence that you collect must remain in your custody until you can give it directly to a law enforcement official to preserve the **chain of evidence**.

As indicated, it is important that you carefully and objectively document all your findings. You may end up defending your words in a court of law. Regardless of the emotions evoked by the call, you must remain a professional at all times.

Finally, you should study the local laws and protocols regarding cases of abuse and assault. All 50 states require health care workers to report suspected cases of child abuse. Some states require EMS personnel to report even a suspicion of abuse or assault. Some states allow minors to seek medical care for sexual assault without parental consent. The Joint Commission mandates that hospital personnel screen incoming patients for abuse. Regardless of where you live, take time to learn the rules and regulations that affect your practice, both for your sake and for the sake of your patients.

identify a person who has escaped the trafficking situation, there are number of organizations to whom the victim could be referred for help with shelter, medical care, legal assistance, and other critical services. The United States National Human Trafficking Resource Center operates a toll-free line, 1-888-373-7888, that is open 24 hours a day and staffed with multilingual personnel to whom you can report a tip or from whom you can request help or services.

Hate Crimes

A **hate crime** is a crime of hatred or prejudice in which the perpetrator targets a particular victim or victims because of the victim's perceived membership in a certain social group. These groups can include racial, religious, sexual orientation, political, disability, and other social groups. The crime is based on bias and sometimes referred to as **bias-motivated crime**. Most hate crimes result from racial bias. This is followed by religious bias, sexual orientation bias, ethnicity/national origin bias, and disability bias. The vast majority of racial hate crimes are against blacks. Most religious hate crimes are directed at Jews. In terms of sexual orientation bias, most hate crimes are motivated by anti-male homosexual bias. Anti-female homosexual hate crimes are much less common. Most ethnicity/national origin hate crimes are directed at Hispanics.[10]

Most hate crimes involve vandalism. Intimidation is also common. Approximately one in three hate crimes involves assault. Certain hate crimes, especially those that are racially motivated, can result in widespread violence. EMS can become involved in any aspect of hate crimes, from simple intimidation to full-fledged riots. Paramedics must recognize that hate crimes and their aftermath are emotionally charged events and paramedics, because of their race, gender, or sexual orientation, can be drawn into the fray. Always treat hate crimes as particularly dangerous situations. Involve law enforcement early and always ensure the safety of you and your partner first.

Summary

The incidence of assault and abuse is more widespread today than ever before. You will encounter more cases during your paramedic career than you can imagine. For the sake of your patients, it is imperative that you learn the hallmarks of partner abuse, elder abuse, child abuse, and sexual assaults. Remember that you have a duty to report these situations, whether you transport the patients or not. By learning to recognize significant physical and emotional assessment findings, as well as characteristics of the victims and assailants, you will be able to provide better treatment of victims of abuse and assault. This includes knowing the legal requirements of your area, protecting evidence, and properly documenting your findings and actions. You may be the only chance a victim has of being saved from further abuse. Be vigilant in your observations and document objectively.

You Make the Call

You and your partner respond to a police request to evaluate an injured child. You find several police officers on the scene of a domestic disturbance. The patient is a three-year-old boy found sitting quietly on the couch. The boy's parents are present and being questioned by the police officers.

You find the patient dressed in underwear with no other clothing, although it is wintertime. He has obvious and different-colored bruises to both his upper arms and his back. During your exam, the boy is silent, not answering your questions or looking toward either of his parents.

1. What do you suspect is taking place?
2. What physical evidence do you have to support this suspicion?
3. What emotional evidence do you have to support this suspicion?
4. What other clues lead you to believe that abuse might be taking place?
5. What are your priorities in this case?

See Suggested Responses at the back of this book.

Review Questions

1. Physical or emotional violence from a man or woman toward a domestic partner is termed ________
   a. child abuse.
   b. spousal abuse.
   c. partner abuse.
   d. transient abuse.
2. The form of partner abuse most obvious to a paramedic or other emergency responder is ________ abuse.
   a. sexual
   b. physical
   c. emotional
   d. psychological
3. Child abuse can occur from infancy to age ________ and can be inflicted by any number of caregivers.
   a. 18
   b. 19
   c. 20
   d. 21
4. To prevent accidental injury, new parents should be instructed to keep children's bathwater below how many degrees Fahrenheit?
   a. 120
   b. 125
   c. 130
   d. 140
5. In children who are abused, common sites of fractures include all of the following *except* the ________
   a. ribs.
   b. nose.
   c. skull.
   d. face.
6. Injuries to which region of the body claim the largest number of lives among abused children?
   a. Chest
   b. Head
   c. Femur
   d. Pelvis
7. Which type of abuse is often the hardest form of abuse to identify?
   a. Verbal
   b. Sexual
   c. Physical
   d. Emotional
8. Soft tissue injuries are common indicators of abuse, especially multiple bruises ________
   a. with distinctive shapes.
   b. in different stages of healing.
   c. in different planes of the body.
   d. on the knees and elbows.
9. You are assessing a child you believe might be a victim of child abuse. You note multiple injuries and bruising to the body. One particular bruise to the back of the neck has a brownish discoloration to it, even though the parents state it occurred yesterday when he "fell." Given the description of the bruise, roughly how old is it?
   a. About 2 days
   b. About 5 days
   c. About 7 days
   d. About 11 days
10. You are completing a PCR regarding an elderly patient whom you suspect is being abused by his daughter-in-law when no one is home. As you provide document on the PCR, you should remember ________
    a. to document your suspicions.
    b. to remain objective in your findings.
    c. to state that you have notified social services.
    d. to state that you have notified the receiving hospital staff of your suspicions.

See Answers to Review Questions at the end of this book.

References

1. Childhelp. *National Child Abuse Statistics.* (Available at http://www.childhelp.org/pages/statistics.)
2. Bureau of Justice Statistics, Office of Justice Programs. *Violent Crime.* (Available at http://bjs.ojp.usdoj.gov/.)
3. Pixley, C. *Domestic Violence: Cracking the Code of Silence.* Los Angeles: Do It Now Foundation, 1995.
4. Weiss, S. J., A. A. Ernst, D. Blanton, et al. "EMT Domestic Violence Knowledge and Results of an Educational Intervention." *Am J Emerg Med* 18 (2000): 168–171.
5. Rinker, A. G., Jr. "Recognition and Perception of Elder Abuse by Prehospital and Hospital-Based Providers." *Arch Gerontol Geriatr* 48 (2009): 110–115.

6. American Academy of Pediatrics, Stirling J., Committee on Child Abuse and Neglect and Section on Adoption and Foster Care, American Academy of Child and Adolescent Psychiatry, Amaya-Jackson L., National Center for Child Traumatic Stress. "Understanding the Behavioral and Emotional Consequences of Child Abuse." *Pediatrics* 122 (2008): 667–673.
7. Her, C. and K. A. Culhane-Pera. "Culturally Responsive Care in Hmong Patients: Collaboration Is a Key Treatment Component." *Postgrad Med* 116 (2004): 39–42.
8. Center for National Victims of Crime. "Statistics." (Available at http://www.ncvc.org/ncvc/main.aspx?dbID=DB_Statistics584.)
9. Meehan, T. J, S. M. Bryant, and S. E. Aks. "Drugs of Abuse: The Highs and Lows of Altered Mental Status in the Emergency Department." *Emerg Med Clin North Am* 28 (2010): 663–682.
10. Federal Bureau of Investigation, Department of Justice. *Hate Crime Statistics*. (Available at http://www2.fbi.gov/ucr/hc2009/incidents.html.)

Further Reading

American Nurses Association. *Culturally Competent Assessment for Family Violence*. Washington, DC: American Nurses Publishing, 1998.

Federal Bureau of Investigation. *Uniform Crime Statistics*. Washington, DC: FBI, 2013.

Giardino, A. P. and E. R. Giardino. *Recognition of Child Abuse for the Mandated Reporter.* 4th ed. St. Louis: STM Learning, 2015.

Hamberger, L. K. and C. Renzetti. *Domestic Partner Abuse.* New York: Springer Publishing, 2004.

Hobbs, C. J. and J. M. Wynne. *Physical Signs of Child Abuse: A Colour Atlas.* 2nd ed. London: W. B. Saunders, 2002.

Kehner, G. *Date Rape Drugs.* Broomall, PA: Chelsea House Publishers, 2004.

Reece, R. M. *Child Abuse: Medical Diagnosis and Management*. 3rd ed. Elk Grove, IL: American Academy of Pediatrics, 2008.

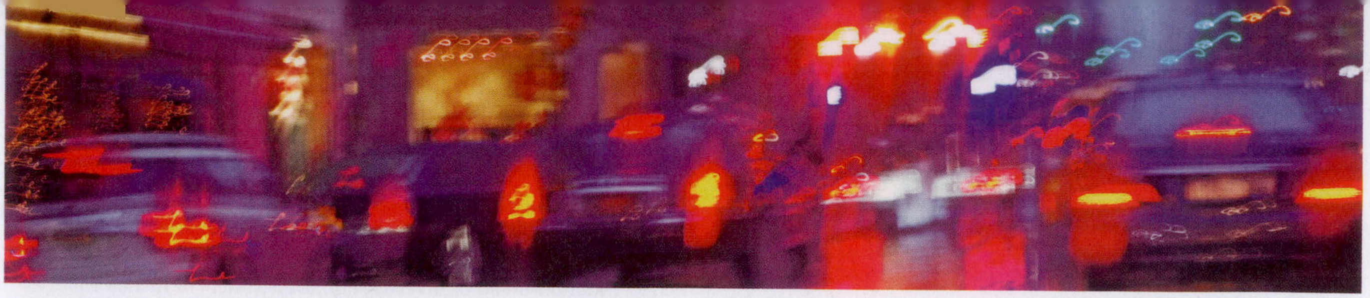

Chapter 7

The Challenged Patient

Bryan Bledsoe, DO, FACEP, FAAEM, EMT-P

STANDARD

Special Patient Populations (Patients with Special Needs)

COMPETENCY

Integrates assessment findings with principles of epidemiology and pathophysiology and knowledge of psychosocial needs to formulate a field impression and implement a comprehensive treatment/disposition plan for patients with special needs.

Learning Objectives

Terminal Performance Objective: After reading this chapter, you should be able to integrate patient assessment findings, patient history, and knowledge of therapeutic communication and medical/legal considerations to recognize and manage patients with a variety of special challenges.

Enabling Objectives: To accomplish the terminal performance objective, you should be able to:

1. Define key terms introduced in this chapter.
2. Identify and discuss the types of physical, mental, emotional, cognitive, and developmental challenges seen in patients whom EMS may encounter in the prehospital environment.
3. Describe the various types of accommodations EMS providers may have to make for patients with physical, mental, emotional, cognitive, and developmental challenges.
4. Discuss how the EMS response to assessment and management is altered relative to patients who are culturally diverse, terminally ill, financially challenged, or have communicable diseases.
5. Given various scenarios, discuss how the paramedic should integrate assessment and management of emergencies in patients with special challenges.

KEY TERMS

aphasia, p. 218
colostomy, p. 221
conductive deafness, p. 216
deafness, p. 216
diabetic retinopathy, p. 217
enucleation, p. 217
glaucoma, p. 217
labyrinthitis, p. 216
mucoviscidosis, p. 225
neutropenia, p. 224
otitis media, p. 216
presbycusis, p. 216
sensorineural deafness, p. 216

Case Study

You sit down for the first meal on your shift at Medic 211, but just as you take out something to eat, you are dispatched to a private residence to aid the victim of a fall. You and your partner look at each other, throw your food back into your lunch bags, and hit the road.

En route to the call, you learn that a 72-year-old woman has fallen out of her wheelchair and is unable to get back up. Dispatch tells you that the door is locked, but the woman has hidden a spare key under a fake rock in the garden near the front door.

Fifteen minutes later, you and your partner gain access to the house. You find a woman lying on her side on the bedroom floor, her wheelchair off to the side behind her. You notice what appears to be a brace on the woman's right leg.

When you introduce yourself, the patient tells you her name is Bonnie Wade. "I was trying to put a dress up in my closet," explains Mrs. Wade, "when I lost my balance and fell."

On further questioning, Mrs. Wade indicates that she is widowed and lives alone. Although she can ambulate for short periods of time, she is, for the most part, wheelchair bound. Mrs. Wade denies losing consciousness and says she feels no neck or back pain and no tingling in her extremities. When asked about pain, she replies, "My left hip and shoulder hurt real bad. I fell so hard that I almost dropped the cell phone. I carry it all the time just in case I ever need help."

During your neurologic exam, you find that the patient is unable to move her right leg. Mrs. Wade responds, "Oh that, I had polio when I was young—long before the vaccination they give to kids today." She also tells you that her left arm is weak from post-polio syndrome.

Your partner goes to the ambulance to get the scoop stretcher. Meanwhile, you put the patient's left arm in a cravat sling. You then explain how the scoop stretcher works and assure Mrs. Wade that it is the safest and most comfortable way to get her off the floor. When Mrs. Wade asks whether her leg brace will be in the way, you tell her that you'd like to keep it in place until a doctor evaluates her.

Once you have packaged the patient in the scoop stretcher, you carefully place her on the ambulance stretcher. Mrs. Wade tells you that the sling has relieved some of the pain in her arm, but asks you to take the bumps slowly because of the pain in her hip. You place her in the back of the ambulance and begin transport to Memorial Hospital.

Introduction

Throughout your EMS career, you can expect to encounter a number of patients who live with a variety of impairments or special challenges. Many will have met these challenges so successfully that you may not notice them right away. For example, people with hearing impairments might lip-read so well that you may not initially realize they cannot hear. People with more obvious challenges, such as paralysis, may have accepted their impairments and built active and rewarding lives. A patient with a history of polio, for example, may have lived with the problem so long that he neglects to tell you about it right away. Instead, the patient talks about a more immediate problem—the reason for summoning EMS.

The one thing that challenged patients share is their variety. They might have any number of physical, mental, or emotional impairments. They might have contracted a pathologic illness that necessitates a special living or working arrangement. They might be suffering from a terminal illness or a communicable disease. They may come from a cultural or financial situation that dictates medical practices contrary to those of the EMS community. The key to treating the "challenged" patient is to understand and recognize the special condition or situation and to make any accommodations that may be needed for proper patient care.

Physical Challenges

A number of physical impairments—conditions that limit the use of one or more parts of the body—can affect patient assessment and/or treatment. These impairments may be the result of accidents, birth injuries, chronic illnesses, aging, and more. Impairments can limit the ability of a patient to hear, see, speak, or move. Patients will react to their impairments in different ways—from acceptance to denial, anger, or shame. It is important that you quickly recognize the impairment and exhibit knowledge and sensitivity to assure the patient that you understand his special needs.

Hearing Impairment

Hearing impairments involve a decrease or loss in the ability to distinguish or hear sounds, particularly those involving speech. An inability to hear is commonly described as **deafness**. A person may be completely deaf or partially deaf. A person may be deaf in one ear or both ears. The condition may be present at birth or may occur later in life as a result of an accident, illness, or aging.

Types of Hearing Impairment

The two basic types of deafness are **conductive deafness** and **sensorineural deafness**. Many forms of conductive deafness can be treated and cured, especially if caught early. Sensorineural deafness, on the other hand, is often incurable.

CONDUCTIVE DEAFNESS Conductive deafness results from any condition that prevents sound waves from being transmitted from the external ear to the middle or inner ear. The condition can be either temporary or permanent.

If an infant or child does not respond to verbal stimulation or questions, rule out the possibility of conductive deafness when performing your assessment of disability. Congenital malformation of the ear is a possible but rare cause of conductive deafness in the neonate. A more common cause of conductive deafness in children is **otitis media**, an infection of the middle ear. This condition often arises from various childhood illnesses, particularly those involving the upper respiratory tract. To prevent hearing loss, children under age six who experience recurrent otitis media may need to take daily prophylactic antibiotics or have tympanostomy (myringotomy) tubes placed.

In addition to infection, a number of other conditions can result in a temporary loss of hearing. Anyone can experience conductive deafness during an airline flight, where changes in air pressure can affect hearing. A deep-water dive can have a similar effect. Impacted cerumen, or earwax, is yet another common and easily treatable cause of conductive deafness.

Other causes might be the temporary blockage of the ear canal by various irritants, such as dust, hair spray, insects, or water ("swimmer's ear"). Patient attempts to clean the canal with cotton applicators may disrupt the ear's natural cleaning process and push the debris deeper into the ear, which sets the stage for bacterial infections and conductive deafness.

Obstructions can also be caused by hematomas, which may result from blunt trauma to the ear. Force to the mandible, such as a fractured jaw, can also produce a temporary loss of hearing and may in fact result in fragments of bone displaced to the ear canal. Although these conditions cannot be treated in the field, they should be taken into account when a trauma patient appears not to respond to, or "hear," your questions.

SENSORINEURAL DEAFNESS Sensorineural deafness arises from the inability of nerve impulses to reach the auditory center of the brain because of damage either to the inner ear or to the brain itself. It is usually a permanent condition.

In the case of infants and children, sensorineural deafness often results from congenital defects or birth injuries. Preterm infants, especially those with severe asphyxia or recurrent apnea in the neonatal period, are particularly at risk for sensorineural deafness. Ototoxic drugs, such as furosemide (Lasix) and gentamicin, can also cause sensorineural deafness if administered to infants in neonatal intensive care units. Finally, many children who develop this type of hearing loss have mothers who contracted rubella (German measles) or cytomegalovirus (CMV) during the first three months of pregnancy.

Diseases such as bacterial meningitis or viral illnesses such as **labyrinthitis** (inner ear infection) can lead to sensorineural deafness at any age. Taking high doses of ototoxic drugs such as aspirin can also cause sensorineural deafness in both children and adults. A common symptom of aspirin toxicity is "ringing in the ears" (tinnitus). Other causes of sensorineural deafness include tumors of the brain or middle ear, concussion, severe blows to the ear, and repeated loud noises such as chain saws, heavy machinery, gunfire, rock music, or sudden blasts of sound.

Conditions associated with aging can also lead to permanent hearing loss. **Presbycusis** is a progressive sensorineural hearing loss that begins after age 20 but is usually significant only in people over age 65. More common in men than women, this type of hearing loss affects high-frequency sounds first, then low-frequency sounds. Eventually, human voices become harder to detect, especially if background noise is present. Elderly people with this condition will often tell others not to "mumble" or will ask them to speak louder.

Recognition of Deafness

As mentioned, it is important to detect deafness early in your assessment. A partially deaf person may ask questions repeatedly, misunderstand answers to questions, or respond inappropriately. Such reactions can easily be mistaken for head injury, leading to misdirected treatment.

The most obvious sign of deafness is a hearing aid. Unfortunately, hearing aids do not work for all types of deafness. In addition, many people do not wear hearing aids, even when they have been prescribed. Furthermore, deaf people may have poor diction due to partial hearing loss or hearing loss later in life. They might use their hands to gesture or use sign language. As noted, deaf people may ask you to speak louder or they may speak excessively loudly themselves. Finally, deaf people will commonly face you so that they can read your lips.

Accommodations for Deaf Patients

When managing a patient with a hearing impairment, you can do several things to ease communication. Begin by identifying yourself and making sure that the patient knows that you are speaking to him. Get the patient's attention by moving so you can be seen or by gently touching the person, if appropriate. By addressing deaf patients face to face, you give them the opportunity to read your lips and interpret your expression.

When talking with a deaf patient, speak slowly in a normal voice. Never yell or use exaggerated gestures. These techniques often distort your facial and body language, making you seem angry or threatening. Keep in mind that nearly 80 percent of hearing loss is related to high-pitched sounds. As a result, you might use a low-pitched voice to speak directly into the patient's ear. Whatever you do, make sure that background noise is reduced as much as possible by turning off the TV, radio, or other sources of sound.

If you are called to a deaf patient's home during the night, you may need to help find or adjust a hearing aid. If you cannot locate the device, you might put stethoscope earpieces into the patient's ears and try speaking into the mouthpiece. Alternatively, you might make use of an "amplified" listener (e.g., an ear microphone).

Don't forget one of the most simple and effective means of communication: use of pen and paper. As long as you do not need to move quickly, you can write out notes for the patient to read and wait for the person to respond by speaking or writing. You can also use a pen and paper to draw pictures to illustrate basic needs or procedures. This approach can ease a patient's anxiety, reducing the fear of miscommunication or lack of control over his treatment.

Finally, many people with hearing impairments know sign language, usually American Sign Language (ASL). If you do not know sign language, try to find an interpreter, such as a family member or even a neighbor. Make sure that you document the name of the person who did the interpreting and the information received. Also, notify the receiving hospital of the need to have an interpreter on hand if the interpreter you have used is unable to accompany you.

Visual Impairments

CONTENT REVIEW

➤ Causes of Visual Impairment
- Injury
- Disease
- Congenital conditions
- Infection
- Degeneration of the retina, optic nerve, or nerve pathways

When caring for the patient with a visual impairment, it is important to note whether the impairment is a permanent disability or a new symptom as a result of the illness or injury for which you were called. It is necessary to understand the causes of blindness before this determination can be made.

Etiologies

Visual impairments can result from a number of causes. Possible etiologies include injury, disease, congenital conditions, infection (such as CMV), and degeneration of the retina, optic nerve, or nerve pathways. Descriptions of each of the etiologies follow.

INJURY A previous injury to the eye can cause a permanent vision loss. An injury to the orbit usually includes injury to the tissue around the orbit as well as to the eye itself. This can cause muscle and nerve damage that may lead to permanent loss of eyesight. Penetrating injuries can result in **enucleation**, which is removal of the eyeball. Chemical and thermal burns to the eye can result in damage to the cornea and can also lead to permanent vision loss if not treated quickly. A temporary loss of vision can result from an injury, such as the chemical burn that may occur with the deployment of an air bag, or from a corneal abrasion. Once treated, these injuries rarely lead to permanent loss of vision.

DISEASE Visual impairments may also be caused by a disease of the eye, or as a secondary result of a primary disease process. **Glaucoma**, for example, is a group of eye diseases that results in increased intraocular pressure on the optic nerve. If not treated, glaucoma leads to loss of peripheral vision and to blindness. The incidence of glaucoma is higher in blacks than in whites. A black person between the ages of 45 and 65 is 15 times more likely to have glaucoma than a white person in the same age group.

Diabetic retinopathy is another disease-related visual impairment. It results from diabetes mellitus, which causes disorders in the blood vessels that lead to the retina. Small hemorrhages in these blood vessels lead to a slow loss of vision and possible blindness.

CONGENITAL AND DEGENERATIVE DISORDERS Cerebral palsy is a congenital disorder that causes visual disturbances. Premature birth can lead to blindness in the neonate. Degeneration of the eyeball, optic nerve, or nerve pathways is most commonly caused by aging and can slowly lead to loss of vision. Cytomegalovirus, an opportunistic infection often seen in AIDS patients, can lead to blindness by causing retinitis, an inflammation of the retina.

Recognizing and Accommodating Visual Impairments

Many people with visual impairments live independent, active lives (Figure 7-1). Depending on the degree of impairment and a person's adjustment to the loss of vision, you may or may not recognize the condition right away. In cases of obvious blindness, identify yourself as you approach the patient so the person knows you are there. Also, describe everything you are doing as you do it.

Many people who are blind have tools to assist them in their activities of daily living. The most obvious is a service dog. When approaching a person with a service dog, *do not* pet the dog or disturb it while the dog is in its harness. For the dog, the harness means that it is working. Ask permission from the patient to touch the dog. Never grab the leash, the harness, or the patient's arm without asking permission. Doing this may place you, the dog, or the owner in danger.[1]

Accommodation must be made for transporting the guide dog with the patient. Circumstances and local protocols will dictate whether you transport the dog in the ambulance with the patient or have the dog transported in another vehicle.

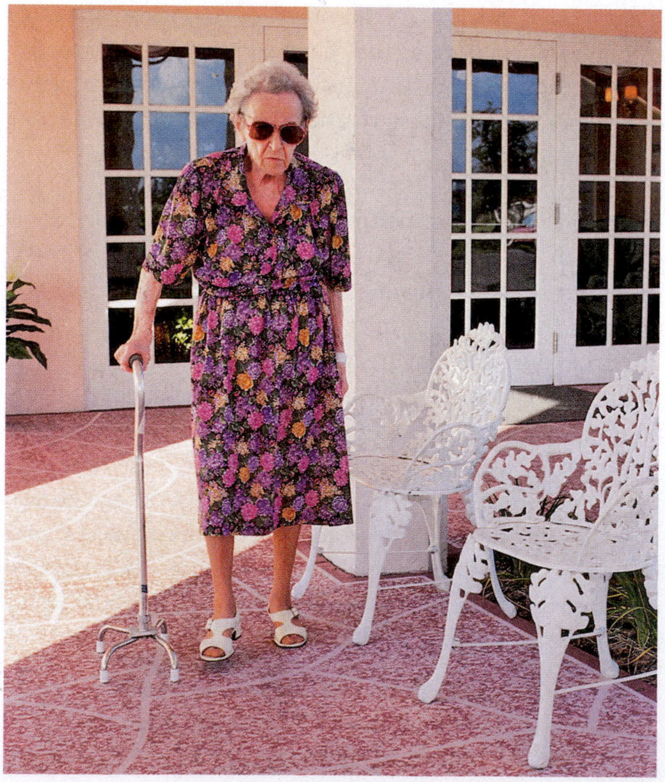

FIGURE 7-1 Individuals who are visually impaired can still maintain active, independent lives.

If your patient does not have a guide dog, inquire about other tools that the person may want brought to the hospital. If the patient is ambulatory, have the person take your arm for guidance rather than taking the patient's arm.

Speech Impairments

When performing an assessment, you may come across a patient who is awake, alert, and oriented, but cannot communicate with you because of a speech impairment. Possible miscommunication can hinder both the treatment you administer and the information that you provide to the receiving facility.

Types of Speech Impairment

You may encounter four types of speech impairment: language disorders, articulation disorders, voice production disorders, and fluency disorders.

LANGUAGE DISORDERS A language disorder is an impaired ability to understand the spoken or written word. In children, language disorders result from a number of causes, such as congenital learning disorders, cerebral palsy, or hearing impairments. A child who receives inadequate language stimulation in the first year of life may also experience delayed speaking ability.

In an adult patient, language disorders may result from a variety of illnesses or injuries. The person may have experienced a stroke, aneurysm, head injury, brain tumor, hearing loss, or some kind of emotional trauma. The loss of the ability to communicate in speech, writing, or signs is known as **aphasia**. Aphasia can manifest itself in the following ways:

- ***Sensory aphasia***—a person can no longer understand the spoken word. Patients with sensory aphasia will not respond to your questions because they cannot understand what you are saying.
- ***Motor aphasia***—a person can no longer use the symbols of speech. Patients with motor aphasia, also known as *expressive aphasia*, will understand what you say, but cannot clearly articulate a response. They may respond to your questions slowly, use the wrong words, or act out answers. It is important to allow such patients to express their responses in whatever way they can.
- ***Global aphasia***—occurs when a person has both sensory and motor aphasia. These patients can neither understand nor respond to your questions. A brain tumor in Broca's region can cause this condition.

CONTENT REVIEW

➤ Types of Speech Impairment
- Language disorders
- Articulation disorders
- Voice production disorders
- Fluency disorders

ARTICULATION DISORDERS Articulation disorders, also known as *dysarthria*, affect the way a person's speech is heard by others. These disorders occur when sounds are produced or put together incorrectly or in a way that makes it difficult to understand the spoken word. Articulation disorders may start at an early age, when the child learns to say words incorrectly or when a hearing impairment is involved. This type of disorder can also occur in both children and adults when neural damage causes a disturbance in the nerve pathways leading from the brain to the larynx, mouth, or lips.

When speaking with people who have articulation disorders, you will notice that they pronounce their words incorrectly or that their speech is slurred. They may leave certain sounds out of a word because they are too difficult for them to pronounce. Again, it is important for you to listen carefully and let the person complete a response.

VOICE PRODUCTION DISORDERS When a patient has a voice production disorder, the quality of the person's voice is affected. This can be caused by trauma or may be due to overuse of the vocal cords or infection. Cancer of the larynx can also cause a speech failure by impeding air from passing through the vocal cords. A patient with a production disorder will exhibit hoarseness, harshness, an inappropriate pitch, or abnormal nasal resonance, or may have a total loss of voice.

FLUENCY DISORDERS Fluency disorders present as stuttering. Although the cause of stuttering is not fully understood, the condition is found more often in men than in women. Stuttering occurs when sounds or syllables are repeated and the patient cannot put words together fluidly. When speaking with patients who stutter, do not interrupt or finish their answers out of frustration. Let patients complete what they have to say, and do not correct how they say it.

Accommodations for Speech Impairments

When speaking to a patient with a speech impairment, never assume that the person lacks intelligence (Figure 7-2). It will be difficult, if not impossible, to complete a thorough interview if you have insulted the patient. Do not rush the patient or predict an answer. Try to form questions that require short, direct answers. Prepare to spend extra time during your interview.

When asking questions, look directly at the patient. If you cannot understand what the person has said, politely ask him to repeat it. Never pretend to understand when you don't. You might miss valuable information about the patient's chief complaint—the reason for the call. If all else fails, give the patient an opportunity to write responses to your questions.

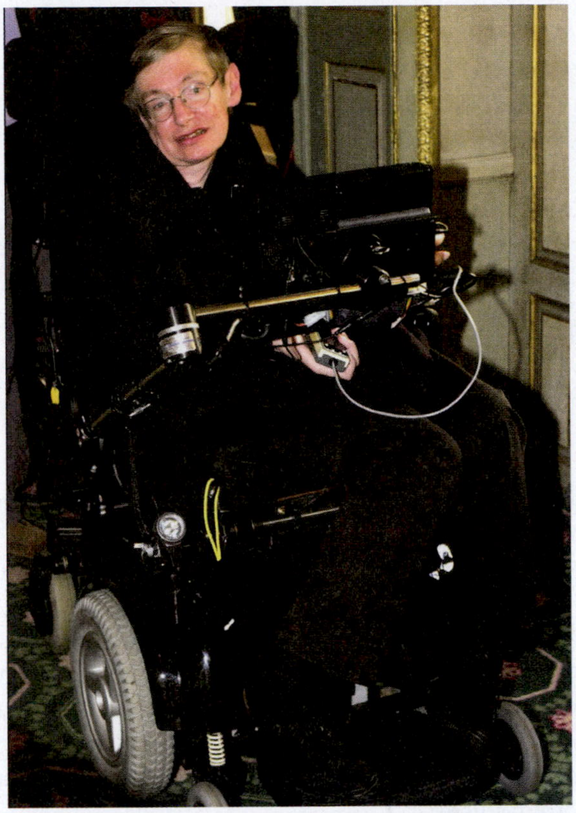

FIGURE 7-2 Physical disabilities do not often impact intellect. Stephen Hawking, the renowned British physicist and mathematician, has done important work despite the crippling effects of amyotrophic lateral sclerosis and the loss of his voice as a result of a tracheostomy.

(© REUTERS/Tobias Schwarz)

Obesity

More than 40 percent of people in the United States are considered obese, and many more are heavier than their ideal body weight. An obese patient can make a difficult job even more difficult for an EMS provider. Besides the obvious difficulty of lifting and moving the obese patient, excess weight can exacerbate the complaint for which you were called. Obesity can also lead to a number of serious medical conditions, including hypertension, heart disease, strokes, diabetes, and joint and muscle problems.

Etiologies

People require a certain amount of body fat to metabolize vitamins and minerals. Obesity occurs when a person has an abnormal amount of body fat and a weight at least 20 to 30 percent heavier than is normal for people of the same age, gender, and height.

Obesity occurs for a number of reasons. In many cases, it happens when a person's caloric intake is higher than the amount of calories required to meet his energy needs. In such cases, diet, exercise, and lifestyle choices play a role in

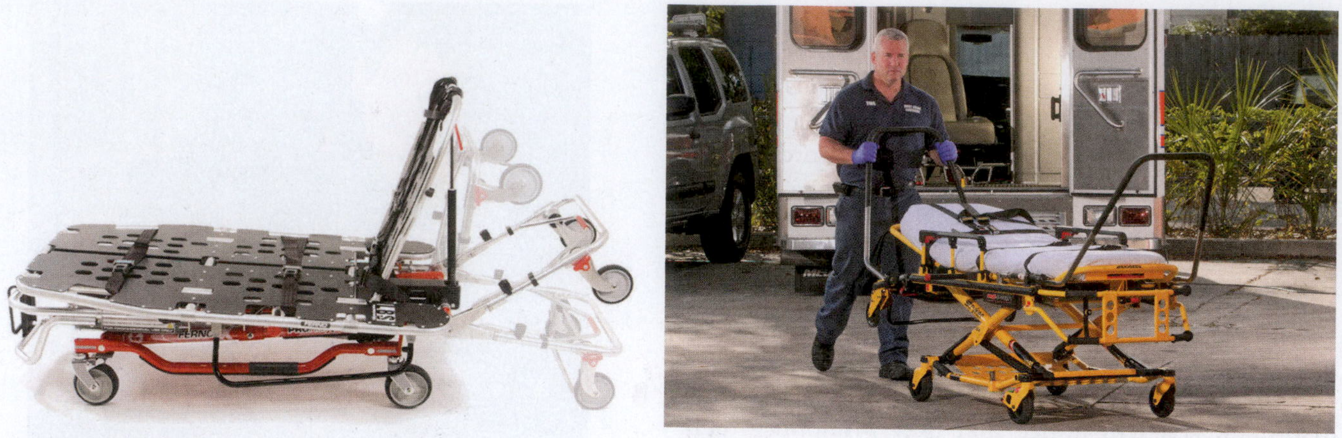

(a)

(b)

FIGURE 7-3 Bariatric cots have been developed that can accommodate obese patients. (a)The Ferno LBS (large body surface) board converts a Ferno cot into a bariatric cot handling up to 1,000 pounds. (b) A variety of manufacturers have developed versions of the bariatric cot.

(Photo a: © Ferno-Washington, Inc.)

the person's condition. Genetic factors may also predispose a patient toward obesity. In rare cases, an obese patient may have a low basal metabolic rate, which causes the body to burn calories at a slower rate. In such cases, the condition may be produced by an illness, particularly hypothyroidism.

Accommodations for Obese Patients

Regardless of the cause of your patient's obesity, your primary responsibility is to provide thorough and professional medical care. Conduct an extensive medical history, keeping in mind the chronic medical conditions commonly associated with obesity.

Obese patients often mistakenly blame signs and symptoms of an untreated illness on their weight. For example, they may quickly dismiss shortness of breath by saying: "When you're as heavy as me, you can't expect to walk up a flight of stairs without some extra breathing." Don't accept such an answer. The shortness of breath may be caused by congestive heart failure. Obtain a complete history of the symptoms and the activities the person was doing when the symptoms appeared. Although the patient usually experiences shortness of breath when climbing stairs, this time the condition may have started while he was sitting down or may have been more severe than usual.

When doing your patient assessment, you may also have to make accommodations for the person's weight. For example, if the patient's adipose tissue presents an obstruction, you may need to place ECG monitoring electrodes on the arms and thighs instead of on the chest. You may also need to auscultate lung sounds anteriorly on a patient who is too obese to lean forward. In assessing an obese patient, flexibility is the key. Keep in mind that no two patients and no two environments will be just alike.[2,3]

Positioning an obese patient for transport may prove especially difficult, because many EMS transportation devices are not designed or rated for heavy weights. Always be sure you have enough lifting assistance for the circumstances. Never compromise your health or safety during the transport process. Another EMS crew or the fire department may be necessary to help move your patient safely. Finally, remember to let the emergency department know that extra lifting assistance and special stretchers will be needed on your arrival (Figure 7-3).

Patho Pearls

Dealing with the Morbidly Obese Patient. Obesity is one of the leading health care problems in the United States today. Several factors can be blamed for this. First, in the 20th century we made a change from a largely agrarian diet to one of processed foods. In the latter half of the 20th century we saw the advent of fast foods. These foods are tasty and readily available—but they contain a large number of calories and saturated fats. In addition, the American lifestyle has become more sedentary, with numerous television channels to watch and numerous video games to play. All these contribute to increasing obesity.

Obesity is often determined using the body mass index (BMI). The BMI incorporates the person's weight and height using the metric system. It is defined as:

$$\text{Body Mass Index (BMI)} = \frac{\text{mass (kilograms)}}{\text{height (meters)}^2}$$

The following definitions of obesity have been established by the World Health Organization based on the BMI:

- Overweight: BMI of 25–29.9 kg/m^2
- Obesity: BMI of 30–39.9 kg/m^2
- Morbid obesity: BMI $\geq$ 40 kg/m^2

The BMI corresponds to the percentage of total body fat. Obesity can also be determined by measuring total body fat;

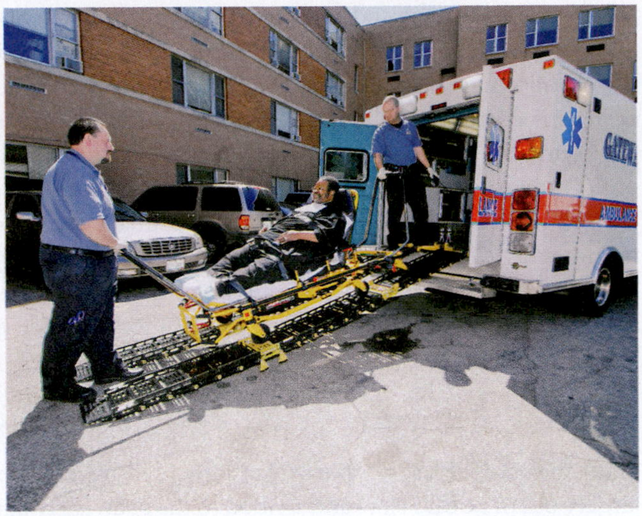

FIGURE 7-4 With an increasing number of morbidly obese patients, many EMS systems have developed specialized bariatric transport units that include bariatric ramp and winch systems.

a male with greater than 25 percent total body fat or a female with greater than 30 percent total body fat is considered obese.

Morbid obesity is defined as being 50 to 100 percent, or 100 pounds or more, above ideal body weight. Morbidly obese persons are at increased risk for diabetes, hypertension, heart disease, stroke, certain cancers (breast and colon), depression, and osteoarthritis. In addition, they tend to develop chronic hypoxemia from inadequate ventilation. This is often complicated by sleep apnea. Morbid obesity is a significant disability, and EMS personnel now encounter the morbidly obese more frequently. Some morbidly obese people can weigh more than 500 pounds and cannot typically be handled by standard ambulance stretchers and equipment. Because of this, several ambulance stretcher manufacturers now manufacture equipment specifically for the morbidly obese. Many ambulance services have developed special ambulances for the obese that contain winches and ramps to ease patient loading.

Moving an obese patient can be a very trying event for all involved. For EMS personnel, it presents several logistical problems. For the patient, it can be a tremendous source of embarrassment. Many of these patients have not been out of their houses in years and now find themselves the center of attention, surrounded by emergency vehicles, often the media, and curious onlookers. Sometimes structural modifications must be made to the house before they can be removed.

Every EMS system must have a protocol and strategy for dealing with the morbidly obese. Many have added bariatric transport vehicles to their fleets (Figure 7-4). They should be treated with the same compassion and care afforded all EMS patients.

Paralysis

Always expect the unexpected in EMS. During your career, you may respond to a call and find that your patient is paralyzed from a previous traumatic or medical event. You will have to treat the chief complaint while taking into account the accommodations that must be made when treating a patient who cannot move some or all of his extremities.

A paralyzed patient may be paraplegic or quadriplegic. A paraplegic patient has been paralyzed from the waist down; a quadriplegic patient has paralysis of all four extremities. In addition, spinal cord injuries in the area of C-3 to C-5 and above may also paralyze the patient's respiratory muscles and compromise the ability to breathe.

If your patient depends on a home ventilator, it is important to maintain a patent airway and to keep the ventilator functioning. Also, a paralyzed patient may have been breathing through a tracheostomy for some time. Therefore, you should keep suction nearby in case the person experiences an airway obstruction. You may also need to use a bag-valve-mask unit to transport the patient to the ambulance if the ventilator does not transport easily. If your ambulance is equipped, use the ventilator with an onboard power supply to save the ventilator's batteries. This is an already anxious time for your patient, so you may need to spend some extra time reassuring the person before making any changes in the life support system.

If the patient has suffered a recent spinal cord injury, halo traction may still be intact. Be sure to stabilize the traction before transport. The patient can probably tell you how to assist with the halo traction; if not, a call to the patient's physician may be necessary.

While performing your physical assessment, you may come across a **colostomy** appliance. This device is necessary when the patient does not have normal bowel function from paralysis of the muscles needed for proper elimination. Be sure to take any other assisting devices, such as canes or wheelchairs, so the patient can get around once out of your care. (For more on acute interventions for people with physical disabilities and other chronic care patients, see the chapter "Acute Interventions for the Chronic Care Patient.")

Mental Challenges and Emotional Impairments

Mental and emotional illnesses present a special challenge to the EMS provider. They may range from psychoses such as schizophrenia to personality disorders to psychological conditions resulting from trauma. Emotional impairments can include such conditions as anxiety or depression. For a detailed discussion of the etiologies, assessment, management, and treatment of these patients, see the chapter "Psychiatric and Behavioral Disorders."

Developmental Disabilities

People with developmental disabilities are individuals with impaired or insufficient development of the brain who are unable to learn at the usual rate. In recent years, a large number of people with developmental disabilities have been mainstreamed into the day-to-day activities of life. They hold jobs and live in residential settings, either on their own, with their families, or in group homes.

Developmental disabilities can have a variety of causes. They can be genetic, as in Down syndrome, or they can be the product of brain injury caused by some hypoxic or traumatic event. Such injuries can take place before birth, during birth, or anytime thereafter.

Accommodations for Developmental Disabilities

Unless a patient has Down syndrome or lives in a group home or other special residential setting, it may be difficult to recognize someone with a developmental disability. The disability may become obvious only when you start your interview, and even then the person may be able to provide adequate information (Figure 7-5). Remember that persons with developmental disabilities can recognize body language, tone, and disrespect just like anyone else. Treat them as you would any other patient, listening to their answers, particularly if you suspect physical or emotional abuse. As mentioned in other chapters, this group has a higher than average chance of being abused, particularly by someone they know.

If a patient has a severe cognitive disability, you may need to rely on others to obtain the chief complaint and history. In this case, plan to spend a little extra time on the physical assessment, because the patient may not be able to tell you what is wrong. In addition, many children or young people with learning disabilities have been taught to be wary of strangers who may seek to touch them. You will have to establish a basis of trust with the patient, perhaps by making it clear that you are a member of the medical community or by asking for the support of a person the patient does trust. Also, some people with developmental disabilities have been judged "stupid" or "bad" for behavior that results in an accident and, therefore, they may try to cover up the events that led up to the call.

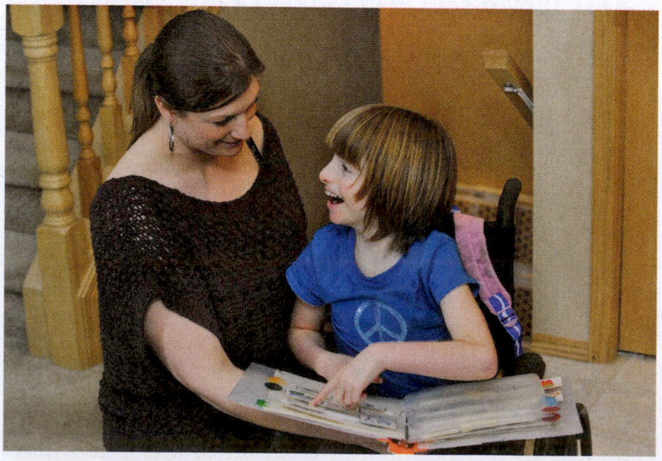

FIGURE 7-5 People with developmental disabilities may have trouble communicating but can often still understand what you say.

At all times, keep in mind that a person with a developmental disability may not understand what is happening. The ambulance, special equipment, and even your uniform may confuse or scare him. In cases of severe disabilities, it will be important to keep the primary caregiver with you at all times, even in the back of the ambulance. Talk to patients with disabilities in terms they will understand and demonstrate what you are doing, as much as possible, on yourself or your partner.

Down Syndrome

Until the mid-1900s, people with Down syndrome lived largely out of public view and tended to die at an early age. Today, people with Down syndrome attend special schools, hold paid jobs, and, because of improved medical care, can live long lives.

Down syndrome is named after J. Langdon Down, the British physician who studied and identified the condition. It results from an extra chromosome, usually on chromosome 21 or 22. Instead of 46 chromosomes, a person with Down syndrome has 47.

Although the cause is unknown, the incidence of this chromosomal abnormality increases with the age of the mother, especially after age 40. It also occurs at a higher rate in parents with a chromosomal abnormality, such as the translocation of chromosome 21 to chromosome 14. In such cases, the parent, usually the mother, has only 45 chromosomes. Theoretically, the chance is one in three that this mother will have a child with Down syndrome.

Typically, Down syndrome presents with easily recognized physical features, including:

- Eyes sloped up at the outer corners
- Folds of skin on either side of the nose that cover the inner corner of the eye
- Small face and features
- Large and protruding tongue
- Flattening of the back of the head
- Short and broad hands

In addition to mild to moderate developmental disability, patients with Down syndrome may have other physical ailments, such as heart defects, intestinal defects, and chronic lung problems. People with Down syndrome are also at risk of developing cataracts, blindness, and Alzheimer's disease at an early age.

When assessing the patient with Down syndrome, consider the level of developmental delay and follow the general guidelines mentioned earlier for dealing with patients who have developmental disabilities (Figure 7-6). Transport to the hospital should be uneventful, especially if the caregiver accompanies you.

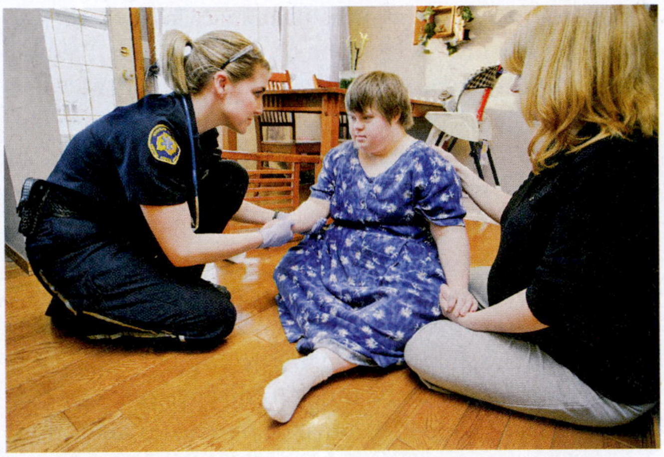

FIGURE 7-6 A patient with Down syndrome may have a mild to moderate developmental impairment.

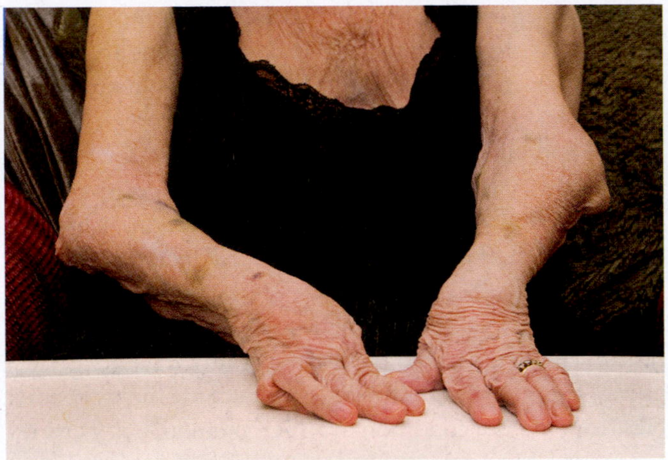

FIGURE 7-7 Rheumatoid arthritis causes joints to become painful and deformed.

Fetal Alcohol Syndrome

Fetal alcohol syndrome (FAS) is sometimes confused with Down syndrome because of similar facial characteristics. Unlike Down syndrome, however, FAS is a preventable disorder, caused by excessive alcohol consumption during pregnancy. Children who suffer FAS have characteristic features, including:

- Small head with multiple facial abnormalities
- Small eyes with short slits
- Wide, flat nose bridge
- Lack of a groove between the nose and lip
- Small jaw

FAS patients often exhibit delayed physical growth, mental disabilities, and hyperactivity. Again, follow the preceding general guidelines when treating children with FAS.

Pathological Challenges

During your career in EMS, you will probably encounter a number of patients with chronic conditions. You should be aware of the most common of these conditions, because chronic care patients require a higher-than-average number of interventions and transports, as discussed in the following sections and in the chapter "Acute Interventions for the Chronic Care Patient."

Arthritis

The three most common types of arthritis are:

- ***Juvenile rheumatoid arthritis (JRA)***—a connective tissue disorder that strikes before age 16
- ***Rheumatoid arthritis***—an autoimmune disorder
- ***Osteoarthritis***—a degenerative joint disease, the most common arthritis seen in elderly patients

All forms of arthritis cause painful swelling and irritation of the joints, making everyday tasks sometimes impossible. Arthritis patients commonly have joint stiffness and limited range of motion. Sometimes the smaller joints of the hands and feet become deformed (Figure 7-7). In addition, children with JRA may suffer complications involving the spleen or liver.

Treatment for arthritis includes aspirin, nonsteroidal anti-inflammatory drugs (NSAIDs), and/or corticosteroids. You should be able to recognize the side effects of these medications because you may be called on to treat a medication side effect rather than the disease. NSAIDs can cause stomach upset and vomiting, with or without bloody emesis. Corticosteroids, such as prednisone, can cause hyperglycemia, bloody emesis, and decreased immunity. You should also take note of all the patient's medications so you do not administer a medication that can interact with the ones already taken by the patient.

When transporting arthritis patients, keep in mind their high level of discomfort. Use pillows to elevate affected extremities. The most comfortable patient position might not be the best position to start an IV, but try to make the patient as comfortable as possible. Special padding techniques may be required because of the patient's arthritis.

Cancer

Entire books have been written about cancer. It is impossible to list here all that a health care provider could learn about this subject. However, some basic points follow that you should keep in mind when treating a patient with cancer.

Cancer is really a blanket term for many different diseases, each with its own characteristics but having in common the abnormal growth of cells in normal tissue. The primary site of origin of the cancer cells determines the type of cancer that the patient has. If the cancer starts in epithelial tissue, it is called a *carcinoma*. If the cancer forms in connective tissue, it is called a *sarcoma*.

It may be difficult for you to recognize a cancer patient, because the disease often has few obvious signs and symptoms. However, treatments for the disease do tend to produce telltale signs, such as alopecia (hair loss) or anorexia (loss of appetite) leading to weight loss. Tattoos may be left on the skin by radiation oncologists to mark positioning of radiation therapy equipment. In addition, physical changes, such as removal of a breast (mastectomy), may be obvious.

Management of the patient with cancer can present a special challenge to the paramedic. Many patients undergoing chemotherapy treatments become neutropenic. **Neutropenia** is a condition in which chemotherapy creates a dangerously low level of neutrophils, the white blood cells responsible for the destruction of bacteria and other infectious organisms. Frequently during chemotherapy the neutrophils are destroyed along with the cancer cells, severely increasing the patient's risk for infection.

If patients have recently undergone chemotherapy, assume that they are neutropenic. Reduce their exposure to infection as much as possible. Remember that, once infected, a neutropenic patient can quickly go into septic shock, sometimes in a matter of hours. For this reason, keep a mask on such patients during both transport and transfer at the emergency department (Figure 7-8).

Also keep in mind that cancer patients' veins may have become scarred and difficult to access as a result of frequent IV starts, blood draws, and caustic chemotherapy transfusions. A patient with cancer may also have an implanted infusion port, found just below the skin, with the catheter inserted into the subclavian vein or brachial artery. This port is accessed for infusion of chemotherapy drugs or IV fluids using sterile technique.

You need special training to use these implanted ports and should not attempt to access them unless you have such training. Local protocols usually dictate whether an EMS provider may access one of these devices. Patients may request that you do not start a peripheral IV if their port can be accessed at the hospital. In such cases, you need to consider if your IV is a lifesaving necessity that cannot wait or if the patient can indeed wait for access at the emergency department.

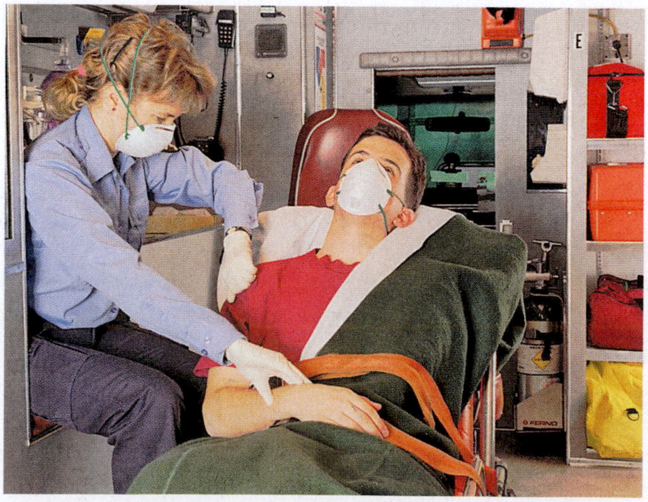

FIGURE 7-8 Make every effort to protect cancer patients from infection. Keep a mask on yourself and the patient during transport and during transfer at the hospital.

Patients with cancer may also have a peripheral access device, such as a Groshong catheter or Hickman catheter, that has access ports that extend outside the skin. In this situation, it may simply be a matter of flushing the line and then hooking up your IV fluids to this external catheter. Whatever you decide to do, involve the patient in the decision-making process whenever possible. Patients with cancer lose much control over their lives during treatment, so it is important for them to maintain as much control over their EMS care as possible.

Cerebral Palsy

Cerebral palsy is a group of disorders caused by damage to the cerebrum *in utero* or by trauma during birth. Prenatal exposure of the mother to German measles can cause cerebral palsy, along with any event that leads to hypoxia in the fetus. Premature birth or brain damage from a difficult delivery can also lead to cerebral palsy. Other causes include encephalitis, meningitis, or head injury from a fall or the abuse of an infant.

Patients with cerebral palsy have difficulty controlling motor functions, causing spasticity of the muscles. This condition may affect a single limb or the entire body. About two-thirds of cerebral palsy patients have a below-normal intellectual capacity, and about half experience seizures. Conversely, a full third of patients with cerebral palsy have normal intelligence and a few are highly gifted.

The three main types of cerebral palsy are spastic paralysis, athetosis, and ataxia. *Spastic paralysis*, which is the most common form of cerebral palsy, forces the muscles into a state of permanent stiffness and contracture. When both legs are affected, the knees turn inward, causing the characteristic "scissor gait." *Athetosis* causes an involuntary writhing movement, usually affecting arms, feet, hands, and legs. If the patient's face is affected, the person may demonstrate drooling or grimacing. *Ataxic cerebral palsy* is the rarest form of the disease and causes problems with coordination of gait and balance.

In treating patients with cerebral palsy, keep this fact in mind: Many people with athetoid and diplegic cerebral palsy are highly intelligent. Do not automatically assume that a person with cerebral palsy cannot communicate with you. Also, as you might expect, many cerebral palsy patients

CONTENT REVIEW

➤ Main Types of Cerebral Palsy
- Spastic paralysis
- Athetosis
- Ataxia

rely on special devices to help them with their mobility. Diplegic patients, for example, may be dependent on wheelchairs.

When transporting patients with cerebral palsy, make accommodations to prevent further injury. If they experience severe contractions, the patients may not rest comfortably on a stretcher. Use pillows and extra blankets to pad extremities that are not in normal alignment. Have suction available if a patient drools. If a patient has difficulty communicating, make sure that the caregiver helps in your assessment. Be alert for patients with cerebral palsy who sign. If you do not know sign language, try to find someone who does and alert the emergency department.

Cystic Fibrosis (Mucoviscidosis)

Cystic fibrosis (CF or **mucoviscidosis**) is an inherited disorder that involves the exocrine (mucus-producing) glands, primarily in the lungs and the digestive system. Thick mucus forms in the lungs, causing bronchial obstruction and atelectasis, or collapse of the alveoli. In addition, the thick mucus causes blockages in the small ducts of the pancreas, leading to a decrease in the pancreatic enzymes needed for digestion. This results in malnutrition, even for patients on healthy diets.

Obtaining a complete medical history is important to the recognition of a patient with cystic fibrosis. A unique characteristic of CF is the high concentration of chloride in the sweat, leading to the use of a diagnostic test known as the "sweat test." A patient with CF may also suffer from frequent lung infections, clay-colored stools, or clubbing of the fingers or toes.

Recent medical advances have extended the lives of patients with CF so that some live well into their thirties. However, because of a poor prognosis, most of the patients with CF that you see will be children and adolescents. In treating these patients, remember that they have been chronically ill for their entire lives. The last thing they may want is another trip to the hospital. For this reason, transport can be difficult for both the patient and family members. To allay their fears, keep in mind the developmental stage of your patient. A child with CF is still a child, so recall everything you have learned about the treatment and comforting of pediatric patients.

Because of the high probability of respiratory distress in a patient with CF, some form of oxygen therapy may be necessary. You may need to have a family member or caregiver hold blow-by oxygen, rather than using a mask, if that is all the patient will tolerate. Suctioning may be necessary to help the patient clear the thick secretions from the airway. CF patients may be taking antibiotics to prevent infection and using inhalers or Mucomyst to thin their secretions. Make sure that you take along all medications so that the hospital staff can continue with the patient's regimen.

Multiple Sclerosis

Multiple sclerosis (MS) is a disorder of the central nervous system that usually strikes between the ages of 20 and 40, affecting women more often than men. The exact cause of MS is unknown, but it is considered to be an autoimmune disorder. Characteristically, repeated inflammation of the myelin sheath surrounding the nerves leads to scar tissue, which, in turn, blocks nerve impulses to the affected area.

The onset of MS is slow. It starts with a slight change in the strength of a muscle and numbness or tingling in the affected muscle. For example, a patient may start to drop things, blaming it on clumsiness. Doctors encourage patients with MS to lead as normal a life as possible, but the patients become increasingly tired. Their gait may become unsteady, and they may slur their speech. Patients with MS may also develop eye problems, such as double vision, owing to weakness of the eye muscles or eye pain due to neuritis of the optic nerve.

The initial signs of MS are usually temporary. However, they return and become more frequent and long lasting. As the symptoms progress, they become more permanent, leading to a weak extremity or paralysis. Over time, some patients may become bedridden and lose control of bladder function. Eventually an MS patient may develop a lung or urinary infection, which may lead to death. As with other chronically ill patients, people with MS may experience mood swings and seek medical attention for their feelings.

Transport of a patient with MS to the hospital may require supportive care, such as oxygen therapy. Make sure the patient is comfortable, by helping to position the person as necessary. Do not expect patients with MS to walk to the ambulance. Even if they normally are ambulatory, they may be in a more weakened state than usual. Again, be sure to bring assistive devices, such as a wheelchair or cane, so the patient can maintain as much independence as possible (Figure 7-9).

Muscular Dystrophy

Muscular dystrophy (MD) is a group of hereditary disorders characterized by progressive weakness and wasting of muscle tissue. It is a genetic disorder, leading to gradual degeneration of muscle fibers. The most common form of MD is Duchenne muscular dystrophy, which typically affects boys between the ages of three and six. It leads to progressive muscle weakness in the legs and pelvis and to paralysis by age 12. Ultimately, the disease affects the respiratory muscles and heart, causing death at

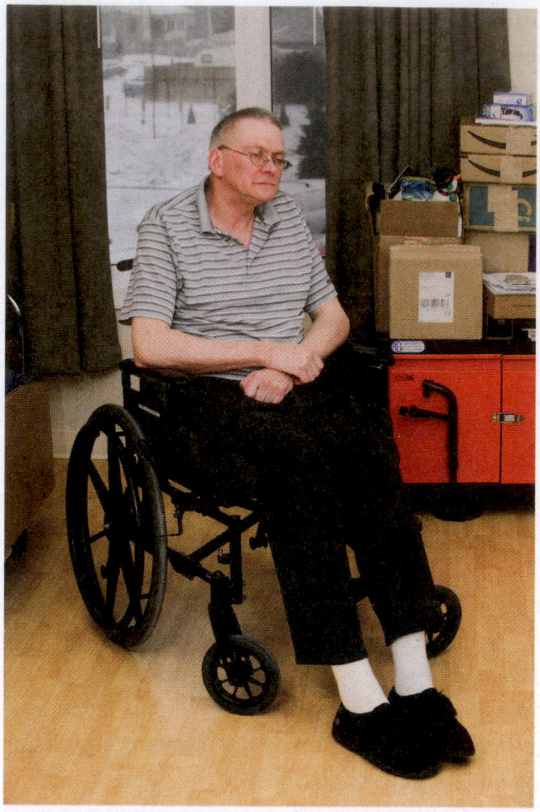

FIGURE 7-9 Patients with multiple sclerosis and muscular dystrophy may need to use wheelchairs.

an early age. The other various MD disorders are classified by the age of the patient at onset of symptoms and by the muscles affected.

Because MD is a hereditary disease, you should obtain a complete family history. You should also note the particular muscle groups that the patient cannot move. Again, because patients with MD are primarily children, choose age-appropriate language. Respiratory support, such as oxygen, may be needed, especially in the later stages of the disease.

Poliomyelitis

Poliomyelitis, commonly called *polio*, is a communicable disease that affects the gray matter of the brain and the spinal cord. Although it is highly contagious, immunization has made outbreaks of polio extremely rare in developed nations. However, it is important to know about polio because many people born before development of the polio vaccination in the 1950s have been affected by the disease.

Typically, the polio virus enters the body through the gastrointestinal tract. It circulates through the digestive tract and then enters the bloodstream. There, it is carried to the central nervous system, where the virus enters and alters the nerve cells. In cases of paralytic poliomyelitis, patients experience asymmetrical muscle weakness that leads to permanent paralysis.

Although most patients recover from the disease itself, they are left with permanent paralysis of the affected muscles. You may recognize a polio victim by the use of assistive devices for ambulation or by the reduced size of the affected limb, which is a result of muscle atrophy. Some patients may have experienced paralysis of the respiratory muscles and require assisted ventilation. Patients on long-term ventilators will typically have tracheostomies.

A related disorder is called *post-polio syndrome*. Post-polio syndrome can develop in patients who suffered severely from polio more than 30 years ago. Although the cause of post-polio syndrome remains unknown, researchers think the condition results from the stress of long-term weakness in the affected nerves. Patients with this condition tire quickly, especially after exercise, and develop an intolerance for cold in their extremities. Unhappily, some persons who survived their original bout with polio die in later years from the effects of post-polio syndrome.

Many patients with polio or post-polio syndrome try to maintain their independence. They may insist on walking to the ambulance but should not be encouraged to do so. The idea of hospitalization will frustrate them, because many polio survivors have memories of spending months or even years in hospitals as children. Unlike other patients with chronic illnesses, most people who have had polio do not require frequent trips to the hospital. Therefore, this may be their first time in the back of an ambulance. Try to alleviate their anxiety as much as possible.

Previous Head Injuries

A patient with a previous head injury may not be recognized easily. You may not notice anything different about the patient until the person starts to speak. A patient who has had a head injury may display symptoms similar to those of a stroke, without the hemiparesis, or paralysis, to one side of the body. The presenting symptoms will be related to the area of the brain that has been injured. The patient may have aphasia, slurred speech, loss of vision or hearing, or a learning disability. Such patients may also exhibit short-term memory loss and may not have any recollection of their original injury.

Obtaining a medical history from these patients is very important, especially if you are responding to a traumatic event. Note any new symptoms the patient may be having or the recurrence of old ones. Conduct the physical assessment slowly. If the patient cannot speak, look for obvious physical signs of trauma or for facial expressions of pain. Transport considerations will depend on the condition for which you were called. However, information about the previous head injury, if you can obtain it, should be an important part of the patient's transfer.

Spina Bifida

Spina bifida is a congenital abnormality that falls under the category of neural tube defects. It presents when there is a defect in the closure of the backbone and the spinal canal. In *spina bifida occulta*, the patient exhibits few outward signs of the deformity. In *spina bifida cystica*, the failure of the closure allows the spinal cord and covering membranes to protrude from the back, causing an obvious deformity.

Symptoms depend on which part of the spinal cord is protruding through the back. The patient may have paralysis of both lower extremities and lack of bowel or bladder control. A large percentage of children born with spina bifida have hydrocephalus, which is the accumulation of fluid in the brain. If the patient has hydrocephalus, a shunt will need to be inserted to help drain off the excess fluid. Permanent disabilities cannot be assessed until the defect is surgically corrected.

When treating patients with spina bifida, keep several things in mind. Recent research has shown that between 18 and 73 percent of children and adolescents with spina bifida have latex allergies. For safety, assume that all patients with spina bifida have this problem. In transporting a patient with spina bifida, be sure to take along any devices that aid the patient. If you are called to treat an infant, safe transport to the hospital should be done in a car seat unless contraindicated.

Myasthenia Gravis

Myasthenia gravis is an autoimmune disease characterized by chronic weakness of voluntary muscles and progressive fatigue. The condition results from a problem with the neurotransmitters, which causes a blocking of nerve signals to the muscles. It occurs most frequently in women between the ages of 20 and 50.

A patient with myasthenia gravis may complain of a complete lack of energy, especially in the evening. The disease commonly involves muscles in the face. You may note eyelid drooping or difficulty in chewing or swallowing. The patient may also complain of double vision.

In severe cases of myasthenia gravis, a patient may experience paralysis of the respiratory muscles, leading to respiratory arrest. These patients will, of course, need assisted ventilations en route to the emergency facility. For patients with less severe cases, accommodations will vary based on presentation.

Other Challenges

In addition to the challenges described in the preceding sections, you can expect to meet a whole range of special situations that will affect the quality of the patient service that you provide. The following are some of the special situations or conditions that you are likely to encounter, if you have not already done so.

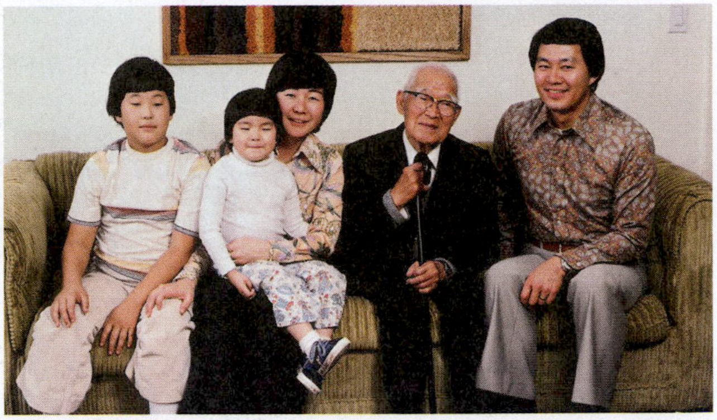

FIGURE 7-10 The population of the United States is becoming increasingly diverse, with the largest number of immigrants coming from Asia and Latin America.

(© Michal Heron)

Culturally Diverse Patients

As a health care provider, you are ethically required to take care of all patients in the same manner, regardless of their race, religion, gender, ethnic background, or living situation. What may make it difficult for you to treat culturally different patients may not be the differences per se but your inability to understand them. Do not consider this a reason for refusing treatment. Rather, consider it a learning experience that will prepare you for a similar situation on another run. With American society becoming more diverse, instead of less diverse, the ability to tolerate cultural differences will become an important part of your professionalism as a paramedic (Figure 7-10).

From time to time, you may encounter a patient who will make a decision about medical care with which you do not agree. For example, Christian Scientists do not believe in human intervention in sickness through the use of drugs or other therapies. You cannot force these patients to accept an IV or to take nitroglycerin if they are having chest pains. Remember, the patient who has decision-making capabilities has a right to self-determination. You should, however, obtain a signed document indicating informed refusal of consent (Figure 7-11).

Accommodation of a culturally diverse population will require patience and, in some cases, ingenuity. If your patient does not speak English, and you do not speak the patient's language, communication may be a problem. You may need to rely on a family member to act as an interpreter or on a translator device, such as a telephone language line, for non-English-speaking people. In such cases, be sure to notify the receiving facility of the need for an interpreter.

REFUSAL OF TREATMENT AND TRANSPORTATION

I, THE UNDERSIGNED, HAVE BEEN ADVISED THAT MEDICAL ASSISTANCE ON MY BEHALF IS NECESSARY AND THAT REFUSAL OF SAID ASSISTANCE AND TRANSPORTATION MAY RESULT IN DEATH OR IMPERIL MY HEALTH. NEVERTHELESS, I REFUSE TO ACCEPT TREATMENT OR TRANSPORT AND ASSUME ALL RISKS AND CONSEQUENCES OF MY DECISION AND RELEASE GOLD CROSS AMBULANCE COMPANY AND ITS EMPLOYEES FROM ANY LIABILITY ARISING FROM MY REFUSAL.

SIGNATURE OF PATIENT

WITNESSED BY

DATE SIGNED

FIGURE 7-11 If a patient refuses care because of cultural or religious beliefs, be sure to have the person sign a refusal of treatment and transportation form.

Terminally Ill Patients

Caring for a terminally ill patient is an emotional challenge. Many times, the patient will choose to die at home, but at the last minute the family will compromise those wishes by calling for an ambulance. In other cases, the patient may call for an ambulance so that a newly developed condition can be treated or a medication adjusted. For more on caring for the terminally ill, either at home or in a hospice situation, see the chapter "Acute Interventions for the Chronic Care Patient."

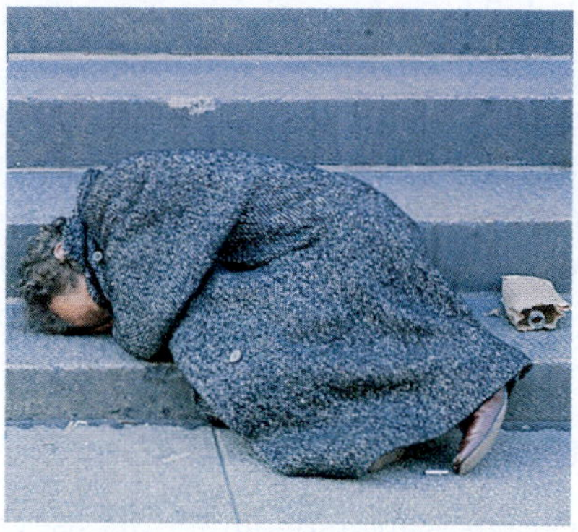

FIGURE 7-12 Homeless people sometimes refuse care, thinking they cannot afford to pay the medical bills. Become familiar with public hospitals and clinics that provide services to the needy.

(© Michal Heron)

Patients with Communicable Diseases

When treating people with communicable diseases, you should withhold all personal judgment. Although you will have to take Standard Precautions just as you would with any patient, keep in mind the heightened sensitivity of a person with a communicable disease. Most of these patients are familiar with the health care setting and understand why you must take certain protective measures. However, you should still explain that you take these measures with all patients who have similar diseases. Also, you do not need to take additional precautions that are not required by departmental policy. The patient will generally spot these extra measures and feel guilt, shame, or anger.

For more information on the etiologies and treatment of communicable diseases, see the chapter "Infectious Disease and Sepsis."

Patients with Financial Challenges

One of the exciting parts of a career in EMS is the opportunity to meet people of all backgrounds. You have the chance to get out into the street and see how people live, work, and play. This allows you to help and educate people who may not otherwise have access to health care. For example, you may get sent to a street corner where a homeless man has fallen and needs medical attention but cannot afford to pay the medical bills. It is your job to help the patient understand that he can receive health care regardless of his financial situation (Figure 7-12).

Become familiar with public hospitals and clinics that provide services to people without money or adequate insurance coverage. Calm a patient's fears by discussing this and providing as much helpful information as you can. In providing care, always keep this guideline in mind: Treat the patient, not the financial condition the patient is in.

Summary

As health care systems improve and make changes, more and more patients with impairments and challenges are beginning to live at home rather than in a medical facility such as a nursing home. EMS is now being summoned to residences for complications with chronic illnesses that were once handled in facilities. Because of this, it is important to be aware of the pathophysiology of diseases that you may encounter and the common complications and treatments seen with them. You will be called for a variety of situations ranging from critical emergencies to simple lifting assistance. In any event, the more you know about the specific situation, the better prepared you will be for the call.

Not all challenges you will face will include chronic illnesses or diseases. Some of these situations may be culturally driven or even financially driven. In any case, keep in mind the legal rights of the patient to accept or refuse treatment, no matter what the reasoning. Keeping patients' best interests in mind includes not only treating their physical being, but also treating their emotional, financial, and spiritual being as well. Remember that it is your responsibility to treat each of your patients with respect and dignity, even if you disagree philosophically with their decisions.

You Make the Call

You and your partner are called to the home of a 56-year-old female patient with a chief complaint of fever. You arrive on the scene to find the door unlocked and a woman calling to you to come to a back bedroom.

She stops you at the door of her bedroom and asks both you and your partner to put on a mask. She tells you that she is undergoing treatment for breast cancer (she has had a mastectomy, she tells you) and that the doctor told her that she shouldn't be around people who are sick because she has an increased risk of infection. She has a scarf around her head and you notice a wig on her bedside table.

She tells you that she has a fever of 102°F and her heart is beating very fast, and this is scaring her. She has had a decrease in appetite and some vomiting. The doctor told her that she should go to the hospital, but she lives alone and didn't have a ride so she called EMS.

Your partner has a cold, so he agrees to drive to the hospital while you ride with the patient. The short transport is uneventful. You arrive at the hospital and transfer patient care to the ED nurse.

1. Why did the patient's doctor tell her that she has an increased risk of infection from communicable diseases?
2. What signs indicate that this patient has cancer?
3. Is it necessary for all three of you to wear a mask? Explain.
4. Will you start a peripheral IV on this patient? Explain.
5. What information will you include in your patient report so the emergency department is prepared for this patient?

See Suggested Responses at the back of this book.

Review Questions

1. Deafness caused by the inability of nerve impulses to reach the auditory center of the brain because of nerve damage either to the inner ear or to the brain is termed ______________
    a. otitis media.
    b. transient deafness.
    c. sensorineural deafness.
    d. conductive deafness.

2. What is the name of the progressive sensorineural hearing loss that begins after age 20 but is significant typically in people over age 65?
    a. Tinnitus
    b. Presbycusis
    c. Labyrinthitis
    d. Otitis media

3. What is the opportunistic infection, often seen in AIDS patients, that can lead to blindness by causing retinitis?
   a. Glaucoma
   b. Enucleation
   c. Diabetic retinopathy
   d. Cytomegalovirus
4. What is said to occur when the patient cannot speak, but can understand what is said?
   a. Visual aphasia
   b. Motor aphasia
   c. Global aphasia
   d. Sensory aphasia
5. A surgical diversion of the intestine through an opening in the abdominal wall where the fecal matter is collected in a pouch is a ____________
   a. stomach.
   b. ileostomy.
   c. colectomy.
   d. colostomy.
6. Down syndrome presents with easily recognized physical features, including all of the following *except* ____________
   a. large face and features.
   b. large and protruding tongue.
   c. short and broad hands.
   d. flattening of the back of the head.
7. The most common form of cerebral palsy is ____________
   a. ataxia.
   b. aphasia.
   c. athetosis.
   d. spastic paralysis.
8. Myasthenia gravis results from a problem with the neurotransmitters and occurs most frequently in women between the ages of ____________
   a. 50 and 60.
   b. 40 and 50.
   c. 10 and 20.
   d. 20 and 50.

See Answers to Review Questions at the back of this book.

References

1. Kom, J. "Servicing the Service Dogs." *Emerg Med Serv* 34 (2005): 56.
2. Haber, C. B. "Bariatric Transport Challenges: Part 1." *EMS Mag* 37(4) (2008): 67–71.
3. Haber, C. B. "Bariatric Transport Challenges: Part 2." *EMS Mag* 37(5) (2008): 73–75.

Further Reading

Barry, P. *Mental Health and Mental Illness*. 7th ed. Philadelphia: Lippincott, 2002.

Dresser, R. *When Science Offers Salvation: Patient Advocacy and Research Ethics*. Oxford, UK: Oxford University Press, 2001.

Early Identification of Hearing Impairment in Infants and Young Children, Program and Abstracts. Bethesda, MD: National Institutes of Health, 1993.

Phipps, W., et al. *Medical-Surgical Nursing: Health and Illness Perspective*. 8th ed. St. Louis: Mosby-Year Book, 2006.

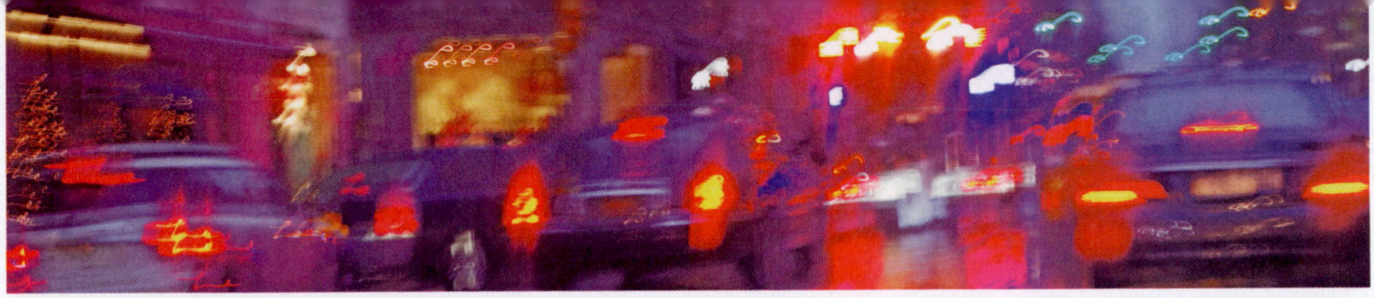

Chapter 8

Acute Interventions for the Chronic Care Patient

Bryan Bledsoe, DO, FACEP, FAAEM, EMT-P

STANDARD

Special Patient Populations (Patients with Special Needs)

COMPETENCY

Integrates assessment findings with principles of epidemiology and pathophysiology and knowledge of psychosocial needs to formulate a field impression and implement a comprehensive treatment/disposition plan for patients with special needs.

Learning Objectives

Terminal Performance Objective: After reading this chapter, you should be able to effectively assess, manage, and take into consideration the psychosocial needs of chronically ill patients encountered in prehospital care.

Enabling Objectives: To accomplish the terminal performance objective, you should be able to:

1. Define key terms introduced in this chapter.
2. Discuss the epidemiology of health care, and describe factors that have contributed to an increase in home health care utilization.
3. Identify reasons that paramedics are summoned to assist patients receiving home health care, and the types of patient complaints that typically accompany these emergencies.
4. Relate the paramedic's role in injury control and prevention by identifying teaching moments as they relate to helping families prepare their home for patient care.
5. Adapt techniques of scene size-up, gathering a patient history and assessment, and providing patient care to patients in the home care setting.
6. Discuss how to integrate history and assessment findings to determine how to care for patients with worsening chronic conditions, or have a malfunction of their home medical equipment.
7. Describe the need to interact with other health care professionals when responding to patients receiving home health care.
8. Identify EMS's role in integrating with hospice and comfort care programs.
9. Given various scenarios, discuss how the paramedic should integrate assessment and management of emergencies in patients with chronic conditions receiving home health care.

KEY TERMS

ARDS, p. 249
BiPAP, p. 243
bronchiectasis, p. 245
cellulitis, p. 237
colostomy, p. 253
cor pulmonale, p. 244
CPAP, p. 243
demyelination, p. 245
emesis, p. 240
exocrine, p. 244
gangrene, p. 235
Guillain-Barré syndrome, p. 235
hemoptysis, p. 244
hospice, p. 238
hypertrophy, p. 235
intermittent mandatory ventilation (IMV) , p. 244
myasthenia gravis, p. 235
PEEP, p. 243
postpartum depression, p. 255
sensorium, p. 236
tracheostomy, p. 247
turgor, p. 237
urostomy, p. 252

Case Study

Desert Springs Paramedic 2 has just ordered a takeout dinner when dispatch reports an "elderly male, short of breath." With a shrug, the crew members cancel dinner and head to the address provided by the dispatcher. On arrival, they find the door slightly ajar and can see the patient sitting on the couch. As they pass through the vestibule, they notice several bottles of oxygen on the floor. They observe that their patient is on a nasal cannula. He is having obvious moderate dyspnea and is using some accessory muscles.

The patient speaks in four- to five-word sentences. He tells the crew that his name is Clarence Casey. Mr. Casey indicates that he is 74 years old. He complains that it has become increasingly difficult for him to breathe. He has used his "puffers" multiple times without relief. Although Mr. Casey says he has no chest pain, he feels as though his breathing has become "heavier."

While the EMT puts together a nebulizer, the paramedic auscultates lung sounds. She notes diminished breathing in all fields with inspiratory and expiratory wheezes. She also observes a prolonged expiratory phase with pursing of lips. The patient is not tripoding and has a respiratory rate of 30 breaths per minute. Use of a pulse oximeter indicates a reading of 86 percent on 4 liters oxygen. The patient's skin is warm, dry, and pale.

On questioning, Mr. Casey tells the crew that he has a history of emphysema, bronchitis, hypertension, and glaucoma, and smoked a pack of cigarettes each day for 60 years. His medications include a Proventil inhaler, a Serevent inhaler, eye drops, and Cardura. He has no allergies. He usually uses oxygen only when walking around the house or doing light chores, such as washing dishes. He lives alone and has home care one day a week. Because of his end-stage COPD, Mr. Casey has authorized a valid prehospital do not resuscitate (DNR) order with his physician, which he shows to the EMS crew.

The paramedic administers nebulized albuterol (2.5 mg/mL) over 15 minutes. She also leaves the patient's nasal cannula at 4 liters per minute. She encourages the patient to take deep breaths. Vital signs indicate a blood pressure of 162/94 mmHg and a pulse rate of 110 beats per minute.

When Mr. Casey is moved to the cot, his dyspnea increases and he becomes more anxious. Reassessment in the ambulance shows that his respiratory rate has increased to 36 and there has been no subjective change in his wheezing. The patient now only speaks in one- to two-word sentences, even though his oxygen saturation has increased to 90 percent. Mr. Casey appears to be growing tired from the work of breathing. The EMT establishes an IV and draws blood. The paramedic contemplates intubating the patient, but the prehospital DNR precludes intubation, so the paramedic is forced to continue pharmacological interventions only.

En route to the hospital, the paramedic administers a second albuterol treatment and continues to encourage Mr. Casey to take deep breaths. Through gentle reassurances, she succeeds in calming him down. During the next 5 minutes, the patient's respiratory rate drops to 30, his wheezes become louder, and tidal volume increases. The patient appears less anxious and the SpO_2 rises slowly to 93 percent.

On arrival at the hospital, the crew administers a third albuterol treatment. The respiratory rate is now 28 breaths per minute, and the patient can again speak in four- to five-word sentences. In the emergency department, the admitting physician gives the patient 125 mg of Solu-Medrol and one more treatment of albuterol. The patient also receives blood tests, chest X-rays, arterial blood gas, and a 12-lead ECG. He is released 5 hours later with a diagnosis of exacerbation of COPD, the acute condition that Mr. Casey treats in a home care setting.

The crew, meanwhile, carefully documents the run and drops off their chart. Luckily, they get a chance to eat dinner before the next call arrives.

Introduction

One of the major trends in modern health care involves the shifting of patients out of the hospital and back into their homes as soon as possible. The result has been a huge increase in home health care needs and services. In 1963, approximately 1,100 home health care agencies existed in the United States. Today, more than 20,000 agencies employ more than 665,000 caregivers: nurses, home health aides, physical therapists, occupational therapists, and other health care professionals. Experts predict that the trend toward home health care will increase in the future. As a result, more and more patients will receive treatment—even of terminal illnesses—in an out-of-hospital setting.[1]

Epidemiology of Home Care

A number of factors have promoted the growth of home care in recent years:

- Enactment of Medicare in 1965
- The advent of health maintenance organizations (HMOs) and patient-centered medical homes (PCMHs)
- Improved medical technology
- Studies showing improved recovery rates and lower costs with home care

Supporters of home health care offer several arguments in its favor. First, they point out that patients often recover faster in the familiar environment of their homes than in the hospital. They also emphasize differences in the cost of home care versus hospital care. With total health expenditures on the rise, the savings promised by home health care continue to speed the dismissal of patients from hospitals and nursing homes.

The shift to home care has important implications for paramedics.[2] As patients and their families assume greater responsibility for their own treatment and recovery, the likelihood of ALS intervention for the chronic care patient increases. Calls may come from the patient, the patient's family, or a home health care provider.

In home care settings, you can expect to encounter a sometimes dizzying array of devices, machines, medications, and equipment designed to provide anything from supportive to life-sustaining care. As a paramedic, you should become familiar with the basic functions of the common home care devices and, just as important, recognize the underlying need for them. The failure or malfunction of this type of equipment has the potential to become a life-threatening or life-altering event. New technologies and machines are being developed constantly. It is your responsibility to stay informed of these changes and the assessment complications that may be involved with the use of each device.

Patients Receiving Home Care

In 1992, the National Center for Health Statistics conducted its first annual National Home and Hospice Care Survey (NHHCS). The survey grew out of the proliferation of home care agencies throughout the United States. The results gave health care professionals their first in-depth look at the home health care population. Key findings from the survey included the following two points:

- Almost 75 percent of home care patients were aged 65 or older.
- Of the elderly home care patients, almost two-thirds were female.

Today some 8 million patients—receiving both acute and chronic care—receive formal health care treatment from paid providers. Millions of others receive unpaid assistance from family members or other volunteers. On average, these informal caregivers give up to 4 hours of assistance per day, 7 days a week. The Balanced Budget Act of 1997 called for a marked reduction in home health expenditures by Medicare. This resulted in a significant reduction in persons receiving Medicare-funded home health care, and thousands of home health agencies folded nationwide. This reduction in the home health care system has put a tremendous load on EMS and is partially responsible for overcrowding of hospital emergency departments. Many EMS systems are now developing innovative programs to deal with this segment of the population.

Patients require home care for a variety of reasons. Some simply do not need to recover from an injury or illness in a hospital or a rehabilitation facility. Their home care is transitory and their conditions usually improve. Other patients have chronic conditions that require varying degrees of home assistance so the patients can live relatively normal lives. These patients usually adjust to their illnesses or disabilities, but never completely recover. Still other patients have terminal illnesses that may or may not involve complicated supportive measures. Their conditions are expected to worsen, and these patients may in fact be waiting to die.

All these situations require sensitivity to the special needs of the patient and consideration of the people involved in the patient's care. Strong emotions may emerge during the call. A previously manageable condition may have suddenly become unmanageable or more complicated. Unlike in a hospital, the patient or home care provider cannot push a button and summon immediate help. Instead, that person often summons you, the ALS provider.

ALS Response to Home Care Patients

A number of situations may involve you in the treatment of a home care patient: equipment failure, unexpected complications, absence of a caregiver, need for transport, inability of the patient or caregiver to operate a device, and more. As already mentioned, you might also be called on to provide emotional support or intervention. Taking responsibility for an illness or an ill family member can be a stressful and overwhelming experience. Some people may be ill equipped to deal with complicated directions, mechanical problems, or the stress of long-term care. Do not minimize their frustrations or allow these frustrations to interfere with your care.

Your primary role as a paramedic is to identify and treat any life-threatening problems. An important source of information is the home care provider, whether that person is a nurse, nurse's aide, family member, or friend. Remember that this person usually knows the patient better than anyone else. The provider will often spot subtle changes in the patient's condition that may seem insignificant to the outsider. In assessing the patient, it is crucial that you listen carefully to what this person says (Figure 8-1).

Home care providers are often health care professionals, but be sensitive in questioning their training or background. You must obtain certain information to care for your patient, and the home care provider may be the only source you have for critical items such as the patient's baseline mental status. If you meet resistance, either from the home care provider's lack of training or from a misunderstanding of your needs, try rephrasing your question or using less technical language. You may also find evidence of neglect or improper patient care by the home care provider. Correct any immediate life threats that you find and document your findings in your patient report. You should also report the situation to your supervisors for corrective action. However, do not confront the home care worker yourself.

CONTENT REVIEW

- ➤ Common Reasons for ALS Intervention
  - Equipment failure
  - Unexpected complications
  - Absence of a caregiver
  - Need for transport
  - Inability to operate a device

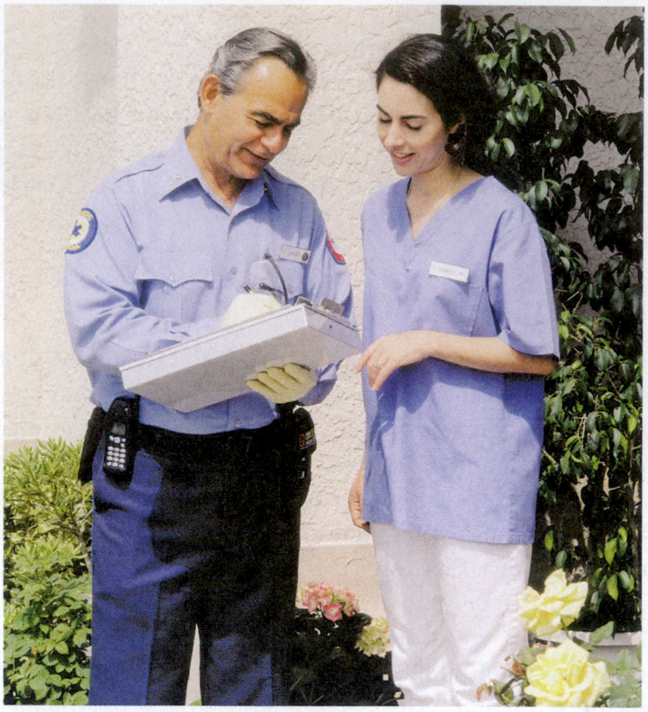

FIGURE 8-1 The home care provider usually knows the patient better than anyone else and will often spot subtle changes in the patient's condition.

At all times, keep in mind the presence of the patient. Involve him in the questioning process. If the caregiver mentions a change or reaction, you might say: "Did you notice this change, too?" "How do you think you reacted?" Your role is to perform as complete and accurate an assessment as possible.

Legal Considerations

Legal Considerations and the Home Care Patient. The line between home care and EMS is becoming increasingly fine. More and more people are cared for in a home setting, and the EMS system is the safety net when a home care patient deteriorates. Numerous legal considerations must be made when dealing with home care patients, especially those who are terminally ill. Various patient self-determination acts have made the terms *living will, durable power of attorney for health care, do not resuscitate order,* and *Uniform Anatomical Gift Act* a part of our vocabulary. These documents often come into play when dealing with a home health care patient or hospice patient. Because of this, it is essential for EMS personnel to understand the intricacies of these documents and any applicable state and local regulations that may apply.

Typical Responses

Many of the medical problems that you will encounter in a home care setting are the same as the ones that you will encounter elsewhere in the field. However, you must always keep in mind that the home care patient is in a more fragile state to begin with. A member of the medical community has already decided that the person needs extra help. A home care patient is likely to decompensate and go into crisis more quickly than members of the general population. As a result, you need to monitor the home care patient carefully and be ready to intervene at all times. Some of the typical responses involve airway complications, respiratory failure, cardiac decompensation, alterations in peripheral circulation, altered mental status, GI/GU crises, infections and/or septic complications, and equipment malfunction. (For more specific information on examples of home care problems requiring acute intervention, see later sections of this chapter.)

AIRWAY COMPLICATIONS The airway is always your paramount concern, and the home care patient is no exception. In the absence of documentation proving the patient's request to withhold intubation and mechanical ventilation, you should protect the airway at all costs. However, even if the patient has a valid DNR order, remember that, in certain situations, you still can use basic airway techniques and suctioning to protect the airway.

Airway compromise can be the result of many different etiologies. Problems that you might encounter include inadequate pulmonary toilet, inadequate alveolar ventilation, and inadequate alveolar oxygenation. (For more on airway problems, see material later in this chapter.)

RESPIRATORY FAILURE As you will read later in this chapter, any number of respiratory problems can be treated in a home care setting. Some of the most common conditions that will lead to respiratory failure or acute crisis include:

- Emphysema
- Bronchitis
- Asthma
- Cystic fibrosis
- Congestive heart failure
- Pulmonary embolus
- Sleep apnea
- **Guillain-Barré syndrome**
- **Myasthenia gravis**

CARDIAC DECOMPENSATION Regardless of the setting, cardiac decompensation is a true medical emergency that can lead to life-threatening shock. This condition requires aggressive identification and treatment. Home care patients who have borderline cardiac output may be placed at risk if their cardiac demand increases from stress or illness and their system cannot compensate. Some other common causes of cardiac decompensation include:

- Congestive heart failure
- Acute myocardial infarction (MI) (Home care patients are at higher risk.)
- Cardiac **hypertrophy**
- Calcification or degeneration of the heart's conductive system
- Heart transplant
- Sepsis

ALTERATIONS IN PERIPHERAL CIRCULATION You already know that the heart circulates blood throughout the body. However, in the case of home care patients, remember that bodily movement also aids in circulation. If a patient has limited mobility, expect the entire circulatory system to be less effective and weaker. As muscle tone declines, so does the flow of blood. When circulation slows, movement becomes more difficult, thus creating a vicious cycle that leads to poorer circulation overall.

Keep in mind that alterations in peripheral circulation can complicate or worsen the course of treatment for a home care patient. Slowed circulation may result in delayed healing, increased risk of infections, or even **gangrene**. Diabetes, a problem that affects some 16 million Americans, commonly results in poor circulation, especially to the extremities. These patients are at high risk of unhealed wounds or ulcers, particularly on the feet.

ALTERED MENTAL STATUS A common ALS response to a home care patient involves some kind of subtle or obvious change in mental status. In the home care patient, always suspect an exacerbation of the condition as well as other causes. Never forget that these patients are at higher risk than the general population of developing new medical problems. Some common causes of altered mental status include:

- Hypoxia (from any number of respiratory or airway problems)
- Hypotension (from any number of cardiac problems or shock)
- Sepsis
- Altered electrolytes or blood chemistries (common in dialysis patients)
- Hypoglycemia (diabetes)
- Alzheimer's disease
- Cancerous tumor or brain lesions
- Overdose
- Stroke (brain attack)

GI/GU CRISES EMS personnel find themselves involved in a number of calls involving home care patients with gastrointestinal or genitourinary problems. The problem often revolves around a misplaced or removed catheter, such as a Foley catheter or a percutaneous endoscopic gastrostomy (PEG) tube. This may not seem like an emergency to you, but the inability to eat or urinate for a period of time can easily compromise an already weakened patient. In addition, home interventions such as peritoneal dialysis can alter fluid balances or electrolytes, creating a subtle but life-threatening problem.

INFECTIONS AND SEPTIC COMPLICATIONS You should always maintain a high index of suspicion for infection in a home care patient with a decreased immune response, either from poor general health or a specific disease. Be particularly alert to infections in patients with indwelling devices such as gastrostomy tubes, peripherally inserted central catheter (PICC) lines, Foley catheters, or colostomies. Also remember that patients with limited lung function or tracheotomies cannot clear their airways easily, putting them at a higher risk of lung infections.

Patients who have decreased **sensorium** from a variety of conditions may have wounds and ulcers that they are unaware of, especially if they have been bedridden or inactive for long periods of time. Surgically implanted drains or wound closures may become infected without the patient realizing it. A bedbound patient may also develop decubitus wounds, pressure sores, or bedsores (Figure 8-2). If these problems are not identified or treated, they can progress from a generalized infection to gangrene and sepsis.

In identifying infections, look for the following general signs:

- Redness and/or swelling, especially at the insertion site of an indwelling device
- Purulent discharge at the insertion site
- Warm skin at the insertion site
- Fever

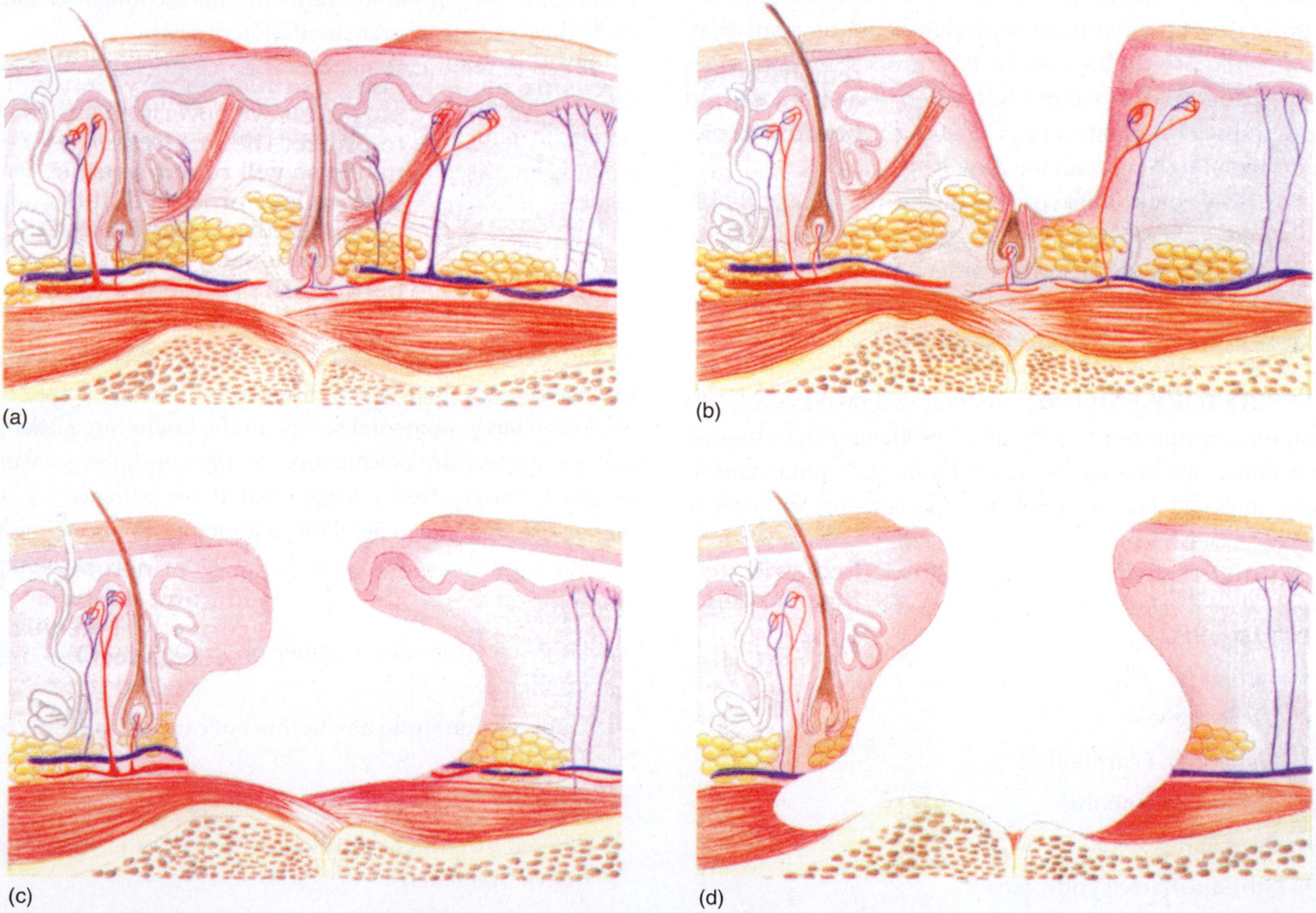

(a) (b) (c) (d)

FIGURE 8-2 Pressure sores are classified by the depth of tissue destruction. (a) **Stage 1:** Inflammation or redness of the skin that does not return to normal after 15 minutes of removal of pressure. Edema is present. It involves the epidermis. Skin may or may not be broken. (b) **Stage 2:** Skin blister or shallow skin ulcer. Involves the epidermis. Looks like a shallow crater. Area is red, warm, and may or may not have drainage. (c) **Stage 3:** Full-thickness skin loss exposing subcutaneous tissue, may extend into the next layer. Edema, inflammation, and necrosis present. Drainage is present, which may or may not have an odor. (d) **Stage 4:** Full-thickness ulcer. Muscle and/or bone can be seen. Infection and necrosis are present. Drainage is present, which may or may not have an odor.

Infection at the cellular level is called **cellulitis** and is not life threatening. When an infection spreads systemically, however, it can lead to sepsis—a serious medical emergency. This may cause a patient's immune system to fail, resulting in septic shock. Signs and symptoms of sepsis include:

- Redness at an insertion site
- Fever
- Altered mental status
- Poor skin color or **turgor**
- Signs of shock
- Vomiting
- Diarrhea

Keep in mind that home care patients may already be receiving treatment for a generalized infection that has, in fact, worsened or spread. Inquire whether a pattern of deterioration has been seen by the caregiver or home care provider. In cases of septic shock, ALS treatment is mainly supportive. Provide fluid for hypotension and necessary airway and oxygen support.

EQUIPMENT MALFUNCTION Home care equipment has the normal limitations of any machine. The power may go out and stop the machine from functioning. The machine may break and/or need maintenance. Some machines, if inoperative, can create a life threat to a patient. Common examples include home ventilators, oxygen delivery systems, apnea monitors, and home dialysis machines.

In cases of equipment malfunction, you may be called on to take the place of a device (such as a ventilator) or to treat problems that have arisen as a result of the malfunction. Even the malfunction of a glucometer can be a difficult situation for some diabetic patients to handle, especially if they suspect hypoglycemia. Your job is to assess the problem and take the appropriate actions.

OTHER MEDICAL DISORDERS AND HOME CARE PATIENTS As already mentioned, you can expect to find a wide variety of problems treated in the home care setting. They can range from an infant on an apnea monitor to progressive dementia in a family member to psychosocial support of the family of a home care patient. Some other conditions that may be treated at home include:

- Brain or spinal trauma
- Arthritis
- Psychological disorders
- Cancer
- Hepatitis
- AIDS
- Transplants (including patients awaiting transplants)

Commonly Found Medical Devices

As previously mentioned, home care patients use a vast number of devices (Figure 8-3). They range from the simplicity of a nasal cannula to the complexity of a home ventilator. If you encounter an unfamiliar device, which may happen at some time in your career, don't panic. Find out what it is used for, and you will then have an idea on how to proceed. Don't be afraid to look foolish by asking questions. You won't. You will be foolish, and endanger the patient, if you pretend to understand a device, but actually do not. Some commonly used devices include:

- Glucometers
- IV infusions and indwelling IV sites
- Nebulized and aerosolized medication administrators
- Shunts, fistulas, and venous grafts
- Oxygen concentrators, oxygen tanks, and liquid oxygen systems
- Oxygen masks and nebulizers
- Tracheostomies and home ventilators

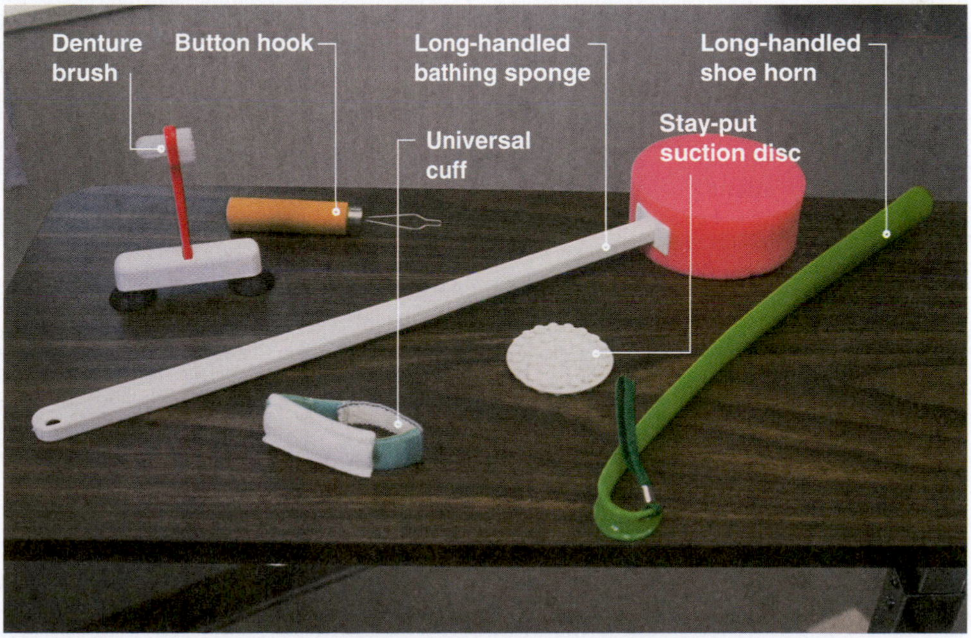

FIGURE 8-3 EMS personnel must become familiar with the common medical devices that they may encounter when providing interventions for the chronic care patient.

- G-tubes, colostomies, and urostomies
- Surgical drains
- Apnea monitors, cardiac monitors, and pulse oximeters
- Wheelchairs, canes, and walkers

Spend some time at the hospital talking with health care personnel about new devices being introduced for the home care setting. Study or make copies of the brochures that come with these devices. You might also talk with manufacturers or vendors, the people who commonly deliver equipment to home care patients.

Intervention by a Home Health Care Practitioner or Physician

Most calls involving home care patients will require acute intervention in problems such as inadequate respiratory support, acute respiratory events, acute cardiac events, acute sepsis, or GI/GU crises. Keep in mind, however, that you may not be the first person to provide intervention. If home care patients have a good relationship with their home health care practitioner or physician, they may contact this person first. In fact, they may be required to do so to receive reimbursement for medical services.

On any call involving a home care patient, be sure to ask whether the patient has called another health care professional. If so, find out what instructions or medications have been issued. Also inquire about written orders from the physician or the physician-approved health care plan. Health care agencies resubmit these plans to physicians at least every 62 days. So check the date to see when the plan was last revised.

In some cases, you may be called to a home care setting in which a home health practitioner or physician must intervene—that is, the scope of the treatment required is beyond your training. In such cases, your role will be mainly supportive. Examples of such conditions include:

- Chemotherapy
- Pain management
- **Hospice** care

Remain especially alert to home care patients receiving medications for pain management. They are at risk for pharmacological side effects and possible overdose. The patient may also be taking nonprescription drugs that could interact with prescribed medications. Substance abuse, especially in critically ill patients, is also a possibility.

Hospice patients have unique psychological needs due to the terminal nature of their illnesses. Although they and their families will have been counseled about the disease process, emotional support is still part of your job. If a call involves a hospice patient, the situation will almost always require intervention by specially trained health care professionals. Find out the names of these people as quickly as possible and determine the advisability of consultation versus rapid transport. (For more on hospice care, see the closing sections of this chapter.)

Injury Control and Prevention

As has been mentioned in the chapters on trauma, the most effective intervention is prevention. Care of the patient begins even before he returns to the home. Some or all of the steps listed in Table 8-1 and Table 8-2 should be taken, depending on the patient's condition. You should also keep in mind a matrix, or strategy, for injury prevention developed by William Haddon in 1972. His 10 steps to injury prevention are essential to all aspects of emergency medicine:

1. Prevent the creation of a hazard to begin with.
2. Reduce the amount of the hazard brought into existence.
3. Prevent the release of the hazard that already exists.
4. Modify the rate of distribution of the hazard from the source.
5. Separate the hazard and that which is to be protected in both time and space.
6. Separate the hazard and that which is to be protected by a barrier.
7. Modify the basic qualities of the hazard.
8. Make that which is to be protected more resistant to the hazard.

Table 8-1 Preparing the Home for Patient Care

Room	Strategies
Bathroom	• Purchase a shower chair and/or tub seat. • Install grab bars. • Install a raised toilet seat. • Hang mirrors, shelves, and racks at wheelchair level. • Set water temperature at a safe level (no higher than 120°F/48.8°C).
Kitchen	• Install easy-to-reach stove dials, countertops, and storage areas. • Provide an easy-to-reach fire extinguisher. • Keep floors dry and nonslippery.
Living Room	• Arrange furniture for free access. • Provide sturdy seating at a suitable height.
Bedroom	• Install a telephone next to the bed. • Obtain a hospital-type bed. • Keep a nightlight or flashlight near the bed. • Keep a bedpan or commode chair within patient reach.
General	• Install smoke alarms. • Provide adequate heating and air conditioning. • Provide good lighting. • Remove all hazards to mobility—throw rugs, electrical wires, etc. • Install wheelchair ramps into house and over doorsills. • Secure all banisters and railings. • Provide a mobile phone.

Table 8-2 Injury Control and Prevention

Organize for Out-of-Hospital Care	• Find out about the patient's condition—length of time for recovery, possible impairments or limitations, prospects for recovery, prescribed treatment plan, frequency of checkups, and possible side effects of medications. • Determine available health care agencies, including home-to-hospital transportation services. • Prepare the home for patient care (see Table 8-1). • Rent or purchase appropriate equipment and learn how it operates. • Arrange for help—Meals on Wheels, visiting nurses, adult day care, and so on.
Provide Proper Bed Care	• Apply restraints—safety vests, safety belts, limb holders, or mitts—as necessary. • Assist in elimination (and safe disposal of wastes). • Encourage exercise. • Look for bedsores or other infections.
Prepare for Emergencies	• Establish a patient baseline. • Learn the danger signs for the patient's particular condition. • Keep a list of emergency numbers at each phone (or program mobile or cell phones). • Notify fire and rescue squads of the patient's condition or special needs. • Obtain necessary Medic Alert identification. • Obtain a Vial of Life and post a decal on the refrigerator door.

9. Counter the damage already done by the hazard.

10. Stabilize, repair, and rehabilitate the object of the damage.

These 10 steps can be used to protect paramedics from the hazards they encounter in the workplace or to protect patients from injuries at home. The steps can be seen in such simple areas as Standard Precautions, the use of side rails to prevent falls, or the use of home rehabilitation to stabilize or repair a patient's injuries.

General System Pathophysiology, Assessment, and Management

Assessment and management of home care patients can be challenging. You can gain confidence by becoming familiar with the pathophysiology of the diseases most commonly found in home care settings. You must also keep in mind the emotional needs of both the home care patient and the caregivers or family members affected by the patient's condition. Some caregivers love what they do and treat the patient's condition as part of their daily lives. Other households feel constant, unremitting stress, and possibly resentment toward the patient's condition.

Getting a feel for the emotional context of a patient's care should be a part of any call. However, in the case of home care patients, you must exhibit extra sensitivity. The way in which you interact with the patient and family can greatly affect the ease and efficiency with which you assess the patient and gather information. Developing a consistent, comprehensive approach to patient assessment and treatment can be your best strategy for dealing with these sometimes complicated responses. The one thing home care calls have in common is their diversity. Be prepared to draw on all your EMS skills and to think quickly as you figure out the most effective management plan.

Assessment

Assessment of the home care patient follows the same basic steps as any other patient: scene size-up, primary assessment, secondary assessment, reassessment, and continued management. However, you will need to modify your mind-set for the home care patient—that is, observe for conditions that you might not ordinarily look for in the general population. This section highlights some of the points you should keep in mind or emphasize when assessing the home care patient. (For more, see the chapters on assessment.)

Scene Size-Up

As with any call, your assessment of the scene begins before you get out of your vehicle. In the case of home care patients, note any special equipment you may observe on entering the home. This will alert you to any possible chronic problems that the patient might have. As you approach the scene, keep the following questions in mind:

- Is there a wheelchair ramp next to the front steps?
- Is oxygen equipment in view?
- Does a trail of oxygen tubing lead into the patient's bedroom?
- Are there infection control supplies on the counter?
- Is there a sharps container present? (This means there are sharps too!)
- Is the patient in a hospital bed?

Introduce yourself to any other medical personnel on the scene—nurse, aide, hospice worker, and so on. By making personal contact, you will help create a health care team that can pool resources and share information. It is a serious mistake to arrive on the scene with a "takeover" mentality that all but eliminates the home care provider from the assessment process.

SCENE SAFETY After you have identified the scene as a home care situation, remain alert for special hazards that might be present. As mentioned earlier, emotions often run high in a home care situation. Evaluate whether any of the people present have a threatening attitude that could be directed toward you. If at any time you don't feel comfortable, withdraw and seek assistance, either from the police or additional personnel. Ask someone to put any pets in another room and have all sources of sound (TV, radio, and so on) turned off so you can work in a quiet, focused environment. As in any patient's home, look for weapons that the patient might use for self-defense, such as firearms, knives, or chemical sprays.

Other special hazards that you may face in a home care situation include infectious wastes, medical supplies such as needles, and potentially dangerous equipment. You would hope that all home care providers would be meticulous with the safe disposal of sharps. However, don't take it for granted. You cannot help any patients if you are on disability because you contracted hepatitis or AIDS from a needle stick. Look around carefully.

In responding to any home care situation, keep in mind the following guidelines:

- Any patient with limited movement may be contaminated with feces, urine, or **emesis**.
- Any bedbound patient may have weeping wounds, bleeding, or decubitus ulcers (bedsores).
- Sharps may be present.
- Collection bags for urine or feces sometimes leak.
- Tracheostomy patients clear mucus by coughing, which can spray.
- Any electrical machine has the potential for electric shock.
- A hospital bed, wheelchair, or walker could be contaminated with body fluid.
- Contaminated medical devices, such as a nebulizer, may be left around unprotected.
- Oxygen in the presence of flame has the potential for fire or explosion.
- Equipment may be in the way and cause you to fall, or it may be unstable and fall on you.
- Medical wastes may not be properly contained or discarded.

Do not minimize the impact of any of these hazards. You can always be contaminated by any patient, but treatment of the home care patient has the potential for a broader range of exposures. Be sure to remove any medical waste you generate so the patient does not return to an unsafe environment. If at all possible, you should also remove any medical waste that is already there for the same reason. Always use Standard Precautions and be careful!

PATIENT MILIEU Another important part of the scene size-up involves an evaluation of the patient's environment. Is the house clean or dirty? Is nutritious food available? Are the sanitary facilities clean? Is the house heated and/or air conditioned? Is there adequate electricity? Is there insect or vermin infestation? The answers to such questions obviously have an impact on the patient's health and ability to recover.

Also note the condition of the patient's specific medical devices. For example, is the nasal cannula clean? Is the wheelchair in good working order? Is the ventilator well situated for safety and effectiveness? Again, these observations provide important clues to the quality of the home care received by the patient and the ability or willingness of the patient to comply with a prescribed treatment regimen.

Remember that you have a responsibility not only to treat the patient, but also to act as an advocate. If a patient is living in a hazardous or unhealthy environment, you have an obligation to notify the proper agency to ensure that the person receives the necessary help. Often, hospital social services will be of assistance. The patient's home care agency or the police might also intervene, depending on the situation.

Remain alert to signs of abuse and/or neglect. In many states, you are required by law to report signs of child or elder abuse. (See the chapters "Pediatrics," "Geriatrics," and "Abuse, Neglect, and Assault.") Know the laws that pertain to the practice of EMS in your state. Home care patients, whether old or young, may be helpless to improve their situations. It is the responsibility of all health care workers to look out for their safety and well-being.

Primary and Secondary Assessments

At this point in your assessment, you may already have a good base of information without actually having seen the patient. As you approach the patient, begin your primary assessment by observing the patient's general appearance, skin color and quality, quality of respiration, and level of distress. Also note any medical equipment that the patient may be currently using.

As you continue to assess the patient for the ABCs, try to ascertain from the primary care provider (if present) a baseline presentation for the patient. Were you called because an existing condition has gotten worse? Or are you here for a new problem? For some home care patients, respiratory distress may be a chronic condition. For example, a patient with chronic obstructive pulmonary disease (COPD) might always have difficulty breathing. Your first impulse may be to reach for your airway supplies, only to find that this is the patient's norm and that you were called to treat an unrelated problem. You must be flexible in your judgments and listen carefully to the report provided by the caregiver or family member who summoned EMS.

As with any patient, treat it as you see it. Once you have established the patient's baseline, assess for changes from the norm. Airway and breathing are always your first concern, followed by circulation. If there are any serious threats to the ABCs, you must treat them. If you are unable to stabilize the patient, complete your rapid assessment and transport immediately. In such cases, your secondary assessment and reassessment will be performed en route to the hospital, if possible.

In noncritical patients, you might take the opportunity to compare vital signs with the bedside records, if they are kept. The focus of your exam should be on the chief complaint and how it might relate to the patient's chronic condition. Be meticulous in your exam, especially with the home care patient. As stated earlier, home care patients are more susceptible to complications than most other patients and can deteriorate rapidly—that is, a noncritical patient can quickly become a critical patient.

In examining a home care patient, be sure to inspect, palpate, and auscultate all potential problem areas. In bedbound patients, look for decubiti (pressure sores or bedsores) on parts of the body subjected to constant pressure or friction. As mentioned, decubiti pose a significant danger to the patient through infection or sepsis and may require surgical debridement.

MENTAL STATUS If your patient has a preexisting altered mental status, such as dementia or Alzheimer's disease, you must have a good understanding of his normal mentation before transport. This information is vital to the physician evaluating and treating the patient at the receiving facility. As stressed in the chapter "Geriatrics," depression can mimic senility and senility can mimic organic brain syndrome. Dementia can also be a sign or symptom of a number of other serious medical problems, such as hypoglycemia or AIDS.

In general, assessment of mental status follows the same general procedure as with other patients. However, you must tailor your questions to the home care setting (Figure 8-4). For example, a person who does not work may be oriented but not know the date or even the day of the week. Also keep in mind the high level of stress in many home care situations and the effect this may have on patient confusion.

To avoid insulting the patient with what may appear to be child-like questions, preface your assessment by saying, "Since I don't know your condition very well, I need to ask you some very basic questions." If patients understand that you are following a systematic assessment, they usually cooperate in what, for them, is often a tedious process.

If a patient cannot or will not answer questions, rely on family members or health care providers to explain why the patient's current mental status is a departure from the norm. For example, belligerent behavior might be normal for a home care patient. If this is the case, find out what is different this time from other times. Perhaps, as pointed out earlier, nothing may be different—the family member or caregiver may have just reached the breaking point and is in need of outside assistance.

Remember that home care patients, especially older or terminal patients, are fearful of being removed from the home environment. This can trigger depression, which in turn worsens a preexisting altered mental status. The key in such cases is tactful questioning combined with your own powers of observation. Pay particular attention to body language and interactions between household members. Note any evidence that the altered mental condition may have been triggered or worsened by a treatable cause and present this information as part of your secondary assessment.

OTHER CONSIDERATIONS In preparing your history, take into account any long-term medical problems (i.e., the conditions that necessitated home care) and the specific events that led to the current crisis. Use the home health history and written orders from the physician, if available. The patient or family may have a discharge sheet with valuable information. As mentioned, talk to the health care provider and to the patient. What changes, if any, have taken place in the patient's life in the recent past? Has patient treatment and/or compliance changed? Are medical devices operating correctly?

Keep in mind that eating habits, fluid intake, and minor illnesses or injuries can have a dramatic effect on a

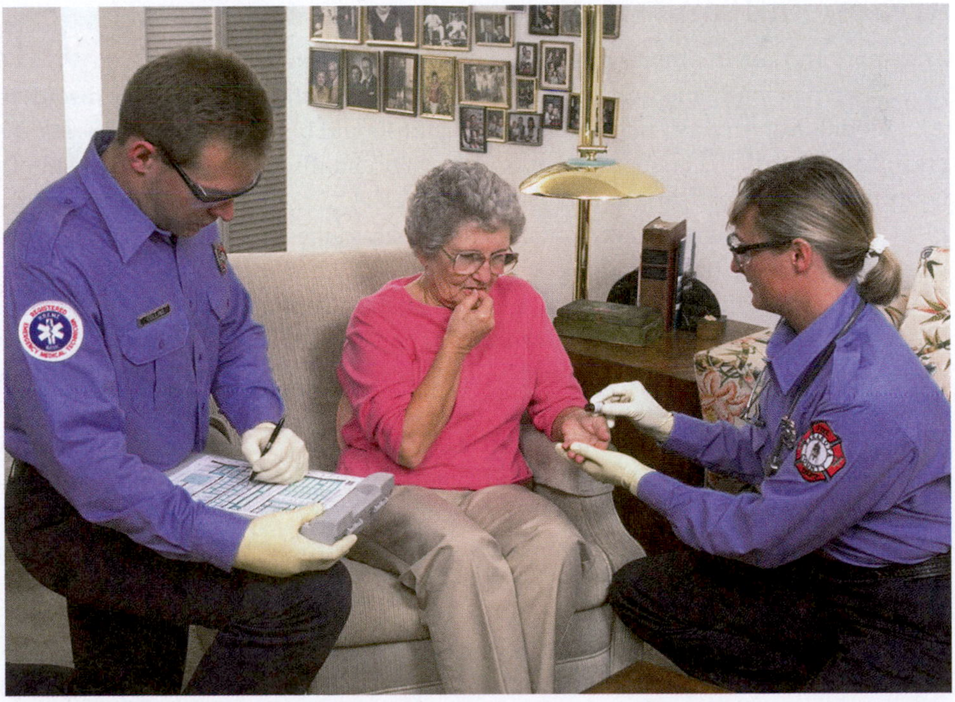

FIGURE 8-4 When assessing a chronic care patient, tailor your questions to the home care setting. Remember that the stress in many home care settings, or fear of removal from the home, can increase patient confusion.

seriously ill homebound patient. Have a high index of suspicion for any new conditions that the patient may be developing. For example, evidence of dementia in an AIDS patient is a serious sign. Correlate this with your physical exam and use this information in developing your treatment plan.

In the case of home care patients, you may more commonly encounter DNR orders, Do Not Attempt Resuscitation (DNAR) orders, living wills, and so on. Ascertain whether these documents are in place before beginning any lifesaving treatments. If that information is unavailable, act in the best interests of the patient. Also, keep in mind that a DNR or DNAR does not mean that you have to withhold *all* treatment. For example, if a congestive heart failure (CHF) patient with crackles and shortness of breath has a DNR, you may still be able to start a line, give nitroglycerin, administer an IV diuretic, and/or transport the patient to the hospital. However, you must read the specific instructions contained within the advance directives and consult with medical control.

Advance directives are designed to prevent unwanted treatment and invasion to the body when natural death or dying occurs. However, many people who have advance directives can be treated in crisis situations and recover. You must use your judgment on a case-by-case basis to determine what qualifies as a resuscitative or life-sustaining measure. (Additional material on advance directives appears later in this chapter.)

Transport and Management Treatment Plan

Transport and/or treatment of a home care patient often involves replacing home health treatment modalities with ALS modalities. Airway and ventilatory support should be straightforward, because EMS providers are usually equipped and trained in the use of most necessary supplies. Some home care interventions, such as Foley catheters, can simply be brought along with the patient. Other interventions, such as PEG tubes, must be flushed and capped, which you may not be trained or equipped to do. In this case, the home care provider should assist you.

In some instances, you may be forced to take the support mechanism on your ambulance if you cannot find a suitable replacement. Certain infusion pumps or other devices may be essential to the patient's well-being and you must bring them along. You should critically assess the risks of discontinuing the home care intervention versus transporting the mechanism. Seek advice from your base physician if you are unfamiliar with the intervention and if the home health provider is unable to help.

When taking a home care patient to a receiving facility, be sure to notify family members and caregivers, if they are not present. Before leaving the scene, secure the home, making sure that doors and windows are locked. In all likelihood, you will need to notify the patient's physician and/or the appropriate health care agency, if you have not already done so.

Document your findings and all care steps carefully. Your run report will become part of the home care patient's record and may, in fact, suggest modifications to the treatment plan. If the patient is not already using a home care agency, provide names of services in your community or refer the person to the proper social service agency. You might also mention nonmedical attendant care, such as housekeeping services and Meals on Wheels. As mentioned earlier, if you suspect the need for intervention in patient care, report your suspicions to the appropriate agency.

Specific Acute Home Health Situations

Although you will undoubtedly intervene in a wide variety of home care situations during your EMS career, you can expect to encounter certain conditions more commonly than others. The chronic care patients that will most likely require acute ALS intervention include those with respiratory disorders, cardiac problems, vascular access devices (VADs), GI/GU disorders, and acute infections. You may also be called on to intervene in the home care of mothers and their newborn infants and to provide assistance in hospice settings. A discussion of each of these situations will help you to prepare for your increasing involvement in the home health care system of the 21st century.

Respiratory Disorders

Respiratory disorders account for more than 630,000 of the hospital patients discharged for home care each year. Nearly 37 percent of patients with simple pneumonia and pleurisy and more than 50 percent of patients with COPD often receive home care within one day of their discharge from the hospital.

Some of the most common home care devices used to treat respiratory disorders include oxygen equipment, portable suctioning machines, aerosol equipment and nebulizers, incentive spirometers, various home ventilators, and tracheostomy tubes and collars. To provide intervention with these devices, you need to review pertinent respiratory anatomy and physiology as it relates to home oxygen and respiratory therapy. (See the chapter "Pulmonology.") You also need to review the pathophysiology of the disorders that most frequently require home respiratory support.

CONTENT REVIEW

➤ Common Acute Home Care Situations
- Respiratory disorders
- Cardiac problems
- Use of VADs
- GI/GU disorders
- Acute infections

Select respiratory disorders and the medical therapy used to treat them are discussed in the following sections. As you read this material, keep in mind earlier comments on the increased risk of airway infections and respiratory compromise in the home care patient.

Chronic Diseases Requiring Home Respiratory Support

Many home care patients have a lung capacity that is minimally able to meet their normal requirements. Sometimes even simple activities, such as climbing stairs, can severely stress their systems. Unlike patients with normal lung capacities, they simply do not have the ability for any increased workload. Even walking from one room to another may require use of oxygen equipment. The following is a review of some of the conditions you may find in the respiratory compromised patient.

COPD As you know, COPD is a triad of diseases: emphysema, chronic bronchitis, and asthma. Some patients may have one, two, or all three disorders. All three are outflow obstructive diseases, impeding the exhalation of air from the lungs. This causes an increase in carbon dioxide and a decrease in oxygenation.

COPD patients work harder to breathe than healthy people do, and they tire quickly. If home equipment fails for any reason, they often panic, thereby worsening their situation. As with any COPD patient, direct your treatment toward increasing oxygen flow. Be prepared to take over their breathing as soon as patients can no longer move enough oxygen to sustain themselves. In some cases, this may mean fixing or replacing home respiratory equipment and/or transport to the hospital (Figure 8-5).

In treating the COPD patient, keep in mind the following disease-specific information.

Bronchitis and Emphysema These two diseases go hand in hand. Most often they result from smoking, but can have other causes as well. Bronchitis involves the chronic overproduction of mucus, which narrows bronchial passages and restricts air flow. Emphysema typically leads to a stiffening and enlargement of the alveoli. This loss of elasticity and compliance requires higher pressures in the lungs to facilitate gas exchanges at the alveolar level. Usually these patients are thin (because breathing takes up a large portion of their daily caloric intake) and barrel chested (due to the retention of air in the lungs as a result of outflow obstruction).

In cases of acute exacerbation, these patients have a difficult time compensating. They may exhibit wheezing with diminished lung sounds, use of accessory muscles, retractions, tripod positioning, and the inability to speak in full sentences. Home treatments that you may see include oxygen, nebulized or aerosol medications, and possibly a ventilator using positive end-expiratory pressure (**PEEP**), continuous positive airway pressure (**CPAP**), or bilevel positive airway pressure (**BiPAP**). PEEP is provided through an endotracheal tube, whereas CPAP and BiPAP are provided through a tightly fitted mask.

When providing intervention, do not forget that home care patients usually have a high dosing regimen, which may make them less responsive to their medications. Always provide these patients with high-concentration oxygen. Medications that may be helpful include:

- Nebulized $beta_2$-specific agonist bronchodilators, such as albuterol or metaproterenol
- IV or oral corticosteroids, such as methylprednisolone (Solu-Medrol)
- Nebulized anticholinergics (ipratropium)

Asthma Asthma, sometimes referred to as *reactive airway disease*, can be seen with patients of any age. A crisis often occurs when some reactant causes an acute constriction of the bronchial passages. Home care patients with asthma can usually handle these episodes on their own. If the episode becomes severe, however, you may be called by a caregiver or parent. (Asthma in children can be especially

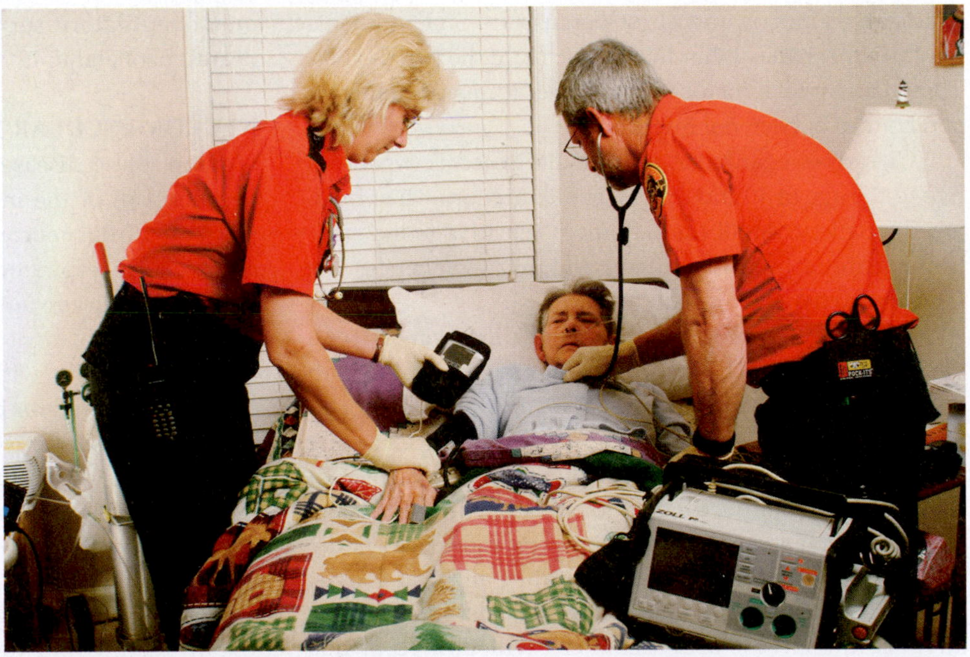

FIGURE 8-5 If the home equipment for a COPD patient fails or is insufficient, you may have to replace it with equipment from the ALS unit.

stressful for the family, so be sure to review its treatment in the "Pediatrics" chapter.)

With asthmatic patients, look for wheezing with diminished lung sounds, use of accessory muscles, and the inability to speak in full sentences. Head bobbing in children is an ominous sign of impending respiratory failure.

Home treatments you may see include oxygen, oral medications, and a variety of nebulizers and/or inhalers. In providing support, always administer high-concentration oxygen. Medications that may be helpful include the same ones used to treat bronchitis and emphysema. You may also consider epinephrine IV or SQ. However, use this medication with caution when treating the elderly or very weak patients.

Long-term care of asthma involves the avoidance or elimination of reactants that can trigger the problem. Try to gather as much information as possible about the cause of the attack so that the physician and patient can take action to avoid future episodes.

CONGESTIVE HEART FAILURE (CHF) CHF often presents as a respiratory problem. For more information on this condition, see "Cardiac Problems" in the chapter "Cardiology."

CYSTIC FIBROSIS (CF) Cystic fibrosis is a genetic disorder usually identified during childhood, sometimes in the late teenage years. It is characterized by chronic and copious overproduction of mucus, inflammation of the small airways and hyperinflation of the alveoli, chronic infections, and erosion of the pulmonary blood vessels secondary to infection. CF is an **exocrine** disease that causes other systemic problems, such as GI disturbances, pancreatic disorders, and glucose intolerance.

Treatment of CF typically involves frequent postural drainage of mucus and chest percussion. Some patients may use mechanical vibrators to facilitate the percussions. They usually take medications aimed at mucus reduction and control of bacterial infection.

CF can be regarded as a terminal disease. Few patients live to the age of 40. Take this fact into account when treating the patient. At all times, remain sensitive to the emotional state of both the patient and any members of the family who may be present.

You may be summoned to help a patient with CF for a variety of reasons. The vigorous coughing associated with the disease can result in **hemoptysis** and pneumothorax. Severe or fatal pulmonary hemorrhage can occur at any time. Patients can also suffer **cor pulmonale**, or right ventricular hypertrophy secondary to pulmonary hypertension.

In treating a patient with CF, ascertain the stage of the disease and inquire about any standing medical orders. Also find out if the patient or family has initiated any advance directives. Your treatment will flow from this information and your own assessment. There is no specific in-field treatment for acute problems stemming from CF. As a general rule, you will provide respiratory support, ventilation, and intubation, if indicated. Be sure to counsel the family or summon the proper counselor to do so, especially if the patient is in the terminal stage of the disease.

BRONCHOPULMONARY DYSPLASIA (BPD) This disease affects primarily infants of low birth weight. It is characterized by an ongoing need for mechanical ventilation in newborns who have been treated for respiratory distress of any cause. These infants may simply fail to wean from mandatory ventilation or from O_2. They are also at increased risk of lower respiratory tract infections, especially viral infections, and may require immediate hospitalization if signs of respiratory infection or increased distress develop.

Home care providers will have been advised to wean infants to lower **intermittent mandatory ventilation (IMV)** settings. However, if the process occurs too quickly, the infant may be at risk of becoming hypoxemic. Arterial oxygenation should be maintained at or above 88 to 90 percent saturation and should be monitored continuously with a pulse oximeter.

Keep in mind that pulmonary congestion and edema may develop in infants with BPD if excessive fluids have been administered. Question caregivers about fluid intake, which may need to be restricted to about 120 mL/kg per day. Inquire, too, about the use of diuretic therapy, which is sometimes prescribed to these patients.

Even after an infant is weaned from a ventilator, supplemental oxygen may still be required for weeks or even months. In such cases, it is usually delivered by nasal cannula.

Remember that BPD is a serious condition in infants. Reduced lung compliance and increased airway resistance may persist for several years. The best treatment is adequate ventilatory support and prompt transport to the nearest neonatal unit.

NEUROMUSCULAR DEGENERATIVE DISEASES As a group, these diseases affect respiratory action through degeneration of the muscles used for breathing. Patients who suffer from neuromuscular degeneration may at some point require respiratory support. Other problems, particularly an inability to ambulate, will have a huge impact on the patient's life.

Many patients with neuromuscular degenerative diseases will be cared for by family members. However, if the condition worsens, professional home care providers may be involved and ALS may be summoned. In cases of respiratory compromise, there is little that you can do other than provide airway and respiratory support and transport. Expect to see all manner of respiratory home care devices, including oxygen and ventilators.

In treating and transporting these patients, keep in mind the following information on the leading neuromuscular degenerative diseases.

Muscular Dystrophy This genetically inherited disorder causes a defect in the intracellular metabolism of muscle cells. (For more details, see the chapter "The Challenged Patient.") The condition leads to degeneration and atrophy of muscles, which are eventually replaced by fatty and connective tissue. There is no cure as yet, and treatment is multidisciplinary because of the many muscle systems involved. These patients have difficulty moving and may need assistance with daily tasks. ALS involvement would almost certainly be for respiratory failure or accidental injuries, usually related to falls.

Poliomyelitis Poliomyelitis is an infectious disease rarely seen today because of effective vaccines. (For more details, see the chapter "The Challenged Patient.") When it does occur, the disease causes destruction of motor neurons, leading to muscular atrophy, muscle weakness, and paralysis. Patients have difficulty ambulating. However, unless respiratory muscles are involved, there may be no systemic effects. Children who contract the disease may suffer permanent crippling or deformity. But once the disease is resolved, further degeneration will cease.

After polio patients recover normal functioning, they sometimes experience a **demyelination** of affected neurons and a return of the disability. This condition is known as *post-polio syndrome* (see the chapter "The Challenged Patient"). Its pathophysiology is unknown.

Guillain-Barré Syndrome This syndrome is thought to be an autoimmune response to a viral (rarely bacterial) infection. It is usually preceded by a febrile episode with a respiratory and/or GI infection. The disease is characterized by muscle weakness leading to paralysis caused by nerve demyelination. It usually starts in the distal extremities and progresses proximally.

Progression of this disorder may take several days. Once it reaches the patient's trunk, respiratory involvement becomes an obvious concern. One way to differentiate Guillain-Barré from a spinal injury is the increased motor involvement. In other words, motor deficits are greater than sensory deficits. As a rule, there is no cognitive or CNS involvement with the disease. With supportive ventilatory care, the patient can be expected to recover.

Myasthenia Gravis Myasthenia gravis is a rare disease that affects the neuronal junction. (For more details, see the chapter "The Challenged Patient.") Because of the breakdown in acetylcholine receptors, nerve impulses are dampened. This disease is characterized by muscle weakness and can be more apparent in muscles proximal to the body than distally.

There is no cure for this disorder, and treatment is aimed at relieving symptoms. If the disease progresses to the diaphragm or intercostal muscles, respiratory compromise can result. Sometimes patients may have an acute exacerbation of the disease brought on by infection or stress. In such cases, intubation or artificial ventilation may be required. These episodes are most commonly preceded by difficulty swallowing or breathing.

SLEEP APNEA Sleep apnea is a complex condition not yet fully understood by experts. It is characterized by long pauses in the respiratory cycle that can be caused by a relaxation of the pharynx or lack of respiratory drive. It can result in hypertension, cardiac arrhythmias, and chronic fatigue.

As a general rule, the muscles of the airway become more relaxed as the mind falls deeper and deeper into sleep. This is what leads to snoring and, in some cases, blockage of the airway. With sleep apnea, decreased oxygen levels cause a partial awakening of the patient. Breathing then resumes and the patient returns to sleep, often with no memory of the incident. Repeated over and over, such interruptions destroy normal sleep patterns and the patient spends much of the sleeping period in a hypoxic state.

People with sleep apnea often suffer alterations in their blood pressure and stroke volume. They loose the normal effect of declining blood pressure as they sleep and their pulse oximetry may fall to 80 percent or less. In patients who have ingested alcohol, the reading can fall to 50 percent.

Treatment of sleep apnea may include surgical alteration of the airway, medications, prescribed loss of weight, avoidance of any CNS depressant or alcohol, or use of a CPAP ventilator.

LUNG TRANSPLANT CANDIDATES Patients receive lung transplants for a variety of cardiopulmonary diseases. Single-lung transplants are performed for pulmonary fibrosis, COPD, or reversible hypertension or cardiac disease. Double-lung transplants are performed for cystic fibrosis, COPD, or **bronchiectasis**. Patients may also receive heart–lung transplants for primary pulmonary hypertension or various congenital diseases. Remember that patients awaiting organ transplants are in the end stages of their diseases and traditional therapies are unlikely to be effective.

Medical Therapy Found in the Home Setting

The treatment of chronic respiratory disorders in the home setting requires a wide range of devices. The following are some of the most common types of medical therapy that you can expect to encounter.

CONTENT REVIEW

➤ Common Home Respiratory Equipment
- Oxygen equipment
- Portable suctioning machines
- Aerosol equipment and nebulizers
- Incentive spirometers
- Home ventilators
- Tracheostomy tubes and collars

HOME OXYGEN THERAPY Oxygen therapy has many advantages for the home care patient. First, it is relatively simple to manage. Second, most patients tolerate it easily. Third, oxygen therapy can add much to the quality of a patient's life. Studies have shown that long-term oxygen use raises the life expectancy of COPD patients considerably. It also prevents hypoxic states that may result in permanent cognitive damage or degeneration.

A medical equipment supplier usually delivers, sets up, and educates patients on the home oxygen delivery systems that they will use. In most cases, the systems include:

- A source of oxygen (e.g., concentrator, cylinder, or liquid oxygen reservoir)
- Regulator–flow meter
- Nasal cannula, face mask, tracheostomy collar, oxygen tubing (large bore for face tents or tracheostomy collars)
- Humidifier
- Sterile water for respiratory therapy (Make sure it is sterile!)

Very few problems arise from the systems themselves. When problems do occur, patients or home care providers can usually correct the situation on their own (Table 8-3). However, you may be called on to provide oxygen while a home system is repaired or to transport the patient to the hospital until the system is replaced. You may also be summoned if a condition unexpectedly worsens and the home oxygen system proves insufficient.

When you arrive at the scene, review the physician's prescription for the type of therapy and the source of the oxygen supply. As already noted, the three sources are:

- ***Oxygen concentrators.*** These systems supply the lowest concentrations of home oxygen. They extract oxygen from room air and add to the flow received by the patient. Home concentrators usually provide no more than 6 liters of oxygen per minute.
- ***Oxygen cylinders.*** Cylinders or tanks are used by patients who may require more than 6 liters per minute or for some reason cannot have a concentrator. Cylinders involve the same technology as that used on EMS portable oxygen systems.
- ***Liquid oxygen.*** Patients who require constant oxygen may have a liquid oxygen system. This allows much more oxygen to be stored in the home. Patients will use this system as a reservoir to fill portable tanks that they may take outside the home.

Although these systems are relatively safe, any high-pressure tank or liquid system has the potential for explosion. In a polite manner, ensure that the patient and home care provider adhere to these safety tips:

- Alert the local fire department to the presence of oxygen in the home.
- Keep a fire extinguisher on hand.
- If a fire does start, turn the oxygen off immediately and leave the house.
- Don't smoke—and do not allow others to smoke—near the oxygen system. (No open flames or smoking should be within 10 feet of oxygen.)
- Do not use electrical equipment near oxygen administration.
- Store the oxygen tank in an approved, upright position.
- Keep oxygen tanks or reservoirs away from direct sunlight or heat.
- Ground all oxygen cylinders.

In terms of the oxygen therapy itself, keep these guidelines in mind:

- Ensure the ability of the patient/home care provider to administer oxygen and to check gauges for supply running low.
- Make sure the patient knows what to do in case of a power failure.
- Evaluate sterile conditions, especially disinfection of reusable equipment.
- As with any patient with chronic respiratory problems, remain alert to signs and symptoms of hypoxemia.

Table 8-3 Common Technical Problems with Oxygen Systems

Problem	Possible Cause	Corrective Action
Oxygen not flowing freely	Faulty tubing	Check for obstruction or replace tubing.
	Dirty or plugged humidifier	Remove from oxygen supply, clean, and refill with sterile water or replace with prefilled bottle.
Buzzer goes off on oxygen concentrator	Unit unplugged	Check plug.
	Power failure	Check fuses, circuit breaker, or, in cases of power outages, use backup oxygen tank until power is restored. (Or call EMS, as necessary.)
Oxygen tank empties too quickly or hisses	Leak in tank	Open all windows, extinguish all flames, and summon help from the fire department, EMS, and/or supplier.

ARTIFICIAL AIRWAYS/TRACHEOSTOMIES Patients who have long-term upper airway problems often have a tracheostomy. A **tracheostomy** is a small surgical opening that a surgeon makes from the anterior neck into the trachea. The tracheostomy may be temporary or permanent. The technique is used on any patient who requires artificial ventilation for a long period of time. (Endotracheal or nasal intubation can be used only on a short-term basis. Pressure on the tracheal tissues, from the inflated cuff, can cause necrosis.) Tracheostomies may also be used on patients who have had damage to their larynx, epiglottis, or upper airway structures from surgery or trauma. They may also be performed on patients who have cancer of the larynx or neck.

The tracheostomy consists of the surgical opening (stoma), an outer cannula, and an inner cannula. The outer cannula keeps the stoma open and is held in place by twill tape or Velcro around the neck. The inner cannula is similar to a mini ET tube and slides down into the trachea a few inches. Because of the small size of the airway, the inner cannula usually has a low-pressure cuff at the end to hold it in place and provide a good seal. In the case of infants, there is no inner cannula because of the small size of infant airways. In addition, the airways of infants are more pliable than those of older patients and more susceptible to blockage.

Tracheostomy patients who have had a laryngectomy may have some ability for speech, and some may have an air connection to the oropharynx or nasopharynx. Keep this in mind if you need to ventilate a person with a tracheostomy. It may be necessary to block off the nose and mouth to prevent air from escaping upwardly instead of being pushed into the lungs.

Patients who are unable to speak will use an artificial larynx. This device looks like a small flashlight. It creates an electronic vibration, which the patient manipulates by pressing the device up against the neck and by changing the shape of his mouth (much as you do when you speak). If the patient does not have an artificial larynx, you will need to resort to writing or signing for communication. Remember that an inability to communicate can create a great deal of stress and frustration for the patient. Try to be part of the solution, not part of the problem.

Routine care of the tracheostomy includes:

- Keeping the stoma clean and dry
- Periodically changing the outer cannula
- Changing and cleaning the inner cannula from every few weeks to every few months, depending on the patient
- For ventilator patients, routine changing of the ventilator hose connections
- Frequent suctioning, because of increased secretions

Remember that a tracheostomy eliminates a large part of the normal air-filtering process. The trapping of bacteria in the nasopharynx and oropharynx no longer occurs; neither does the humidification and heating of air by the nasal passages. This means that bacteria have a more direct route to the lungs, and the air received in the lungs is drier and cooler than normal. Therefore, people with a tracheostomy have a higher incidence of lung infections, mucus production, and irritation. Because they have less control over their airway, it is also more difficult for them to clear blocked airways.

If a patient is not currently using a tracheostomy, it may be closed with a Trach-Button™. This device or a similar one simply plugs up the opening until it is needed again.

Common Complications—The most common problems faced by tracheostomy patients include blockage of the airway by mucus and a dislodged cannula. The patient can usually clear the obstructing mucus by coughing. (Be careful—the mucus can fly out of the stoma for quite a distance.) Sometimes suctioning, either by the patient or by the caregiver, will suffice. Cannulas can become dislodged by patient movement, or, in the case of children, by their growth. In assessing a child with a cannula problem, find out when it was last changed. Maybe the child is ready for the next size. Children can also have their stoma blocked by foreign objects that enter by accident or are put there by a sibling. Other complications include infection of the stoma, drying of the tracheal mucus leading to crusting or bleeding, and tracheal erosion from an overinflated cuff (causing necrosis).

Management—If EMS has been called, it means that neither the patient nor the caregiver has been able to solve the problem. If the tracheostomy patient is on a ventilator, you must rapidly determine if the problem is with the ventilator or with the airway itself. If the problem is simply a loose fitting or disconnected tube, fix it. If the problem is not immediately apparent, do not waste time trying to troubleshoot the machine, unless you are qualified and authorized by local protocols to do so. Your bag-valve device will connect directly to where the ventilator tubing connects. Remove the tubing, connect the bag-valve device to the trach connector, and ventilate (Figure 8-6).

If the problem is with the patient's airway, you will need to clear it. If the patient is hypoxic, always hyperventilate before suctioning. Be sure to evaluate any postural or positional considerations. If the patient is slumped over, straighten him up. Remember to ensure that ventilations are directed downward into the lungs, not upward into the mouth. (Ask the home care provider if there is a connection from the trachea to the upper airway.)

If you are unable to ventilate, clearing the airway is your first priority. Visualize as much of the airway as possible and check for obstructions. If none are visible, introduce a suction catheter and suction while withdrawing—no more than 10 to 15 seconds for an adult, 5 seconds for a child. Again, always hyperventilate before and after suctioning.

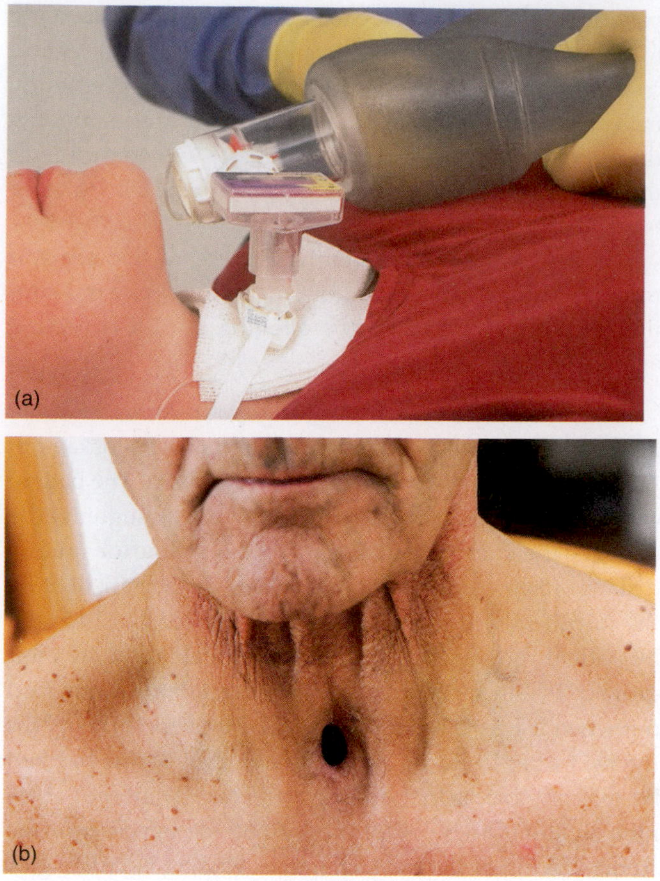

FIGURE 8-6 (a) Artificial ventilation can be accomplished in the patient with a tracheostomy tube by attaching the bag-valve device directly to the tube. (b) Photo shows the site of the stoma.

If it appears that the inner cannula is blocked or dislodged, you may remove it. If cuffed, you must first deflate the cuff. Connect a 10-mL syringe to the cuff valve and withdraw the air. If a syringe is unavailable, you can cut off the valve and the air will escape. You can then remove the inner cannula, hyperventilate, and continue to suction as needed.

If necessary, you may intubate the stoma. The inner cannula must always be removed first. Use an appropriately sized tube to pass through the outer cannula, and advance so the ET cuff (if a cuffed tube is used) is 1 to 2 cm inside the trachea. Inflate the cuff and verify placement by auscultating the epigastrium and both lungs. Add an end-tidal CO_2 device to the end of the tube. Pulse oximetry should also be used to monitor patient oxygenation.

Once the airway is secure, you may proceed with the rest of your assessment. It is inappropriate to proceed until you have protected the airway.

HOME VENTILATION Although you will see positive-pressure ventilators with most home care patients, you may also encounter negative-pressure ventilators. Both devices are used to ventilate patients for a wide variety of diseases and conditions.

Some of the most common reasons patients may be on a ventilator include:

- Decreased respiratory drive
  - Spinal cord injury
- Ventilatory muscle weakness
  - Muscular dystrophy
  - Poliomyelitis
  - Myasthenia gravis
  - Guillain-Barré syndrome
- Obstructive pulmonary disorders
  - COPD
  - Sleep apnea
  - Cystic fibrosis
  - Bronchopulmonary dysplasia
- Other disorders
  - Pediatric sleep apnea
  - Chest wall deformities

Ventilators provide ventilation in several different ways. They also have a number of operating controls and options, depending on the manufacturer. Volume-cycled ventilation, for example, has long been the standard type of ventilatory support for all forms of severe respiratory failure. All modern ventilators can provide this feature as well as several other modes that vary in ventilatory waveform, method of terminating the machine-aided cycle, and so on.

Positive-Pressure Ventilators—According to current practice, positive-pressure ventilation (PPV) is the recommended form of support for acute respiratory disorders. A positive-pressure ventilator pushes air into the lungs, through either a face mask, nasal mask, or tracheostomy. Features of this type of ventilator include variations in tidal volume, respiratory rate, flow rate, and pressure. Optional connectors will be available for oxygen and a humidifier.

There are too many types of positive-pressure ventilators to list here. However, any home care provider should be familiar with a patient's particular machine, including the small ventilators that attach to a mobile patient's wheelchair.

Negative-Pressure Ventilators—Ventilators that apply negative pressure to the chest—tank, cuirass, or poncho-wrap—require a rigid structure to support the vacuum compartment. When they expand, they pull on the chest, causing it to expand and allowing air to flow into the lungs. This mimics the normal breathing process.

The iron lung is one of the best known examples of negative-pressure ventilators. However, some home care patients may also be fitted with a poncho-wrap, which is a suit that is sealed at all openings. Patients most commonly use this device at night.

PEEP, CPAP, AND BiPAP These three ventilator options add pressure at various times in the respiratory cycle. They may be used by full-time or part-time ventilator patients. Keep in mind that the danger of pneumothorax exists because of the increased pulmonary pressure. Take this into account during your assessment of PEEP.

PEEP Positive end-expiratory pressure (PEEP) is used to keep alveoli from collapsing. It works by providing a little back pressure at the end of expiration. This option can be used for newborns—usually premature ones—who have insufficient surfactant to keep the alveoli inflated or in adults who have surfactant washout from acute pulmonary edema, **ARDS**, or drowning.

PEEP also has a use in treating COPD. However, because of stiffening and degeneration of the alveoli in emphysema, patients require higher diffusion pressures for gas exchange. If you ever see COPD patients pursing their lips as they exhale, they are providing their own PEEP. By blowing against a slight resistance, they will keep their alveoli open. A COPD patient who is getting worse may deteriorate to the point at which he needs occasional assistance from a ventilator with PEEP.

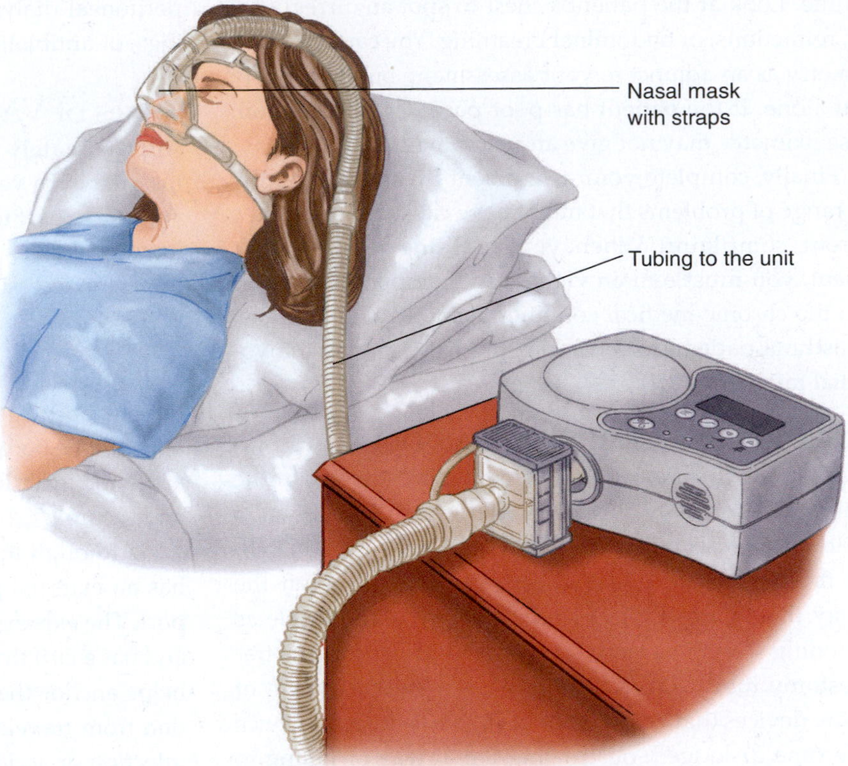

FIGURE 8-7 Sleep apnea patients will often use continuous positive airway pressure (CPAP) to keep their airways open.

CPAP Continuous positive airway pressure (CPAP) is used to keep pharyngeal structures from collapsing at the end of a breath. This option is often prescribed for sleep apnea patients who need help in keeping their airways open. Most of these patients will use nasal CPAP, which is a mask that encompasses the nose (Figure 8-7). In these cases, patients must learn to keep their mouths closed for the mask to work correctly. Otherwise, the pressure will be lost. The idea behind mask CPAP or nasal CPAP is the same as PEEP, except that CPAP is provided via a mask, whereas PEEP is provided via an endotracheal tube.

BiPAP Bilevel positive airway pressure (BiPAP) provides two levels of pressure, one on inspiration and one on exhalation. This option is used for patients who require more or higher levels of pressure than CPAP. Although the settings on the patient's home ventilator may be useful to the ED or to follow-up patient care, they are not essential to your assessment. Try to gather this information at the scene, but don't let it delay your management of any serious airway or breathing problems.

As you may already have inferred, a home care patient with a chronic respiratory problem might eventually progress from home oxygen to occasional ventilator support (PEEP, CPAP, BiPAP) to full ventilator dependency. Knowing each stage of the illness and how it relates to the various ventilatory options will give you a more complete understanding of the patient's clinical progress.

GENERAL ASSESSMENT CONSIDERATIONS Assessment of the respiratory patient should focus on the patient's entire respiratory apparatus. Any deficit found in the system must be rapidly identified and managed.

As you approach the patient, look at the effort required to breathe. Observe for head bobbing, retractions, respiratory rate, tripod posturing, pursed lips, quality and effort of speech, cyanosis, and depth of respiration. Listen for sounds of wheezing or crackles. Note any devices or medications that the patient is currently using.

Immediately assess the patient's mental status by talking to him as you approach. Patients will indicate understanding with their eyes even if they are unable to speak as a result of dyspnea. Note the number of words the patient can speak without stopping for a breath. Rapidly confirm the patient's baseline respiratory effort and mental status from the home care worker, if present.

Next, auscultate the lungs to identify the type of problem that the patient may be having and to determine tidal volume. Look at the patient's chest to spot any irregularities, retractions, or abdominal breathing. You can use pulse oximetry as an adjunct to your assessment, but do not rely on it alone. If the patient has poor peripheral circulation, pulse oximetry may not give an accurate reading.

Finally, complete your assessment by considering the full range of problems that might have caused the patient's current complaint. Whenever assessing a home care patient, you must remain vigilant for complications other than the chronic medical condition being treated at home. An asthma patient, for example, might be having a myocardial infarction (MI).

GENERAL MANAGEMENT CONSIDERATIONS As always, your first considerations when intervening in the care of a chronically ill patient center on the ABCs. In the absence of documentation or a valid prehospital DNR, you must maintain a patent airway or improve on the airway that is already in place. This may be as simple as suctioning secretions from an airway device, such as a tracheostomy tube. You should also assess the placement of airway devices that you did not insert. It is easy for a device to become dislodged, obstructing the airway or failing to ensure patency. You may be forced to remove home airway devices and replace them with your own interventions, such as endotracheal tubes.

Ventilatory problems are traditionally easy to fix in the prehospital environment. If a home ventilator fails, you should begin manual PPV immediately. The failure may be easy to remedy, such as in the case of unplugged power cords or a temporary loss of electricity. If you are trained to work with the ventilator, you can adjust the settings to restore or improve ventilations. However, if you are unfamiliar with the ventilator, play it safe and support ventilations with your own equipment.

As with ventilation, oxygenation problems are also generally easy for EMS providers to fix. First, assess the patency of the patient's home oxygen delivery system. The power may be off, the tubing damaged, or the oxygen supply depleted. You can adjust the flow rate of an intact home oxygen delivery system or replace it with your own system.

Whatever interventions you choose, you will have to make arrangements for the devices to be transported with you to the hospital. Flexibility is the key to transporting home care patients. You should reassure patients that you will properly care for their needs, because they will be physically as well as psychologically dependent on their home care systems.

Vascular Access Devices

Vascular access devices (VADs) are used to provide any parenteral treatment on a long-term basis. The type of device and treatment depend on the disease process involved. Patients may have chemotherapy, hemodialysis, peritoneal dialysis, total parenteral nutrition (TPN) feedings, or antibiotic therapy provided through a VAD.

Types of VADs

Approximately 500,000 long-term therapy catheters are inserted each year. Some of the most common VADs that you can expect to find in the home are described in the following sections. Consult your local protocols and procedures for accessing VADs.

HICKMAN, BROVIAC, AND GROSHONG CATHETERS These catheters may have single, double, or triple lumens and can be inserted into any central vein in the trunk of the body. The subclavian vein is the most common anatomic insertion site, because it is usually easy to locate and secure.

Although these catheters have slight differences, each has an external port that looks like a typical intravenous port. The external hub of the catheter is sutured to the skin and has a cuff that promotes fibrous ingrowth. This growth helps anchor the catheter to the body and prevents infection from traveling down the catheter. The highest risk of infection or accidental removal of the catheter occurs during the first two weeks after insertion. Care of these devices consists of keeping the site clean and dry and administering anticoagulant therapy to prevent clot formations.

PERIPHERALLY INSERTED CENTRAL CATHETERS Peripherally inserted central catheters, or PICC lines, are inserted into a peripheral vein, such as the median cubital vein in the antecubital fossa. These veins are easily accessible and allow a physician to thread a catheter from the insertion site into central venous circulation. PICC lines are inserted under fluoroscopy by radiology rather than in an operating room. As a result, the procedure has a relatively low complication rate (Figure 8-8).

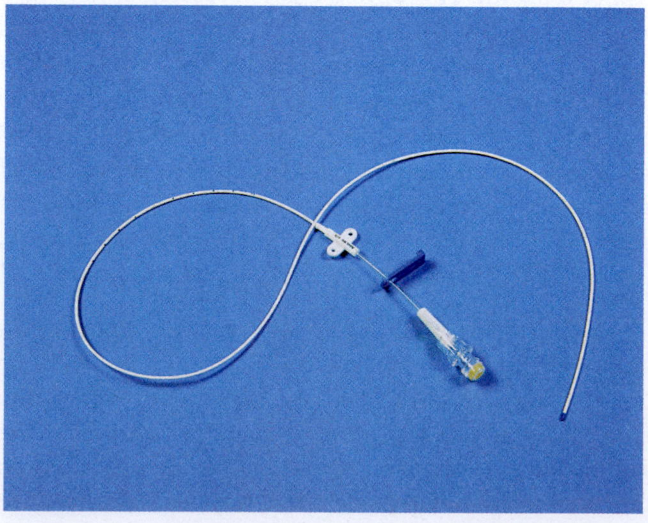

FIGURE 8-8 A peripherally inserted central catheter (PICC). These are usually inserted through an antecubital vein and advanced into the central circulation.

SURGICALLY IMPLANTED MEDICATION DELIVERY SYSTEMS Surgically implanted devices, such as the Port-A-Cath or Medi-Port, are similar to Hickman-style catheters. However, the infusion port is implanted completely below the skin. These devices are disk-shaped and have a diaphragm that requires a specially shaped needle, such as the Huber needle, to access. They are typically found in the upper chest and can be felt through the skin.

Never access a surgically implanted port unless local protocols allow you to do so. If such protocols exist, only properly trained personnel with proper equipment should complete the procedure. A regular intravenous catheter or needle will permanently damage an implanted port. Surgically implanted medication delivery devices should only be accessed using sterile technique.

DIALYSIS SHUNTS Dialysis shunts are used for patients undergoing hemodialysis to filter their blood. An A-V shunt is a loop connecting an artery and a vein, usually in the distal arm, where the dialysis apparatus draws out and returns blood (Figure 8-9). A fistula connects an artery and a vein, creating an artificially large blood vessel for access. It is also usually found in the upper extremity.

Both shunts and fistulas are created surgically and are very delicate. As a result, you should avoid vascular access and application of blood pressure cuffs in the extremity where they are located. (Some jurisdictions allow shunt access by paramedics during life-threatening emergencies.) You will be able to see the shunt in the extremity, and you should be able to auscultate a bruit over the area. Failure to auscultate a bruit over the shunt area may indicate an obstruction, either a thrombus that has formed or an embolus that has lodged there.

Anticoagulant Therapy

Patients with VADs will be on some type of anticoagulant therapy. The most commonly found anticoagulants are those used to flush the device to prevent clot formation. Some patients may be on systemic anticoagulants as well. Because VADs are artificial, the body's natural clotting mechanism must be suppressed to ensure that the devices function properly. As a result, these patients will be much more prone to bleeding disorders. The most common sites for hemorrhage are GI bleeding, strokes, and extremity bruising.

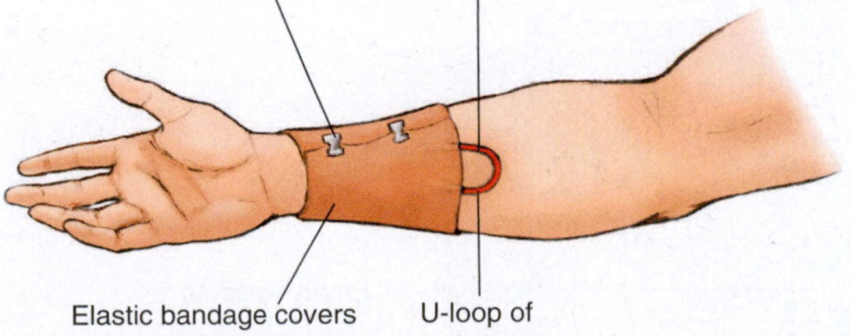

FIGURE 8-9 An A-V shunt is a loop connecting an artery and a vein, usually in the distal arm, where the hemodialysis apparatus draws and returns blood. It is used in home care patients requiring hemodialysis.

VAD Complications

In treating patients with VADs, keep in mind possible complications. The most common complications result from various types of obstructions. A thrombus may form at the catheter site, or an embolus may lodge there after formation elsewhere in the body. Inactivity increases the risk for clot formation. Other obstructive problems include catheter kinking or catheter tip embolus.

With central venous access devices, you should always be aware of the potential for an air embolus. The devices provide a clear pathway for air to enter central circulation. Signs and symptoms of an air embolus include:

- Headache
- Shortness of breath with clear lungs
- Hypoxia
- Chest pain
- Other indications of myocardial ischemia
- Altered mental status

Of course, any device implanted in the body has a risk of infection or hemorrhage. Look for redness, swelling, tenderness, localized heat, or discharge at a potentially infected catheter site. Because these catheters provide a channel into the central circulation, patients may quickly become septic, especially if they are weakened or immunosuppressed.

Cardiac Conditions

Many chronic care patients receive treatment for a wide variety of cardiac conditions. You may be called to intervene in the following situations:

- Post-MI recovery
- Postcardiac surgery
- Heart transplant
- Congestive heart failure (CHF)
- Hypertension
- Implanted pacemaker
- Atherosclerosis
- Congenital malformation (pediatric)

Home care for the cardiac patient can consist of oxygen, monitoring devices, and regular visits by a home health care provider. You can expect to find a variety of medications associated with the specific cardiac problem: bedside cardiac monitors (for adults and children), diagnostic devices such as a halter monitor, and possibly a defibrillator. For a review of the assessment, treatment, and management of cardiac problems, see the chapter "Cardiology."

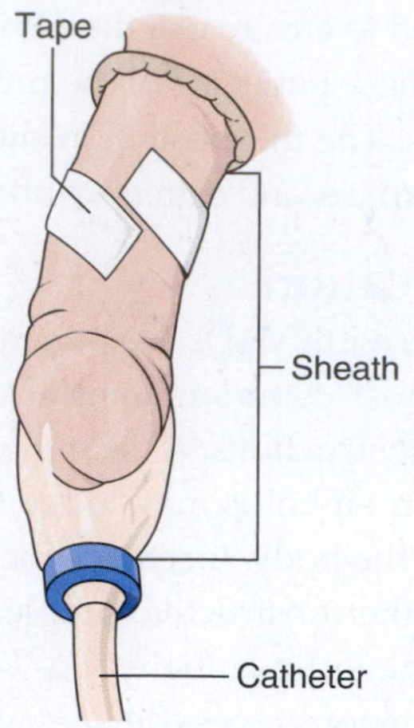

FIGURE 8-10 A condom catheter.

GI/GU Crisis

Patients with various long-term devices to support gastrointestinal or genitourinary functions may need ALS intervention. Your response may be directly related to a problem with the GI or GU device, or you may simply need to be aware of the device and support during transport.

Urinary Tract Devices

Various medical devices have been designed to support patients with urinary tract dysfunction. External devices, such as Texas catheters (also called condom catheters), attach to the male external genitalia to collect urine (Figure 8-10). Because these devices are not inserted into the urethra, they reduce the risk of infection. However, they do not collect urine in a sterile manner, nor are they adequate for long-term use.

Internal catheters, such as Foley or indwelling catheters, are the most commonly used devices for urinary tract dysfunction. They are long catheters with a balloon tip that is inserted through the urethra into the urinary bladder. The balloon is then inflated with saline to keep the device in place (Figure 8-11). Internal catheters are well tolerated for long-term use and are frequently found in hospitals, skilled nursing facilities, or home care situations.

Suprapubic catheters are similar in purpose to internal catheters. However, they are inserted directly through the abdominal wall into the urinary bladder. Suprapubic catheters may be used instead of indwelling catheters in the event of surgery or other problems with the genitalia or bladder.

A **urostomy** is a surgical diversion of the urinary tract to a stoma, or hole, in the abdominal wall. A collection device will be attached to the stoma outside the body to collect urine. Urostomies are used when the bladder is unable to collect urine effectively.

Urinary Device Complications

Most complications related to urinary tract support devices result from infection or device malfunctions. Infection is a very common problem with urinary tract devices because the area is rich with pathogens and because the catheter provides a pathway directly into the body. Remain alert to foul-smelling urine or altered urine color, such as tea-colored, cloudy, or blood-tinged urine. Also look for signs and symptoms of systemic infection, or urosepsis, because urinary infections can quickly spread in the immunocompromised patient. Suprapubic catheters or urostomies may also have infections at the abdominal wall site. You should note redness, swelling, heat, discharge, or loss of skin integrity.

Device malfunctions typically include accidental displacement of the device, obstruction, balloon ruptures in devices that use a balloon as an anchor, or leaking collection devices. Changes in the patient's anatomy, such as a shortened urinary tract or tissue necrosis, can also cause malfunctions. Ensure that the collection device is empty

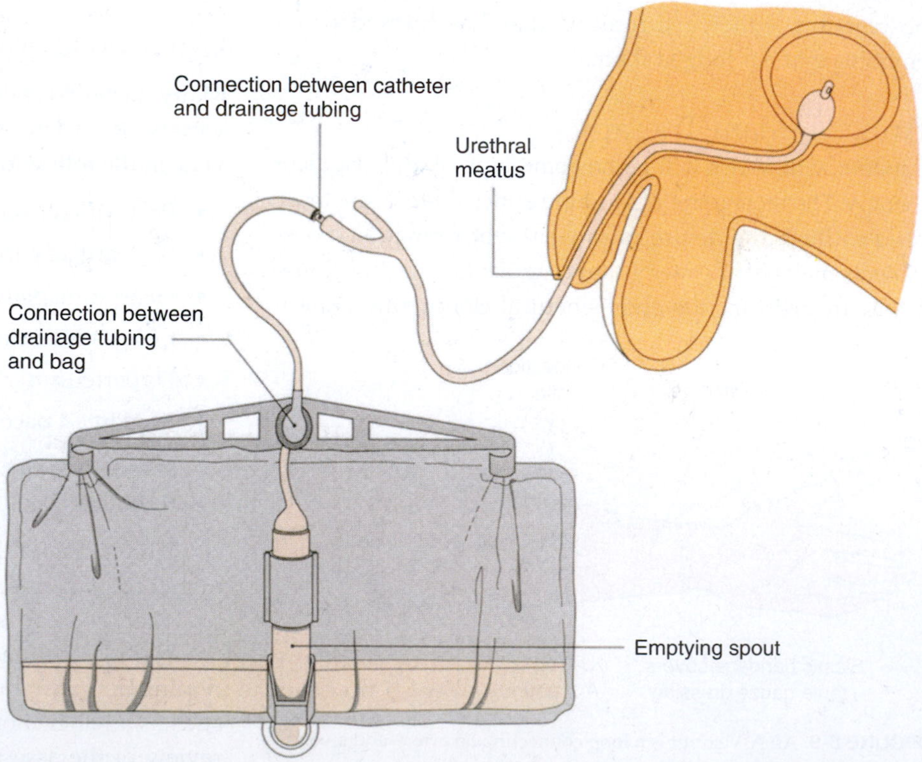

FIGURE 8-11 An indwelling Foley catheter with balloon. Note sites where bacteria can enter.

and record the amount of urine output. Look for kinks or other obstructions in the device, and make sure that the collection bag is placed below the patient.

Gastrointestinal Tract Devices

You can expect to encounter a wide variety of devices to support the gastrointestinal tract. Nasogastric (NG) tubes are commonly seen by EMS personnel because they are often used to decompress gastric contents in the prehospital environment (Figure 8-12). NG tubes may also be used to lavage the GI system in various situations, such as GI bleeding or substance ingestion. NG tubes are not usually long-term devices, because they cause discomfort and may lead to tissue necrosis in the nasal passages if left intact for an extended period.

Feeding tubes are more substantial than NG tubes and come to rest in either the duodenum or jejunum. Often they are weighted to help them pass through the pyloric sphincter and have a steel filament to facilitate insertion. Feeding tubes are used for supplemental nutrition when a person cannot swallow because of dysphagia, paralysis, or unconsciousness.

For longer-term supplemental nutrition, a gastric tube may be inserted through the abdominal wall into the small intestine (Figure 8-13). Indications for a gastrostomy tube include Alzheimer's disease, neurologic deficits from strokes or head trauma, or mental retardation. Gastrostomy tubes come in many forms, such as percutaneous endoscopic gastrostomy tubes, surgical gastrostomy tubes,

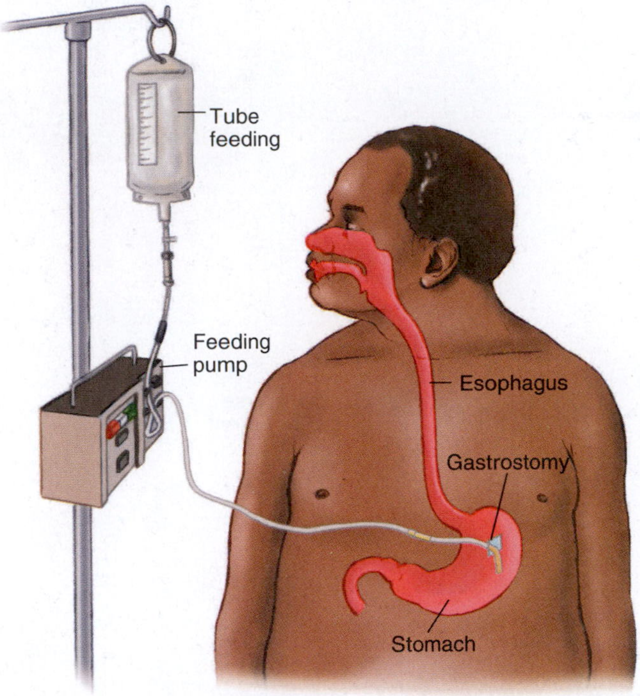

FIGURE 8-13 A gastrostomy feeding tube.

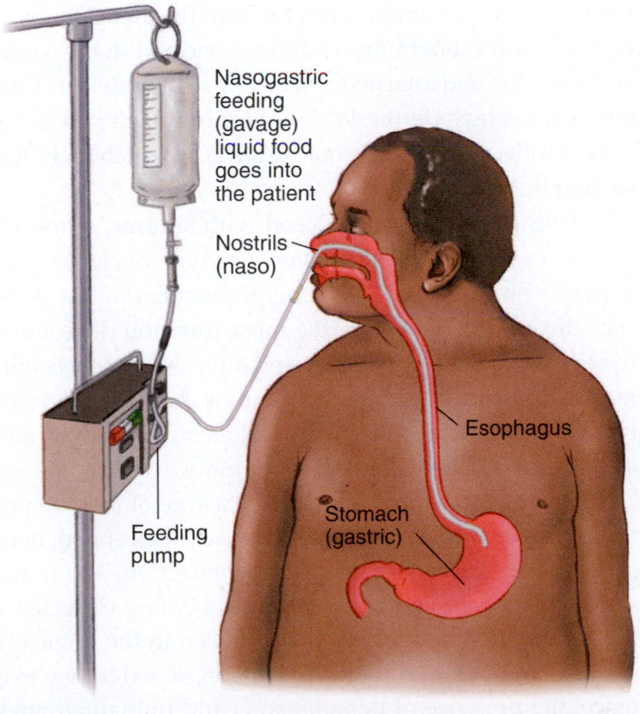

FIGURE 8-12 A nasogastric feeding tube.

and jejunal tubes, to name a few. These tubes have different means of insertion (surgical vs. endoscopic), location (stomach vs. duodenum), and function (feeding vs. aspiration prevention).

A **colostomy** is used to bypass part of the large intestine and allow feces to be collected outside the body in a collection bag, either on a temporary or permanent basis. Indications for a colostomy include cancer of the bowel or rectum, diverticulitis, Crohn's disease, or trauma. A surgical connection of the bowel to an ostomy created in the skin results in diversion of feces into the collection bag (Figure 8-14).

Gastrointestinal Tract Device Complications

Complications from GI tract devices include tube misplacement, obstruction, or infection. Because misplaced tubes can obstruct the airway or GI system, you should always ensure device patency if you have doubts about placement of the tube. First, have the patient speak to you. If he cannot speak, the tube may be in the airway and need to be removed. Second, to ensure patency of an NG tube, use a 60-mL syringe to insert air into the stomach. Use your stethoscope to listen over the epigastrium for air movement within the stomach. A low-pitched rumbling should be heard. You may also note stomach contents spontaneously moving up the tube, or they may be aspirated with a 60-mL syringe. In such cases, patients may be repositioned to return patency, or the device may be reinserted.

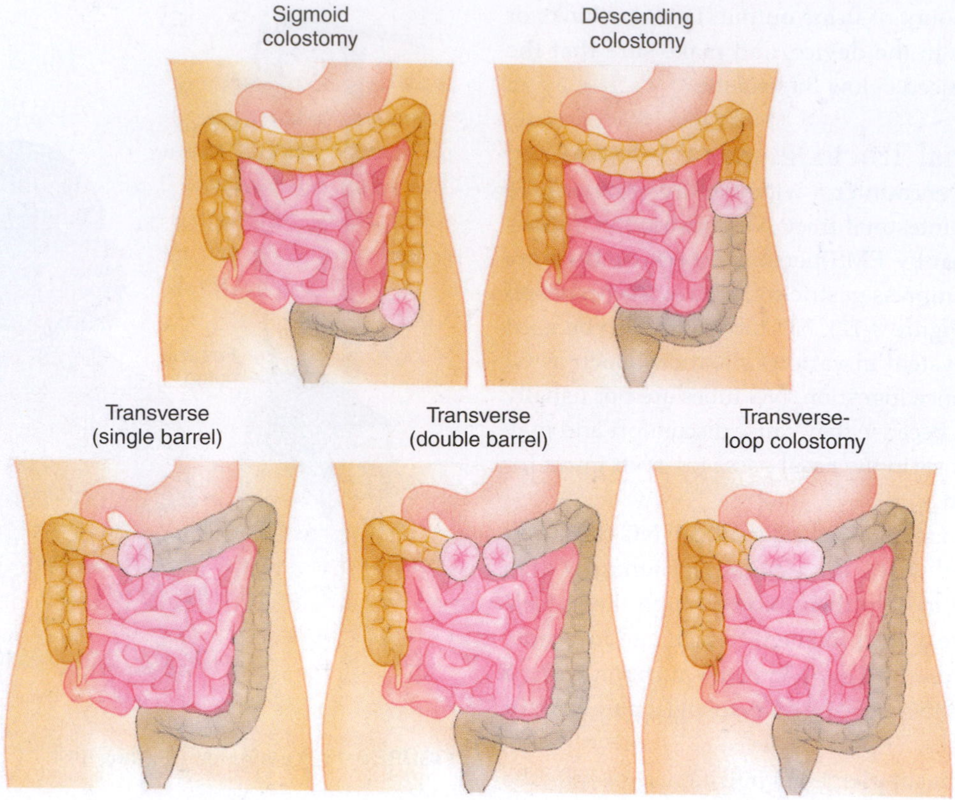

FIGURE 8-14 Examples of colostomy stoma locations.

Tubes are also prone to obstructions. Colostomies may become clogged or otherwise obstructed. Feeding tubes can become clogged because of the thick consistency of supplemental feedings or pill fragments. As a result, the tubes may require irrigation with water. In addition, the thick consistency of food may cause bowel obstructions or constipation.

As might be expected, ostomies can become infected (or lose skin integrity from pressure). Look for signs and symptoms of skin or systemic infection. In addition, remember that digestive enzymes may leak from various ostomies and begin to digest the skin and abdominal contents.

Psychosocial Implications

Many patients with GI or GU support devices lead active and otherwise normal lives. These patients may be understandably self-conscious about their conditions and many experience embarrassment, avoidance, anger, or discomfort when questioned. You should be sensitive to the patient's emotions during your patient assessment and treatment.

Acute Infections

After physicians or hospital personnel treat open wounds, they typically release patients to home care. These wounds may be surgical wounds or loss of skin integrity for other reasons. In such instances, you may see dressings covering wounds to protect against infection, absorb drainage, or immobilize the wound area. Gauze packing may also be inserted in infected spaces to absorb drainage.

Drains may sometimes be inserted in a wound site to remove blood, serum bile, or pus from the area. Drains are typically soft rubber tubes that have one end in the wound and the other end attached to a bag or suction device. Common drains include the Penrose drain, which is a simple rubber tube, and the Jackson-Pratt drain, which includes a suction bulb.

Wounds are typically closed with sutures, wires, staples, or cyanoacrylate adhesives. The type of closure used depends on the wound and the preferences of the physician closing it. Sutures are the most common device used to secure a wound, but staples and adhesives are becoming more widespread because of their ease of use. Wires are typically used to secure musculoskeletal structures, such as ribs or the sternum after a sternotomy.

In assessing wounds, always be aware of the potential for improper wound healing. As already mentioned, home care patients are at increased risk of infection. The immunologic response and rate of wound healing expected in the general population are compromised in the home care patient by poor peripheral perfusion, a sedentary existence, the presence of percutaneous and implanted medical devices, the existence of chronic diseases, and more.

An infected superficial wound may quickly lead to major infections or sepsis in the immunocompromised or weakened patient. Keep in mind that chronically ill or homebound patients, particularly the elderly, often have a decreased ability to perceive pain or to perform self-care. Pay particular attention to signs of infection in wounds found in home care patients. If you inspect a wound, be sure to use sterile technique and redress the wound.

Maternal and Newborn Care

Today, many women who deliver their babies in a hospital will be discharged in 24 hours or less. This trend, fueled by rising health care costs, greatly shortens the transition time from hospital to home. Some parents, especially first-time parents, may not yet be emotionally prepared to care for a new baby. Rapid discharge may also leave a mother or newborn with an unrecognized problem or complication stemming from delivery. As a result, you, the ALS provider, might be summoned to the home and called on to use the neonatology and pediatrics skills that you learned in the "Neonatology" and "Pediatrics" chapters.

Common Maternal Complications

For the mother, postpartum bleeding and embolus (especially after a Caesarean section) are the most common complications. Management of an embolus would be the same as with any patient with a similar complaint. Postpartum bleeding can be a serious condition. Management steps include:

- Massage of uterus, if it has not already contracted
- Administration of fluids to correct hypotension
- Administration of certain medications, such as Pitocin (if ordered)
- Rapid transport to the hospital, if necessary

Mothers may also experience **postpartum depression**. In such cases, women may have difficulty caring for both themselves and their newborns. In extreme cases, babies have been neglected or even harmed.

When entering the home, be sensitive to the needs of the parents. First-time mothers and/or fathers may be inexperienced in child rearing and may call EMS for what a more experienced parent might regard as normal. It is important that you always take any parent's concerns seriously, and if no medical support is needed, provide emotional reassurance. If you suspect neglect or abuse of the newborn, take the actions recommended in the "Neonatology," "Pediatrics," and "Abuse, Neglect, and Assault" chapters.

Common Infant/Child Complications

As pointed out in the "Neonatology" chapter, newborns must rapidly adapt to a new environment and may well not have reached a state at which they can thrive on their own. Newborns must be positioned properly to breathe, their noses must be clear (newborns are nose breathers), and they must be kept warm because of immature thermoregulation. Newborns also have immature immune systems and can develop rapid, life-threatening infections or septicemia.

Infants with recognized problems may already be receiving home care. They may have cardiac or respiratory abnormalities or other congenital defects. Premature or low-birth-weight babies, as well as babies with any number of respiratory disorders, are at risk for sleep apnea. Such babies may wear apnea monitors around their chests so that an alarm sounds at any pause in their breathing pattern. Some infants may also be on pulse oximetry. If you are summoned because of an alarm and find a normal breathing pattern, still encourage the parents or caregivers to have the baby examined as soon as possible.

As noted, newborns may also be discharged from the hospital with an undetected cardiac or respiratory condition. Signs and symptoms of cardiac or respiratory insufficiency include:

- Cyanosis
- Bradycardia (<100 beats per minute)
- Crackles
- Respiratory distress

In such cases, resuscitation should be initiated immediately. Management should be toward respiratory support with a bag-valve-mask (BVM) unit or intubation, as necessary. If any newborn has a heart rate <80 beats per minute despite 30 seconds or more of oxygenation, start CPR. Preserve warmth and obtain a record from the parents of feeding intake since birth. If the infant has not been feeding or has been vomiting with diarrhea, the infant may be dehydrated. In this case, a fluid bolus of 20 mL/kg is indicated. If a peripheral IV cannot be obtained in two attempts or 2 minutes, obtain access via the intraosseous route. If blood sugar is below 80 mg/dL, administer $D_{10}W$ at a dosage of 0.5 mg/kg.

For a newborn with infection or septicemia, look for fever, tachycardia, and irritability. If septicemia progresses to septic shock, you should initiate resuscitation as previously described.

Children who have serious, long-term health problems are usually cared for by their parents at home, with or without the help of a home care professional. Commonly found medical therapies for children who are home care patients include:

- Mechanical ventilators
- IV medications or nutrition
- Oxygen therapy
- Tracheostomies
- Feeding tubes

- Pulse oximeters
- Apnea monitors

Education of the parents or caregivers by doctors and nurses forms a critical component in their ability to deal with a crisis. Some people adapt well to the task and can deal with their child's chronic problems in a professional manner. Others, however, may become panicked or, either through misunderstanding or denial, have little comprehension of the situation. As with any difficult call, maintain a professional demeanor at all times.

When dealing with children, remember to keep the parents or caregivers informed of your assessment and treatment plans. Children quickly pick up on a person's emotions. As a result, it is part of your job to act in a supportive and controlled manner. Calming a child could make a huge difference in the long-term effects of the current episode.

Hospice and Comfort Care

Today more than 5,000 hospice providers—and hundreds of volunteer agencies—provide support for the terminally ill and their families. Initially philanthropic, these programs are now covered by Medicare. Most states also include them under Medicaid. Most programs are home based, with Medicare and Medicaid stipulating that at least 80 percent of an agency's care be provided to patients in their homes.[3]

Up to 450,000 patients per year receive services from hospices funded by Medicare or Medicaid. (Thousands more receive help from private or volunteer agencies.) Although the majority of Medicare patients are age 70 and older (Table 8-4), children receive benefits, too. Reimbursement is extended to patients with a life expectancy of six months or less.

The goal of hospices is to provide palliative or comfort care, rather than curative care. This is a very different role from that of most other branches of the health care profession, including EMS. For an ALS team, care is usually geared toward aggressive and lifesaving treatment. A hospice team, on the other hand, seeks to relieve symptoms, manage pain, and give patients control over the end of their lives. It is important to remember that these patients have, for the most part, exhausted or declined curative resources.

Table 8-4 Percentage of Hospice Patients by Age

Age	Percentage
Less than 45 years	8.1
45–54 years	7.9
55–64 years	14.8
65–69 years	8.7
70–74 years	15.6
75–79 years	14.5
80–84 years	12.3
85 years and older	16.4

Source: National Center for Health Statistics, Centers for Disease Control and Prevention.

ALS Intervention

Involvement in a hospice situation can be a difficult and stressful call. In most cases, family members, caregivers, and health care workers have been instructed to call a hospice rather than EMS. However, you may be summoned for intervention, particularly in situations involving transport. You should always keep in mind that the hospice patient is in the end stages of his disease and has already expressed wishes to withhold resuscitation. However, even a valid DNR order should not prevent you from performing palliative and/or comfort care.

Common diseases that you can expect to see in hospice include:

- CHF
- Cystic fibrosis
- COPD
- AIDS
- Alzheimer's disease
- Cancer

In some instances, particularly with cancer, you may also be confronted with patients on high dosages of pain medications. In cases of cancer, for example, morphine is the drug of choice. It is important for you to know that patients using morphine (often taking doses of up to 3,000 mg a day) will have few side effects other than constipation. They will have grown used to the drug and normal side effects will not be seen. Other drugs that may be administered include hydromorphone (Dilaudid), oxycodone (Percocet, Oxycontin), or a fentanyl (Duragesic) patch. Some patients may also have a portable pump that provides a continuous infusion of medication through a PICC line. The pumps can be small and hidden by clothing.

In a hospice, you need to establish communication with the home health care worker as quickly as possible. Your inclination may be to intubate, start a line, or administer medications. However, as noted, palliative care supersedes curative care. A hospice worker, when faced with the end stage of a disease, may do nothing, in accordance with the patient's wishes. Therefore, it is vital that you gain a clear understanding of these wishes, whether through a family member or a written document. If you are called to the house, it is your responsibility to respect the wishes of the patient and the ideals of hospice care.

In a hospice situation, family members might panic at a patient's imminent death and appropriate care might involve support for the family rather than resuscitation of the patient. Local protocols may also vary with respect to DNRs, DNARs, living wills, and durable power of attorney documents. Be sure that you are familiar with these legal statements and their implications for care of the terminally ill. (See "Medical–Legal Aspects of Prehospital Care.")

Terminally ill patients who are not involved in a hospice present a potentially gray area. Remember that although hospice prepares families for the impending death of their loved ones, families without hospice may be ill prepared for the end stages of life. Don't assume that all terminally ill patients are under hospice care. A simple question to determine the presence of hospice may alter your course of treatment and approach to the family.

Regardless of whether a patient is in hospice or not, keep in mind the stages of the grief process: denial, anger, depression, bargaining, and acceptance. Remember that both the patient and the family will go through these stages, and, in the case of the terminally ill, the patient may have reached acceptance well ahead of those who remain behind.

CONTENT REVIEW

➤ Stages of Response to Death and Grief
- Denial
- Anger
- Depression
- Bargaining
- Acceptance

Summary

The shift toward home health care is one of the most important trends of the early 21st century and will have a great impact on the ALS profession. You can expect in your career to provide acute intervention for a growing number of chronic care patients of all ages and in all stages of the disease process. These calls will challenge you to use all of your assessment skills in developing an effective management plan, which in many cases will be based on input from an extended team of home health care workers.

You Make the Call

Pridemark Paramedic 4 receives a call to assist a patient who has fallen out of a wheelchair. En route to the scene, dispatch informs the crew that the patient is a 32-year-old woman with possible head injuries. A home health care worker is with the patient.

On arrival, the crew finds the patient supine on the floor, A/O × 3, with a relatively minor amount of blood caked into her hair over the left temple. The health care worker introduces herself as the nursing assistant who regularly visits the patient. When she arrived for her normal visit about 20 minutes earlier, she knocked on the door and heard the patient call out for help. She then opened the door with a key and found the patient on the floor.

While the EMT assesses the patient, the paramedic interviews the home care worker for a complete history and baseline presentation. During this time, the fire department arrives with three firefighters to assist per local protocol. The Pridemark crew notes that the patient's apartment is messy and dirty.

The home care worker explains that the patient has a left-sided neurologic deficit from a right-sided head injury caused by a motor vehicle crash when the patient was 18 years old. The patient does have sensation on her left side, but movement is limited. Her left arm is normally contracted, and she has a left-sided facial droop. The home care worker shows the paramedic where the patient keeps her medications, but does not know what they are. Examination of the bottles reveals that the patient takes Tegretol, Glucophage, and Zoloft.

Firefighters offer further history because they know the patient from past runs. They explain that the patient smokes heavily, uses marijuana, and can be hostile at times.

Members of the Pridemark crew meet to share what they have learned. The EMT reports that the patient fell out of her wheelchair last night, approximately 14 hours before the crew's arrival. She apparently lost her balance and was not dizzy, weak, or sick. She complains of being cold and demands a cigarette. There is blood on the left side of her temple, but the wound cannot be visualized due to matted hair. The patient denies loss of consciousness and does not want to go to the hospital. Blood pressure is 110/84 mmHg; pulse is 72, normal and regular; and respirations are normal and unlabored. Skin is cool, dry, and normal in color. The patient's eyes are equal and reactive. The abdomen is soft and nontender. No other injuries are noted.

The EMT reports that the patient is lying in a pool of urine. The home care worker states that the patient is normally incontinent. However, she seems quieter than usual.

Although the patient has no neck or back pain, C-spine stabilization is taken. The paramedic talks to the patient and attempts to get her consent for treatment and transport. After explaining that she could have a possible C-spine injury, the patient changes her mind and gives her approval. Although C-spine clearance is allowed in the local protocol, the paramedic feels that, due to the patient's baseline neurologic deficits, more caution is required.

The crew applies a rigid cervical collar. They then log-roll the patient onto a long spine board and secure her in place. En route to the hospital, the crew conducts a secondary assessment with no new findings. On further questioning, the patient vehemently denies a history of diabetes or seizures, despite medications to the contrary. She repeatedly states, "I am normal!" She also denies allergies. A blood glucose test is not done because of the patient's strong emotional response to the procedure.

At the emergency department, the crew gives a full report and transfers care of the patient to the hospital staff. The patient is later released from the hospital with a butterfly bandage for a 1-inch head laceration and returned home by wheelchair van.

1. What does the condition of the apartment tell you?
2. Why is it important to immediately interview the home care worker?
3. What are some of the causes of urinary incontinence?
4. How can you rule out spinal injury to this patient?
5. Why do you think the patient denies a history of diabetes and seizures if she takes Tegretol and Glucophage?
6. Why is it acceptable to defer the glucose test when patient medications indicate a possible blood sugar problem?
7. Was there any need for an IV?
8. Should the patient have been placed on oxygen?

See Suggested Responses at the back of this book.

Review Questions

1. Diabetes commonly results in poor circulation, especially to the ____________
   a. head.
   b. neck.
   c. trunk.
   d. extremities.
2. Infection at the cellular level, which is often not life threatening, is called ____________
   a. sepsis.
   b. necrosis.
   c. cellulitis.
   d. gangrene.
3. Pressure sores are classified by ____________
   a. the degree of necrosis present.
   b. the depth of tissue destruction.
   c. the amount of drainage present.
   d. the number of blisters around the area.
4. Some of the most common home care devices used to treat respiratory disorders include ____________
   a. oxygen equipment.
   b. incentive spirometers.
   c. various home ventilators.
   d. all of the above.

5. Which of the following findings in children with dyspnea is an ominous sign of impending respiratory failure?
   a. Retractions
   b. Head bobbing
   c. Use of accessory muscles
   d. Abdominal breathing
6. Which genetically inherited disorder causes a defect in the intracellular metabolism of muscle cells and leads to degeneration and atrophy of muscles?
   a. Poliomyelitis
   b. Myasthenia gravis
   c. Muscular dystrophy
   d. Guillain-Barré syndrome
7. According to current practice, what type of ventilator is recommended for acute respiratory disorders that require ongoing mechanical ventilation?
   a. Positive pressure ventilator
   b. Negative pressure ventilator
   c. Continuous positive airway pressure
   d. Positive end-expiratory pressure
8. Which option is often prescribed for sleep apnea patients who need help in keeping their airways open?
   a. PPV
   b. CPAP
   c. BiPAP
   d. PEEP
9. Which vein is the most common anatomic insertion site for a central catheter, such as a Hickman, Broviac, or Groshong catheter?
   a. Cephalic
   b. Subclavian
   c. Saphenous
   d. External jugular
10. You arrive on scene for a patient with a preexisting traumatic brain injury who has a trach tube inserted and is on a home ventilator. The family states that the home ventilator was just replaced with a new one, and shortly afterward, it started to alarm, so the family summoned EMS. As you look at the ventilator, you note multiple red lights flashing and a loud audible alarm. What should you do first?
    a. Remove the ventilator tubing and attempt to ventilate the patient with a BVM.
    b. Call the company that installed the ventilator and ask for guidance.
    c. Rapidly load the patient into the ambulance and initiate transport.
    d. Remove the tracheostomy tube and intubate the patient through the ostomy.

See Answers to Review Questions at the end of this book.

References

1. Centers for Disease Control and Prevention. *Home Health Care.* (Available at http://www.cdc.gov/nchs/fastats/homehealthcare.htm.)
2. Arendts, G., M. Sim, S. Johnston, and R. Brightwell. "ParaMED Home: A Protocol for a Randomized Controlled Trial of Paramedic Assessment and Referral to Access Medical Care at Home." *BMC Emerg Med* 8 (2011): 7.
3. National Hospice and Palliative Care Organization. *Advancing Care at the End of Life.* (Available at http://www.nhpco.org.)

Further Reading

Neal, L. J. and S. E. Guillet. *Care of the Adult with a Chronic Illness or Disability: A Team Approach.* St. Louis, MO: Mosby-Year Book, 2004.

Redman, B. K. *Patient Self-Management of Chronic Disease: The Health Care Provider's Challenge.* Sudbury, MA: Jones and Bartlett Publishers, 2003.

Spratt, S. J., et al., eds. *Home Health Care: Principles and Practices.* Delray Beach, FL: GR/St. Lucie Press, 1997.

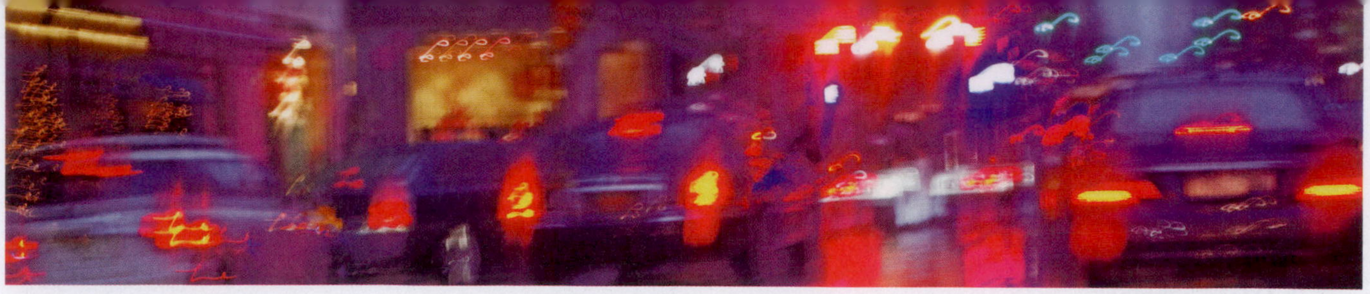

Chapter 9
Ground Ambulance Operations

Bryan Bledsoe, DO, FACEP, FAAEM, EMT-P

STANDARD

EMS Operations (Principles of Safely Operating a Ground Ambulance)

COMPETENCY

Applies knowledge of operational roles and responsibilities to ensure patient, public, and personnel safety.

Learning Objectives

Terminal Performance Objective: After reading this chapter, you should be able to place patient care tasks in the context of ground ambulance operations to safely respond to calls and transport patients.

Enabling Objectives: To accomplish the terminal performance objective, you should be able to:

1. Define key terms introduced in this chapter.
2. Describe administrative rules and regulations, standards, and trends that affect the design of ambulances and the equipment they carry.
3. Identify typical components of an ambulance checklist and the responsibilities of the paramedic in checking the ambulance at the beginning of each shift.
4. Describe considerations in ambulance deployment and staffing configurations.
5. Discuss how to implement safety measures related to reducing the risk of ambulance collisions, safe driving practices, safely parking the ambulance, and techniques to safely load/unload the ambulance.

KEY TERMS

demographic, p. 264
deployment, p. 261
DOT KKK 1822F specs, p. 261
due regard, p. 267
essential equipment, p. 261
gold standard, p. 261
minimum standards, p. 261
peak load, p. 264
primary area of responsibility (PAR), p. 264
reportable collisions, p. 266
reserve capacity, p. 265
spotter, p. 266
system status management (SSM), p. 265
tiered response system, p. 265

Case Study

It's 6:00 A.M., the start of another shift. You and your partner have just arrived to relieve the overnight crew. As you check and sign out the narcotics with the outgoing paramedic, the tones go off for a priority one call on the other side of town. You quickly finish the paperwork and rush out the door. As you load your personal protective equipment, you shout to the outgoing crew, "How's the rig?" The paramedic responds, "Fine. We just restocked."

You feel confident that the ambulance has everything you will need. Your service is dedicated to ensuring that each shift fills in ambulance checklists and that replacement supplies are easily obtained. In this case, you arrive at the scene to find that the patient is having difficulty breathing, most likely from an acute exacerbation of asthma. The call runs smoothly, and the patient actually improves en route to the hospital.

You quickly wrap up the paperwork and return to the station. On the way, you and your partner recall the haphazard ambulance operations of a few years ago. The former management team looked the other way when some medics failed to restock the supplies and equipment that they used. Imagine not having enough oxygen or a bronchodilator for an asthma patient. You and your partner both agree—things have gotten a lot better since the new management has insisted that crews take the tour checklists seriously.

Introduction

Good ambulance operations involve some of the knowledge and skills that you have already established in your EMT training and through field experience. However, because the safety of so many people—the EMS team, the patient, and bystanders—depends on effective ambulance maintenance and operation, it is important for you to review this information regularly so it becomes second nature. In addition to the communication and dispatch skills learned in the chapter "EMS Systems and Communications," you should keep in mind these topics: ambulance standards, maintenance of ambulance equipment and supplies, ambulance stationing, and safe ambulance operations.

Ambulance Standards

Various standards, as well as administrative rules and regulations, influence the design of ambulances and the medical equipment carried on each unit. Similar guidelines determine staffing levels and **deployment** of EMS agencies (see information later in this chapter).

Because the oversight for EMS usually falls to state governments, many of the requirements for ambulance service are written in state statutes or regulations. However, national standards and trends do have an influence on the development of these laws. Typically, state laws are broad, whereas corresponding regulations provide more specific guidelines or rules. For example, a public health law may authorize the state department of health to issue regulations through its EMS bureau. These regulations, known as the "state EMS code," might then handle such matters as the **essential equipment** to be carried on every ambulance.

In most cases, state standards tend to be generic enough that they are "palatable," affordable, and politically feasible to all EMS agencies throughout the state. State standards usually set **minimum standards**, rather than a **gold standard**, for operation. In other words, they establish the lowest level at which units will be allowed to operate. When local and/or regional EMS systems get involved in regulation, their lists tend to be much more detailed and often approach a gold standard, which is the goal when ample resources are provided.

Ambulance Design

The U.S. General Services Administration's Automotive Commodity Center issues the federal regulations that specify ambulance design and manufacturing requirements. These specifications, known as the **DOT KKK 1822F specs**, attempt to influence safety standards as well as standardize the look of ambulances.[1]

Over the years, the "KKK specifications" have had a significant influence on ambulance manufacturing. The specs describe the following three basic ambulance designs:

- *Type I*—conventional truck cab-chassis with a modular ambulance body
- *Type II*—standard van, forward control integral cab-body ambulance
- *Type III*—specialty van, forward control integral cab-body ambulance

In addition to these three designs, there is also a medium-duty ambulance rescue vehicle (Figure 9-1) that is designed to handle heavier loads and has a gross weight of approximately 24,000 pounds.

The federal specifications not only provide standards for the purchase of ambulances used by the federal government, but they also provide guidelines for the states to follow. Massachusetts, for example, refers to the federal specifications in its own state regulations. In such cases,

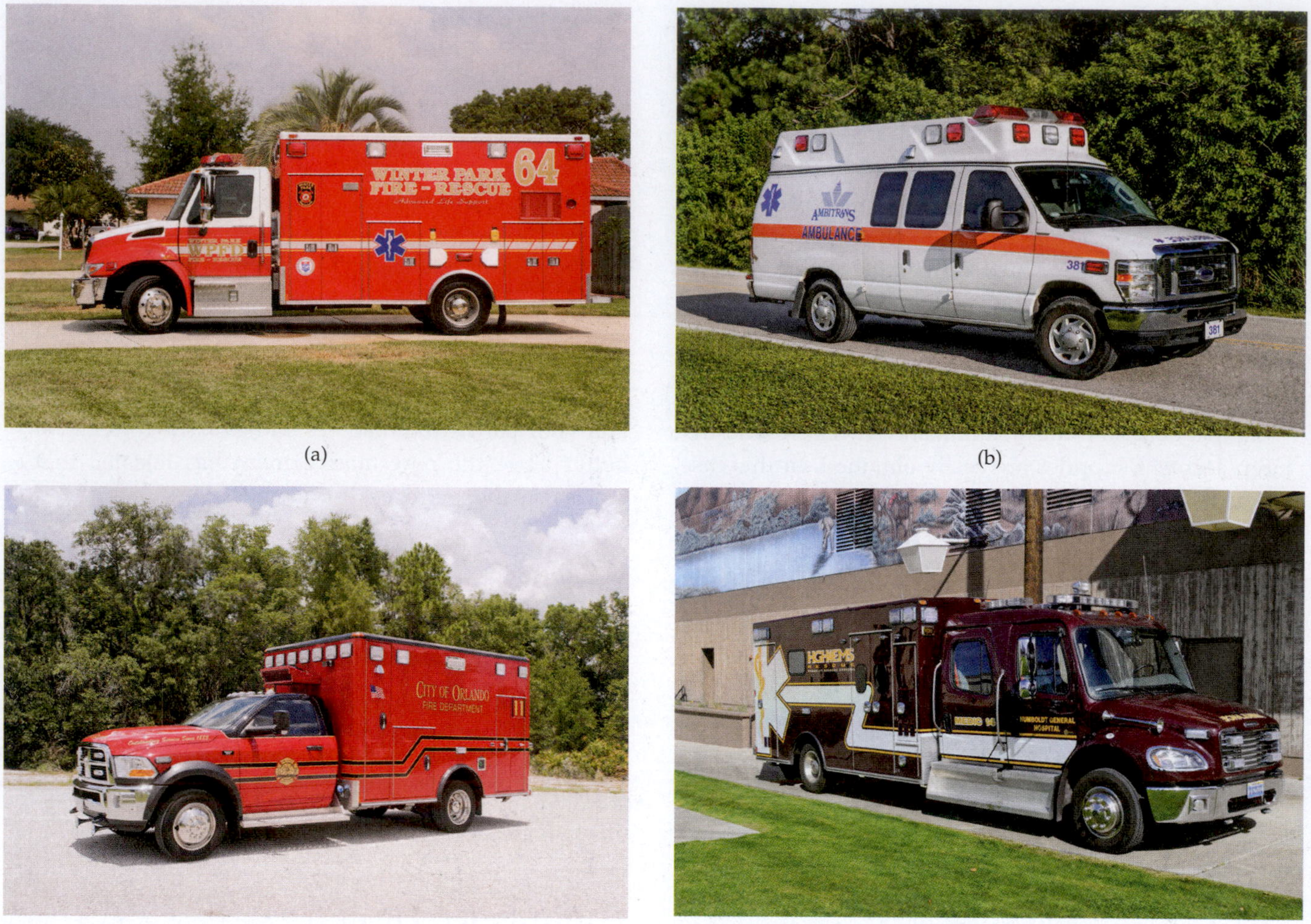

(a) (b) (c) (d)

FIGURE 9-1 Four types of ambulances. (a) Type I, (b) Type II, (c) Type III, and (d) medium-duty rescue vehicle.

(Photo d: © Pat Songer)

the federal specifications become the state standard for ambulance services to follow when purchasing vehicles.

Some states, including Connecticut, Vermont, and New Jersey, have chosen to develop their own standards. Often, these states use the federal specifications as the basis or starting point for their own regulations. A few states, such as New York, use neither federal nor state specifications. Instead, the decisions for ambulance purchases are determined on a local or regional basis.

There has been a recent push over the past decade to improve the safety of ground ambulances. The National Highway Traffic Safety Administration (NHTSA) and the National Institute for Occupational Safety and Health (NIOSH) are collaborating on a four-year research-based project to improve existing standards to make patients and EMS workers safer in the rear compartment of ambulances. Several ambulance manufacturers and EMS operators have developed concept vehicles to explore and test new ambulance safety systems and designs (Figure 9-2).

In addition to the U.S. Department of Transportation (DOT), other federal agencies and national organizations influence standards. Air ambulance standards, for example, are usually designed with input from representatives of the Air and Surface Transport Nurses Association (ASTNA), the International Association of Flight and Critical Care Paramedics (IAFCCP), and the Association of Air Medical Services (AAMS). The Federal Communications Commission (FCC), which is discussed in the "EMS Systems and Communications" chapter, specifies the radio bands and types of equipment that may be used in ambulances.

Medical Equipment Standards

With increases in the presence of hazardous materials and awareness of infectious diseases, the Occupational Safety and Health Administration (OSHA) has become more and more involved in ambulance standards. As the agency charged with protecting worker safety, OSHA has helped ensure the use of equipment lists calling for disinfecting agents, sharps containers, red bags, HEPA masks, and personal protective equipment. NIOSH has established similar standards.

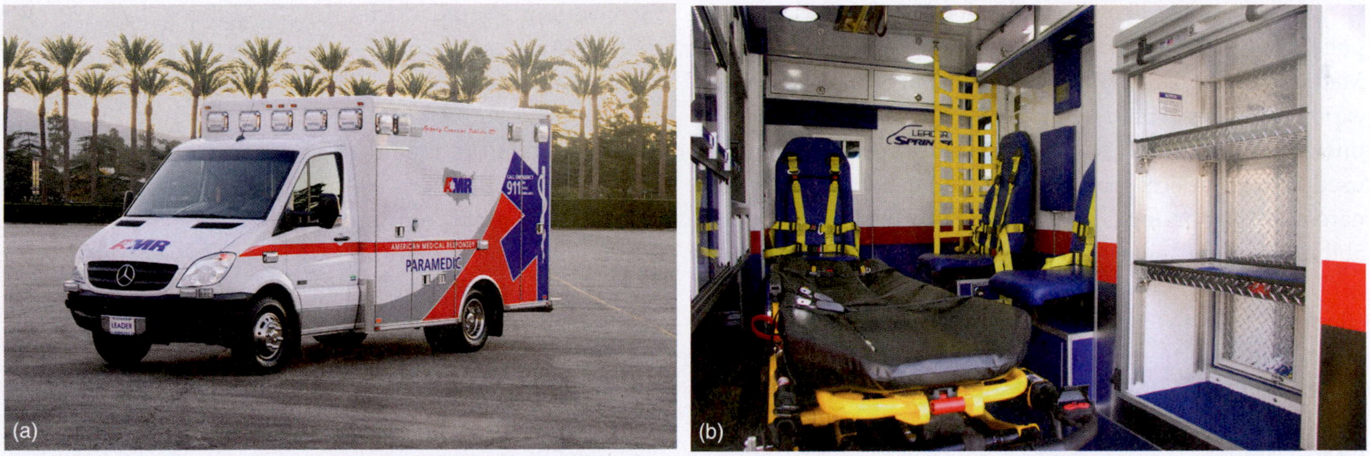

FIGURE 9-2 Many safety concept ambulances are under evaluation as safety becomes a paramount concern for EMS. (a) Exterior view. (b) Interior view with safety harness.

(Photos courtesy of American Medical Response and American Emergency Vehicles)

Other voluntary standards have been set by peer organizations, such as the National Fire Protection Association (NFPA). In many cases, these standards are referenced in local ordinances and thus have become the standard for a given municipality.

In addition to city, county, and/or district ambulance ordinances, local medical direction boards sometimes list the medications that paramedics can carry. These boards, which issue indirect medical direction, may also list the specific advanced life support (ALS) equipment and supplies that should be on every ambulance. For example, in areas where the paramedics are trained to obtain a 12-lead ECG, the medical direction board may have specified the actual brand of equipment in an effort to standardize care on a system-wide or regional basis.

Additional Guidelines

At the national level, the Commission on Accreditation of Ambulance Services (CAAS) provides a voluntary "gold standard" for the EMS community to follow. CAAS requires that onboard medical equipment and supplies comply with state and local guidelines. In the absence of these guidelines, CAAS requires services to develop guidelines that meet or exceed those established by the American College of Surgeons (ACS). The ACS Committee of Trauma issued its first list of "essential equipment" to be carried on ambulances in 1970 and revised the list in 1994. Of note is that as long ago as 1970 the list included the ALS equipment, emergency drugs, and fluids commonly used on ALS calls today.

Checking Ambulances

On each shift, an essential part of a paramedic's duties includes completion of the ambulance equipment and supply checklist. Aside from reminding the personnel exactly where all equipment and supplies are stored on the ambulance, the shift checklist helps ensure that all equipment and supplies will be available and in working order when needed for patient care. The checklist also makes the work environment safer by ensuring mechanical maintenance and the availability of personal protective equipment.

The components of a typical vehicle/equipment checklist include the following:

- Patient infection control, comfort, and protection supplies
- Initial and focused assessment equipment
- Equipment for the transfer of the patient
- Equipment for airway maintenance, ventilation, and resuscitation
- Oxygen therapy and suction equipment
- Equipment for assisting with cardiac resuscitation
- Supplies and equipment for immobilization of suspected bone injuries
- Supplies for wound care and treatment of shock
- Supplies for childbirth
- Supplies, equipment, and medications for the treatment of acute poisoning, snakebite, chemical burns, and diabetic emergencies
- ALS equipment, medications, and supplies
- Safety and miscellaneous equipment
- Information on the operation and inspection of the ambulance itself

Routine detailed shift checks of the ambulance can minimize the issues associated with risk management. Many services, for example, hold a "stretcher day" once a week. By performing and documenting preventive maintenance on stretchers, it is less likely that a faulty stretcher will cause a patient to be dropped or EMS personnel to injure their backs. Medications carried on the paramedic unit expire. Therefore, expiration dates should be checked each shift, and the older, unexpired drugs marked appropriately so that they will be used first. In services that use scheduled medications such as narcotics, the paramedics should sign for these medications at the beginning and at the end of each shift.

As mentioned, the vehicle itself should be regularly checked so that it is always in safe working order. If the ambulance or any equipment needs repair, it is your responsibility to report the failure to your supervisor in a manner prescribed by the standard operating procedures (SOPs) for your service.

To meet OSHA requirements, you must also make sure that the ambulance has been properly disinfected after the transport of any patients with potentially communicable diseases (Figure 9-3). Most services routinely clean the ambulance after every call, and some agencies document the procedure. All services are required, either by OSHA or the state equivalent of OSHA, to have an exposure control plan that specifies cleaning requirements and the methods of cleaning up blood spills in the ambulance. If there is no specific SOP in your agency, you should document cleaning and disinfecting on the shift checklist.

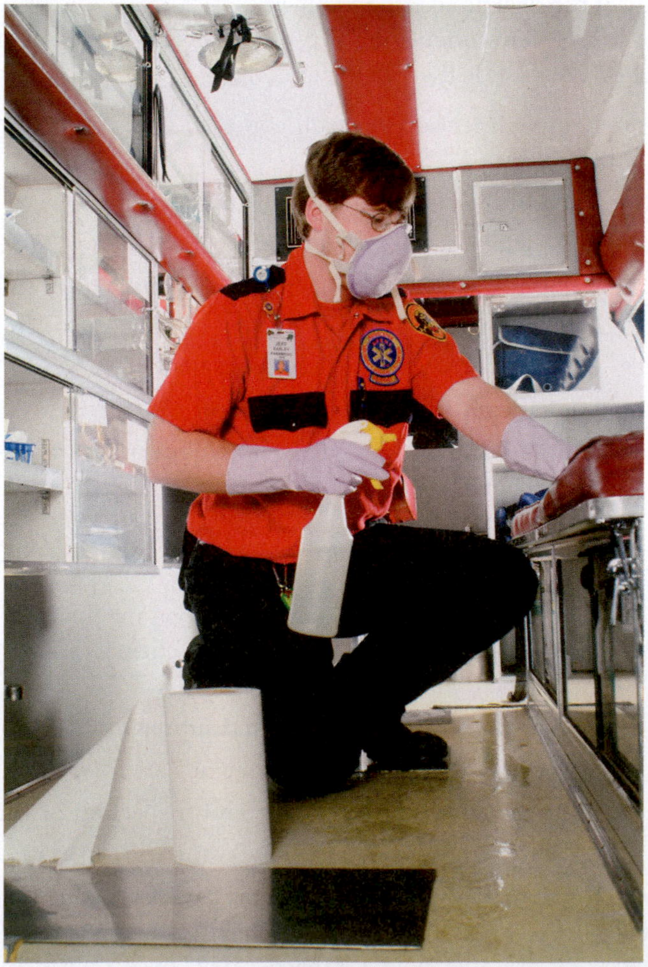

FIGURE 9-3 Disinfecting the ambulance.

Finally, you should do all scheduled tests, maintenance, and calibrations on specific medical equipment. Items that should be regularly checked include:

- Automated external defibrillator (AED)
- Glucometer
- Cardiac monitor
- Capnograph
- Oxygen systems
- Automated transport ventilator (ATV)
- Pulse oximeter
- Suction units
- Laryngoscope blades
- Lighted stylets
- Penlights
- Any other battery-operated equipment

CONTENT REVIEW

➤ Deployment Factors
- Location of facilities to house ambulances
- Location of hospitals
- Anticipated volume of calls
- Local geographic and traffic considerations

Ambulance Deployment and Staffing

The strategy used by an EMS agency to maneuver its ambulances and crews in order to reduce response times is known as *deployment*. Deployment is based on a number of factors: location of the facilities to house ambulances, location of hospitals, anticipated volume of calls, and the specific geographic and traffic considerations of your area.

Most services must develop deployment strategies based on current station locations. Few agencies are in a position to move their stations to better locations. Such moves require years of budgeting, land acquisition, community education, building design, and financing of a capital construction project.

The ideal deployment decisions must take into account two sets of data: past community responses and projected **demographic** changes. The highest volume of calls, or **peak load**, should be described both in terms of the day of the week and the time of day.

In communities that do not have multiple strategically located stations, services often deploy ambulances to wait for calls at specific high-volume locations. Such stationing locations are known as **primary areas of responsibility (PARs)**. These ambulances may be relocated throughout the day as the population moves—to work or to school—and as other ambulances in the community respond to calls. The size of a PAR can vary from a few city blocks to a larger location, such as "northeast sector of town." The PAR size depends on the number of ambulances available and the expected call volume.

Some technologically sophisticated systems use computers to assist the dispatch center in relocating the ambulances. Vehicle tracking systems tell the computer exactly where each ambulance is located at a given time.

Traffic Congestion

In determining deployment strategies, traffic congestion must be taken into account, as well as special situations such as a ground-level railroad. Some communities, for example, must station an ambulance on the other side of the tracks before a freight train splits the town in half for perhaps 15 minutes or more. Other special deployment considerations include the ongoing daily activities within the community, especially commuter traffic and school bus schedules. Additional vehicles and crews may be required for these time periods. Other traffic (and potential patient) considerations include sporting events, VIP appearances, mass gatherings, and community days.

One deployment strategy that has become popular in recent years is known as **system status management (SSM)**. SSM is a computerized personnel and ambulance deployment system designed to meet service demands with fewer resources and to ensure appropriate response times and vehicle locations.

The EMS response time can make the difference between life and death for the citizens of a community—especially in the setting of cardiac arrest. However, recent research has shown that only response times of less than 4 minutes are associated with improved outcomes.[2] Several studies have shown that an 8-minute response time, a de facto industry standard, is not uniformly associated with better patient outcomes overall.[3,4,5] In most areas, a routine response time of 4 minutes is either impossible or cost prohibitive. Thus, appropriate response times must be determined by each community and its available resources.[6] A system's standards for reliability must take into account the time frames for such high-priority calls. The medical director should have direct input into setting these standards. An example of such a reliability standard might be response within 4 minutes to 90 percent of the priority-one calls (cardiac arrests, respiratory complaints, and motor vehicle collisions).

To meet reliability standards, many communities use a **tiered response system** in which public safety agencies trained as first responders carry an AED to a patient's side. The first tier of response, which helps ensure arrival within the 4-minute window, is then backed up by a second tier that brings an ALS unit to the patient within 8 minutes. Some communities add a third tier of response by separating their paramedics from their ambulances. No one system works best for all communities. The system that is ideal for your specific area will depend on such considerations as available personnel, available training, and many other factors.

Operational Staffing

For as long as paramedics have been trained, controversy has existed over the number of paramedics who should be assigned to a unit. This is a complex decision. Clearly, an ambulance with two paramedics onboard is limited in the amount of care that these two highly trained personnel can provide if they are the only available responders to cardiac arrests (meaning no backup for simultaneous additional emergencies). As a result, some communities prefer to combine an Advanced EMT with a paramedic to make an ALS unit. Other communities, such as New York City, specify that an ALS unit must have two paramedics so that they can back up one another in making on-scene decisions. Because communities and available resources vary so widely, the controversy will, in all likelihood, be settled locally based on particular needs and available resources.

In general, ambulance staffing should take into account the peak load of the system. Some services vary shift times to ensure ample coverage for the busiest days of the week and the busiest times of the day. Services should also take into account the need for **reserve capacity**—the ability to muster additional crews when all ambulances are on call or when a system's resources are taxed by a multiple-casualty incident. Some services fulfill this need by asking off-duty personnel to carry pagers or to volunteer for backup. Whatever plan is adopted, each system must consider how it will deal with establishing a reserve of paramedics.

Finally, each service needs to determine standards for ambulance operators (drivers) and for driving the vehicle itself. As a rule, these standards are usually spelled out at the local service level.

Safe Ambulance Operations

Patients, family members, motorists, and EMS providers are injured—sometimes fatally—in ambulance collisions. In addition to personal injuries, ambulance collisions exact a high toll: vehicle repair or replacement, lawsuits, downtime from work, increased insurance premiums, and damage to your agency's reputation in the community.

No national database has been set up to provide statistics on ambulance collisions in all 50 states. As a result, it is difficult to establish any form of "acceptable" ambulance collision rate per number of calls or miles driven. Furthermore, few scientific studies have been published that attempt to prove what, if any, strategies effectively reduce ambulance collisions. However, you can be certain of one thing: If your agency does experience a serious ambulance collision, questions will undoubtedly arise about the agency's training of drivers and its collision prevention program.[7,8]

Educating Providers

The first part of any proactive collision prevention program is the recognition and definition of the problem. In the absence of a national database, this is easier said than done. However, some states do keep data, and their examples can provide a starting point. The following statistics come from an analysis of 22 years of **reportable collisions**—collisions involving more than $1,000 in vehicle damage or a personal injury—in New York State. The data are not intended to be scientific evidence that can be generalized to the other 49 states. The data also do not include many of the crashes that have resulted from backing up the ambulances, resulting in crashes that could be avoided by use of a **spotter**. Rather, the data, which come from a large number of cases, are used for purposes of illustration.

There has been a marked increase in the frequency of ground ambulance accidents over the past decade. The exact cause is unclear, although several theories have been proposed. First, modern automobiles are better sealed and more soundproof than cars of even a decade ago. This can make it difficult for persons to hear an approaching ambulance. In addition, ambulances have increased in size and weight. The performance that is characteristic of modern ambulances is quite different from those of older models. Modern ambulances tend to be on a truck chassis and have characteristics more consistent with a large truck than a car. They accelerate poorly, are less responsive, and have a much greater braking distance. Also, the center of gravity is quite different from that of automobiles. Although the first rule in medical practice is "Do no harm," collisions by these emergency vehicles have harmed a considerable number of people.[9]

An analysis of the data collected by New York provides a profile of the typical ambulance collision. Inclement weather accounted for a relatively small number of the accidents. About 18 percent occurred on rainy days, 16 percent on cloudy days, and 6 percent on days with snow, sleet, hail, or freezing rain. The majority of collisions (55 percent) took place on clear days. Of all the collisions, some 67 percent took place during daylight hours.

Although head-on collisions can be very serious, they accounted for only 1 percent of the accidents. The largest number of collisions (41 percent) occurred when the ambulance struck another vehicle laterally or at a right angle, or was struck itself. Approximately 21 percent of the collisions resulted from sideswiping or overtaking another vehicle. Another 12 percent occurred while making a right or left turn.

Probably the most important observation from the data is that nearly three-quarters (72 percent) of all collisions took place at intersections. Most safety-minded ambulance operators agree that the days of "blowing through" an intersection at high speeds with lights blaring and siren blasting have come and gone. However, nearly half of all accidents took place at locations with a traffic control device. Another third took place at locations with no traffic device or sign at all.

Based on the statistics from New York, the profile of a typical ambulance collision might read as follows: *a lateral collision that takes place on a dry road during daylight hours on a clear day in an intersection with a traffic light*. Typically, when ambulance operators respond in poor weather conditions, they try to drive with a bubble of safety around the vehicle. Perhaps the bubble should be there all the time, instead of reserving it for poor road conditions when ambulance collisions rarely occur!

Reducing Ambulance Collisions

What is your EMS agency doing to reduce ambulance collisions? Do you have an aggressive, proactive driver training program? Or does the agency follow a "we'll deal with it when it becomes a problem" kind of approach? All too often, the latter approach can result in news bulletins such as this one from the Associated Press: "Ambulance collides with car, killing three small children and seriously injuring their mother and sister; ambulance driver arrested on three counts of manslaughter."

As mentioned, such situations can be prevented by determining when and where they are most likely to occur. That is why the New York profile—or better yet, a profile from your own state—can be helpful in directing your own personal attitudes and training. Instead of confining your practice to skidding around wet or snowy parking lots, consciously practice safe driving under normal conditions.[10]

If you have the opportunity to develop programs to reduce ambulance collisions in your community, consider implementing the following actions or standards:

- Routine use of driver qualification checklists and driver's license checks, either through the local police or the Department of Motor Vehicles
- Demonstrated driver understanding of preventive mechanical maintenance, including a vehicle operator checklist and a procedure for reporting any problems found during the check or while driving the vehicle
- Provision of adequate hands-on driver training, using experienced and qualified field officers. (A 10,000- to 24,000-pound ambulance has a much longer stopping distance than the 2,500-pound pickup truck that an operator drove to work. One goal, for instance, would be to prevent an inexperienced driver from being stopped by a light pole—or another car—after sliding through an intersection [Figure 9-4].)

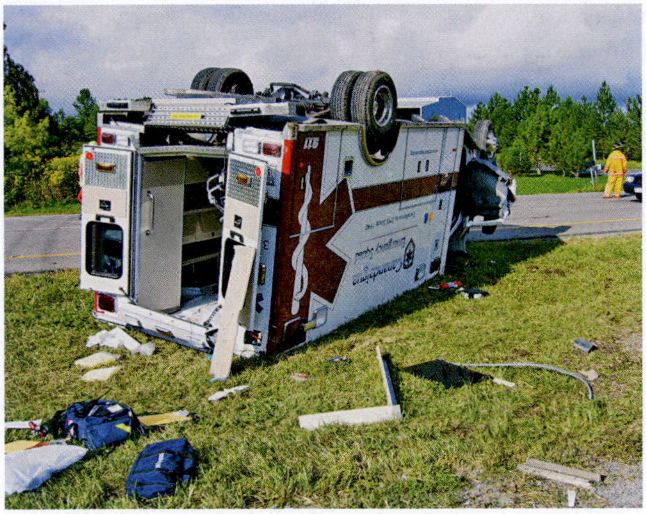

FIGURE 9-4 Ambulance collision.
(© Canandaigua Emergency Squad)

- Implementation of a slow-speed course to ensure that operators know how to use mirrors, back up, park, and handle ambulance-sized vehicles, including accurate estimation of braking distance and turn radius
- Training that ensures operators know how to react to emergency situations such as the loss of brakes, loss of power steering, a stuck accelerator, a blown-out tire, or a vehicle breakdown
- Demonstrated driver knowledge of both the primary and backup routes to all hospitals in your service response area
- Demonstrated driver understanding of the rules, regulations, and laws that your Department of Motor Vehicles has established for drivers in general and for ambulance operators in particular

Standard Operating Procedures

Each EMS agency should have standard operating procedures pertaining to the operation of its vehicles. At a minimum, SOPs should spell out the following:

- Procedure for qualifying as an ambulance operator
- Procedure for handling and reporting an ambulance collision
- Process for investigating and reviewing each collision
- Process for implementing quality assurance in the aftermath of a collision
- Method for using a spotter when backing up a vehicle (Figure 9-5)
- Use of seat belts in the ambulance, and the procedure for transporting a child passenger under 40 pounds
- Guidelines on what constitutes an emergency response and the exemptions that may be taken under state laws

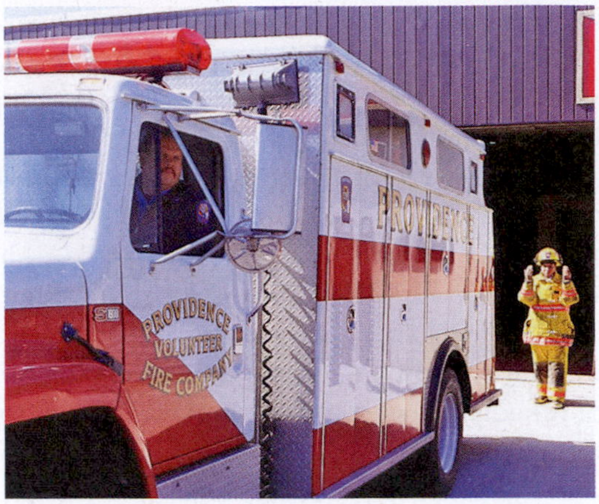

FIGURE 9-5 Use of a spotter.

- Guidelines on prudent speed; proper travel in, and the circumstances for using, oncoming lanes; and safe negotiation of intersections
- Circumstances and procedures for use of escorts
- A zero-tolerance policy for driving the vehicle under the influence of alcohol or any drugs

The Due Regard Standard

The motor vehicle laws enacted by most states are based on a model law. As might be expected, state laws pertaining to ambulance operation tend to be similar. One similarity centers on the legal concept of **due regard**. Essentially, due regard exempts ambulance drivers from certain laws but at the same time holds them to a higher standard.

State laws typically exempt ambulance drivers who are operating in an emergency from posted speed limits, posted directions of travel, parking regulations, and requirements to wait at red lights. There are, however, certain situations from which ambulances are rarely or never exempt. They include passing over a railroad crossing with the gates down and passing a school bus with flashing red lights. In the latter case, you should wait until the bus driver secures the safety of the children and turns off the red lights. Only then should you proceed past the bus.

Although the laws are often liberal in their exemptions, they place the responsibility for deciding when and where these exemptions should be applied squarely on the shoulders of drivers. The laws often say, for example, "the foregoing provisions and exemptions do not relieve the operator of an emergency vehicle from acting with due regard for the safety of all persons." Such language sets a higher standard for ambulance operators than for almost any other driver on the road. Nowhere in the motor vehicle laws are other drivers held accountable for the safety of all other motorists!

To see how this higher standard might affect you, consider a situation that could occur in any community. It's

7:00 P.M. in a suburban neighborhood. After a dry, clear, warm day, the sun has started to set. A five-year-old child takes one last ride on a Big Wheel, a low-profile, plastic tricycle. The child pedals down a slightly inclined driveway past a pine tree obstructing the view of oncoming motorists and rolls into the street. A midsized car with four adults on their way to dinner and a movie is headed toward the driveway. The driver is sober, traveling at the speed limit, and having a normal conversation. Suddenly the child darts into view from behind the pine tree. The driver immediately steps on the brakes, but it is too late. The car strikes the child, who later dies from multiple trauma in the emergency department.

When the police arrive, they take statements from all involved, ensure that the driver is sober, make sure the vehicle's inspection sticker is up to date, and measure skid marks. In all likelihood, they issue no tickets. The family of the child may decide to sue the driver for the loss of their child, but the police usually take no action unless a specific motor vehicle law has been violated.

Now imagine the same situation, except it is your ambulance headed toward the child while on an emergency call. You have lights on, siren off, and are not exceeding the posted speed limit. As you and your partner search for house numbers, a child suddenly darts into view. You strike the brakes immediately, but unfortunately the child instantly dies from multiple trauma.

When the police arrive, they take statements from all involved, ensure you are sober, check the vehicle's inspection documentation, and measure the skid marks. They then turn the case over to the county grand jury for further investigation. You will appear before the jury, which may scrutinize your personal and professional driving record, service SOPs, rules of the road, and perhaps even your personal habits. In the meantime, the local newspaper has run a front-page story, complete with your name and that of your service. The headline implies that you killed the child as you raced through town in your ambulance.

By now, some of your neighbors have begun to throw dirty looks at you while you empty your mailbox. The reputation of your service has been indelibly tarnished in the public's mind. Members of other crews say their patients have questioned the safety of riding in your service's ambulances. But you can't really respond. Your service has suspended you from driving pending the results of the hearing.

After more than a week of deliberations, the grand jury clears you of all responsibility. It has found that you were sober, attentive, and doing your job. There was nothing you could have done, says the jury, to have prevented the child's death. If the newspaper even carries the final chapter of the story, it appears inside the paper in a small follow-up piece.

The moral is this: As an ambulance driver, you will always be held to a higher standard than other drivers. You must be attentive and prepared to shoulder the responsibilities that come with the profession that you have chosen.

Lights and Siren: A False Sense of Security

As a general rule, do not rely solely on lights and siren to alert other motorists of your approach. Studies have shown that most motorists do not see or hear your ambulance until it is within 50 to 100 feet of their vehicles. Even so, the siren is the most commonly used—and abused—audible warning device. Before you decide to turn on the siren, consider the following points:

- Motorists are less inclined to yield to an ambulance when the siren is sounded continuously.
- Many motorists feel that the right-of-way privileges given to ambulances are abused when sirens are sounded.
- Inexperienced motorists tend to increase their driving speeds by 10 to 15 miles per hour when a siren is sounded.
- The continuous sound of a siren can possibly worsen the condition of sick or injured patients by increasing their anxiety.
- Ambulance operators may also develop anxiety, not to mention the possibility of hearing problems, from sirens used on long runs.

Some states and services have specific laws and/or SOPs that address the use of sirens. Consider these useful guidelines:

- Use the siren sparingly and only when you must.
- Never assume that all motorists will hear your siren.
- Assume that some motorists will hear your siren but choose to ignore it.
- Be prepared for panic and erratic maneuvers when drivers do hear your siren.
- Never use the siren to scare someone.

Whenever the ambulance is on the road, day or night, turn on the headlights to increase its visibility. Alternating headlamps should be used at night only if they are installed in a secondary lamp. Probably the most useful light is the one in the center of the cowling on the front hood. This light can usually be easily seen in the rearview mirror of the car in front of you.

Each corner of the ambulance should have large flashers that blink in tandem or unison to help oncoming vehicles identify the location and size of the ambulance. Although the controversy over the use of strobes continues, consider the latest research on the subject when designing or choosing the lighting on your ambulance. At present, recommendations lean toward the use of single-beam bulbs and strobes instead of relying on one type of lighting system. The most important point is visibility. The vehicle must be clearly visible from 360 degrees to all other motorists and pedestrians.

Interestingly, several studies have shown that the use of lights and sirens reduced response times only a modest amount—an amount that may not be clinically significant. Because of the risk associated with lights and siren usage, EMS must ensure that the potential benefits afforded the patient by a lights and siren response are not offset by the risks imposed on the crew and the public.[11,12,13]

Escorts and Multiple-Vehicle Responses

Most EMS agencies no longer suggest the use of a police escort for ambulances, except in circumstances in which the ambulance is providing service to an unfamiliar district and needs to be taken to the patient and/or the hospital. There are several reasons for this. First, ambulances and police cars have different braking distances. If an ambulance follows a police car too closely, it can easily rear-end the car if they both stop quickly. Second, the two vehicles have different acceleration speeds. As a result, an ambulance operator may have trouble keeping up with a police car. A gap often develops, allowing other vehicles to pull in between. Finally, other motorists are not likely to realize that the two emergency vehicles are traveling together. After the police car speeds by, a vehicle may pull in front of an ambulance, assuming the coast is clear.

In multiple-vehicle responses, the dangers are the same as for an escort. In addition, another danger occurs when two emergency vehicles approach an intersection at the same time. Besides totally confusing motorists and pedestrians, the potential for an intersection collision increases dramatically. Motorists often fail to yield the right of way to the first emergency vehicle, the second emergency vehicle, or, in some instances, both vehicles.

It is a good idea to pay attention to other calls taken in your district. However, do not assume that you know all the responses that are taking place. To avoid warning the perpetrators of crimes, for example, the police often respond to incidents without announcing their approach. As a general rule, always negotiate an intersection assuming that you may meet another emergency vehicle.

Parking and Loading the Ambulance

Whenever you arrive first at the site of a motor vehicle collision, take steps to size up the scene for potential hazards to you, your crew, and the patients. Consider establishing a danger zone, parking at least 100 feet from the wreckage upwind and uphill (if possible) to avoid fire or any escaping hazardous liquids or fumes. If there are no fire or escaping liquids or fumes, park at least 50 feet from the wreckage. If possible, assign a member of the crew to handle traffic until the police arrive to take control of the task.

If your ambulance is the first emergency vehicle on the scene, make sure you park in front of the wreckage so your warning lights can alert approaching motorists. Then set up flares, or nonincendiary warning devices, as quickly as possible.

If the scene has already been secured, park beyond the wreckage to prevent your ambulance from being exposed to traffic (Figure 9-6). If command has already been established by an on-scene EMS unit, you may receive prearrival instructions. In the case of multiple-casualty incidents, for example, the commander may tell you where to park and whom you should report to.

Always be aware of potential traffic hazards at the scene of a call. Many EMS providers have been seriously injured—and some even killed—after being struck by passing motorists. As much as possible, try not to expose either your crew or your patient to traffic. Keep in mind that the rear ambulance doors often obstruct the warning lights when they are opened to load the patient. Also remember that studies have shown that red revolving lights attract drunk or tired drivers. Consider pulling off the road, turning off your headlights, and using just the amber rear sealed blinkers that flash in tandem or in unison. These lights, as noted, will help oncoming motorists to identify both the size and the location of your vehicle.

The Deadly Intersection

Recall that New York statistics reveal that 72 percent of all ambulance collisions occur in intersections. Clearly the intersection is a very unsafe, if not deadly, place to be. Exercise extreme caution whenever you approach one of these hazards. Keep in mind the braking distance of your ambulance, the effectiveness of lights and siren, the rules of the road, the SOPs of your service, the acceleration needed to get through the intersection safely, and more. Helpful tips for negotiating an intersection include the following:

- Stop at all red lights and stop signs and then proceed with caution.
- Always proceed through an intersection slowly.
- Make eye contact with other motorists to ensure that they understand your intentions.
- If you are using any of the exemptions offered to you as an emergency vehicle, such as passing through a red light or a stop sign, make sure you warn motorists by appropriately flashing your lights and sounding the siren.

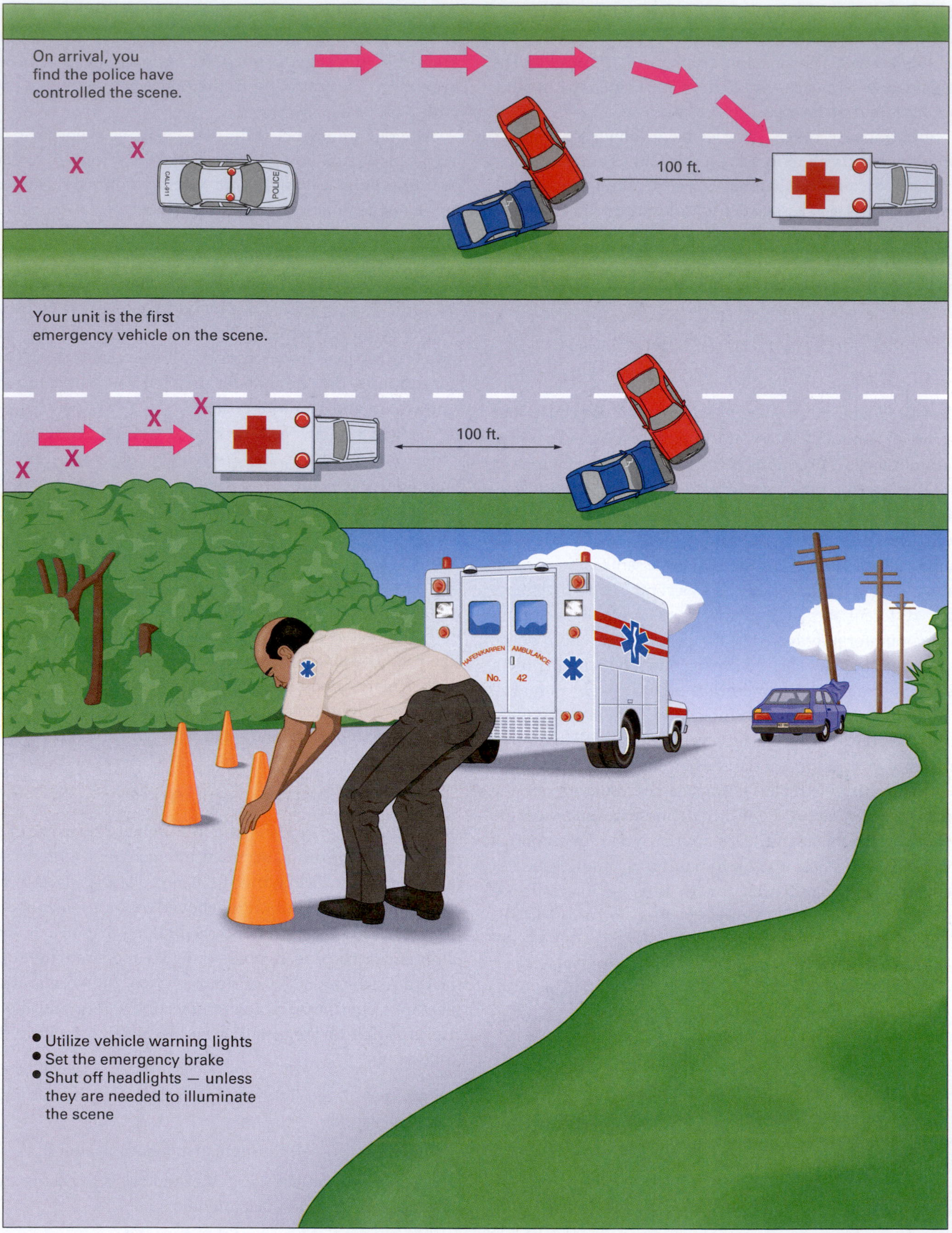

FIGURE 9-6 Parking the ambulance.

- Remember that lights and siren only "ask" the public to yield the right of way. If the public does not yield, it may be because they misunderstand your intentions, cannot hear the siren because of noise in their own vehicles, or cannot see your lights. Never assume that other motorists have a clue to what you plan on doing at the intersection.
- Always go around cars stopped at the intersection on their left (driver's) side. In some instances, this may involve passing into the oncoming lane, which should be done slowly and very cautiously. You invite trouble when you use a clear right lane to sneak past a group of cars at an intersection. If motorists are doing what they should do under motor vehicle laws, they may pull into the right lane just as you attempt to pass.
- Know how long it takes for your ambulance to cross an intersection. This will help you judge whether you have enough time to pass through safely.
- Watch pedestrians at an intersection carefully. If they all seem to be staring in another direction, rather than at your ambulance, they may well be looking at the fire truck headed your way.
- Remember that there is no such thing as a rolling stop in an ambulance weighing more than 10,000 pounds or a medium-duty vehicle weighing some 24,000 pounds. Even at speeds as slow as 30 miles per hour, these vehicles will not stop on a dime. When negotiating an intersection, consider "covering the brake" to shorten the stopping distance.

Patho Pearls

Rooting EMS Practice in Sound Science During the development of emergency medical services, most practices were based on common sense, current medical practices, or rational conjecture. In the late 1990s, the National Highway Traffic Safety Administration (NHTSA), in conjunction with the Health Resources and Services Administration, developed *The EMS Agenda for the Future*, published by the NHTSA in 1996. *The EMS Agenda for the Future* provided an opportunity to examine what had been learned during the past three decades and created a vision for the future. This opportunity has come at an important time—when the agencies, organizations, and individuals that affect EMS are evaluating their role in the context of a rapidly evolving health care system. See the introductory chapter, "EMS Systems," for a more extensive discussion of *The EMS Agenda for the Future*.

Furthermore, the government and third-party payers (Medicare, Medicaid, private insurance companies) are going to pay only for prehospital care interventions that can be proven to improve patient care and patient outcome. Because of this, all current EMS practices must come under scrutiny. For example, medical helicopters may not provide the patient benefit once thought. The quality of prehospital care has improved to a degree that there is often little difference between the quality of care a helicopter crew can provide when compared to a ground EMS crew. Likewise, we are learning that speed makes a difference for very few patients. Because of this and other issues, it is important that we specifically define the role and utilization criteria for expensive resources such as medical helicopters and similar interventions. This is all a part of the natural evolution of modern EMS.

Summary

Even though you have learned about ambulance operations in your EMT training and in your everyday experience, good safety habits grow stronger with review and practice. As a paramedic, you should be familiar with standards that influence ambulance design, equipment requirements, and staffing. You should also regularly complete all checklists, whether they apply to the vehicle, onboard equipment, or essential supplies. Be aware of items that require routine maintenance or calibration, as well as the expiration dates on all drugs. Keep in mind OSHA requirements that promote the safety of personnel and patients and know how to report equipment problems or failures to your supervisor.

As you know, ambulance operators have a special responsibility whenever they take the wheel. It is your professional duty to recognize the profile of a typical ambulance collision and to develop strategies for preventing it from occurring. You should also be aware of the issues surrounding the staging and staffing of ambulances and determine your agency's policies on these matters.

You Make the Call

You and your partner are working on Medic Ambulance 622 covering the west portion of town. It's your turn to drive when a call comes in for an automobile collision. Responding priority one, lights and siren, you travel eastbound on Central Avenue, approaching the intersection of Wolf Road. You know that this is probably one of the busiest intersections in town. It has two through lanes and two turn lanes in each direction. As a result, there are almost always two moving lanes of traffic.

About 250 feet from the intersection, you notice that the light has turned red. Cars have stopped in both of the left turn lanes. There are a few cars in the center lane, and no cars at all in the right lane. As usual, there are a number of cars traveling northbound through the intersection. There are also southbound cars waiting to turn left and proceed eastbound.

1. Should you drive down the open eastbound right lane with your lights and siren on? Explain.
2. Should you enter the oncoming traffic by going around the left side of the vehicle that is currently stopped in the left-hand, eastbound lane? Explain.
3. How can you best deal with this very dangerous intersection?

See Suggested Responses at the back of this book.

Review Questions

1. State EMS agencies establish state standards that are characterized to be what type of standards for ambulance operation?
   a. Gold
   b. Optimal
   c. Minimum
   d. Maximum
2. Which of the following describes a Type II ambulance design?
   a. Medium-duty ambulance rescue vehicle
   b. Standard van, forward control integral cab-body ambulance
   c. Specialty van, forward control integral cab-body ambulance
   d. Conventional truck cab-chassis with a modular ambulance body
3. Which agency is charged with protecting worker safety in the job environment?
   a. ASTNA
   b. FCC
   c. OSHA
   d. CAAS
4. At the national level, what organization provides a certification for EMS entities that can adhere to a grouping of guidelines and standards that meet or exceed state and local guidelines for EMS operations?
   a. ACS
   b. NHTSA
   c. OSHA
   d. CAAS
5. The strategy used by an EMS agency to maneuver its ambulances and crews in order to reduce response times is known as ______________
   a. assignment.
   b. calibration.
   c. deployment.
   d. maintenance.
6. ______________ is a common computerized personnel and ambulance deployment system designed to meet service demands with fewer resources and to ensure appropriate response time and vehicle location.
   a. SSM
   b. PAR
   c. SAR
   d. AED
7. Regarding the laws that govern the EMS person who is driving the ambulance with the emergency lights and siren in operations, who is assigned the highest responsibility for ensuring that an accident does not occur?
   a. The EMS provider driving the ambulance
   b. The driver of the car in front of the ambulance
   c. All drivers of vehicles within seeing and hearing distance of the ambulance warning devices
   d. No increased responsibility is placed on anyone.
8. As a general rule, at least how far upwind from the scene of an accident in which there may be a danger of hazardous liquids or fumes should the ambulance be parked?
   a. 50 feet
   b. 100 feet
   c. 150 feet
   d. 200 feet
9. Where do the majority of ambulance crashes that occur while operating emergency lights and sirens happen?
   a. On freeways
   b. On rural roads
   c. In city intersections
   d. Within 3 miles of the hospital

See Answers to Review Questions at the end of this book.

References

1. United States General Services Administration. *Federal Specification for the Star-of-Life Ambulance (KKK-A-1822F)*. Washington, DC: Government Printing Office, 2007.
2. De Maio, V. J., I. G. Stiell, G. A. Wells, D. W. Spaite, Ontario Prehospital Advanced Life Support Study Group. "Optimal Defibrillation Response Intervals for Maximum Out-of-Hospital Cardiac Arrest Survival Rates." *Ann Emerg Med* 42 (2003): 242–250.
3. Pons, P. T., J. S. Haukoos, W. Bludworth, T. Cribley, K. A. Pons, and V. J. Markovchick. "Paramedic Response Time: Does It Affect Patient Survival?" *Acad Emerg Med* 12 (2005): 594–600.
4. Blackwell, T. H., J. Kline, J. Willis, et al. "Lack of Association between Prehospital Response Times and Patient Outcomes." *Prehosp Emerg Care* 11(1) (2007): 115.
5. Vukmir, R. and L. Katz, Sodium Bicarbonate Study Group. "The Influence of Urban, Suburban, or Rural Locale on Survival from Refractory Cardiac Arrest." *Am J Emerg Med* 22 (2004): 90–93.
6. Valenzuela, T. D., D. J. Roe, G. Nichol, L. L. Clark, D. W. Spaite, and R. G. Hardman. "Outcomes of Rapid Defibrillation by Security Officers after Cardiac Arrest in Casinos." *N Engl J Med* 343 (2000): 1206–1209.
7. Berger, E. "Nothing Gold Can Stay? EMS Crashes, Lack of Evidence Bring the Golden Hour Concept under New Scrutiny." *Ann Emerg Med* 56 (2010): A17–A19.
8. Studnek, J. R. and A. R. Fernandez. "Characteristics of Emergency Medical Technicians Involved in Ambulance Crashes." *Prehosp Disaster Med* 23 (2008): 432–437.
9. Custalow, C. B. and C. S. Gravitz. "Emergency Medical Vehicle Collisions and Potential for Preventive Intervention." *Prehosp Emerg Care* 8 (2004): 175–184.
10. De Grave, K., K. F. Deroo, P. A. Calle, et al. "How to Modify the Risk-Taking Behaviour of Emergency Medical Services Drivers." *Eur J Emerg Med* 10 (2003): 111–116.
11. Marques-Baptista, A., P. Ohman-Strickland, K. T. Baldino, M. Prasto, and M. A. Merlin. "Utilization of Warning Lights and Siren Based on Hospital Time-Critical Interventions." *Prehosp Disaster Med* 25 (2010): 335–339.
12. Brown, L. H., C. L. Whitney, R. C. Hunt, M. Addario, and T. Hogue. "Do Warning Lights and Sirens Reduce Ambulance Response Times?" *Prehosp Emerg Care* 4 (2000): 70–74.
13. Hunt, R. C., L. H. Brown, E. S. Cabinum, et al. "Is Ambulance Transport Time with Lights and Siren Faster Than That Without?" *Ann Emerg Med* 25 (1995): 507–511.

Further Reading

Limmer, D. and M. F. O'Keefe. *Emergency Care*. 13th ed. Upper Saddle River, NJ: Pearson/Prentice Hall, 2015.

Lindsey, J. T. and R. W. Patrick. *Emergency Vehicle Operations*. Upper Saddle River, NJ: Pearson/Prentice Hall, 2007.

Mistovich, J. J. and K. J. Karren. *Prehospital Emergency Care*. 10th ed. Upper Saddle River, NJ: Pearson/Prentice Hall, 2013.

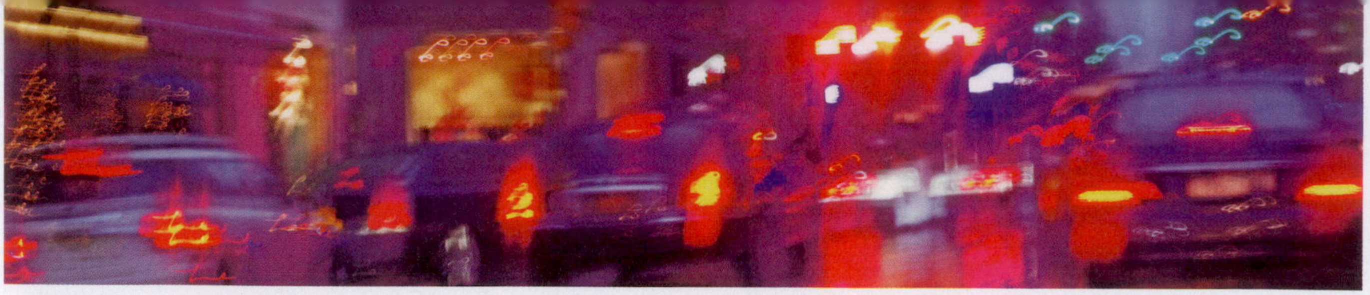

Chapter 10

Air Medical Operations

Bryan Bledsoe, DO, FACEP, FAAEM, EMT-P
Mike Abernethy, MD, FAAEM
Ryan J. Wubben, MD, FAAEM

STANDARD

EMS Operations (Air Medical)

COMPETENCY

Applies knowledge of operational roles and responsibilities to ensure patient, public, and personnel safety.

Learning Objectives

Terminal Performance Objective: After reading this chapter, you should be able to place patient care tasks in the context of air ambulance operations to safely interact with or operate within air medical services to respond to calls and transport patients.

Enabling Objectives: To accomplish the terminal performance objective, you should be able to:

1. Define key terms introduced in this chapter.
2. Identify the multiple ways in which helicopters and fixed wing aircrafts have contributed to modern-day EMS practice and health care.
3. Describe the evolution of air medical transport over time, including key events that led to the development of air medical transport as it exists today.
4. Describe the characteristics and capabilities of fixed-wing and rotor-wing aircraft, to include the use of various types of flight rules.
5. Discuss the indications, limitations, concerns, and controversies about the use of air medical transport.
6. Given a scenario involving air medical response, discuss the actions needed to ensure effective and safe ground operations.
7. Given a scenario involving air medical response, obtain and communicate information needed for safe and effective interaction between the air medical crew and ground personnel.

KEY TERMS

ADAMS, p. 285
fixed-wing aircraft, p. 278
instrument flight rules (IFR), p. 280
night vision goggles (NVG), p. 276
rotor-wing aircraft, p. 278
visual flight rules (VFR), p. 280

Case Study

On a rural Nevada highway, approximately 75 miles north of Las Vegas, a small sports car pulls around a slow-moving recreational vehicle (RV) to pass. However, as the driver is alongside the RV, he sees a motorcycle approaching quickly in the oncoming lane. He hits the brakes and tries to return to his prior position behind the RV, but he is unable to get back before striking the motorcycle. The motorcyclist, seeing the impending accident, tries to avoid a head-on collision by laying the bike on its side. Thus, at approximately 60 miles per hour, the bike and the motorcyclist are tumbling down the highway. The bike hits the sports car and the motorcyclist tumbles into the desert.

The driver of the sports car screeches to a halt. The elderly couple in the RV see the accident in their rearview mirrors and return to the scene. The motorcyclist is about 30 meters off the road. He is unresponsive, with gurgling respirations. Despite the fact that he is wearing a helmet and leathers, he has sustained multiple significant injuries. The couple from the RV and the driver involved in the accident run to the victim. Unsure of what to do, they retrieve a small first aid kit from the RV. The driver of the sports car tries to use his cell phone but cannot get a signal. The couple in the RV try as well—to no avail. About this time, another motorcyclist arrives. He is a friend of the victim. He cannot get a cell phone signal either. He decides to drive down the road to a roadside emergency phone and summon the police and EMS.

After about 20 minutes, a volunteer fire department staffed with first responders arrives. After a quick look, they summon a medical helicopter because the closest hospital is about an hour away by ground. They provide initial stabilizing care and, along with the highway patrol, establish a safe landing zone for the incoming helicopter.

The helicopter lands and the medical crew assesses the patient. The crew members perform a rapid secondary assessment and rapidly prepare the patient for transport. The patient is moved to the helicopter and transported to a trauma center in Las Vegas. On arrival at the trauma center, the patient is treated promptly. He is found to have a subdural hematoma, multiple facial fractures, a fractured spleen, and multiple lower-extremity fractures. He is taken immediately to surgery for an exploratory laparotomy and splenectomy. He requires 8 units of blood. He remains intubated and on mechanical ventilation in the trauma ICU for four days. He is eventually extubated and transferred to a standard floor bed. He undergoes numerous operations to repair his facial fractures and orthopedic injuries. Finally, after six weeks in the hospital, he is discharged to return to his home in Montana. His prognosis is very good.

Introduction

The use of aircraft for emergency patient transport has become a critical component of modern EMS practice. Both helicopters and airplanes (fixed wing) have proved to be vital assets in the emergent transport of the ill or injured patient. Their uses include:

- ***Scene responses.*** The first major use of aircraft, specifically helicopters, was for flying directly to an incident scene and then transporting the patient to a definitive care facility (Figure 10-1). Scene responses may be primary (the air medical crew is first on the scene) or secondary (summoned by ground personnel).[1,2]
- ***Interfacility transport.*** One of the most rapidly expanding areas of air medical transport is the emergent transfer of patients between health care facilities (Figure 10-2). In the rural setting, patients often require

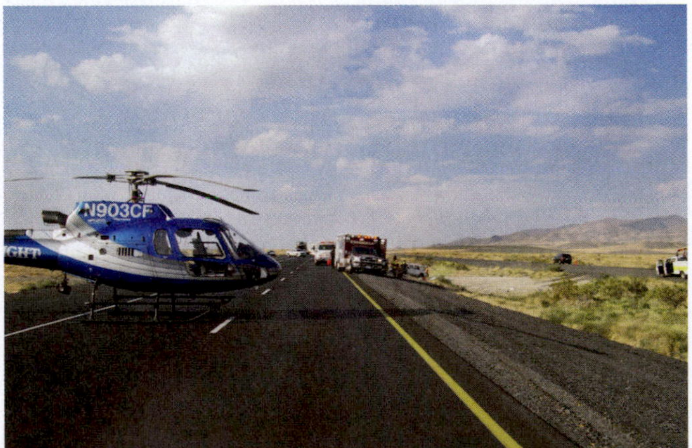

FIGURE 10-1 A helicopter can fly directly to an incident scene and transport a patient to a definitive care facility.

(© Pat Songer)

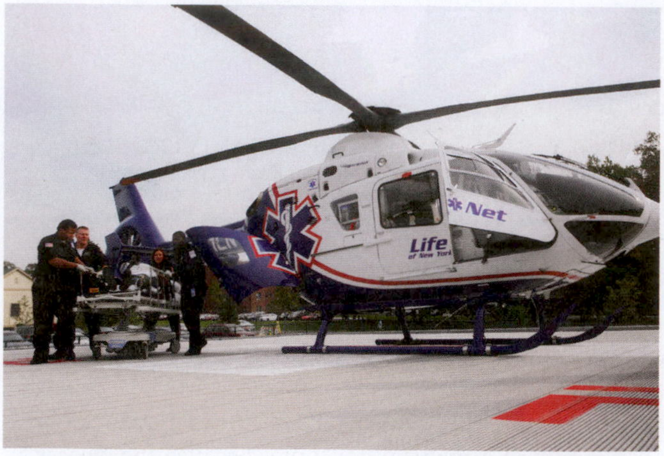

FIGURE 10-2 A rapidly expanding area of air medical transport is the emergent transfer of patients between facilities.

(© Mark Foster)

a level of specialty care that is unavailable locally. When dealing with critically ill patients, significant prehospital time can be minimized through air transport. The type of aircraft used is based on the distance to be traveled and the patient's condition. Generally speaking, helicopters are limited to distances less than 150 to 200 miles.[3–5]

- ***Specialty care.*** Air medical transport can bring specialty teams to community hospitals for care of selected patients (Figure 10-3). The most common example is that of neonatal transport. Neonates, especially preterm infants, can require sophisticated specialized care. In some systems, a neonatal team is transported to the community hospital where initial stabilization is completed. Following that, transport may or may not be by aircraft. In some systems, the neonatal team is transported to the community hospital by helicopter but return to the tertiary care facility is often by ground ambulance.[6,7]
- ***Organ procurement.*** The transplantation of human organs has evolved significantly over the past two decades. The procurement of human organs is a time-sensitive endeavor. Because of this, organ procurement teams often use aircraft to respond to the site of the donor and subsequently transport the organs back to the transplant center.
- ***Search and rescue.*** The use of aircraft for search and rescue has been a part of aviation virtually since its inception. Medical aircraft, including both fixed-wing aircraft and helicopters, are sometimes used in search-and-rescue operations. Although this can be system dependent, it is not an uncommon practice. Medical helicopter pilots and crews are often intimately familiar with local geography and can provide much-needed assistance in search-and-rescue operations. The addition of technology such as high-intensity spotlights, forward-looking infrared (FLIR), and **night vision goggles (NVG)** makes helicopters a valuable asset in these situations (Figure 10-4).
- ***Disaster assistance.*** Disaster situations often impact or destroy the infrastructure of the community and region affected. In many instances, ingress and egress are restricted because of the destruction of roads. This is commonly seen following both earthquakes and hurricanes. However, it is also seen in tornadoes and similar events. Aircraft, particularly helicopters, can provide access to disaster regions not accessible by ground ambulances. The role of helicopters proved crucial and lifesaving, for example, following Hurricane Katrina, which struck New Orleans and southern Louisiana as well as adjoining states in the 2005 Atlantic hurricane season.[8]

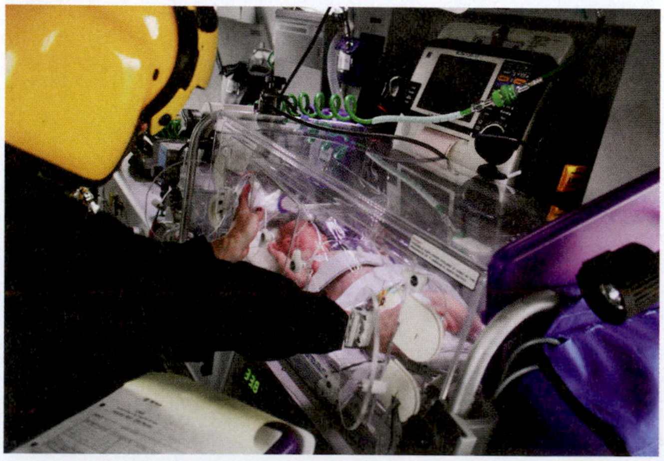

FIGURE 10-3 Helicopters can bring neonatal specialty teams to community hospitals.

(© Austin/Travis County STARFlight)

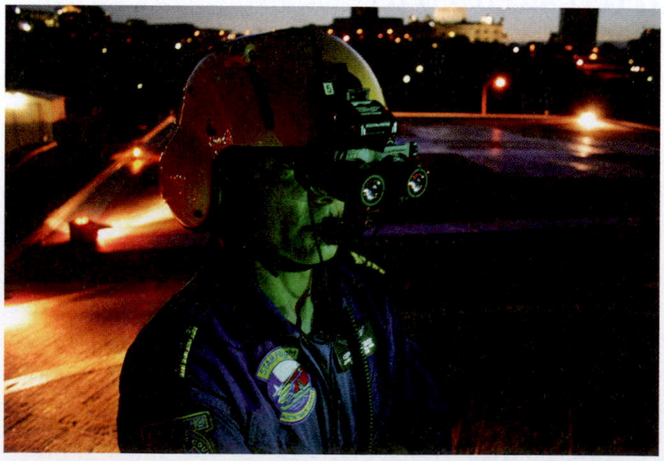

FIGURE 10-4 Night vision goggles are useful in helicopter search-and-rescue operations.

(©Austin/Travis County STARFlight)

Air medical transport is an important asset to any EMS system. It should be considered a medical procedure with benefits and risks. These risks and benefits must be weighed. However, like any other asset or tool, air medical transport must be used responsibly. EMS providers should be familiar with local medical capabilities and those protocols for usage.

History

Like most aspects of emergency medicine, air medical transport's origins and development are deeply rooted within the military. The first recorded use of an airplane to evacuate wounded casualties was during World War I by a French aircraft in Serbia. Later in that same war, the British used aircraft to evacuate casualties in the Turkish theater. Subsequently, a fully organized air ambulance operation was used by both the French and British during the African and Middle Eastern colonial wars of the 1920s. During Germany's involvement in the Spanish Civil War, casualties from its "Condor Legion" expeditionary force were evacuated by Junkers Ju-52 trimotors back to Germany for care.

The first successful operational helicopter was the Sikorsky YR-4, built in the United States in 1942. These were then deployed in an experiment to Burma by the U.S. Army in 1944–1945. Initially they were intended to be used in a search-and-rescue function for downed aircrew, but on January 26, 1945, the first documented medical evacuation by helicopter took place in the jungles of Burma that would have taken 10 days on foot to accomplish.

By the time the United States entered the Korean War in 1950, helicopter usage had become more common both as an aerial observation platform and for the medical evacuation of infantry casualties. In Korea, patients were evacuated from the battlefield to Mobile Army Surgical Hospital (MASH) units and battalion aid stations for emergency medical and surgical care. As the patients were transported on the skids of the aircraft, medical care during transport was nonexistent. Critically ill or injured casualties were later transported to well-equipped hospital ships for definitive care and repatriation.

By 1960, the mass production of more powerful gas turbine engines allowed the design of larger, more powerful helicopters. For the first time, battlefield casualties could ride inside the helicopter and receive in-flight care from medical personnel.

The helicopter in the military serves several nonmedical roles. Medical evacuation of battlefield casualties by helicopter, often referred to as "dust off," was heavily used during the Vietnam War and was responsible for a significant improvement in the outcome of wounded soldiers (Figure 10-5). In modern warfare, medical evacuation by both helicopter and fixed-wing aircraft plays an important role in the safety of military personnel.[9]

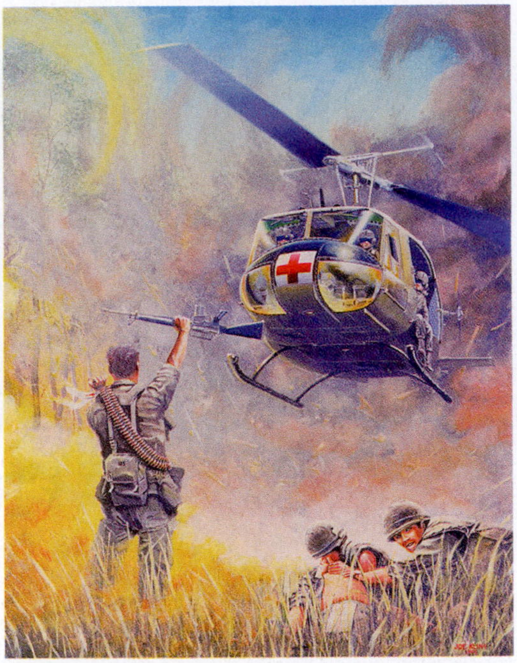

FIGURE 10-5 The medevac (also called the "dust-off") helicopter played a major role in decreasing mortality in Vietnam by rapidly moving injured soldiers from the battlefield to definitive care.

(Dustoff © 2000, Joe Kline Aviation Art)

The civilian use of aircraft for medical evacuation and care was initiated in rural areas, such as those in Australia and Canada. Most notably, Australia developed the Royal Flying Doctor Service (RFDS), which provided medical care to the inhabitants of rural Australia. The RFDS continues to operate today. The first dedicated air ambulance service in the United States was begun by Schaeffer Ambulance Service in Los Angeles. The service opened in 1947 and was the first to use Federal Aviation Administration (FAA)-certified aircraft in an ambulance role. By the late 1960s, the helicopter had proven itself as an effective means of transport for critically injured military casualties. However, this lifesaving technology saw little, if any, use in the civilian sector.

In 1970, Congress passed legislation creating the Military Assistance to Safety and Traffic (MAST) program. This authorized the U.S. military to use the battle-proven system of simultaneous helicopter evacuation and medical care to augment existing U.S. civilian EMS. MAST programs were established at 12 active army bases, as well as several National Guard and Army Reserve installations.

In 1970, the Maryland State Police established the first nonmilitary helicopter medical evacuation program. Two years later, St. Anthony's Hospital in Denver founded the first civilian helicopter air ambulance (HAA) program, called Flight for Life (Figure 10-6).

Over the next 30 years, there was a gradual, expected growth in the HAA industry. The majority of the new programs were hospital based, mainly because of the cost of

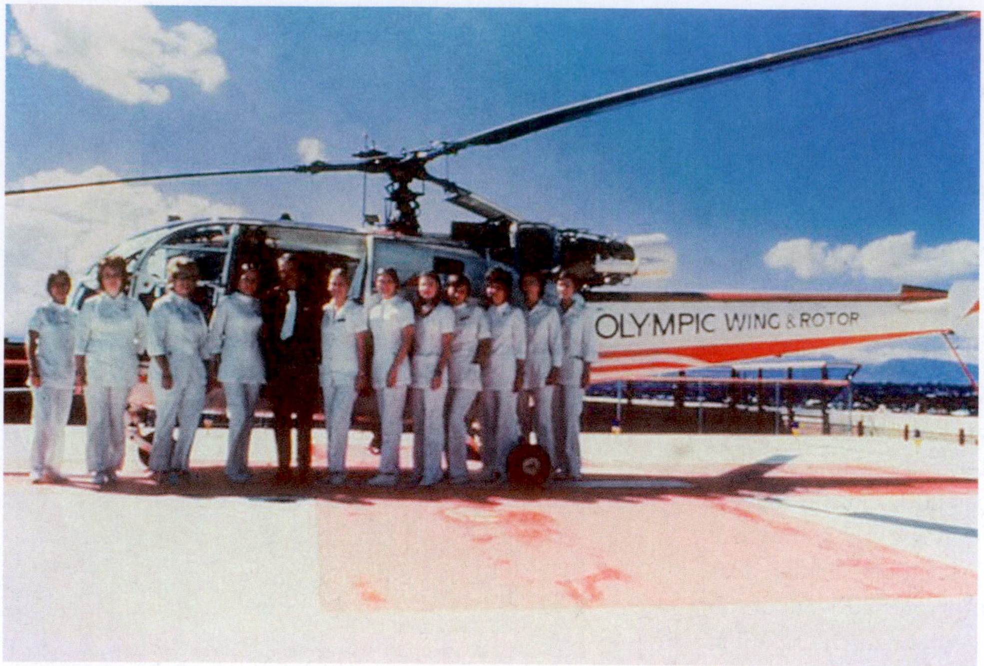

FIGURE 10-6 The first U.S. civilian helicopter devoted exclusively to patient care was St. Anthony's Flight for Life in Denver.

(© Flight For Life Colorado)

such an endeavor. In 2001, Medicare increased the reimbursement for HAA transport, allowing a huge growth in the community (nonhospital)-based sector of the industry. As of 2010, there were approximately 730 HAA bases with 900 aircraft in the United States.

In 2015, the FAA determined that the previously used term "helicopter EMS (HEMS)" was obsolete and the term "helicopter air ambulance (HAA)" should be used. The reasoning stated was that even though a critical life and death medical emergency may exist, air ambulance flights are not operated as an emergency. Pilots and operator management personnel should make flight decisions based not on the condition of the patient, but rather on the safety of the flight.

Aircraft

The types of aircraft used in air medical transport have changed considerably over the past several decades. Much of this was in response to developments and improvements in aviation technology. The two types of aircraft used in air medical transport are **fixed-wing aircraft** (airplanes) and **rotor-wing aircraft** (helicopters). Fixed-wing aircraft provide comfort, speed, and significant range, especially when compared with ground ambulances. Rotor-wing aircraft can access hard-to-reach situations and provide transport that is often quicker than that available in ground ambulances. The choice of aircraft type is usually based on the distance of transport, medical needs, patient condition, and availability.

Fixed-Wing Aircraft

Fixed-wing aircraft, commonly referred to as airplanes, are vehicles capable of flight that use fixed wings to generate lift (Figure 10-7). Generally speaking, the speed of an airplane is greater than that of most helicopters. Either a turbine engine or a piston engine typically powers fixed-wing aircraft. Some turbine-powered airplanes have a propeller (turboprop) to provide propulsion, whereas others are jet powered. In the turboprop system, most of the energy derived from the turbine goes to power the propeller. In the jet propulsion system, the turbine powers a rotary air compressor that compresses incoming air and exhaust gases and ejects these via a duct. The ejected gases generated by the turbine are the propulsion used to move the aircraft.

Most air ambulances are turbine powered and usually have at least two engines. Many fixed-wing aircraft contain pressurized cabins that allow safe and comfortable travel at altitudes that are inaccessible by aircraft without a pressurized cabin. Generally, fixed-wing aircraft are somewhat larger than helicopters, with many being capable of transporting several patients at the same time. Jet airplanes have a much greater range and speed than helicopters.

The limitation of airplanes as air ambulances is that they must land and take off from established airports. Such airports are not always in close proximity to the patient or

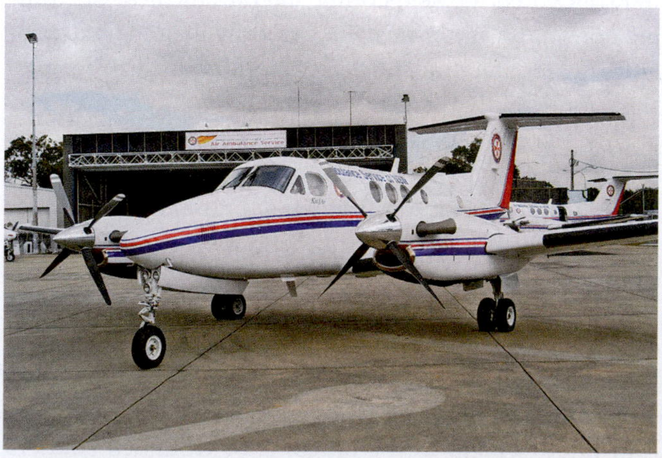

FIGURE 10-7 Fixed-wing fleet operated as part of the New South Wales, Australia, ambulance service.

(© Dr. Bryan E. Bledsoe)

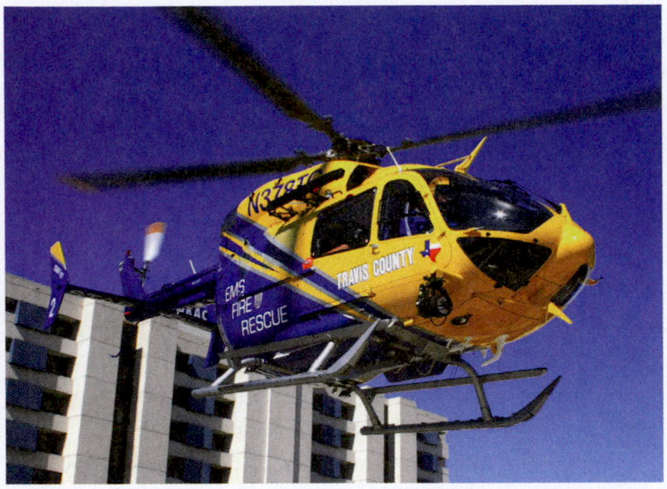

FIGURE 10-8 Helicopters (rotary-wing aircraft) are commonly used in modern EMS.

(© Austin/Travis County STARFlight)

hospital. Thus, the patient must also be transported by ground ambulance to the airport to meet the aircraft, which incurs delays to definitive care.

Rotor-Wing Aircraft

Helicopters, which by definition are rotary-wing aircraft, are commonly used in modern EMS (Figure 10-8). Helicopters use rotating blades, referred to as a *rotor*, to provide lift and propulsion. The main rotor system is supplemented by a tail rotor to counteract the natural torque produced by the rotor; without the tail rotor, the cabin and fuselage would spin in the opposite direction from the main rotors. Essentially, all helicopters used in an EMS role in the United States are powered by a turbine (jet) engine. As of 2009, 46 percent of the EMS helicopter fleet had single engines, whereas 54 percent used twin-engine aircraft.[10] Most EMS helicopters are considered small to medium in size (Figures 10-9 through 10-13).

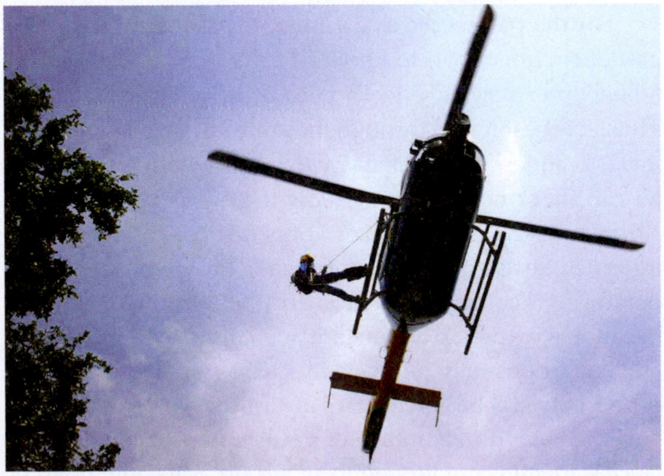

FIGURE 10-9 Eurocopter EC135 helicopter.

(©Austin/Travis County STARFlight)

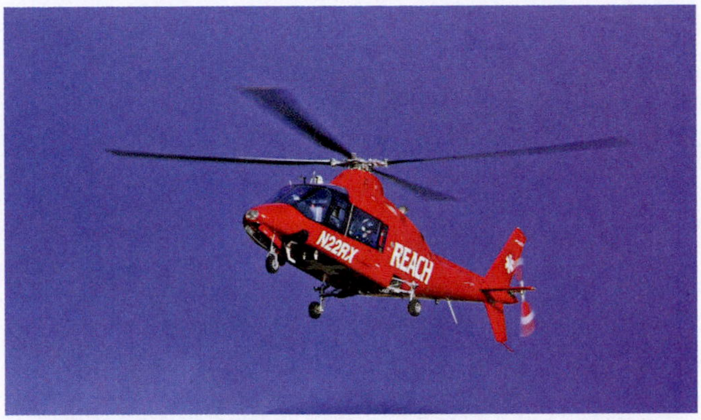

FIGURE 10-10 Agusta 109 Power helicopter.

(REACH Air Medical Services)

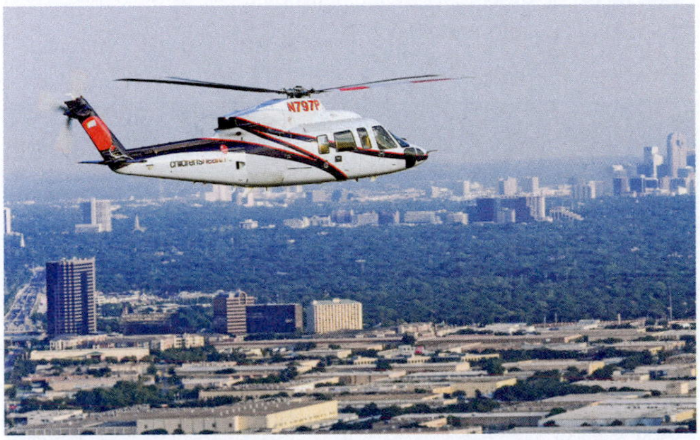

FIGURE 10-11 Sikorsky S76 helicopter.

(Courtesy of Children's Medical Center, Dallas)

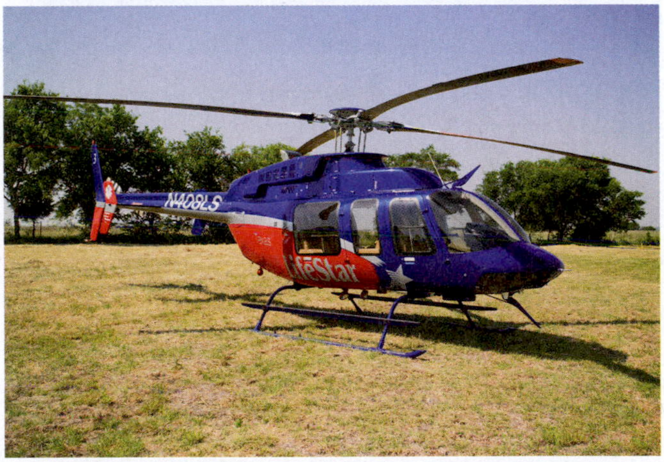

FIGURE 10-12 Bell 407 helicopter.

(© Mark Foster)

Others use a larger airframe (Figure 10-14). In the United States, most EMS helicopters have a single pilot. Some medical helicopters in the United States are capable of instrument flight rule usage.

One of the most significant limitations that all helicopters face is the weather. There are very specific rules that all pilots must follow in regard to the weather when making decisions to fly or to continue flying once they are in the

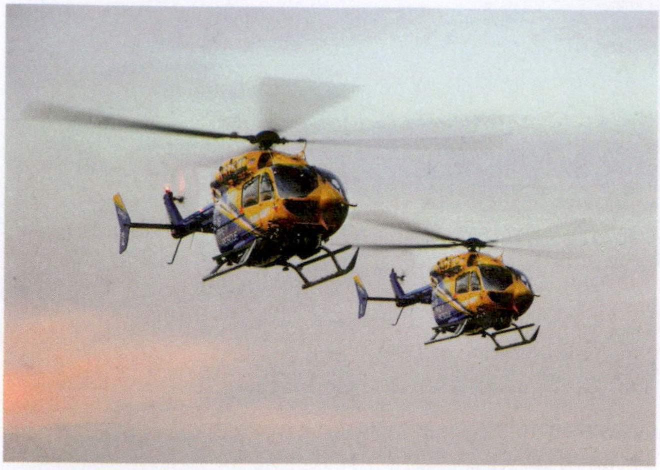

FIGURE 10-13 Eurocopter EC145 helicopter.
(©Austin/Travis County STARFlight)

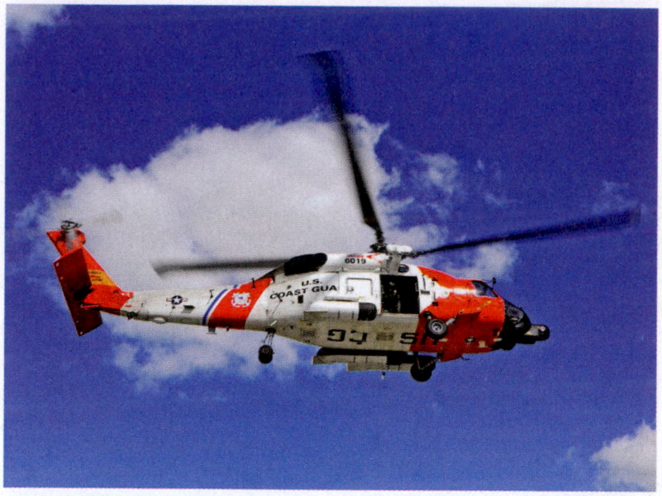

FIGURE 10-14 The U.S. Coast Guard uses larger-frame helicopters.
(US Coast Guard)

air. The basic dichotomy is between flying under **visual flight rules (VFR)** or under **instrument flight rules (IFR)**. The difference between the two is whether the pilot can fly visually (without instruments) and be able to see a visible horizon for orientation. This is contrasted with conditions such as flying in the clouds or in marginal weather and relying on aircraft instruments and direction from the FAA's Air Traffic Control (ATC) system.

Most programs in the United States are limited to flying under VFR conditions at all times and train to fly on instruments in an emergency only when poor weather conditions are inadvertently encountered. A few helicopter EMS programs in the United States have made the investment to train their pilots and equip their aircraft to fly in IFR conditions intentionally with patients on board. The vast majority of EMS helicopters in the United States only have one pilot, which then requires sophisticated autopilot and global positioning system (GPS) navigation systems to fly safely in the clouds.

The weather conditions that an EMS helicopter requires before it can fly safely vary from program to program and vary with the expected terrain that will be encountered, lighting (day or night), distance from home base, and so on. For example, a VFR helicopter program may need to have at least 3 miles of horizontal visibility and there must be at least 1,000 feet of clearance between the ground and lowest level of clouds before it will accept a flight. All the variables mentioned here can change the minimum conditions required before a pilot can accept a flight. All aircraft must give thunderstorms a wide berth; in certain parts of the country at certain times of the year, these storms can be a common problem, limiting the ability to fly.

Even helicopter programs that have the capability and training to fly under IFR conditions have significant limitations. For example, most civilian helicopters are not certified by the FAA to fly knowingly in conditions in which ice may form on the airframe of the helicopter (which adds weight and drag, seriously degrading aircraft performance and handling), making this a significant safety issue that has caused many accidents. In northern climates, this may mean that flights may be prohibited whenever there are clouds in winter, or when the temperatures at altitude are below freezing and precipitation may be encountered. Programs that fly IFR are also limited in where they can fly under ATC direction. Specifically, these aircraft usually are able to fly only from airport to airport, or from hospital to hospital if the hospital is near an airport or has an approved instrument approach directly to the hospital.

Helicopters are also not generally able to fly on instruments to random points on the ground, such as accident scenes on the highway, because of the limitations of current technology and the ATC system. In this situation, it may be best as the paramedic on the ground to transport your patient to the nearest hospital. Despite these limitations, the ability to fly IFR provides far more options should weather conditions change, and affords an added layer of safety in a constantly changing environment.

For the paramedic in the field, it is difficult under the best of circumstances to know all the variables that go into a helicopter service's decision to accept or deny a flight. Thus, it is best to call through the appropriate channels and make a request, rather than try to guess whether a helicopter can fly or not. This will allow the pilot to evaluate the situation using the resources at his disposal and make an informed decision. Even if there is fog, driving snow, thunderstorms, or tornadoes, it is still best to make the call because weather is a constantly changing phenomenon and conditions may improve in a time frame when a helicopter may still be able to provide assistance.

The obvious advantage of a helicopter as an air ambulance is that it is not limited to an airport as its only point of takeoff or landing. Thus, helicopters have become an important part of the modern trauma system. Weather permitting, they can land almost anywhere, retrieve a patient, and transport directly to a trauma center or hospital. In many instances, this can shorten the patient's out-of-hospital time.

Role in EMS

In many EMS systems, air medical transport has been an important part of system operation for decades. Most Australian ambulance services, for instance, have air medical divisions. These operations are often a mix of airplanes and helicopters. Because Australia is such a rural nation, these aircraft are used on a daily basis to move patients between rural areas and the major cities. In the coastal states of Australia, helicopters are used primarily for rescue. In London, the helicopter service is intimately linked with the ground EMS system.

The use of helicopters and airplanes in the U.S. EMS system has evolved in the past 40 years. In the 1970s, several hospitals and other entities established air medical operations. By the mid-1980s, virtually every major community had access to an air ambulance. Most of these operations were hospital based, whereas some, such as the Maryland State Police, were government operations. Because of poor reimbursement, without the backing of a large medical institution or government, it was extremely difficult for independent for-profit programs to exist.

In 2001, the federal government changed the reimbursement scheme for air medical transport. This resulted in a significant increase in the number of air ambulances in the United States. Following this, there has been a transition from a hospital-based model to a community-based model. With that, there has been a transition from hospital-operated models to for-profit models as well.

Uses

There is no doubt that air medical transport plays an important role in the modern EMS system. However, the exact role that helicopter EMS plays in the United States is somewhat loosely defined and unregulated. Because of the rapid growth of air medical operations in the United States and the shift from hospital-based to for-profit models, there has been a proportionate increase in usage. There has been a recent push to better determine and define the role of air ambulances.

The initial use of medical helicopters in EMS was for trauma care. Much of this was based on the work and writings of Dr. R. Adams Cowley, the founder of the Shock Trauma Center in Baltimore. As Dr. Cowley developed the Maryland system, he introduced two concepts that have helped to drive modern trauma care. One was the concept of the "Golden Hour."[11,12] The second was the establishment of a network of helicopters, operated by the Maryland State Police, who would transport trauma patients from the scene directly to the Shock Trauma Center in Baltimore. These two principles became a fundamental tenet of modern trauma care. However, subsequent research has shown that these two factors are less important than originally thought. Despite this, recent research has demonstrated that a specific subset of patients—those with significant injuries—appears to benefit from helicopter transport.[13–19]

Today, there is no doubt that medical helicopters still play a critical role in the prehospital management of trauma. However, they are now also used for nontrauma situations. Although scene responses have remained a major and important use of medical helicopters, there has been a significant expansion of medical helicopter usage for interfacility transport. Much of this has resulted from the specialization of hospitals. The concept of a general hospital is now uncommon. Thus, it has become common practice to move patients, even those who are seriously ill or injured, between facilities. Many institutions have found air medical transport an effective, efficient, and timely method of moving these patients to minimize the inherently risky out-of-hospital time. This is particularly true in the care of patients with a recent stroke and for patients suffering a more severe, identifiable type of acute myocardial infarction (STEMI).[20]

Several studies have shown limited benefit from many helicopter transports. Strategies are being investigated to help prehospital and hospital personnel identify which patients stand to benefit from air medical transport. The American College of Emergency Physicians (ACEP) has endorsed a strategy to guide decision making in regard to selecting a medical helicopter for patient transport (Table 10-1). This statement supplements a prior position paper that defines criteria, developed by the National Association of EMS Physicians (NAEMSP) and ACEP, under which air medical dispatch might be considered (Table 10-2). Table 10-2 does not, however, reflect utilization criteria. One must not confuse the criteria for transfer to a trauma and/or burn center with the need for air transport to those facilities. Simply because a patient needs the care of a specialized center does not necessarily mean that the patient must be transported by helicopter or airplane. In addition, patients with traumatic cardiac arrest have such a poor prognosis that helicopter transport is generally not warranted.

The benefits of air medical transport include speed, decreased out-of-hospital time, and, in some instances, better quality of care. Patients who do not need rapid transport or a reduced out-of-hospital time, or who can receive adequate quality of care by ground transport personnel, should be transported by ground units, if available. If patients need a decreased out-of-hospital time, quality of care that is unavailable by ground transport, or rapid access to specialty care, air medical transport should be considered seriously.

Table 10-1 Appropriate and Safe Utilization of Helicopter Emergency Medical Services*

We believe:

- That patients benefit from the appropriate utilization of Helicopter Emergency Medical Services (HEMS).
- That EMS and regional healthcare systems must have and follow guidelines for HEMS utilization to facilitate proper patient selection and ensure clinical benefit.

Clinical benefit may be provided by:

- Meaningfully shortening the time to delivery of definitive care to patients with time-sensitive medical conditions;
- Providing necessary specialized medical expertise or equipment to patients before and/or during transport;
- Providing transport to patients otherwise inaccessible by other means of transport.

That the decision to utilize HEMS is a medical decision, separate from the aviation determination whether a transport can safely be completed.
Physicians with specialized training and experience in EMS and air medical transport must be integral to HEMS utilization decisions, including guideline development and HEMS quality improvement activities.
Federal Aviation Administration approved Safety Management Systems must be developed, adopted, and adhered to by air medical operators when making decisions to accept and continue each and every HEMS transport.
That HEMS must be fully integrated within the local, regional, and state emergency healthcare system.
HEMS programs cannot operate independent of the surrounding health care environment.
The EMS and health care system must be involved in the determination of the number of HEMS assets necessary to provide appropriate coverage for their region.
Excessive resources may lead to competitive practices that can impact utilization and ultimately affect safety.
Inadequate resources will result in delayed receipt of definitive care.

We further believe that:

- National guidelines for appropriate utilization of HEMS must be developed. These guidelines should be national in scope yet allow for local, regional, and state implementation
- A National HEMS Agenda for the Future should be developed to address HEMS utilization and availability, and to identify and support a research strategy for ongoing, evidence-based refinement of utilization guidelines.

*American College of Emergency Physicians, National Association of EMS Physicians, American Academy of Emergency Medicine, and Air Medical Physicians Association. Policy Statement Approved 2016;.

Table 10-2 Guidelines for Air Medical Dispatch

Guidelines for Air Medical Dispatch*

1. General
   a. Patients requiring critical interventions should be provided those interventions in the most expeditious manner possible.
   b. Patients who are stable should be transported in a manner that best addresses the needs of the patient and the system.
   c. Patients with critical injuries or illnesses resulting in unstable vital signs require transport by the fastest available modality, and with a transport team that has the appropriate level of care capabilities, to a center capable of providing definitive care.
   d. Patients with critical injuries or illnesses should be transported by a team that can provide in transport critical care services.
   e. Patients who require high-level care during transport, but do not have time-critical illness or injury, may be candidates for ground critical care transport (i.e., by a specialized ground critical care transport vehicle with level of care exceeding that of local EMS) if such service is available and logistically feasible.
2. Comparative considerations for air transport modes
   a. Rotor-wing
      i. Advantages
         1. In general, decreased response time to the patient (up to approximately 100 miles distance depending on logistics such as duration of ground transfer leg)
         2. Decreased out-of-hospital transport time
         3. Availability of highly trained medical crews and specialized equipment
      ii. Disadvantages
         1. Weather considerations (e.g., icing conditions, weather minimums)
         2. Limited availability as compared with ground EMS
   b. Fixed-wing
      i. Advantages
         1. In comparison with rotor-wing, decreased response time to patients when transport distances exceed approximately 100 miles
         2. In comparison with ground transport, decreased out-of-hospital transport time
         3. Availability of highly trained medical crews and specialized equipment
         4. In comparison with rotor-wing, less susceptibility to weather constraints
      ii. Disadvantages
         1. Requires landing at airport, with two extra transport legs between airports and the patient origin and destination
         2. In comparison with ground transport, more subject to weather-related unavailability (e.g., icing, snow)
         3. Overall, less desirable as a transport mode for severely ill or injured patients (though extenuating circumstances may modify this relative contraindication to fixed-wing use)
3. Logistical issues that may prompt the need for air medical transport
   a. Access and time/distance factors
      i. Patients who are in topographically hard-to-reach areas may be best served by air transport.
         1. In some cases patients may be in terrain (e.g., mountainside) not easily accessible to surface transport.
         2. Other cases may involve the need for transfer of patients from island environs, for whom surface water transport is not appropriate.
      ii. Patients in some areas (e.g., in the western United States) may be accessible to ground vehicles, but transport distances are sufficiently long that air transport (by rotor-wing or fixed-wing) is preferable.
   b. Systems considerations
      i. In some EMS regions, the air medical crew is the only rapidly available asset that can bring a high level of training to critically ill/injured patients. In these systems, there may be a lower threshold for air medical dispatch.

Table 10-2 Guidelines for Air Medical Dispatch (*Continued*)

ii. Systems in which there is widespread advanced life support (ALS) coverage, but such coverage is sparse, may see an area left "uncovered" for extended periods if its sole ALS unit is occupied providing an extended transport. Air medical dispatch may be the best means to provide patient care and simultaneously avoid deprivation of a geographic region of timely ALS emergency response.

iii. Disaster and mass casualty incidents offer important opportunities for air medical participation. These roles, too complex for detailed discussion here, are outlined elsewhere.

4. Clinical situations for scene triage to air transport (also known as "primary" air transport) are outlined below. In some cases (e.g., flail chest), the diagnosis can be clearly established in the prehospital setting; in other cases (e.g., cardiac injury suggested by mechanism of injury and/or cardiac monitoring findings), prehospital care providers must use judgment and act on suspicion. Absent unusual logistical considerations as an overriding factor, scene air response involves rotor-wing vehicles rather than airplanes. As a general rule, air transport scene response should be considered more likely to be indicated when use of this modality, as compared with ground transport, results in more rapid arrival of the patient to an appropriate receiving center or when helicopter crews provide rapid access to advanced level of care (e.g., when a ground basic life support team encounters a multiple trauma patient requiring airway intervention).

a. Trauma: Scene response to injured patients probably represents the mode of helicopter utilization with the best supporting evidence.

i. General and mechanism considerations
1. Trauma Score <12
2. Unstable vital signs (e.g., hypotension or tachypnea)
3. Significant trauma in patients <12 years old, >55 years old, or pregnant patients
4. Multisystem injuries (e.g., long-bone fractures in different extremities; injury to more than two body regions)
5. Ejection from vehicle
6. Pedestrian or cyclist struck by motor vehicle
7. Death in same passenger compartment as patient
8. Ground provider perception of significant damage to patient's passenger compartment
9. Penetrating trauma to the abdomen, pelvis, chest, neck, or head
10. Crush injury to the abdomen, chest, or head
11. Fall from significant height

ii. Neurologic considerations
1. Glasgow Coma Scale score <10
2. Deteriorating mental status
3. Skull fracture
4. Neurologic presentation suggestive of spinal cord injury

iii. Thoracic consideration
1. Major chest wall injury (e.g., flail chest)
2. Pneumothorax/hemothorax
3. Suspected cardiac injury

iv. Abdominal/pelvic considerations
1. Significant abdominal pain after blunt trauma
2. Presence of a "seatbelt" sign or other abdominal wall contusion
3. Obvious rib fracture below the nipple line
4. Major pelvic fracture (e.g., unstable pelvic ring disruption, open pelvic fracture, or pelvic fracture with hypotension)

v. Orthopedic/extremity considerations
1. Partial or total amputation of a limb (exclusive of digits)
2. Finger/thumb amputation when emergent surgical evaluation (i.e., for replantation consideration) is indicated and rapid surface transport is not available
3. Fracture or dislocation with vascular compromise
4. Extremity ischemia
5. Open long-bone fractures
6. Two or more long-bone fractures

vi. Major burns
1. >20% body surface area
2. Involvement of face, head, hands, feet, or genitalia
3. Inhalational injury
4. Electrical or chemical burns
5. Burns with associated injuries

vii. Patients with near drowning injuries

b. Nontrauma: At this time the literature support for primary air transport of noninjured patients is limited to logistical considerations. It is conceivable that clinical indications for scene air response may be identified in the future. However, at this time prehospital providers should incorporate logistical considerations, clinical judgment, and medical oversight in determining whether primary air transport is appropriate for patients with nontrauma diagnoses.

5. Clinical situations for air transport in interfacility transfers are best summarized as being present when (1) patients have diagnostic and/or therapeutic needs which cannot be met at the referring hospital, and (2) factors such as time, distance, and/or intratransport level of care requirements render ground transport nonfeasible.

a. Trauma: Injured patients constitute the diagnostic group for which there is best evidence to support outcome improvements from air transport.

i. Depending on local hospital capabilities and regional practices, any diagnostic consideration (suspected, or confirmed as with referring hospital radiography) listed above under "scene" guidelines may be sufficient indication for air transport from a community hospital to a regional trauma center.

ii. Additionally, air transport (short- or long-distance) may be appropriate when initial evaluation at the community hospital reveals injuries (e.g., intra-abdominal hemorrhage on abdominal computed tomography) or potential injuries (e.g., aortic trauma suggested by widened mediastinum on chest x-ray; spinal column injury with potential for spinal cord involvement) requiring further evaluation and management beyond the capabilities of the referring hospital.

b. Cardiac: Due to regionalization of cardiac care and the time-criticality of the disease process, patients with cardiac diagnoses often undergo interfacility air transport. Patients with the following cardiac conditions may be candidates for air transport:

i. Acute coronary syndromes with time-critical need for urgent interventional therapy (e.g., cardiac catheterization, intra-aortic balloon pump placement, emergent cardiac surgery) unavailable at the referring center

ii. Cardiogenic shock (especially in presence of, or need for, ventricular assist devices or intra-aortic balloon pumps)

iii. Cardiac tamponade with impending hemodynamic compromise

iv. Mechanical cardiac disease (e.g., acute cardiac rupture, decompensating valvular heart disease)

(*Continued*)

Table 10-2 Guidelines for Air Medical Dispatch (*Continued*)

c. Critically ill medical or surgical patients: These patients generally require a high level of care during transport, may benefit from minimization of out-of-hospital transport time, and may also have time-critical need for diagnostic or therapeutic intervention at the receiving facility. Ground critical care transport is frequently a viable transfer option for these patients, but air transport may be considered in circumstances such as the following examples:
- **i.** Pretransport cardiac/respiratory arrest
- **ii.** Requirement for continuous intravenous vasoactive medications or mechanical ventricular assist to maintain stable cardiac output
- **iii.** Risk for airway deterioration (e.g., angioedema, epiglottitis)
- **iv.** Acute pulmonary failure and/or requirement for sophisticated pulmonary intensive care (e.g., inverse-ratio ventilation) during transport
- **v.** Severe poisoning or overdose requiring specialized toxicology services
- **vi.** Urgent need for hyperbaric oxygen therapy (e.g., vascular gas embolism, necrotizing infectious process, carbon monoxide toxicity)
- **vii.** Requirement for emergent dialysis
- **viii.** Gastrointestinal hemorrhages with hemodynamic compromise
- **ix.** Surgical emergencies such as fasciitis, aortic dissection or aneurysm, or extremity ischemia
- **x.** Pediatric patients for whom referring facilities cannot provide required evaluation and/or therapy

d. Obstetric: In gravid patients, air transport's advantage of minimized out-of-hospital time must be balanced against the risks inherent to intratransport delivery. If transport is necessary in a patient in whom delivery is thought to be imminent, then a ground vehicle is usually appropriate, although in some cases the combination of clinical status and logistics (e.g., long driving times) may favor use of an air ambulance. Air transport may be considered if ground transport is logistically not feasible and/or there are circumstances such as the following:
- **i.** Reasonable expectation that delivery of infant(s) may require obstetric or neonatal care beyond the capabilities of the referring hospital
- **ii.** Active premature labor when estimated gestational age is <34 weeks or estimated fetal weight <2,000 grams
- **iii.** Severe preeclampsia or eclampsia
- **iv.** Third-trimester hemorrhage
- **v.** Fetal hydrops
- **vi.** Maternal medical conditions (e.g., heart disease, drug overdose, metabolic disturbances) exist that may cause premature birth
- **vii.** Severe predicted fetal heart disease
- **viii.** Acute abdominal emergencies (i.e., likely to require surgery) when estimated gestational age is 34 weeks or estimated fetal weight <2,000 grams

e. Neurologic: In addition to those with need for specialized neurosurgical services, this category is being expanded to include patients requiring transfer to specialized stroke centers. Examples of neurologic conditions where air transport may be appropriate include:
- **i.** Central nervous system hemorrhage
- **ii.** Spinal cord compression by mass lesion
- **iii.** Evolving ischemic stroke (i.e., potential candidate for lytic therapy)
- **iv.** Status epilepticus

f. Neonatal: Regionalization of neonatal intensive care has prompted the development of specialized (air and/or ground) services focusing on transport for this population. Given the fact that, in neonates, rapid transport is often less of a priority than (time-consuming) stabilization at referring institutions, some systems have found that the best means for incorporating air vehicles into neonatal transport is to use them to rapidly get a stabilization/transport team to the patient; the actual patient transport is then performed by a ground vehicle. In some systems, patients are transported (usually with a specialized neonatal team) by air when the ground transport out-of-hospital time exceeds 30 minutes. Examples of instances where air medical dispatch may be appropriate for neonates include:
- **i.** Gestational age <30 weeks, body weight <2,000 grams, or complicated neonatal course (e.g., perinatal cardiac/respiratory arrest, hemodynamic instability, sepsis, meningitis, metabolic derangement, temperature instability)
- **ii.** Requirement for supplemental oxygen exceeding 60%, continuous positive airway pressure (CPAP), or mechanical ventilation
- **iii.** Extrapulmonary air leak, interstitial emphysema, or pneumothorax
- **iv.** Medical emergencies such as seizure activity, congestive heart failure, or disseminated intravascular coagulation
- **v.** Surgical emergencies such as diaphragmatic hernia, necrotizing enterocolitis, abdominal wall defects, intussusception, suspected volvulus, or congenital heart defects

g. Other: Air medical dispatch may also be appropriate in miscellaneous situations such as the following:
- **i.** Transplant
  - **1.** Patient has met criteria for brain death and air transport is necessary for organ salvage.
  - **2.** Organ and/or organ recipient requires air transport to the transplant center in order to maintain viability of time-critical transplant.
- **ii.** Search-and-rescue operations are generally outside the purview of air medical transport services, but in some instances helicopter EMS may participate in such operations. Since most search-and-rescue services have limited medical care capabilities, and since most air medical programs have similarly limited search-and-rescue training, cooperative effort is necessary for optimizing patient location, extrication, stabilization, and transport.
- **iii.** Patients known to be in cardiac arrest are rarely candidates for air medical transport.
  - **1.** A previous NAEMSP position paper has addressed situations in which resuscitation efforts should be ceased in the field for adult nontraumatic cardiac arrest victims. In such cases air transport should not be considered an alternative to discontinuing (futile) efforts at resuscitation.
  - **2.** In situations where patients are in cardiac arrest and do not meet local criteria for cessation of resuscitative efforts, or in jurisdictions in which prehospital providers cannot cease such efforts, air transport is an option only in very rare cases (e.g., pediatric cold-water drowning where helicopter transport to a cardiac-bypass center is considered).

*Excerpt, Policy Resource and Education Paper, of the National Association of EMS Physicians (NAEMSP); American College of Emergency Physicians (ACEP), 2006.

Limitations

Despite the potential benefits, air medical transport has its limitations. First and foremost, especially with regard to helicopter operations, flights may be impossible during periods of inclement weather, as described earlier. In these cases, ground transport may be the only option.

Air medical transport is an expensive endeavor. Costs routinely exceed $30,000 to $40,000 per transport. Insurance may cover some of these costs, but it is not uncommon for patients and their families to bear the full burden if they are uninsured or underinsured. The expense is derived from the high costs of aircraft maintenance, initial and recurrent training for medical and aviation crew, 24/7 staffing and availability, fuel, and insurance. Thus, it is incumbent on providers to ensure that air medical transport is used only for patients who stand to benefit from such care.

There are significant space limitations within most small to medium-sized helicopters, which are markedly smaller than even the smallest ground ambulance. In some instances, and on some airframes, the ability to carry morbidly obese patients is quite limited, not so much from the weight itself (as in the case of one of the most popular light twin EMS helicopters in use, the Eurocopter EC-135) but from the girth that prevents safe loading through clamshell doors at the rear of the fuselage. Unfortunately, our population is slowly becoming more obese. Patients who are morbidly obese may not be candidates for medical transport. Likewise, depending on the aircraft type, patients who are quite tall or who have a traction splint applied may not fit into the helicopter. Providers should be familiar with local weight restrictions and limitations of the services that provide air medical transport in their service areas. In some aircraft, access to parts of the patient is limited. In these situations, ground transport may afford better access and room.

Staffing

The staffing and crew configurations of air ambulances vary significantly—both in the United States and around the world. In most instances, modern medical helicopters are staffed by a three-person crew consisting of the pilot and two medical providers. In some operations, two pilots are used, increasing the crew size to four. In the United States, approximately 95 percent of HAA programs use a crew configuration consisting of a paramedic and a nurse. However, there are multiple variations of crew staffing, ranging from nurse–nurse to nurse–respiratory therapist, nurse–doctor, or two paramedics. Occasionally, in specialty care situations, specifically trained personnel, such as a pediatric respiratory therapist or a neonatal nurse, will replace one of the regular flight crew members. In some rare instances in the United States, certain flight programs have a nurse–physician crew configuration. Most commonly, these are emergency physicians or emergency medicine residents functioning under the direction of an attending-level emergency physician.[21–24] A crew consisting of a pilot and a single medical provider (nurse, paramedic, or physician) is generally inadequate except for the transport of extremely stable patients.

The physician–nurse staffing model is much more common outside the United States, including in Europe, Australia, Japan, and South Africa—where the physicians are often anesthesiologists, intensivists, emergency physicians, or general practitioners. In some helicopter EMS operations in the United Kingdom and New Zealand, ground providers will staff medical helicopters as the need arises. Typically, staffing is based on local tradition and availability. It is very much country and system specific.

Controversies

Even though air medical transport, especially helicopter EMS, has become a fixture in modern EMS systems, it has not been without controversy. Significant concern has been raised by many, including the National Transportation Safety Board, regarding a perceived increase in the rate and incidence of crashes involving medical helicopters.

As of 2009, there were almost 900 helicopters in service in the United States, according to the most up-to-date information from the **ADAMS** (Atlas and Database of Air Medical Services) database. This brisk expansion has come under increasing scrutiny in recent years, as many helicopters are based in close proximity to one another, raising significant questions of medical necessity. There has also been increasing concern about this near-exponential expansion outside the medical community. Specifically, even federal transportation agencies, such as the National Transportation Safety Board (NTSB), have begun to look into the number of helicopters with growing concern that competition may lead to poor aeronautical decision making or subliminal pressures that influence the decision to accept a flight.[25,26] Although many of these aircraft are flying in very rural areas with long distances between the scene of an accident and the hospital, or between rural hospitals and tertiary higher-level care, many helicopter programs are being developed in areas of the country that already have adequate air medical coverage.

Another area of significant concern arose following a series of crashes in 2008 that marred the safety record of helicopter EMS. That year, there were 13 accidents that resulted in 29 fatalities (Figure 10-15). This was a significant increase in the accident and fatality rate when compared with the previous year.[27] There was also an initiative from within the air medical community to develop and embrace strategies to improve the safety of helicopter EMS. As a result, the Patient First Air Ambulance Alliance (PFAA), a grassroots organization of medical and aviation providers, was formed. The organization is committed to ensuring that critically ill and injured patients have access to the safest and highest quality air medical system possible.[28]

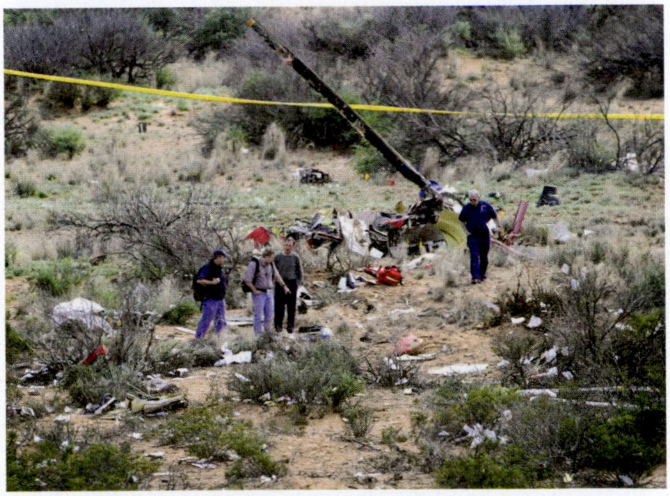

FIGURE 10-15 Medical helicopter operations have come under greater scrutiny because of an increased incidence of accidents.

(© AP Images/Odessa American, Paul Zoeller)

In many respects, the HAA industry has been the beneficiary of tools developed in the military to aid their mission. Specifically, more and more programs are using night vision goggle (NVG) technology, especially for night scene responses. In the past several years, in response to accidents in which helicopters have collided with terrain, the adoption of GPS-based helicopter-specific terrain avoidance warning systems (HTAWS) and enhanced ground proximity warning systems (EGPWS), as well as radar altimeters that precisely measure the aircraft's altitude from the ground, are all tools that improve safety. Even in 2011, however, none of these tools was mandated by the FAA to be on all EMS helicopters.

Unlike the fairly heavily regulated ground EMS industry, local and state governments have little, if any, authority to regulate air ambulances. The authority to regulate operation of air ambulances (helicopter and fixed-wing) is exclusively that of the FAA. Air ambulances fall under the authority and purview of the Airline Deregulation Act, which was signed into law in 1978. As a direct result of this act, states have been prohibited from overseeing the "quality, accessibility, availability, and acceptability" of air ambulance services. This has prevented local and state governments from developing rules and regulations for air ambulance usage. Currently, there is no one uniformly recognized certifying organization for the air medical industry. Air ambulance services (as well as critical care ground services) can be accredited by the Commission on Accreditation of Medical Transport Services (CAMTS), a private nongovernmental entity.

Scene Operations

The decision to summon a medical helicopter should be made early in scene operations. If it is later determined that the patient or patients do not require helicopter transport, then the inbound aircraft can be canceled, frequently at no charge to anyone. It is vital to notify local air medical services as soon as possible, as it takes several minutes to check the weather, prepare to fly, and cover the distance to the scene of the accident. Unlike ground EMS and fire operations, which are often dispatched with an urgency that results in only seconds or minutes before they are out the door, flight crews must be careful to properly assess all the variables, such as weather, hazards, and terrain, before accepting a flight.

Initial Information

Most EMS agencies will be familiar with the requirements and needs of their local HAA providers. However, the following general concepts apply to most EMS systems:

- Location of scene:
    - GPS coordinates (longitude and latitude), including degrees, minutes, and decimals of minutes (e.g., 37 14.50 N and 115° 48.50 W). There are several conventions with regard to how GPS coordinates are displayed, so check with local programs to determine the local convention, whether degrees/minutes/decimals of minutes (the convention in the aviation world) *or* degrees/minutes/seconds and decimals of seconds.
    - Closest cross street or roads. Many helicopter communication centers have commercially available computer mapping programs (Delorme) that will automatically show GPS coordinates when the cursor is hovered over an intersection or spot on the computer screen.
    - Closest city/town.
    - Actual address of location.
    - Well-known landmarks (e.g., water tower, high school, local airports).
- Launch information:
    - Requesting agency identity, contact radio frequencies, and a call-back cell phone number on location, if possible.
    - Local weather conditions.
    - Presence of hazardous materials.
    - Number of patients and basic medical description (e.g., rollover with ejection, 30-foot fall with LOC, GSW to chest).

Landing Zone

The early establishment of a landing zone (LZ) is important. As a part of NIMS and the ICS, an LZ officer should be designated. The LZ officer should coordinate the incoming aircraft operations with the incident commander (IC). The responsibilities of the LZ officer include:

- Selection of site
- Site preparation
- Site protection and control
- Air-to-ground communications with incoming aircraft
- Updating IC on estimated time of arrival (ETA) of aircraft

When establishing an LZ, look for an area that is (ideally) 100 feet by 100 feet square (Figure 10-16). An LZ of this size will accommodate most EMS helicopters. There should be little, if any, slope to the LZ, and it should be clear of any readily visible debris or obstructions. If the area is dusty, consider wetting the area with a light water fog pattern to prevent blowing dust (brownout) from obscuring the pilot's view during landing. It is never necessary to routinely have a charged fire hose pointing at the aircraft, as is the custom with some fire services at LZs (and makes many flight crews nervous). In most circumstances, the approach and landing will be made as near into the wind as practical,

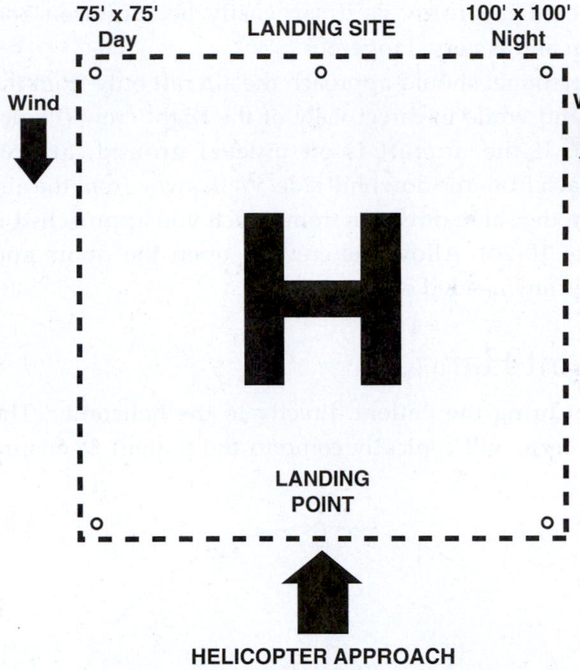

FIGURE 10-16 The helicopter landing zone should be at least 100 × 100 feet (at night) and clear of obstacles.

keeping in mind obstructions and terrain. A marker on the upwind side of the LZ (such as a cone or strobe) is conventional practice (Figure 10-17).

Mark the LZ with cones (day) and strobes (night). As an alternative to strobes, consider laying the cones down, pointing toward the center of the LZ, with a flashlight placed inside each cone. Avoid shining lights up toward the approaching aircraft. Lights should be directed across the LZ away from the approaching aircraft (Figure 10-18). Different services may use different-colored strobes for night scene operations, but it should be kept in mind that certain colored strobes (green and blue) are difficult to see with NVGs. Red and white strobes are much easier to see at night with NVGs. Aircraft equipped with NVGs may actually ask that bright scene lights be turned off, as they may interfere with their ability to see the periphery of the lit area where wires, trees, and poles may hide. Avoid using flares.

LZ security is of critical importance from the time of initial approach until the aircraft departs. Nonessential personnel and all vehicles and equipment must be kept clear of the LZ during this period. Have personnel walk the LZ looking for debris, obstructions, or other dangers. The mnemonic HOTSAW is sometimes used to remind crews of potential hazards:

- Hazards
- Obstructions
- Terrain
- Surface
- Animals
- Wind/Weather

It is also important not only to look around an LZ, but also to look up! Many forget that aircraft work in a three-dimensional environment and are of course approaching from above, so be sure to look up and assess the LZ for any obstructions above, such as wires, poles, and trees.

Helicopter Approach

The LZ officer should remain in contact with the incoming aircraft and respond to any requests made by the pilot. Ideally, during night landings, as the helicopter approaches, ensure that you do the following:

- Turn off flashing white lights (the pilot may request that other lights be turned off).

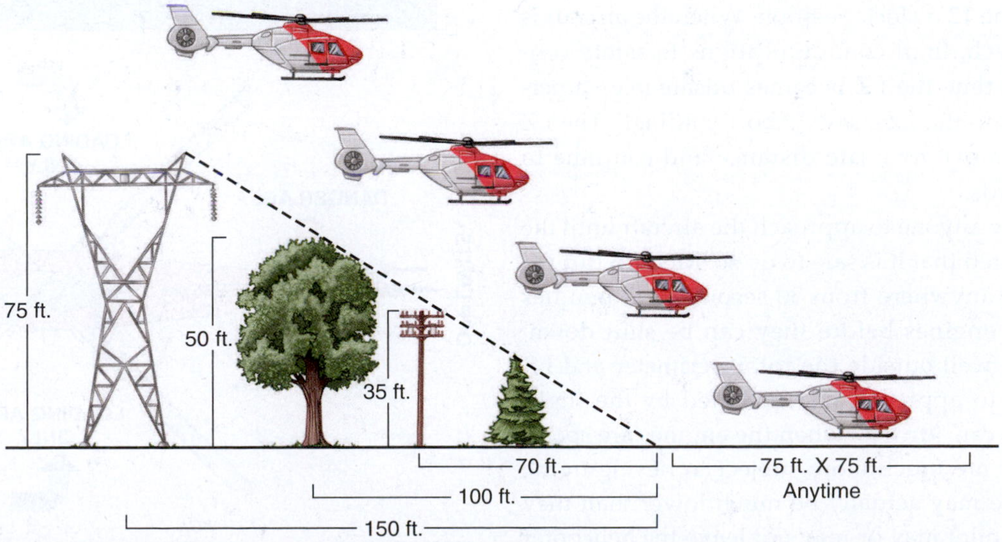

FIGURE 10-17 When selecting a landing zone, always consider wind direction and nearby obstacles such as trees, buildings, towers, and other structures.

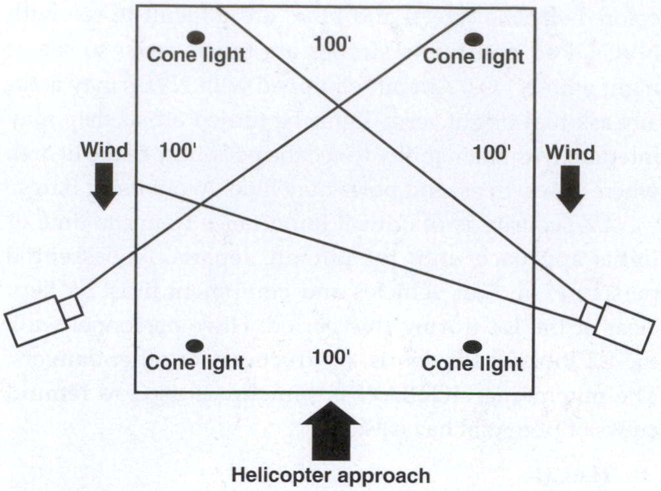

FIGURE 10-18 Lighting of helicopter landing zones must not interfere with the pilot's vision. Never point lights up toward the approaching aircraft.

- Use spotlights to mark any possible obstacles (e.g., overhead wires, trees, poles).
- Do not shine lights (or lasers) at the helicopter.

Many medical helicopters use night vision imaging systems (i.e., NVGs) during night operations. These devices significantly increase visible light. If these are being used, the crew may request that many scene lights be turned off to ensure a safe landing.

Generally, the crew of the inbound aircraft will notify you when they are close to the scene (usually 5 minutes out). In turn, notify them when you hear the aircraft and when you are able to see it. Although you can see the aircraft, its crew may not be able to see you.

If necessary to provide guidance to the approaching aircraft, use clock-based directional terms. Always consider the point of reference for the pilot (the nose of the aircraft) to be the 12 o'clock position. When the aircraft is on final approach, limit communications to safety concerns. If at any time the LZ becomes unsafe (e.g., a person wanders onto the LZ), say, "Abort landing!" The LZ officer should move to a safe distance and continue to watch for hazards.

Never allow anyone to approach the aircraft until the crew has indicated that it is safe to do so. Modern turbine aircraft require anywhere from 30 seconds to 2 minutes to cool off the engines before they can be shut down. Always remain well outside the rotor perimeter and LZ until it is safe to approach (as indicated by the flight crew), as rotors can "droop" when the engines are spooling down; they are much more subject to flexing in the wind and hence may actually be much lower than they are at rest. The pilot may or may not leave the helicopter running. Under no circumstances should anyone approach the tail of a helicopter, even if it has a shrouded or ducted tail rotor, as it can easily be forgotten and unseen and is very dangerous.

Personnel should approach the aircraft only from the front and while in direct view of the flight crew (Figure 10-19). If the aircraft is on unlevel ground, always approach from the downhill side. Walk away from the aircraft in the same direction from which you approached it (Figure 10-20). Allow the crew to open the doors and remove any needed equipment.

Patient Handoff

Do not bring the patient directly to the helicopter. The flight crew will typically come to the patient to ensure

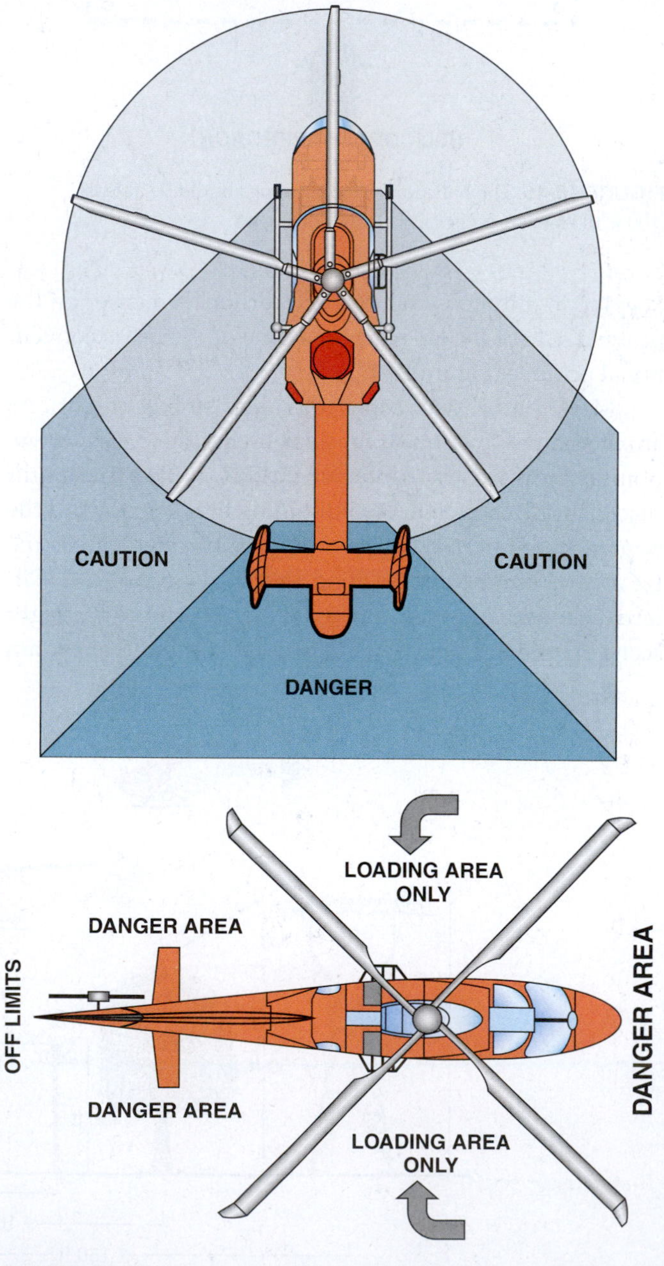

FIGURE 10-19 Personnel should approach the aircraft when requested to do so by the flight crew. They should approach only from the front and while in direct view of the flight crew.

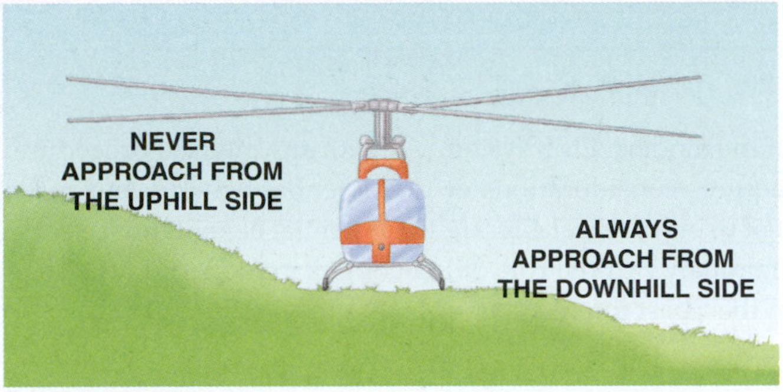

FIGURE 10-20 Always approach a helicopter from the downhill side if the landing zone has an incline.

adequate assessment and packaging for transport. After exiting the aircraft, the helicopter flight crew should be directed to the patient. The primary caregiver (paramedic) should give a brief, concise report of the patient's condition, describe any care provided, and detail the response to such care. It is important to report which medications were administered (e.g., fentanyl, sedatives, paralytics), the dose provided, and when the medications were given. If possible, provide a copy of the patient's identification, vital signs, and any other physiologic data (e.g., ECG, capnography). Other important details to relay to the flight crew include the best GCS and neuro exam if the patient has been intubated, what paralytics were given and when, any episodes of hypotension for a trauma patient, and the mechanism of injury. If a patient was intubated, relate the size of the tube used and the location (how many centimeters at the lip).

Aircraft Loading

If asked to do so, assist the flight crew in loading the patient. Again, follow all safety rules for approaching and leaving the aircraft. Do not hold any equipment above shoulder height. Always follow any directions of the flight crew. Some helicopters load from the side, whereas others load from the rear (Figures 10-21 and 10-22). Keep an eye on the crew, as verbal communications are often difficult because of the noise. Allow the crew to close and secure the doors and any outside compartments. Again, it is critically important to avoid the tail of the aircraft at all times.

If an ambulance is used to move the patient to the aircraft, it should never get closer than 25 feet to the aircraft. If any vehicle contacts any portion of the helicopter or blades, that helicopter will be considered inoperable until inspected by a mechanic.

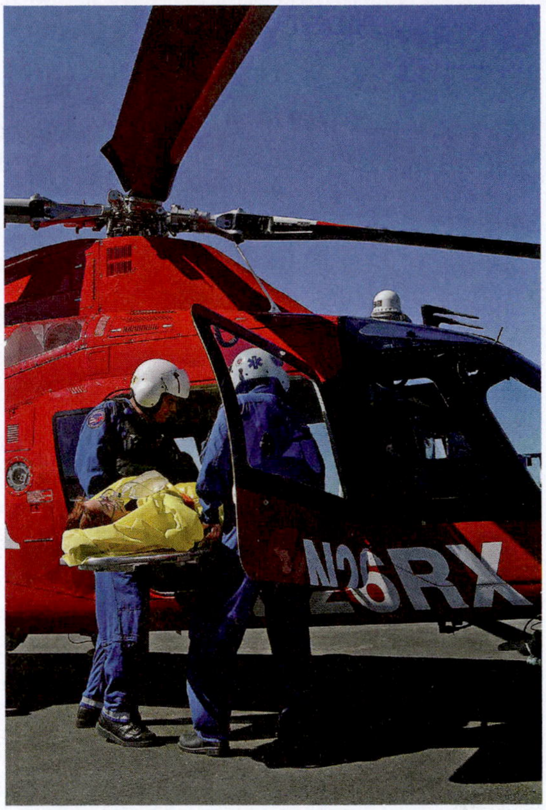

FIGURE 10-21 Loading a patient from the side of the helicopter.

Aircraft Departure

Once the crew has secured the patient, leave the LZ and remain at a safe distance. Assist the crew by being alert for open doors or compartments. Look for any straps left hanging out. Immediately notify the pilot of any new or unseen hazards. Remain in contact with the aircraft until it is well clear of the area.

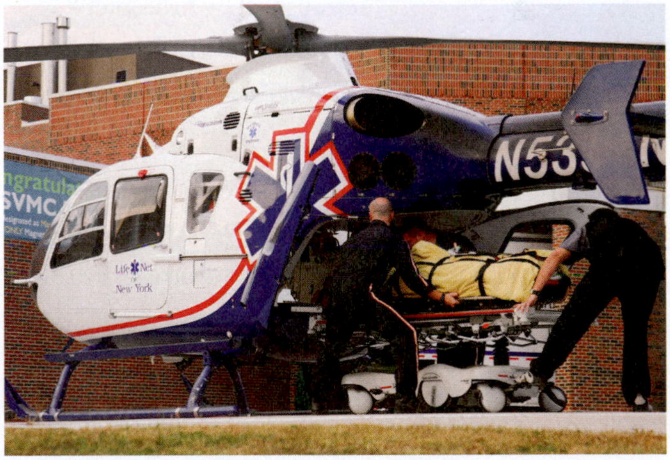

FIGURE 10-22 Loading a patient from the rear of the helicopter.

(© Mark Foster)

Summary

Air ambulances are an important part of the modern EMS system. As with any medical procedure, transporting a patient by helicopter requires considerations of the potential benefits and risks. Because of the inherent danger and cost of using medical aircraft, the potential benefit must clearly outweigh the risks. Patients will be unfamiliar with the role of helicopters in modern EMS. They depend on you, the paramedic, to act in their best interest.

You Make the Call

You and your partner are responding to an injured-person call in a remote part of the county. Little additional information is known. You know that the local first responders, the Red Canyon Volunteer Fire Department, are already en route to the scene. You turn onto a rural road and see the flashing lights of the fire department in the distance. You pull up to the scene and park behind the fire truck. The house is a small rural frame house that is well kept. One of the first responders meets you and your partner and leads you to the patient.

The patient is a 72-year-old woman who tripped over a throw rug and fell. She is complaining of left hip pain. The patient's husband is at her side and is holding her hand. You complete your primary and secondary assessments and feel that the patient is suffering an isolated left hip fracture. You send one of the first responders to the front yard to retrieve your ambulance stretcher. The first responder gives you somewhat of an inquisitive look and states, "We have the helicopter coming." You look at him and ask, "You have a helicopter coming for her?" He replies that the crew felt that the patient would be more comfortable in a helicopter as opposed to the 20-minute transport in your ground ambulance. Besides, the husband told the first responders that he had a subscription to one of the local helicopter services.

You and your partner both know that this patient does not require a medical helicopter. However, you want to maintain good relations with the volunteer fire department. Based on the scenario, answer the following questions:

1. Would you go ahead and allow the patient to be transported by helicopter when her condition clearly does not warrant helicopter transport?
2. What would you tell her husband and the first responders to explain your decision to not transport by helicopter?
3. What options are available to you to assist in dealing with the situation?

See Suggested Responses at the back of this book.

Review Questions

1. The first recorded use of aircraft to evacuate casualties was during ____________
   a. World War I.
   b. World War II.
   c. the Korean War.
   d. the Vietnam War.
2. One of the most significant limitations faced by all helicopters is ____________
   a. distance to fly.
   b. ambient light conditions.
   c. patient condition.
   d. weather conditions.
3. An aircraft can fly intentionally in weather with poor visibility only if the pilot and aircraft have been equipped to fly under which flight rules?
   a. IFR
   b. VFR
   c. V4R
   d. GPS

4. Benefits of air medical transport include which of the following?
   a. Less expensive mode of transport
   b. Transporting patients in all weather conditions
   c. Shortened time to deliver the patient to the hospital
   d. Better quality of care
5. A patient with which of the following conditions is the best candidate for air transport by helicopter?
   a. Diving emergency
   b. Cardiac arrest
   c. Hazmat exposure
   d. Acute stroke
6. You are on scene of a head-on collision with entrapment. Your patient is pinned in the vehicle and has a massive head injury and altered level of consciousness. Which of the following factors may prevent the patient from being accepted by air medical services?
   a. Head injury
   b. Patient size
   c. Spinal injury
   d. Altered level of consciousness
7. Which of the following is a GPS-based helicopter-specific terrain warning system designed to help pilots avoid flying into terrain?
   a. HTAWS
   b. GPSWS
   c. FAA-NVG
   d. NVG
8. The initial information you provide when requesting an air ambulance should include ____________
   a. distance to the scene.
   b. patient weight.
   c. your supervisor's name
   d. closest body of water.
9. The landing zone officer is responsible for site preparation and selection, updating the incident commander on ETA of aircraft, and ____________
   a. ground response to the scene.
   b. air-to-ground communications.
   c. rescue scene safety.
   d. patient preparation.
10. Ideally, a landing zone (LZ) should be free from debris; have a minimum slope, if any; and be physically how large?
    a. 50 feet by 50 feet
    b. 75 feet by 75 feet
    c. 100 feet by 100 feet
    d. 150 feet by 150 feet
11. During a night landing, the perimeter of the LZ should be marked with ____________
    a. flashing white lights.
    b. spotlights on overhead obstacles.
    c. flares in a cross-like pattern.
    d. lasers fixed on the aircraft.
12. You are talking in an approaching aircraft. Which of the following statements would be correct for giving the pilot directions?
    a. "The LZ is to the left of Belmont Road."
    b. "The LZ is marked with Captain Jones' pickup truck on the right edge."
    c. "I have you in sight; the LZ is 50 yards north of my location."
    d. "The LZ is marked with cones on each corner and is at your 3 o'clock position."
13. The most dangerous direction to approach an aircraft while the engines and rotor systems are engaged is ____________
    a. from the downhill side.
    b. from the front.
    c. from the pilot's side.
    d. from the rear.
14. If the flight crew were to ask for assistance with a "hot" loading of a trauma patient, you should ____________
    a. allow the crew to direct you to the aircraft.
    b. remove all patient clothing.
    c. approach from the uphill side.
    d. wait for the copilot to throttle down the engines.
15. If any debris or foreign object comes in contact with the aircraft, the aircraft must ____________
    a. be rendered inoperable until checked out by a mechanic.
    b. be delayed 20 minutes while the pilots check out the aircraft.
    c. automatically shut down for a 45-minute cool-down.
    d. cool down for 20 minutes before additional patient care.

See Answers to Review Questions at the end of this book.

References

1. Karanicolas, P. J., P. Bhatia, J. Williamson, et al. "The Fastest Route between Two Points Is Not Always a Straight Line: An Analysis of Air and Land Transfer of Nonpenetrating Trauma Patients." *J Trauma* 61 (2006): 396–403.
2. Talving, P., P. G. Teixeira, G. Barmparas, et al. "Helicopter Evacuation of Trauma Victims in Los Angeles: Does It Improve Survival?" *World J Surg* 33 (2009): 2469–2476.
3. Svenson, J. E., J. E. O'Connor, and M. B. Lindsay. "Is Air Transport Faster? A Comparison of Air versus Ground Transport Times for Interfacility Transfers in a Regional Referral System." *Air Med J* 25 (2006): 170–172.
4. Diaz, M. A., G. W. Hendey, and H. G. Bivins. "When Is the Helicopter Faster? A Comparison of Helicopter and Ground Ambulance Transport Times." *J Trauma* 58 (2005): 148.
5. Fan, E., R. D. MacDonald, N. K. Adhikari, et al. "Outcomes of Interfacility Critical Care Adult Patient Transport: A Systematic Review." *Crit Care* 10 (2006): R6.
6. Werman, H. A. and B. N. Neely. "One-Way Neonatal Transports: A New Approach to Increase Effective Utilization of Air Medical Resources." *Air Med J* 15 (1996): 13–17.
7. Berge, S. D., C. Berg-Utby, and E. Skogvoll. "Helicopter Transport of Sick Neonates: A 14-Year Population-Based Study." *Acta Anaesthesiol Scand* 49 (2005): 999–1003.
8. Thomas, S. H., T. Harrison, S. K. Wedel, and D. P. Thomas. "Helicopter Emergency Medical Services Roles in Disaster Operations." *Prehosp Emerg Care* 4 (2000): 338–344.
9. Martin, T. *Aeromedical Transport: A Clinical Guide.* 2nd ed. Williston, VT: Ashgate Publishing, 2006.
10. Atlas and Database of Air Medical Services (ADAMS). (Available at http://www.aams.org/AAMS/Media_Room/ADAMS_Database/aams/MediaRoom/ADAMSDatabase/ADAMS_Database.aspx?hkey=4cccf748-2bc7-4bb9-b41a-c710366c51dc.)
11. Lerner, E. B. and R. M. Moscati. "The Golden Hour: Scientific Fact or Medical 'Urban Legend'?" *Acad Emerg Med* 8 (2001): 758–760.
12. Newgard, C. D., R. H. Schmicker, J. R. Hedges, et al. "Emergency Medical Services Intervals and Survival in Trauma: Assessment of the 'Golden Hour' in a North American Prospective Cohort." *Ann Emerg Med* 55 (2010): 235–246.
13. Brown, J. B., N. A. Stassen, P. E. Bankey, A. T. Sangosanya, J. D. Cheng, and M. L. Gestring. "Helicopters and the Civilian Trauma System: National Utilization Patterns Demonstrate Improved Outcomes after Traumatic Injury." *J Trauma* 69 (2010): 1030–1034; discussion 1034–1036.
14. Schiller, J., J. E. McCormack, V. Tarsia, et al. "The Effect of Adding a Second Helicopter on Trauma-Related Mortality in a County-Based Trauma System." *Prehosp Emerg Care* 13 (2009): 437–443.
15. Butler, D. P., I. Anwar, and K. Willett. "Is It the H or the EMS in HEMS That Has an Impact on Trauma Patient Mortality? A Systematic Review of the Evidence." *Emerg Med J* 27 (2010): 692–701.
16. Bledsoe, B. E., A. K. Wesley, M. Eckstein, T. M. Dunn, and M. F. O'Keefe. "Helicopter Scene Transport of Trauma Patients with Nonlife-Threatening Injuries: A Meta-Analysis." *J Trauma* 60 (2006): 1257–1265; discussion 1265–1266.
17. Black, J. J., M. E. Ward, and D. J. Lockey. "Appropriate Use of Helicopters to Transport Trauma Patients from Incident Scene to Hospital in the United Kingdom: An Algorithm." *Emerg Med J* 21(3) (2004): 355–361.
18. Thomas, S. H., F. Cheema, S. K. Wedel, and D. Thomson. "Trauma Helicopter Emergency Medical Services Transport: Annotated Review of Selected Outcomes-Related Literature." *Prehosp Emerg Care* 6 (2002): 359–371.
19. Thomas, S. H. "Helicopter EMS Transport Outcomes Literature: Annotated Review of Articles Published 2004–2006." *Prehosp Emerg Care* 11 (2007): 477–488.
20. Bayley, R., M. Weinger, S. Meador, and C. Slovis. "Impact of Ambulance Crew Configuration on Simulated Cardiac Arrest Resuscitation." *Prehosp Emerg Care* 12 (2008): 62–68.
21. Burney, R. E., L. Passini, D. Hubert, and R. Maio. "Comparison of Aeromedical Crew Performance by Patient Severity and Outcome." *Ann Emerg Med* 21 (1992): 375–378.
22. Burney, R. E., D. Hubert, L. Passini, and R. Maio. "Variation in Air Medical Outcomes by Crew Composition: A Two-Year Follow-Up." *Ann Emerg Med* 25 (1995): 187–192.
23. Ray, A. M. and D. P. Sole. "Emergency Medicine Resident Involvement in EMS." *J Emerg Med* 33 (2007): 385–394.
24. Garner, A., S. Rashford, A. Lee, and R. Bartolacci. "Addition of Physicians to Paramedic Helicopter Services Decreases Blunt Trauma Mortality." *Aust N Z J Surg* 69 (1999): 697–701.
25. National Transportation Safety Board. Public Hearing: Helicopter Emergency Medical Services, February 3–6, 2009.
26. Federal Aviation Administration. *Fact Sheet–Helicopter Emergency Medical Services Safety.*
27. National Transportation Safety Board. *EMS Helicopter Safety: Is It an Oxymoron?* (Available at http://www.ntsb.gov/doclib/speeches/sumwalt/aamt.pdf.)
28. Patient First Air Ambulance Alliance. (Available at http://www.patientfirstalliance.org/.)

Further Readings

Air and Surface Transport Nurses Association. *ASTNA Patient Transport: Principles and Practices.* St. Louis: Mosby, 2009.

Bledsoe, B. E. and R. W. Benner. *Critical Care Paramedic.* Upper Saddle River, NJ: Pearson/Prentice Hall, 2006.

Deschamp, C. *Introduction to Air Medicine.* Upper Saddle River, NJ: Pearson/Prentice Hall, 2006.

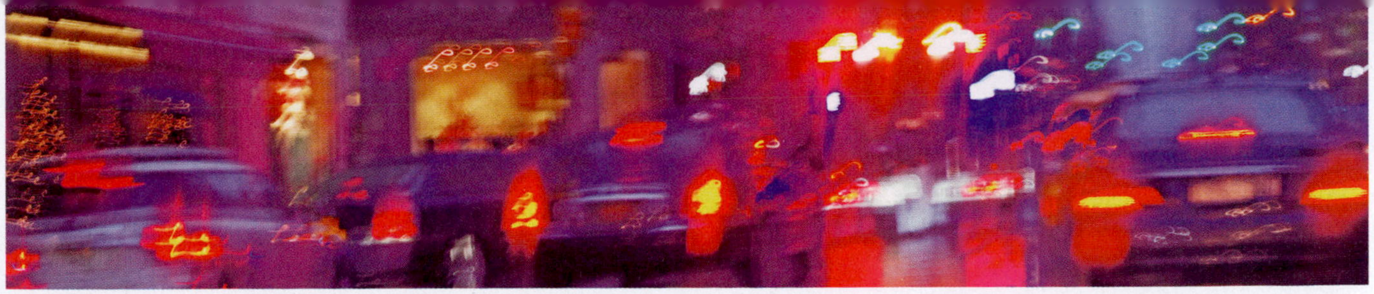

Chapter 11

Multiple-Casualty Incidents and Incident Management

Bryan Bledsoe, DO, FACEP, FAAEM, EMT-P

Louis Molino, NREMT-I

STANDARD

EMS Operations (Multiple-Casualty Incidents)

COMPETENCY

Applies knowledge of operational roles and responsibilities to ensure patient, public, and personnel safety.

Learning Objectives

Terminal Performance Objective: After reading this chapter, you should be able to effectively perform the expected functions of EMS personnel in a multiple-casualty incident.

Enabling Objectives: To accomplish the terminal performance objective, you should be able to:

1. Define key terms introduced in this chapter.
2. Anticipate situations that can result in low-impact, high-impact, and disaster-related multiple-casualty incidents (MCIs).
3. Describe the origins and purposes of incident command or incident management systems, and describe the components of the National Incident Management System (NIMS).
4. Identify and describe the purpose and function of each of the five major functional areas of NIMS or Incident Command System (ICS).
5. Describe the purpose of a mutual aid coordination center (MACC).
6. Discuss the roles of various personnel within each of the five major functional areas of NIMS/ICS.
7. Identify the functional groups within an EMS branch of an IMS process.
8. Discuss the various functions expected of EMS personnel in the triage, treatment, and transport branch or group in a multiple-casualty incident.
9. Identify the components of the START and JumpSTART systems, and discuss what each component of each entails.
10. Discuss the four stages of disaster management and how disasters can impact typical MCI.
11. Anticipate common problems that occur in MCIs and disasters, and discuss the importance of preplanning, drills, and critiques with regard to MCI and disaster response.
12. Describe the role of disaster mental health services.

KEY TERMS

branches, p. 305
C-FLOP, p. 299
closed incident, p. 300
command, p. 299
command staff, p. 303
consensus standards, p. 297
demobilized, p. 303
Department of Homeland Security (DHS), p. 297
disaster management, p. 316
domestic incidents, p. 298
emergency operations center (EOC), p. 298
EMS communications officer, p. 316
extrication, p. 315
facilities unit, p. 304
finance/administration section, p. 304
incident command post (ICP), p. 301
Incident Command System (ICS), p. 297
incident commander (IC), p. 299
Incident Management System (IMS), p. 297
information officer (IO), p. 304
liaison officer (LO), p. 304
logistics section, p. 304
medical supply unit, p. 304
morgue, p. 313
morgue officer, p. 313
multiple-casualty incident (MCI), p. 294
mutual aid agreements, p. 305
mutual aid coordination center (MACC), p. 298
National Incident Management System (NIMS), p. 297
open incident, p. 300
operations section, p. 305
planning/intelligence section, p. 305
primary triage, p. 306
rapid intervention team, p. 316
safety officer (SO), p. 303
SALT (sort–assess–lifesaving interventions–treatment/transport) triage, p. 308
scene-authority law, p. 297
secondary triage, p. 299
section chief, p. 303
sector, p. 305
singular command, p. 300
situational awareness, p. 299
span of control, p. 299
staff functions, p. 303
staging area, p. 314
staging officer, p. 314
START, p. 307
transportation unit supervisor, p. 315
treatment group supervisor, p. 313
treatment unit leader, p. 314
triage, p. 306
triage group supervisor, p. 306
triage officer, p. 300
unified command, p. 300
windshield survey, p. 299

Case Study

A charter bus carrying 29 elementary school children is headed northbound on County Road 219 when the driver loses control of the vehicle on a patch of "black ice." The bus swerves off the roadway and strikes a thickly wooded stand of pine trees at approximately 45 miles per hour on the left shoulder of the county road. The bus driver is able to use his cell phone to call the county 911 public safety answering point (PSAP). The PSAP notifies the local police, fire, and EMS agencies, and notifies the school district's administrative headquarters via landline.

The first ambulance arrives shortly after the first police unit. The paramedic in the passenger seat does a windshield survey. She then relays her size-up to dispatch: "Central, Ambulance 21 on scene, assuming County Road 219 Command, we have a school bus that veered off the road into a heavily wooded area on the shoulder of the road, severe damage to the vehicle with a probable extrication problem. Ambulance 21 will be County Road 219 Command." The dispatcher acknowledges the message, "OK, Ambulance 21, you're on scene at 0723 hours, establishing County Road 219 Command."

The lead paramedic, now acting as the incident commander (IC), assigns her partner to be the triage officer. The IC then performs a 360-degree perimeter walk of the scene to assess the entire area, surveying for hazards to responders, rescue problems, and locations for the future staging of incoming resources. Meanwhile, the triage officer, after donning his personal protective equipment (PPE), enters the bus through the rear emergency entrance, as the main entry door is damaged and obscured by debris from the woods. He does a rapid patient count and finds 30 patients—all of whom are children, except for the bus driver. He relays this to the IC via radio. Using the START/JumpSTART system, the triage officer moves quickly from patient to patient, making a rapid assessment of each and tagging each patient while keeping a running count of the patient totals.

The triage officer completes his primary triage and reports to the IC that they have 30 patients in total: 7 red tags, 12 yellow tags, 11 green tags, and 0 black tags. Three patients, including the bus driver, are heavily entrapped.

Outside the bus, the IC calls the dispatcher and reports: "Central, County Road 219 Command, we have a full-size school bus that has run into a heavily wooded area on the left side of County Road 219 about one mile north of State Highway 34. We have a total of 30 patients. All are children except for the bus driver. We have a significant MCI at this location. I am requesting at least ten additional transport units, as well as more fire, heavy rescue, and police units. Have the next due unit establish a staging area on the opposite side of County Road 219 near the open field and have everyone keep the center lane clear for transport units to exit the scene."

The senior dispatcher at the PSAP activates the county's Mutual Aid Coordination Center (MACC) and activates the regional MCI and disaster plan. Additional EMS, fire, police, and other response agencies are mobilized for scene response as well as back-fill coverage for empty stations to ensure adequate coverage for normal call volume. Several mutual aid agencies initiate call-backs of off-duty personnel to staff additional units and provide fill-in coverage. All local hospitals are notified of the incident through use of phones and radio and pager systems and are asked to update the MACC with up-to-date counts of their available beds and specialty beds of all types.

More ambulances arrive and begin to treat the critical patients, focusing their care on life-threatening conditions only, until more resources can reach the scene. Fire and rescue units arrive a short time later, initiating hazard control and rescue operations for the severely entrapped patients. The on-duty EMS field supervisor arrives and meets with the IC, who provides a situation report and then transfers command to the EMS Field Supervisor. She alerts dispatch, "Central, County Road 219 Command. Transferring command from Ambulance 21 to EMS-1." The paramedic from Ambulance 21 is then assigned to the operations section chief position.

As additional EMS units arrive, the operations section chief assigns various functions, such as safety officer, treatment unit manager, and transport unit manager; other personnel provide patient care, gather supplies, or transfer patients to waiting ambulances. Operations run smoothly, with all the various incident management system elements communicating with each other and personnel performing their assigned tasks.

Ambulances transport the first critical patients off the scene at 7:49, just 26 minutes after the first arriving unit established command. The transportation officer distributes patients evenly among the three local hospitals, with the patient loads determined by the types of injury and with appropriate care centers such as the designated trauma center receiving the most critical trauma patients. The last patients depart the scene 53 minutes after Ambulance 21 established command. Although the emergency response phase of the incident is now terminated, several units remain on the scene to assist in the investigation of this incident.

During this incident, other EMS units in the county responded to eight emergencies, including one multiple-vehicle collision, which created another smaller-scale MCI event. Although some minor delays were reported on the routine call load, neither of the two multiple-casualty incidents in any way significantly compromised either response times or patient care within the county EMS system.

Introduction

Traditional paramedic education focuses on the relationship between one or two patient care providers and a single patient. In this setting, a paramedic has the ability to concentrate on the assessment and treatment of the patient. Occasionally, however, paramedics are called on to treat more than one patient at a time. The multiple-patient incident may result from a motor vehicle collision (MVC), an apartment fire, a gang fight, or any number of other scenarios. During your career as a paramedic, you can also expect to respond to a much larger **multiple-casualty incident (MCI)**, also known as a *mass-casualty incident*. The MCI can involve "everyday" incidents, such as the school bus collision described in the opening case study, or disasters such as tornadoes, train wrecks, airline crashes, or even a terrorist event (Figures 11-1 through 11-3). Definitions of an MCI vary from agency to agency and may even vary on a district level within a single jurisdiction or agency. Some agencies define an MCI as any incident involving three or more patients. Other agencies set the level for an MCI at five, seven, or more patients. In situations involving a disaster, the number of patients can reach into the hundreds or thousands. In general practice, the accepted definition of an MCI is any incident that depletes the available on-scene resources at any given time. Using this criterion, a single ambulance with two paramedics that arrives at an MVC with four patients who are all in need of advanced life support (ALS) care would be an MCI by definition.

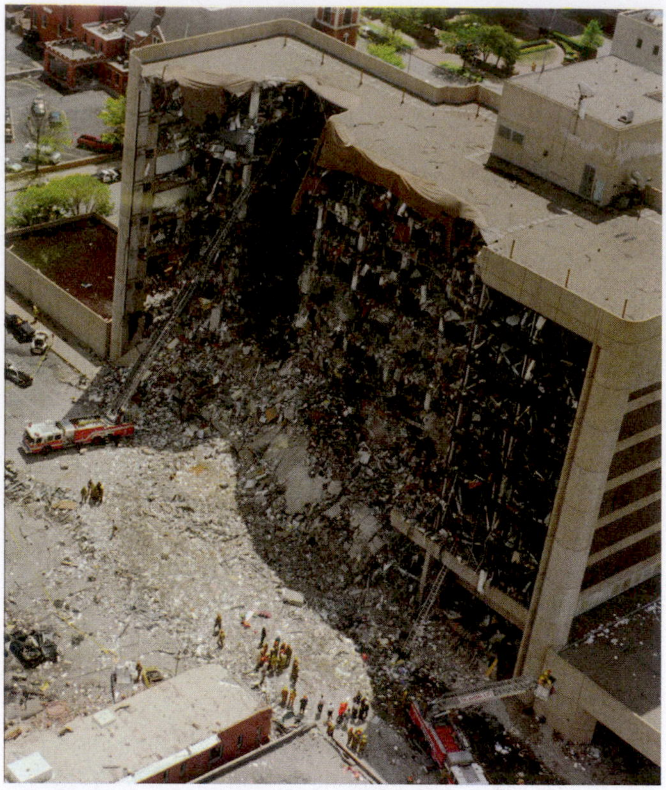

FIGURE 11-1 The scene of the April 19, 1995, bombing of the Alfred P. Murrah Federal Building in Oklahoma City.

(© AP Images)

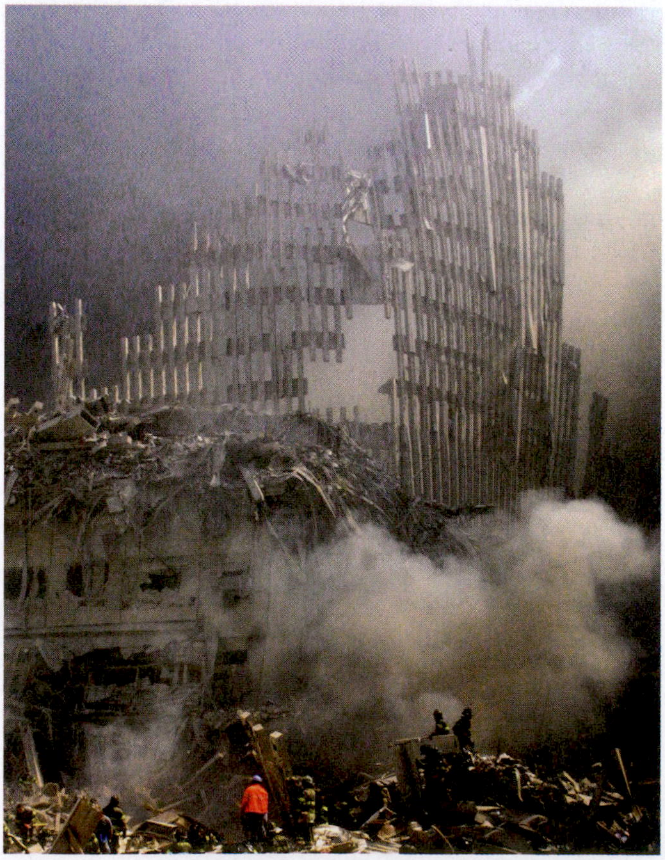

FIGURE 11-2 The attacks on the World Trade Center and the Pentagon on September 11, 2001, will forever change the way mass-casualty incidents are handled.

(© AP Images/Shawn Baldwin)

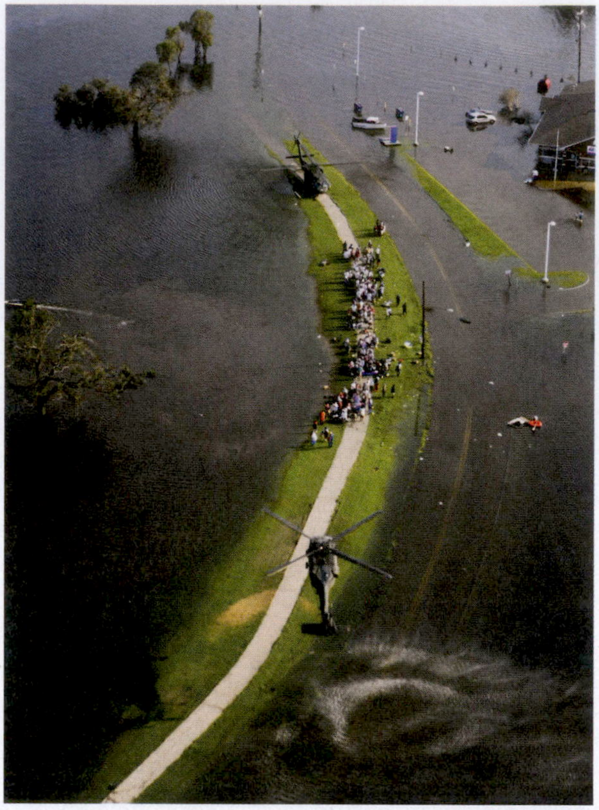

FIGURE 11-3 Hurricane Katrina, which struck the central Gulf coast on August 29, 2005, was one of the worst natural disasters in U.S. history. It also exposed flaws in the national disaster support system.

(© AP Images/David J. Phillip)

Each EMS system has a relatively finite capacity to manage an MCI. Some large urban departments can easily manage an MCI that would overwhelm a smaller department. However, generally, an MCI can be classified as follows:

- ***Low-impact incident.*** A low-impact incident is one that can typically be managed by local emergency personnel. It may tax the local EMS system, but typically will not overwhelm it. Examples include a motor vehicle collision with multiple victims, a shooting with multiple victims, or similar scenarios.
- ***High-impact incident.*** A high-impact incident is one that stresses local emergency resources including fire, police, and EMS as well as local hospitals. Examples include tornadoes, structural collapse, floods, and similar scenarios.
- ***Disaster.*** A disaster is an event that overwhelms regional emergency response resources. Examples include hurricanes, earthquakes, and major floods. Terrorist acts can also result in disaster situations.

In this chapter, you will learn about the EMS response to MCIs as well as response to disasters in general, which may or may not generate casualties. The same techniques and tools used to respond to a multiple-patient MVC will be used to manage a more extensive MCI. Command-and-control concepts that have evolved during the past 25 years to help facilitate the organization and eventual control of such responses are discussed. The special considerations involved in disaster management appear near the end of the chapter.

Origins of Emergency Incident Management

Based on the confusion surrounding several major fires and other large-scale incidents in the 1970s, the fire service, particularly in the Southern California area, took the lead in organizing responses to large-scale emergencies. This later evolved into a statewide system that became known as FIRE SCOPE. This system then began to be exported into other major areas around and throughout the United States. Each area had its own way of doing things and more or less adopted the basic tenets of the system that had become known as the **Incident Command System (ICS)**. In essence, ICS is a management system or philosophy that takes the basic tenets of good, sound management and adapts them to the needs of the emergency scene. ICS was designed for controlling, directing, and coordinating emergency response resources in, as much as possible, an effective manner. Although the ICS was originally developed for use at major fires, a standardized ICS, or **Incident Management System (IMS)**, has been adopted by law enforcement, EMS, hospitals, and industry.

In recent years, particularly in the months since the terrorist attacks against the United States on September 11, 2001, the various versions of the ICS or IMS in use in the United States have been merged into the comprehensive, standardized **National Incident Management System (NIMS)**. NIMS was prescribed by way of a Homeland Security Presidential Directive (HSPD), which will, in time, require that all emergency services agencies develop and implement a comprehensive IMS that adopts the standards as prescribed by the **Department of Homeland Security (DHS)**. Since the NIMS was formally introduced to the United States response community, much guidance and direction have been provided to all manner of response agencies for compliance with the requirements of NIMS.

All EMS agencies need to be aware of the requirements for NIMS compliance because, in the future, federal funding for disaster response and other federal funding may be withheld from any jurisdiction that fails to adopt such a system for response to emergencies. The Internet and the speed at which information can now flow is a great tool to learn the needs of your agency's efforts to remain in compliance with the NIMS and to get your agency to the point at which you are able to integrate with any level of response needed, whether it be to a large-scale local-level MCI, such as the school bus accident described in the case study, or an "incident of national significance" such as Hurricanes Katrina and Sandy, or a terrorist event such as the Boston Marathon bombing or the San Bernardino shooting, or a potential event of the magnitude of the World Trade Center attack.

Regulations and Standards

The uniform practices followed in incident management stem from a variety of sources. Prior to Homeland Security Presidential Directive #5 (HSPD5), which prescribed the National Incident Management System, the only federal requirement for use of IMS fell under the Occupational Safety and Health Administration (OSHA) regulations requiring "the use of a site-specific ICS" during an emergency response to the release of hazardous substances, more often known as a hazmat response.[1] The OSHA regulations were mirrored by Environmental Protection Agency regulations that forced the adoption of this type of management system by all states, regardless of their OSHA status.

In addition, various states have passed laws requiring the use of the IMS. As a paramedic, you should research whether such laws exist in your state. Pay particular attention to the presence of a **scene-authority law**, a legal statute specifying who has ultimate authority at an incident.

National **consensus standards**, or widely agreed-on guidelines, have been developed by the National Fire Protection Association (NFPA) and other such entities. Although these standards are not laws or regulations, some of these may recommend practices for use at MCIs. Many of these standards, with which you should be familiar, include the ones that relate to hazardous materials incidents (as discussed in the chapter "Hazardous Materials"), health and safety, and disaster management. Such standards are being continually reviewed in the post-September 11 world because the rules of the game have changed seemingly overnight with regard to the response to such incidents. To be more prepared for a large-scale event, a robust day-to-day response system needs to be developed and must be practiced in order to be effective when needed.

Although there is no true national standard curriculum for implementing an IMS, several model curricula are available, such as those taught by the National Fire Academy in Emmitsburg, Maryland, and further by the National Wildland Coordinating Group (NWCG), a consortium of wildland firefighting service members from throughout the United States. The reason that many of the concepts of IMS have evolved from the wildland world is simply that the incidents they tend to respond to get very large very fast and then, once controlled, require a rapid fold-up of operations. The use of a solid and standardized IMS allows for the easy and rapid escalation of a response to a large-scale incident.

Legal Considerations

The National Incident Management System. Following the attacks on the United States on September 11, 2001, and with the establishment of a federal Department of Homeland Security, it became clear that we needed an IMS that was effective for, and understood by, all agencies who might respond to a disaster or MCI. The National Incident Management System (NIMS) was developed to provide a common system that emergency service agencies can use at local, state, and federal levels. It is a model for an IMS that is driven by Homeland Security Presidential Directive #5 (HSPD5), as discussed in the text. This directive was issued on February 28, 2003, and was intended to enhance the ability of the United States to manage **domestic incidents** by establishing a single, comprehensive National Incident Management System.

NIMS consists of five major subsystems that collectively provide for a total system approach to all hazards and risk management:

- *The Incident Management System (IMS)*—includes operating requirements, eight interactive components, and procedures for organizing and operating an on-scene management structure
- *Training*—standardized teaching that supports the effective operations of NIMS
- *Qualifications and certification system*—provides for personnel across the nation to meet standard training, experience, and physical requirements to fill specific positions in the ICS
- *Publications management*—includes development, publication, and distribution of NIMS materials
- *Supporting technologies*—includes satellite remote imaging, sophisticated communications systems, and geographic information systems that support NIMS operations

The U.S. Department of Homeland Security has recognized the value that incident management provides in the response both to natural disasters and to potential large-scale terrorist acts. They have used the experiences of the fire and other emergency services to produce and refine a standardized and national approach to major incident response. The concept of a national standard for incident response ensures that when services respond to disasters distant from their normal service area, all parties will be using the same terminology and the same response structure.

NIMS ensures that interservice and incident-wide communications are standardized so agency managers can get an accurate and complete picture of the incident's nature and scope. Additionally, NIMS ensures that communication with the public is timely, accurate, and appropriate. Because much of NIMS is derived from the concepts of the more established IMS and incorporates much of the ICS currently used by the nation's fire and emergency services, this should mean little change for most EMS providers participating in incident responses.

NIMS has the ability to place all members of the response continuum—including those not usually involved in emergency services activities in a field mode, such as public health—on the same page with a common system of command, control, communications, and coordination of emergency incidents.

Since the publication of HSPD5, many pieces of guidance and direction have been issued by the DHS related specifically to the training requirements for the implementation of NIMS. Many pre-September 11 courses have been updated and/or otherwise revised so they are now seen as NIMS compliant. Much of that guidance may be found online at the NIMS Integration Center (NIC) website. This site (http://www.fema.gov/emergency/nims/index.shtm) should be reviewed periodically by every emergency responder to determine what changes have been made to NIMS and the related compliance documents that are found on the site.

A Uniform, Flexible System

With its uniform terminology and approach, the National Incident Management System has a number of advantages over the multitudes of currently existing IMSs that developed during past decades. First, NIMS recognizes that an incident can, and will, cross jurisdictional and geographic boundaries, and the use of a standardized and compatible management system will permit a well-organized response to routine and large-scale emergencies. The single best example of this was the devastating hurricane season of 2005, with Hurricanes Katrina and Rita. Many states were affected by these two storms and, in fact, by the end of the response to both of these events all 50 states and all 6 U.S. territories would be integrated into the massive responses. Recovery from those events is still not complete. Second, the NIMS has the flexibility to respond to emergencies in both the public and private sectors and incorporates concepts of business continuity and crisis management employed by the private sector to ensure the necessary continuity and continuance of critical operations.

Also, remember that a key element in the management of any incident that spans jurisdictions is the **mutual aid coordination center (MACC)**, formerly referred to as the **emergency operations center (EOC)**. The MACC is a site from which civil government officials (e.g., municipal, county, state, and/or federal) exercise direction and control in an emergency or disaster. From this site, management and support personnel carry out coordinated emergency response activities. The MACC may be a dedicated facility or an office, conference room, or other predesignated location having appropriate communications and informational materials to carry out the assigned emergency response mission. When possible, the MACC should be located in a secure and protected location.

To familiarize yourself with the concepts, structure, and practices of both NIMS and the ICS, which is the fundamental tenet of NIMS, the following sections of this chapter will focus on the major functional areas of NIMS and ICS. Use the mnemonic **C-FLOP** to keep these areas in mind as you read. The letters stand for:

C—Command

F—Finance/administration

L—Logistics

O—Operations

P—Planning

Command

The most important functional area in the Incident Management System is **command**. The **incident commander (IC)** is the individual who essentially runs the entire incident. The IC has the full legal authority and, in most cases, all of the associated liabilities of dealing with this incident.

The most critical concept to grasp about command is this: *The ultimate authority for decision making rests with the incident commander. The IC is responsible for coordinating the many activities that occur on the emergency scene. Because it would be too confusing or impossible for all on-scene personnel to report directly to the IC, the person charged with command delegates certain functions and responsibilities to others.* In this way, the IC maintains a reasonable **span of control**, or number of people or tasks that a single individual can monitor. Depending on the complexity of a given operation, the overall scope of the incident, and the resources that are available to the IC, the span of control may range from three to seven people, with the optimal span of control for most emergency operations being five.

The important thing to bear in mind regarding span of control is that the more risky any given task or operation is, the more tightly must be the span of control. Tasks that put operational personnel in the greatest physical danger *must* be supervised by both qualified and competent persons who *must* have the right numbers of the right qualified and competent personnel operating under them to ensure that all operations are conducted in an environment that is as safe as possible.

Establishing Command

As already mentioned, the determination of when to establish command and when to declare an MCI will vary from agency to agency. The formal declaration of an MCI may occur as soon as an incident reaches a certain patient count or when some other predetermined condition has been met

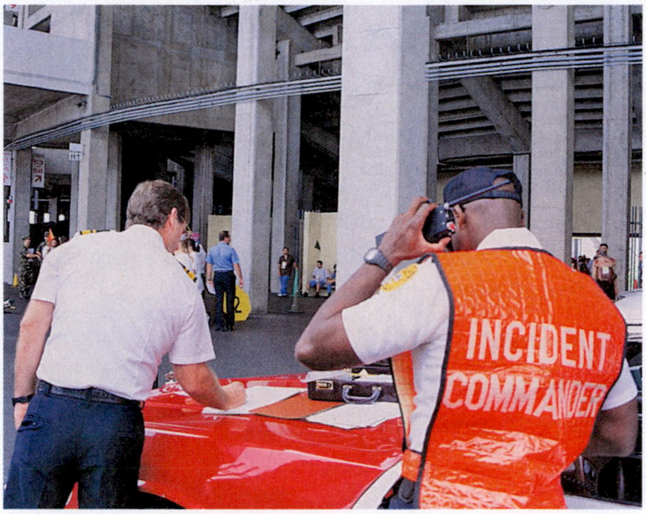

FIGURE 11-4 The first on-scene unit must assume command and direct all rescue efforts at a multiple-casualty incident.

that makes scene management challenging or significantly taxes the available resources of a system. Generally, when any two or more units respond to an emergency, when casualties include two or more patients, or if multiple agencies are involved in response to the incident, you should implement IMS.

As a rule, the first-arriving public safety unit should establish command (Figure 11-4). This may or may not be the first-arriving EMS unit, and it may or may not be from the agency that has the legal authority to establish command for the type of incident in question. On arrival, the IC will do a **windshield survey** of the scene. As you already know, EMS providers should never exit their vehicle until they have identified any and all potential hazards of the incident to the extent possible from inside their vehicle. At an MVC, for example, do not miss the vehicle partially hidden in the woods or the pool of gasoline near your vehicle. Once you have determined the visible scope of an incident and any obvious hazards, relay this information to dispatch and all other responding units and agencies.

Incident Size-Up

Size-up is a concept that is widely taught to fire personnel. However, it is often not taught to EMS personnel in this context. Regardless, it has application in any emergency response situation. A size-up is simply a formal evaluation of the situation surrounding an incident. It is an integral part of establishing command at any incident and is an integral component of the management of an MCI. The initial size-up, as well as ongoing size-ups, are key in ensuring that both the operational personnel and the IC have a high level of **situational awareness**. This will keep personnel out of danger and help keep them aware of the hazards that they are likely to encounter on an incident scene. It is

CONTENT REVIEW

➤ Incident Priorities
- Life safety
- Incident stabilization
- Property conservation

vital that EMS responders maintain a good operational picture and situational awareness at all times when operating on any emergency scene.

During the initial and ongoing size-ups, you must keep in mind the three main priorities of all emergency services operations:

- Life safety
- Incident stabilization
- Property conservation

Life Safety

Life safety is always the top priority in response to any incident. If you arrive first on the scene of a high-impact incident, you must observe and protect all rescuers, including yourself, from hazards. Then and only then will you attend to patients who are in immediately life-threatening situations. At this point, keep in mind that the needs of the many usually outweigh the needs of the few. If you commit to caring for the first patient you encounter, you may neglect 10 other critical patients lying nearby—some of whom may be more salvageable than the first one you came across.

If you are the IC, remember that responsibility for triage belongs to the **triage officer**. At a small-scale incident, the IC may end up triaging some patients. Even so, the triage officer assumes the main responsibility for sorting patients into categories based on the severity of their injuries.

Depending on the scope of the incident and local protocols, you and your partner will most likely fill the roles of incident commander and triage officer if you are the first public safety unit on the scene. These designations will remain in place at least until other units arrive.

Never forget the importance of establishing command early in an incident.

Incident Stabilization

While attending to the first priority, life safety, all response personnel should also keep in mind the second priority—incident stabilization. To achieve this goal, quickly identify whether the situation is an open incident or a closed incident. An **open incident**, also known as an *uncontained incident*, has the potential to generate more patients at any time. A fire that traps people inside an office building is an example. You may find only a few patients when you arrive on scene. However, other patients, including firefighters injured during incident operations, may soon appear. Consequently, the IC must anticipate the need for additional resources. Whenever you find yourself in command of an open incident, remember this point: It is better to call too many resources than too few; you can always send them home.

In the case of a **closed incident**, or *contained incident*, the injuries have usually already occurred by the time you arrive on scene. An example might be a multiple-vehicle collision. However, even a so-called closed incident carries the potential for additional hazards, such as an undetected gas leak, a distraught family member who rushes into traffic, further injury to patients wandering about the scene and, of course, injuries to responders during the course of incident operations. As a result, it makes sense for an IC to expend effort in stabilizing an incident. Preventing further injuries, either of patients or of rescue personnel, helps to ensure smoother and more successful management of an MCI.

Property Conservation

As with any other call, the third priority of an IC is conservation of property. At no time during an operation should rescue personnel damage property unless it is absolutely necessary for achieving the first two priorities—life safety and incident stabilization. Property conservation should include protection of the environment where operations are staged.

Most MCIs are "won or lost" in the first 10 minutes. Without the establishment of incident command, emergency personnel may begin to "freelance." They may fail to prioritize patients, underestimate the severity of the incident, or delay requesting additional resources. Successful handing of any MCI involves coordination of all key personnel, whether 2 people or 20.

Singular versus Unified Command

Most agencies have a single person who is the agency's highest-ranking official. That person carries the authority to administer the agency in full on a day-to-day basis, without question. However, in the case of nearly all evolving incidents, command is established by the first-arriving public safety official. This will generally be the way things work at all smaller-scale incidents with limited jurisdictional issues. This type of command is called **singular command**, and it usually works out well for all concerned. Singular command incidents usually have a smaller scope than an MCI and usually do not involve outside agencies. For example, a traffic collision may involve the local fire department, EMS, and police department. Prior to the incident, the three agencies involved might have agreed that the fire department will assume overall command of this type of incident, thus creating a singular command situation.

In many incidents, however, a singular command will not be feasible because of overlapping responsibilities or jurisdictions. Instead, a **unified command** will be established. Examples of incidents in which unified command is used include terrorist attacks, explosions, sniper or hostage situations, and large-scale natural disasters. In each of these examples, the managers from several agencies, such as law enforcement, fire, and EMS at multiple jurisdictional levels of government (local, state, and federal), will coordinate their activities and share command responsibilities for the overall incident while also maintaining control of their respective agencies.

In establishing a unified command, the managers of the respective agencies and jurisdictions try to achieve balanced decision making. Together, they identify and access the appropriate agencies or specialized organizations that might be needed at the scene, such as the American Red Cross, the local health department, or public works. They also create divisions of labor on the basis of reasonable and accepted spans of control.

Finally, the incident commander determines the need for an information officer to interact with the media as well as a liaison officer to deal with all the agencies and organizations that will undoubtedly respond to any incident of significance. At any complex incident that, in time, will involve multiple agencies and may well be multijurisdictional in nature, the issue of command will be complicated. The decision to remain in a singular command structure or to move to a unified command structure will depend greatly on the scope and nature of the incident and may well be dictated by legislation—as is usually the case in incidents known to be or suspected to be related to terrorism—or the decision may be dictated by a preexisting disaster plan. (The importance of planning is discussed later in this chapter.)

When an incident is of such a magnitude that the incident commander deems it necessary, he may direct that an **incident command post (ICP)** be established on or near the incident scene. The ICP provides a place where representatives and officers from the various agencies involved in the incident can meet with one another and make relevant decisions. Because an ICP may operate continuously for days or weeks, the site for the ICP should be selected carefully. Access to telephones, restrooms, and shelters should be taken into account. The command post should be close enough to the scene that officers can easily monitor scene operations but far enough away so that they are outside the direct operational area. Persons operating on the scene, members of the media, and bystanders should not have routine access to the ICP.

Identifying a Staging Area

Identification of a staging area goes hand in hand with the scene assessment. At MCIs involving hazardous materials or structural fires, for example, you must note wind speed and direction. The IC must ensure that the staging area and ICP lie well beyond the reach of any fumes, smoke, water, chemicals, or other hazardous materials.

Once you establish command of an MCI, you should also designate both a primary and a secondary staging area. In picking a primary site, keep in mind the main purpose of a staging area: organization of resources in one place for quick and easy deployment throughout the incident. Position the primary staging area as close to the scene as possible without compromising the safety of the responders and resources placed in staging. Make sure the site has good access and exit points to ensure the flow of emergency vehicles.

If required, the secondary staging area should ideally be located in a different area from the primary staging area. This will provide the IC with a contingency plan in case the primary staging area becomes unusable. Conditions that may force a change in staging areas include altered traffic patterns, shifts in wind direction, or restricted access due to the deployment of fire hoses or other special equipment.

Incident Communications

Communications forms the cornerstone of the IMS. Once command is established, the IC has a responsibility to relay this information to dispatch. Then, as soon as possible, the IC should transmit a preliminary report that includes the following data: type of incident, approximate number of patients by priority, request for additional resources, staging instructions, and a plan of action. If a fixed incident command post has been set up, the IC should communicate the location of this site as well.

Once an MCI has been declared, further communications should be moved to a secondary, or tactical, channel. The IC must be able to supply the information necessary to coordinate resources. That is the whole purpose of the IMS. Use of a secondary channel will also prevent an IC from interfering with the communications by other jurisdictions and agencies or from overwhelming the primary EMS channel. Communications and interoperability issues are generally cited as the main reasons for problems in both exercises of disaster plans and in actual incidents.

When you act as an IC, remember that communications will involve units from different jurisdictions and perhaps different districts. One of the foundations of any incident management is the use of a common terminology. When communicating, you should eliminate all radio codes and use only plain English. A radio code may have different meanings in different places. As an IC, you must eliminate any unnecessary confusion in an already complicated situation. In fact, it may be preferable to avoid radio codes even in routine operations. Then there will be no need to even think about switching to plain English when you assume command of an MCI.

Resource Utilization

Few EMS departments have the resources to handle an MCI without outside help. Regardless of the nature of an incident, most units will need additional ambulances, personnel, equipment, and medical supplies. In many cases, they will also require specialized equipment and perhaps the help of public or private agencies.

The primary role of an IC is the strategic deployment of all necessary resources at an incident. Development of a strategy means setting goals and determining the tactics needed to accomplish these goals. Because of the complicated nature of an MCI, the IC must continually assess the effectiveness of a given strategy or plan.

To ensure flexibility, an IC should radio a brief progress report to the dispatcher approximately every 10 minutes until the incident has been stabilized. The report should state established goals, tactics, and resources being used to meet these goals, and any progress or lack of progress. This forces an IC to monitor an operation, to adapt tactics or resources to changing circumstances, and to eliminate ineffective tactics entirely. Subordinates should deliver similar reports to the IC so he can properly evaluate the overall operation.

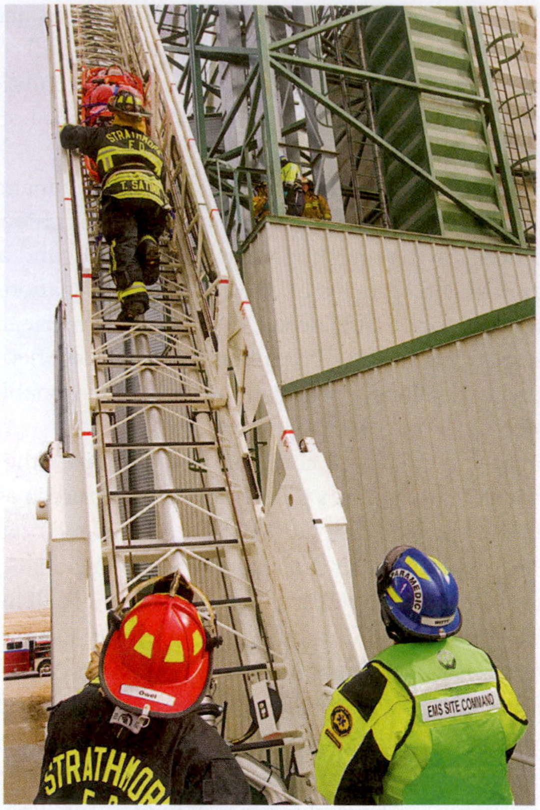

FIGURE 11-5 Using a command vest at a multiple-casualty incident makes it easier to identify personnel. The incident commander directs the response and coordinates resources.

(© Kevin Link/Science Source)

Command Procedures

Several procedures help an IC manage an MCI. First and foremost, all personnel must be able to recognize the IC and the ICP once it is established. At smaller, single-agency events, everyone may know the IC simply by his voice over the radio. However, at medium or large-scale incidents, such recognition is often impossible. As a result, the IMS calls for the IC and other officers to wear special reflective vests (Figure 11-5). The vests can be color coded to functional areas and may have the officer's title on the front and back. Such vests should be worn whenever IMS is used, even at smaller incidents. By making a basic set of vests available on every response unit—especially for command and triage—personnel will get in the habit of wearing and/or recognizing the vests prior to a major incident.

An IC can also benefit from the use of a worksheet or clipboard, two useful tools for tracking decisions and actions (Figure 11-6). An IMS worksheet should include basic information on the incident, a small area to sketch the scene, and a checklist of important items to remember. It might also include a section to record the on-scene units and personnel, their assignments, and relevant patient information, particularly transport data. Many commercial products are

COLONIE EMS *Incident Tactical Worksheet*

Location________
Med. Command________

____ Establish unified command with fire & police
____ Place 2 cones on command vehicle
____ Put bib on
____ Designate triage office
____ Advise inbound units where to stage
____ Advise crews to stay with units until given instructions
____ Advise units to switch to EMS Admin., 265 or 715

LEVEL 1 *(3-10 Patients)*	LEVEL 2 *(11-25 Patients)*	LEVEL 3 *(over 25 Patients)*	FIRE	RESCUE
___ Declare MCI	___ Declare MCI	___ Declare MCI	___ Assess # of Units Needed	___ Establish Perimeter
___ EMS All Call	___ EMS All Call	___ EMS All Call	___ EMS All Call Req. 619	___ Request Specialty Units
___ Request # of Units Needed	___ Request # of Units Needed	___ Request # of Units Needed	___ Designate Triage	___ Triage Officer Handles Inner Circle
___ Cover Town/Sr. Medic Act 615	___ Cover Town/Sr. Medic Act 615	___ Cover Town/Sr. Medic Act 615	___ Set up Rehab at Air Bank	
___ Roll Call Hospitals	___ Roll Call Hospitals	___ Roll Call Hospitals	___ Use 619 as ALS Unit	
___ Transport Officer?	___ Get Mutual Aid Units	___ Get Mutual Aid Units	**HAZ-MAT**	
	___ Designate Treatment Officer	___ Designate Treatment Officer	___ Req. # of Units Needed	___ Medical Baseline Assessment of Team
	___ Designate Transport Officer	___ Designate Transport Officer	___ EMS All Call	___ Don Protective Barriers
	___ Designate Staging Officer	___ Designate Staging Officer	___ Est. Command in Cold Zone	___ Assist With Decontamination
	___ REMO MD to Scene	___ REMO MD to Scene	___ Designate Triage	___ Rehabilitate
	___ Consider Rehab & CISD	___ Request Bus to Scene	___ Identify Agent	
			___ Research Decontamination	
(2-5 Amb. Needed)	*(6-13 Amb. Needed)*	*(over 13 Amb. Needed)*	___ Research Med.	

HOSPITAL ROLL CALL	AMCH	St. PETERS	MEMORIAL	VA	ELLIS	St. CLARE'S	LEONARD	St. MARY'S	SAMARITAN
CAN TAKE									
# PATIENTS SENT									

# OF PATIENTS BY PRIORITY				
1 *(Red)*	2 *(Yellow)*	3 *(Green)*	0 *(Black)*	TOTALS

UNITS RESPONDING

620 621 622
630 631 632
640 641 642
650 651 652
610 611 605
TSU-1 TSU-2
619
Guild.
CPHM
Albany
Mohawk
Empire

UNITS IN STAGING

620 621 622
630 631 632
640 641 642
650 651 652
610 611 605
TSU-1 TSU-2
619
Guild.
CPHM
Albany
Mohawk
Empire

FIGURE 11-6 An incident tactical worksheet from the Town of Colonie (New York) EMS.

currently available for this purpose, including programs for generating worksheets by computer.

You will find a worksheet especially useful when transferring command, as often happens when higher-ranking officers arrive on scene. Command is transferred only face to face, with the current IC conducting a short but complete briefing on the incident status. A higher-ranking officer does not become IC simply by his arrival; a briefing must take place. The worksheet serves as an outline for the briefing.

Termination of Command

As the incident progresses, resources will be reassigned or released. For example, an IC who transfers command to a higher-ranking officer may become an aide to the new IC or be assigned to a totally new IMS role. Eventually resources will be **demobilized**, or released for use elsewhere in the EMS system. Once the incident has progressed to the point at which the IMS is no longer needed, command should be terminated. A final progress report should be delivered to the communications center. All units will then return to routine rules of operation.

The point at which command terminates depends on the incident. Some high-impact incidents, such as natural disasters or terrorist events, may last for weeks. However, not all agencies may have a significant presence for the long term. EMS may have a strong initial response, for example, but may simply have a single ambulance stand by for the long term. Other agencies may be released entirely from the incident if their services are no longer needed.

Support of Incident Command

As noted earlier, incident command—the C in C-FLOP—is supported by four sections or functional areas:

- Finance/administration
- Logistics
- Operations
- Planning

Each section has a place within the IMS and is headed by a **section chief**. All these areas have functions that will in some way, shape, or form be fulfilled in every emergency response, even in a day-to-day-type response. However, all four areas may not be formally established at every incident. At small- or medium-sized incidents, for example, operations may be the only section implemented. At large-scale or long-term incidents, the IMS may activate the areas of finance/administration, logistics, and planning. Depending on the type of incident and the structure of command, these sections may not be filled with EMS

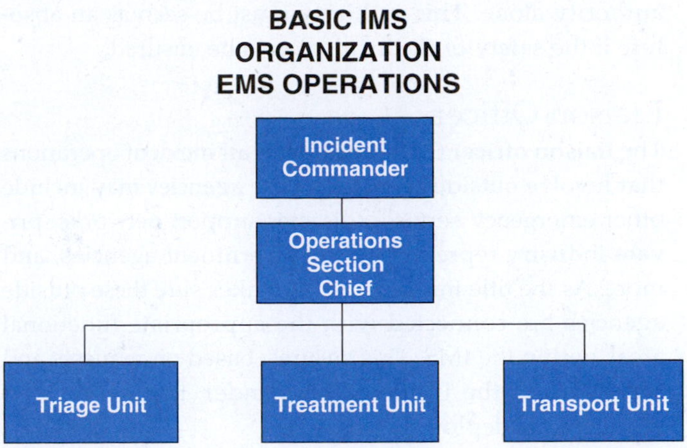

FIGURE 11-7 Basic Incident Management System organization for a small- to medium-sized incident.

personnel. However, they may help coordinate some EMS activities.

In addition, several important officers may report directly to the incident commander. These officers handle information, safety, outside liaisons, and mental health support. Together they are known as the **command staff**. The combination of command staff and section chiefs comprises and carries out what are called **staff functions**.

As a paramedic, it is more important for you to know how the IMS works than to be an expert in specific job functions. Figure 11-7 and the following sections give you a quick overview of the basic elements of the IMS.

Command Staff

The establishment and role of command have already been described. However, the command staff can play an important role in supporting the incident commander, particularly at major incidents or disasters. Therefore, you should be familiar with the roles of the following command staff officers.

Safety Officer

The **safety officer (SO)** may hold the most important role at an MCI. This person or, in some cases, team of people monitors all on-scene actions and ensures that they do not create any potentially harmful conditions. Because almost anything that happens at an incident is potentially harmful, the SO assumes an enormous responsibility. Some of the areas that must be monitored for safety compliance include infection control, use of personal protective equipment, crowd control, lifting of patients and equipment, and quality of scene lighting. Under the IMS, the SO has the authority to stop any action that is deemed an immediate life threat with no further action needed. In other words, the SO may at any time terminate any operations at the incident on his authority alone. This authority must be seen as an absolute if the safety of the incident is to be ensured.

Liaison Officer

The **liaison officer (LO)** coordinates all incident operations that involve outside agencies. These agencies may include other emergency services, disaster support networks, private industry representatives, government agencies, and more. As the title implies, the LO makes sure these outside agencies are connected with the appropriate functional areas within the IMS. This ensures, based on requests and reports from the incident commander, that specialized resources are deployed effectively.

Information Officer

The **information officer (IO)** collects data about the incident and releases it to the press, as well as to other agencies, on an as-needed and appropriate basis. Although you may not have a preexisting relationship with the media in your community, a major incident will put your unit in the public spotlight. Your department's image depends on favorable exposure in the media. More important, the safety and reassurance of the public may depend on their receiving timely and accurate information about the event. As a result, it is important for an IMS to have an effective IO. In any large-scale, high-impact incident where a large press presence can be expected, appointment of a specific public information officer (PIO) may also be made; in that instance, the PIO would report to the IO for coordination of information flow.

Mental Health Support

A large incident has the capacity to overwhelm resources and tax personnel, both physically and mentally. Thus, it is important to continually rotate personnel in and out of the event to allow adequate rest. Personnel should be evaluated periodically to ensure that they are not exhibiting signs or symptoms of excessive stress or abnormal stress reactions. Persons exhibiting abnormal stress should be removed from service. Critical incident stress management is no longer recommended. Instead, support and mental health personnel should provide "psychological first aid." This entails simply providing for the rescuer's immediate needs (food, water, rest)—not attempting to provide therapy or forcing personnel to talk.

All EMS agencies should have a licensed mental health professional affiliated with the organization. For large-scale events, it would be prudent to have this person respond and assist in screening personnel for excessive stress. The mental health professional must understand the work and the culture and be able to screen personnel who are showing maladaptive stress reactions and refer them to competent mental health personnel for additional evaluation and care.

The following general guidelines are recommended for organizational response to stressful events.

SMALL INCIDENTS The mental health needs of those involved in small incidents, including those that result in the death of colleagues, should be handled by competent mental health personnel, as follows:

- Psychological first aid should be provided.
- Debriefing and defusing should not be provided.
- Mental health personnel should screen affected personnel for up to two months following the incident for abnormal responses to stress.
- Personnel not adapting normally should be referred to competent personnel for accepted forms of therapy.

MAJOR INCIDENTS/DISASTERS The stress of major events can be mitigated by several strategies:

- Proper use of the IMS
- Rotating personnel in and out of the disaster scene
- Providing psychological first aid
- Not providing debriefing or defusing
- Constant surveillance of personnel by competent mental health personnel for signs of stress
- Postincident surveillance of involved personnel by competent mental health personnel

Finance/Administration

The **finance/administration section** rarely operates on small-scale incidents, even though financial considerations are obviously important in all day-to-day incidents. However, for large-scale or long-term incidents, the finance/administration staff supports command by assuming responsibility for all accounting and administrative activities. This section keeps personnel and time records. It also estimates costs, pays claims, and handles procurement of items required at the incident. These functions are usually performed by the jurisdictional government where the incident has occurred. The need for accuracy in the work of this unit cannot be overstressed, because a large-scale response may be eligible for reimbursements from federal or other disaster funding sources. Such reimbursements will depend directly on the ability of the agencies involved to document expenses, particularly those that are above and beyond normal operational expenditures.

Logistics

The **logistics section** supports incident operations. One of its most critical functions is operating the **medical supply unit**. This unit coordinates procurement and distribution of equipment and supplies at an MCI. Depending on the structure of the IMS used, other units may also be established by the logistics section. The **facilities unit**, for example, selects and maintains areas used for command and rehabilitation. It makes sure that adequate food, water, restrooms, lighting, power, and so on are available to support incident operations. Other units might be set up to manage field communications, on-scene medical care for workers, and other functions.

Operations

Whatever work needs to be performed at an incident takes place under the **operations section**. This section carries out tactical objectives, directs front-end activities, participates in planning, modifies the action plan, maintains discipline, and accounts for personnel. In short, the operations section gets the job done.

As will be explained later in the chapter, the operations section may have many **branches**, which are functional levels based on primary roles or geographic locations. Branches organized by role might include sections within the various jurisdictions at an incident: EMS, rescue, fire, law enforcement, and so on. Branches based on geography might include operations at various locations. The IMS structure used at the 1993 bombing of the World Trade Center, for example, assigned a branch of operations to each building in the complex.

Planning/Intelligence

The **planning/intelligence section** provides past, present, and future information about an incident. The planning section helps formulate the overall incident action plan (IAP) and oversees changes in that plan. It collects information such as weather reports, documents incident actions, and develops contingency plans. It ensures that written standard operating procedures (SOPs) for **mutual aid agreements** that govern sharing of departmental resources are activated or fulfilled.

The planning/intelligence section operates according to the principle of "anything that can go wrong will go wrong." The staff uses past incidents to anticipate trouble that might arise at the current incident. The section then acts accordingly. When the command and operations sections must change tactics, the planning section stands ready to provide the necessary strategic support.

Division of Operations Functions

As already noted, getting organized quickly and early is essential to the success of any IMS operation. There are several ways to divide functions at an incident. The choice of organization depends on the scope of an incident and its associated strategic goals, the structure of your department, the implementation of singular or unified command, and so on.

If you are an incident commander, one of your jobs will be to organize line functions—that is, operations—in the most effective manner. To do this, you should become familiar with the basic functional levels within the IMS.

Branches

The incident commander or the comanagers of a unified command incident may choose to establish any number of branches. As mentioned, these branches may be organized by primary role or by geography. Branches are supervised by branch directors, who report to the section chief for that particular functional area. The EMS branch director supervises all operations involved with patient care and transportation. Figure 11-8 shows the functional levels within a typical EMS branch. Depending on the system and the scope and magnitude of the incident, rescue may be an independent branch or it may report to the director of the EMS or fire branch.

Groups and Divisions

Branches may be further organized into groups and divisions—working areas of an incident where specific job tasks are accomplished. Groups are based on function, whereas divisions are based on geography. As an example, think of triage as a group and the responders working on the third floor of a multiple-floor incident as a division. Groups and divisions are managed by supervisors who, in turn, report to the branch director.

Units

Groups and divisions can be broken into even more task-specific groups known as *units*. They are supervised by unit leaders, who report to the supervisor of a group or division.

Sectors

Depending on the type of IMS used in your area, you may hear the term **sector** used. A sector is an interchangeable name for a branch, group, or division. However, it does not designate a functional or geographic area. Although there is no formal name for individuals who supervise a sector, they are often called sector officers.

Functional Groups within an EMS Branch

The IMS operates under the so-called toolbox theory: Do not remove a tool from the toolbox unless you actually need to use it. The flexibility of IMS is founded on the ability to implement only the areas of IMS that are needed at an incident. This theory holds for all areas of IMS, including branches, groups, sectors, divisions, and specific areas

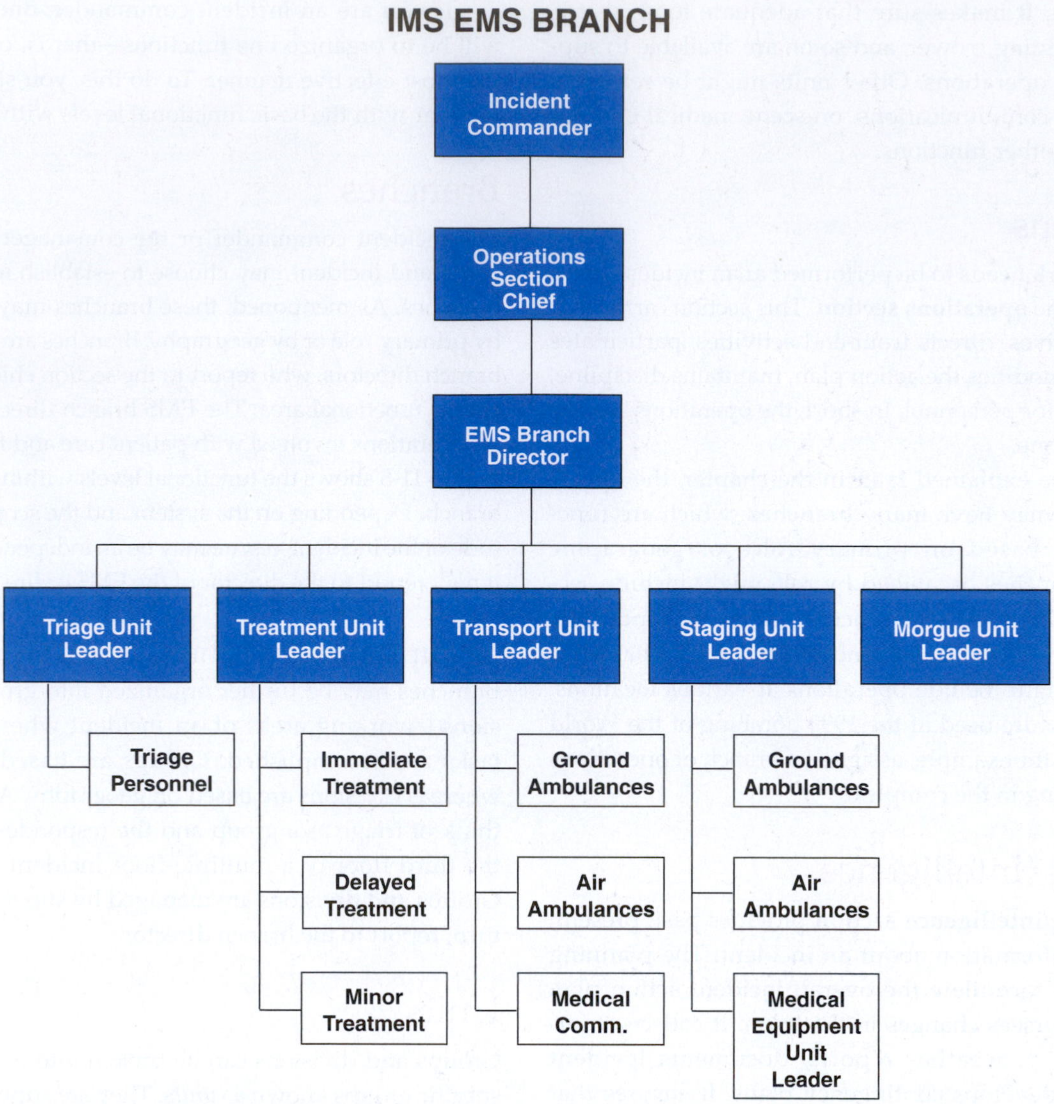

FIGURE 11-8 Example of branches that may operate during a major incident.

where EMS operates. At many EMS incidents, the basic IMS organization—triage, treatment, and transport (review Figure 11-7)—will be all the "tools" you need.

Triage

As you have read, **triage** is the act of sorting patients based on the severity of their injuries. The objective of emergency medical services at an MCI is to do the most good for the most people. For this reason, you need to determine which patients need immediate care to live, which patients will live despite delays in care, and which patients will die despite receiving medical care.

Because triage will drive subsequent incident operations, it is one of the first functions performed at an MCI. As a result, all personnel should be trained in triage techniques and all response units should carry triage equipment. The **triage group supervisor** may act independently or may supervise the triage group or triage sector.

Primary and Secondary Triage

Triage occurs in phases. **Primary triage** takes place early in the incident, when you first contact patients. The action provides a basic categorization of sustained injuries. It must be done quickly and efficiently so that command can determine on-site treatment needs and resources. Universally recognized triage categories include the following:

Category	Color	Priority
Immediate	Red	Priority-1 (P-1)
Delayed	Yellow	Priority-2 (P-2)
Minimal	Green	Priority-3 (P-3)
Expectant	Black	Priority-0 (P-0)

The category names have the following meanings: *Immediate* means the patient should receive immediate treatment; *delayed* means the patient's treatment may safely be delayed; *minimal* means the patient requires minimal or no treatment; *expectant* means the patient is expected to die or is deceased.

Secondary triage is ongoing and takes place throughout the incident as patients are collected, moved to treatment areas, given appropriate medical care, and, finally, transported off scene. A patient's condition may change over time, requiring you to upgrade or downgrade his triage category.

The START System

The most widely used triage system is **START**, an acronym for **S**imple **T**riage **a**nd **R**apid **T**ransport.[2–4] The system was developed at Hoag Memorial Hospital in Newport Beach, California. START's easy-to-use procedures allow for rapid sorting of patients into the categories listed earlier. START does not require a specific diagnosis on the part of the responder. Instead, it focuses on these areas (Figure 11-9):

- Ability to walk
- Respiratory effort
- Pulses/perfusions
- Neurologic status

CONTENT REVIEW

➤ Signs in START
- Can get up and walk
- Open airway; respirations over 30/minute
- Radial pulse
- Follows commands

ABILITY TO WALK You initiate the START system by asking patients who can walk to get up and come to you. Any patients who can complete these acts, despite their injuries, will be categorized Priority-3 or "green." Either you or another member of the triage group should place the appropriate tag on these patients. Because patients who can walk will walk, you should make every effort to confine them to one site. There is already enough confusion at an

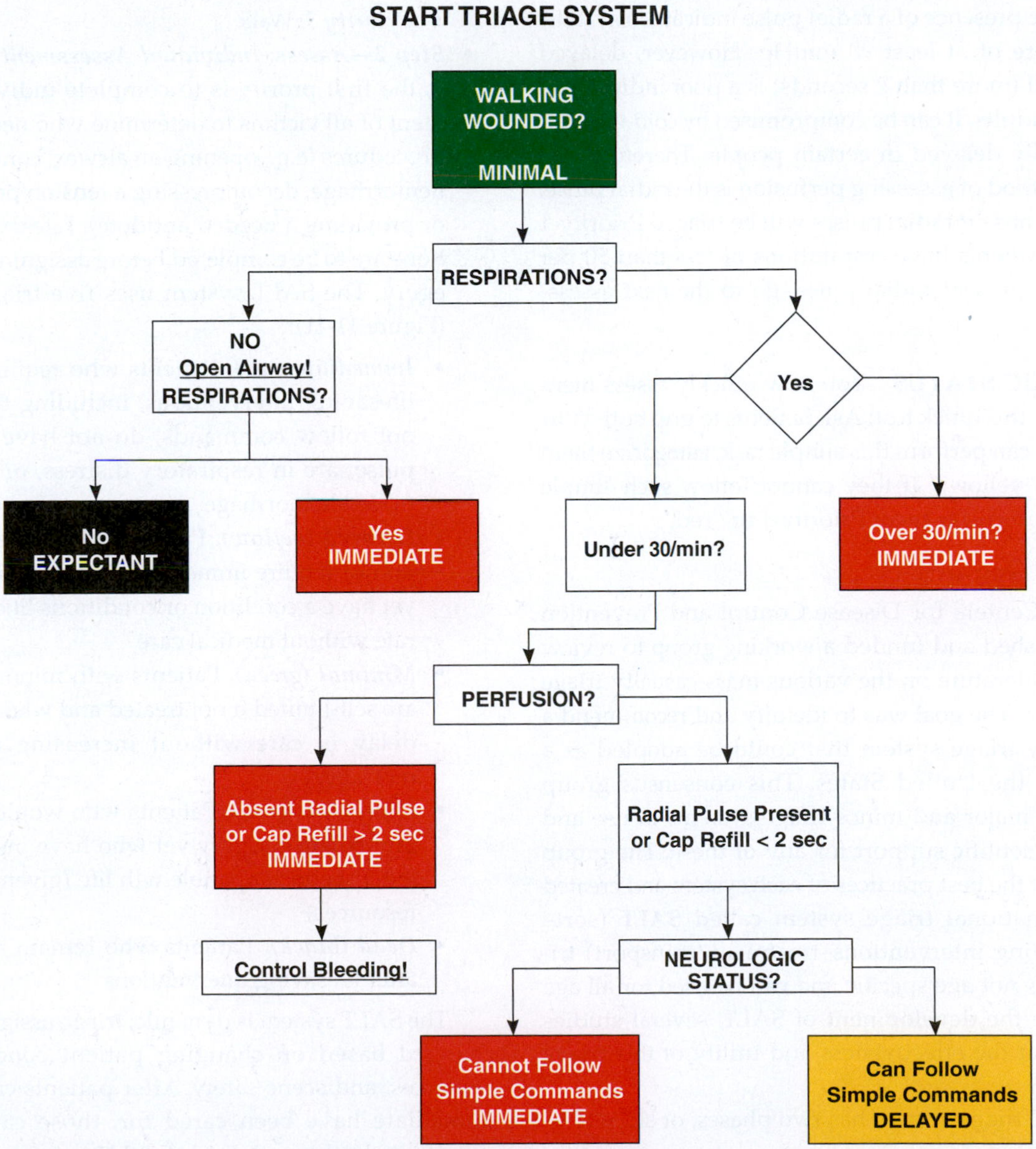

FIGURE 11-9 Operation of the START system, the most widely used triage system.

MCI without having the "walking wounded" wandering around the scene.

RESPIRATORY EFFORT Next, you begin to triage the nonwalking patients. Remember to keep the focus on tagging patients. Your only treatment effort should be directed toward correction of airway problems and severe bleeding.

Begin by assessing breathing effort. If patients are not breathing, open their airways manually. Categorize those patients who start to breathe spontaneously as Priority-1 or "red." Tag those who fail to respond as Priority-0 or "black." For those patients who are breathing, quickly assess their respiratory rates. Patients with respirations above 30 per minute should be tagged "red." If respirations are less than 30 per minute, go to the next assessment step.

PULSE/PERFUSION Assessment of circulatory status can be accomplished in two ways: radial pulses and capillary refill. The presence of a radial pulse indicates a systolic blood pressure of at least 90 mmHg. However, delayed capillary refill (more than 2 seconds) is a poor indicator of perfusion in adults. It can be compromised by cold weather or be normally delayed in certain people. Therefore, the preferred method of assessing perfusion is the radial pulse. Patients with absent radial pulses will be triaged Priority-1 or "red." If patients have respirations of less than 30 per minute *and* a present radial pulse, go to the next assessment step.

NEUROLOGIC STATUS You now quickly assess mental status. Use this quick test: Ask patients to grip both your hands. If they can perform this simple task, categorize them Priority-2 or "yellow." If they cannot follow such simple commands, categorize them Priority-1 or "red."

The SALT System

In 2006, the Centers for Disease Control and Prevention (CDC) established and funded a working group to review the scientific literature on the various mass-casualty triage systems in use. The goal was to identify and recommend a mass-casualty triage system that could be adopted as a standard for the United States. This consensus group reviewed the major and minor triage systems in use and found little scientific support for any of these. The group then looked at the best practices of each system and created a proposed national triage system called **SALT** (sort–assess–lifesaving interventions–treatment/transport) triage.[5,6] SALT is not age specific and can be used for all age groups. Since the development of SALT, several studies have looked at the effectiveness and utility of this triage scheme.

The SALT triage system has two phases, or steps (Figure 11-10):

- ***Step 1—Sort: Global Sorting.*** The SALT triage system begins with a global sorting of patients to prioritize them for individual assessment. First, patients should be asked to walk to a designated area. Those able to walk are given the lowest priority (3rd) for individual assessment. Those who remain after the first group have walked away are asked to wave (or follow a similar command) or be observed for purposeful movement. Those who do not move (e.g., remain still) and those with obvious life threats (e.g., uncontrolled hemorrhage) are made the highest priority (1st) and should be assessed first. Those who could wave, yet who were unable to walk away, are given the intermediate (2nd) priority. In summary, step 1 should result in the following categorization:
    - ***Priority 1:*** Still/obvious life threat
    - ***Proirity 2:*** Wave/purposeful movement
    - ***Priority 3:*** Walk
- ***Step 2—Assess: Individual Assessment.*** During step 2, the first prority is to complete individual assessment of all victims to determine who needs lifesaving procedures (e.g., opening an airway, controlling major hemorrhage, decompressing a tension pneumothorax, or providing a needed antidote). Lifesaving interventions are to be completed before assigning a triage category. The SALT system uses five triage categories (Figure 11-11):
    - ***Immediate (red).*** Patients who require immediate lifesaving interventions, including those who do not follow commands, do not have a peripheral pulse, are in respiratory distress, or have uncontrolled hemorrhage
    - ***Delayed (yellow).*** Patients who have injuries that do not require immediate lifesaving interventions, yet have a condition or conditions likely to deteriorate without medical care
    - ***Minimal (green).*** Patients with minor injuries that are self-limited if not treated and who can tolerate a delay in care without increasing their risk of mortality
    - ***Expectant (gray).*** Patients who would fall into the immediate category yet who have injuries that are felt to be incompatible wth life (given the available resources)
    - ***Dead (black).*** Patients who remain nonbreathing after lifesaving interventions

The SALT system is dynamic; triage assignment can be changed based on changing patient condition, scene resources, and scene safety. After patients categorized as immediate have been cared for, those categorized as expectant, dead, or minimal should be reassessed, as some

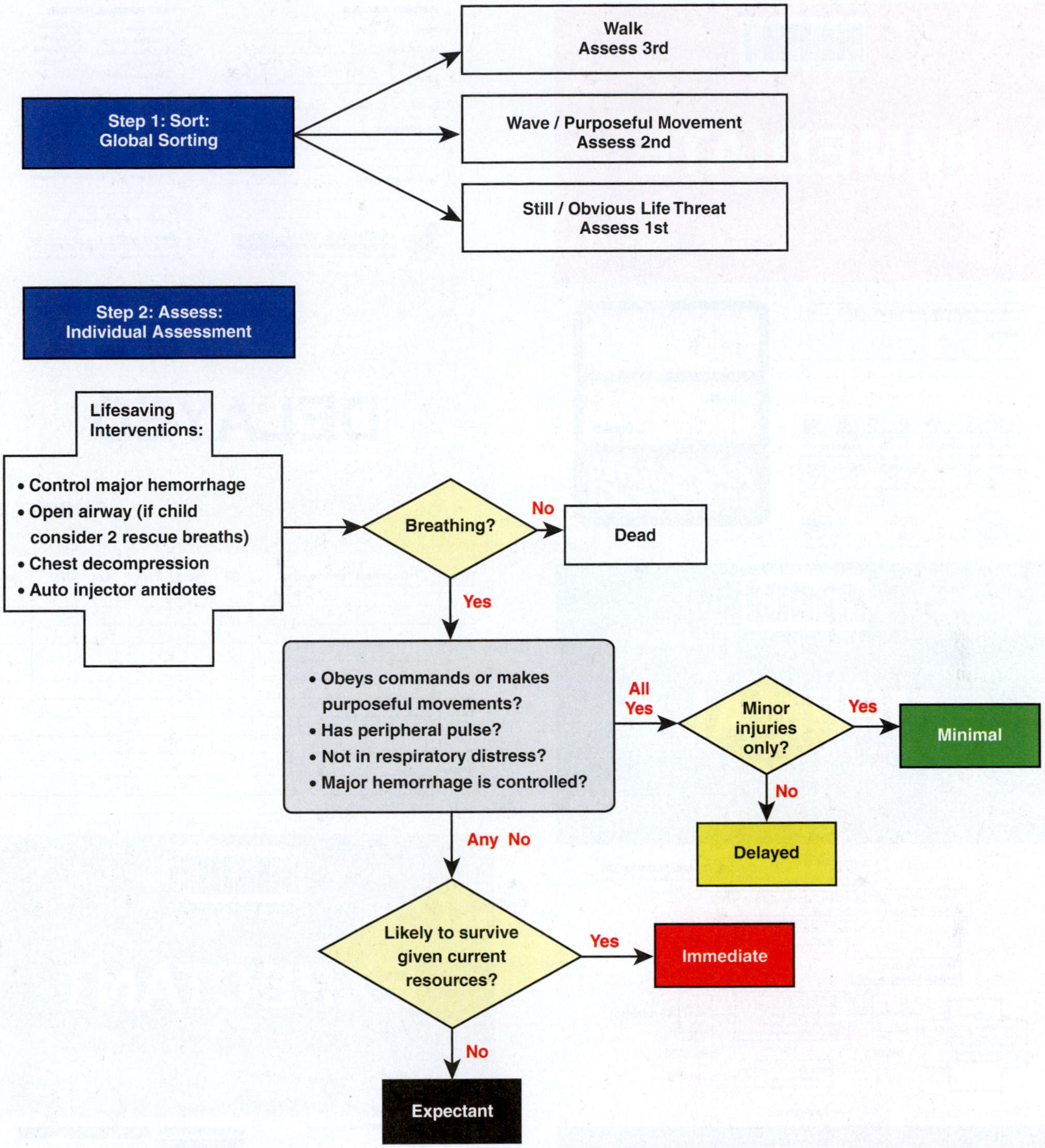

FIGURE 11-10 The SALT triage system.

patients may improve, whereas others may deteriorate. Treatment/transport should be provided in the following order:

1. Immediate
2. Delayed
3. Minimal
4. Expectant (if resources permit)

The effectiveness and utility of the SALT triage system remains to be seen. Unfortunately, until a national (or international) triage system is developed, paramedics may need to be familiar with more than one triage system.

The JumpSTART System

The JumpSTART Pediatric MCI Triage Tool is an objective tool developed specifically for the triage of children in the

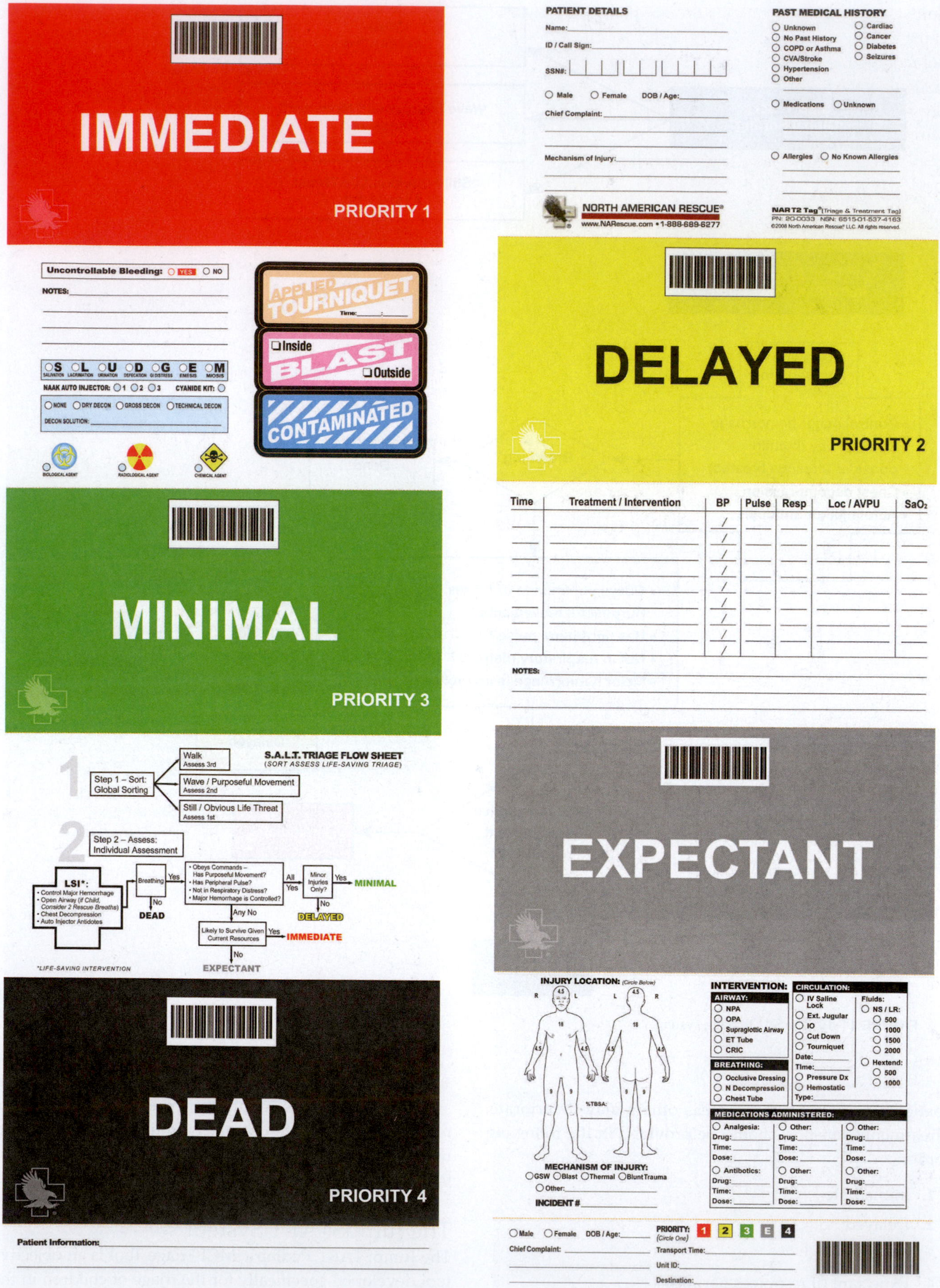

FIGURE 11-11 Triage tags for use with the SALT triage system.

multicasualty/disaster setting and was designed to parallel the structure of the START system, the adult MCI triage tool most commonly used in the United States.[7] The JumpSTART system takes into consideration the anatomic and physiologic differences found in children. The objectives of JumpSTART are:

1. To optimize the primary triage of injured children in the MCI setting
2. To enhance the effectiveness of resource allocation for all MCI victims
3. To reduce the emotional burden on triage personnel who may have to make rapid life-or-death decisions about injured children in chaotic circumstances

JumpSTART provides an objective framework that helps to ensure that injured children are triaged by responders using their heads instead of their hearts, thus reducing overtriage that might siphon resources from other patients who need them more and result in physical and emotional trauma to children from unnecessary painful procedures and separation from loved ones. Undertriage is addressed by recognizing the key differences between adult and pediatric physiology and using appropriate pediatric physiologic parameters at decision points (Figure 11-12). The JumpSTART system readily integrates with the START system (Figure 11-13).

Triage Tagging/Labeling

As already mentioned, you should attach a color-coded tag to each patient that you have triaged. Tagging offers these advantages:

- Alerts care providers to patient priorities—that is, provides organization of treatment
- Prevents retriage of the same patient
- Serves as a tracking system during transport and/or treatment

Commercial tags are available, such as the METTAG (Figure 11-14) or the SALT tag. However, you can also use colored surveyor's tape. Each has its advantages and disadvantages. Tags provide tear-off strips that help you count patients in each triage category. Tags also make it easier to track patients, record treatment information, and indicate a patient's location in a transportation accident. However, tags can be damaged in wet weather, and tear-off strips can make it difficult to change patient categories. Surveyor's tape costs less money but does not allow you to count patients during triage. Furthermore, black tape cannot easily be seen at night.

Some systems combine the use of tags and tape. Others use tags only when immediate transport is unavailable and/or when patients need to be sorted into separate treatment areas. Whatever method of tagging you use, it must meet these two criteria:

- Be easy to use
- Provide rapid visual identification of priorities

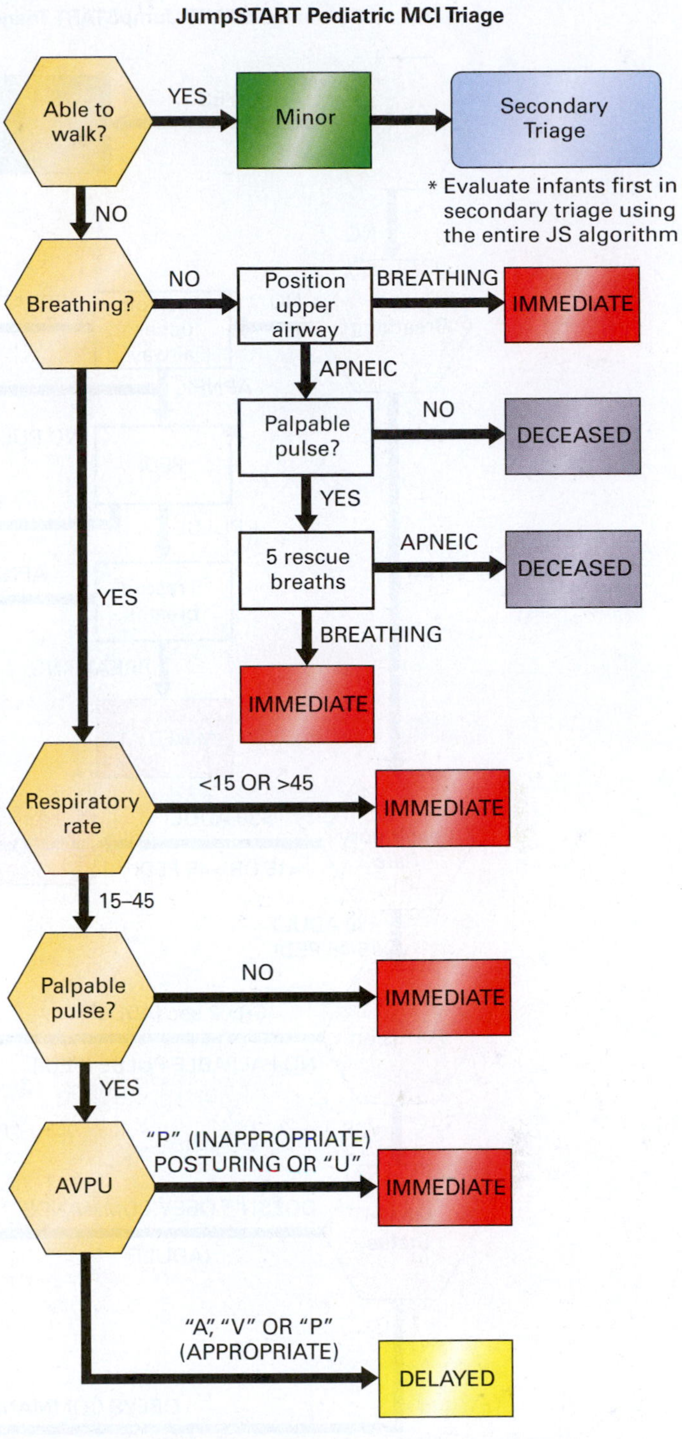

FIGURE 11-12 The JumpSTART pediatric triage system.

The Need for Speed

As stated on several occasions, you must not become committed to one-on-one patient care during triage. However, that does not mean that you do nothing. Simple care, such

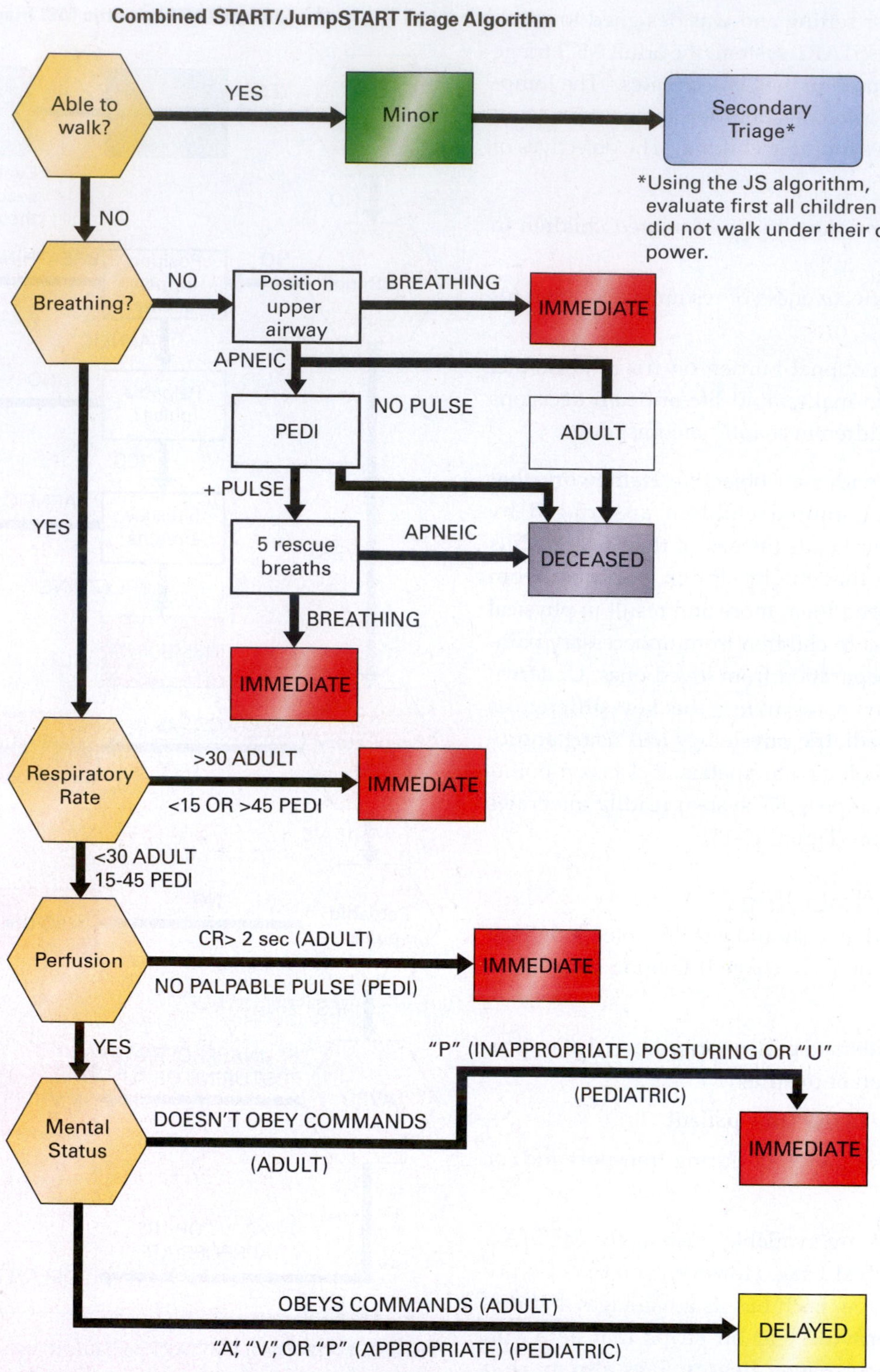

FIGURE 11-13 Algorithm showing integration of the START and JumpSTART triage systems.

as opening airways and applying direct pressure on profuse bleeding, can save lives early in an incident. As a result, the triage officer should carry certain medical equipment: infection control supplies, oral airways, and trauma dressings. Other essential items for the triage officer include tags or tape, a portable radio to communicate with the incident commander, a command vest, and a flashlight (at night).

Ideally, it will take you less than 30 seconds to triage each patient. However, that means it will take you 5 minutes to triage 10 patients, more than 20 minutes to triage 40 patients, and so on. As a result, other personnel will often assist the triage officer in MCIs with a large number of patients. The simple decision to add personnel can dramatically reduce triage time and speed treatment and transport. Triage personnel can act individually or be assigned to units. Either way, they

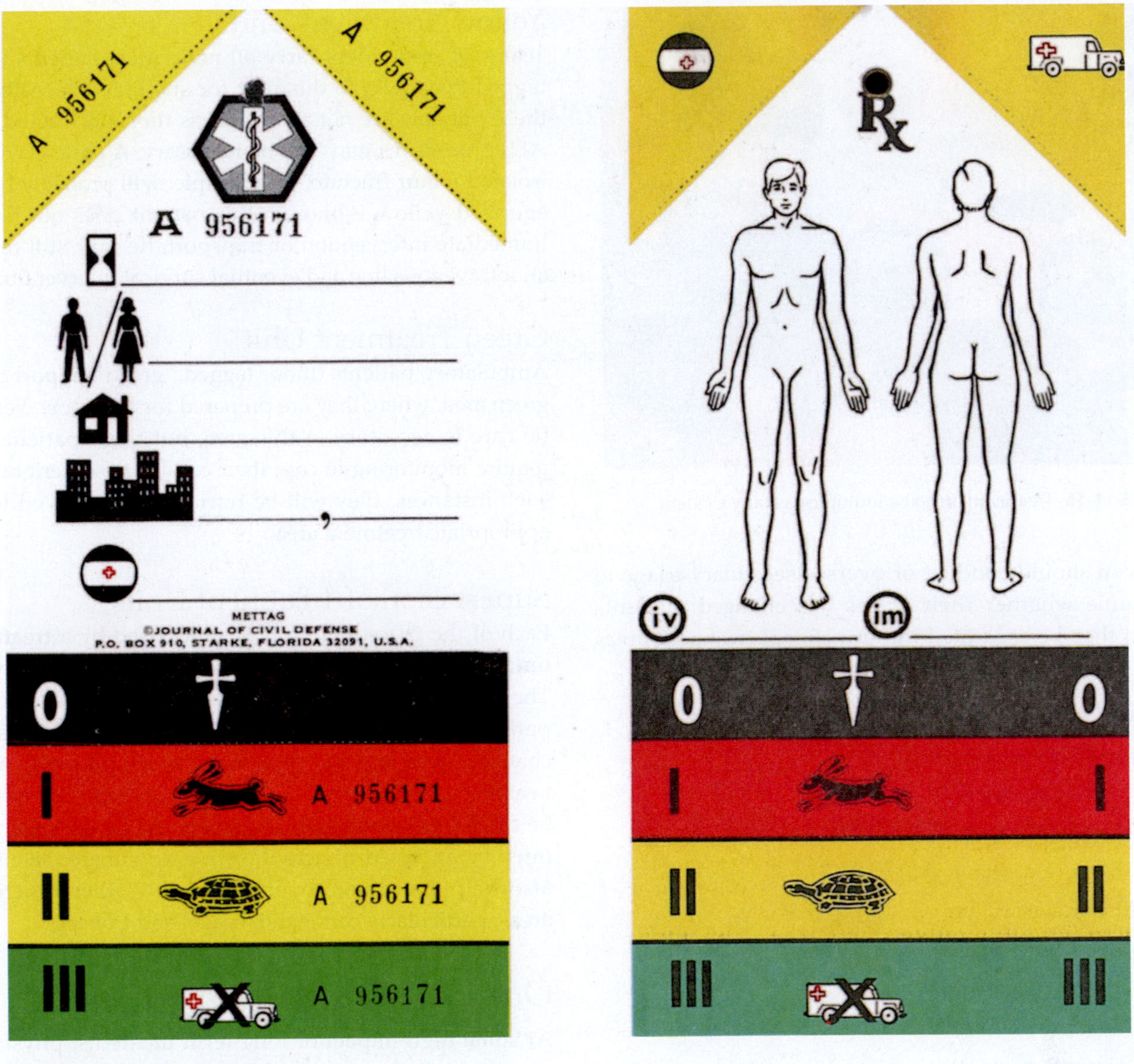

FIGURE 11-14 The METTAG.

(Copyright © by METTAG. Used by permission of American Civil Defense Association)

report to the triage officer, who in turn relays necessary information to the IC. After completing the task of triage, personnel can be reassigned to other units, such as treatment.

Morgue

You should collect patients who are triaged "black" or expectant (Priority-0) in an area away from treatment. Access to this area, known as the **morgue**, should be controlled so that bystanders or the media cannot enter it. In determining the disposition of the deceased, you will need to work closely with the medical examiner, coroner, law enforcement, and other appropriate agencies. (If possible, delay dealing further with the deceased who have been gathered in the morgue area until a decision and plan for the disposition of their bodies can be determined.)

Once a morgue is established, it will be supervised by a **morgue officer**. This person may report to the triage officer or the treatment officer. In many cases, these supervisors will assist in selecting and securing an area for the morgue.

Keep in mind the importance of having a preexisting plan for managing situations with large numbers of fatalities. Special facilities may be required to care for the victims. In addition, responders may require the support of counselors or members of the clergy.

Treatment

When the number of patients exceeds the number of ambulances available for transportation, you will need to collect patients into treatment areas (Figure 11-15). The **treatment group supervisor** controls all actions in the treatment group/sector. The responders who carry patients to the treatment area should be organized into teams of four to prevent lifting injuries. As patients arrive in the treatment

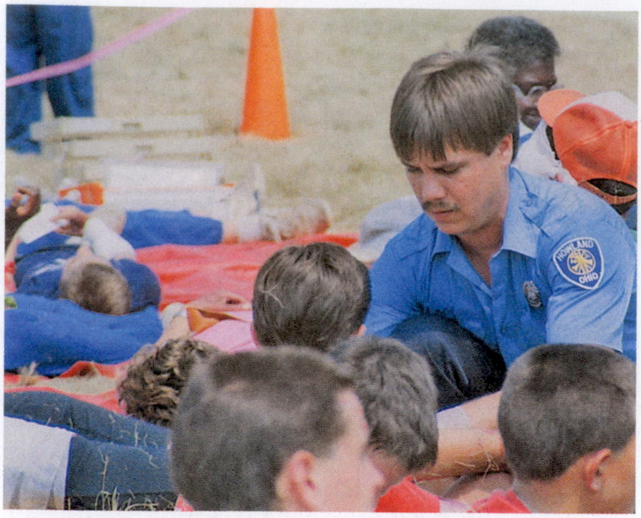

FIGURE 11-15 Treatment area at a multiple-casualty incident.

area, you should conduct or oversee secondary triage to determine whether their status has changed. Patients should then be separated into functional treatment areas based on their category:

- START Triage system:
  - Red (Immediate, P-1)
  - Yellow (Delayed, P-2)
  - Green (Minimal, P-3)
  - Black (Expectant, P-0)
- SALT Triage system:
  - Red (Immediate)
  - Yellow (Delayed)
  - Green (Minimal)
  - Gray (Expectant)
  - Black (Dead)

You will also need medical equipment to operate a treatment area properly. Essential equipment includes airway maintenance supplies, oxygen and delivery devices, bleeding control supplies, and burn management supplies. In addition, you will need patient immobilization and transportation devices, such as stretchers and long spine boards.

Red Treatment Unit

This area provides care for all critical patients—that is, those tagged "red." As a result, command and/or logistics will assign the bulk of medical resources to this unit. Providers with ALS skills usually report to the red treatment area so they can stabilize patients and prepare them for transport. Because medical resources can be used up quickly, a supply system is necessary to support this operation. Finally, this is the place where any on-scene physicians or nurses should be used.

Yellow Treatment Unit

Teams of responders carry all noncritical patients (those tagged "yellow") to this unit for stabilization. Although these patients are not as critical as those in the red area, ALS procedures may still be necessary. A patient with an isolated femur fracture, for example, will probably be categorized yellow. Although this patient does not require immediate intervention or transport, he may still require an intravenous line and eventual surgical intervention.

Green Treatment Unit

Ambulatory patients (those tagged "green") report to the green area, where they are prepared for transport. Very little care is necessary in this area, but these patients still require monitoring in case their conditions deteriorate. In such instances, they will be retriaged and moved to the appropriate treatment area.

Supervision of Treatment Units

Each of the preceding units is supervised by a **treatment unit leader** who reports to the treatment group supervisor. The leader's job requires extreme flexibility to ensure that patients receive adequate care. Patient conditions can change and responders, equipment, or supplies may not be available in the subarea. As a result, communications must be carefully coordinated. The treatment group supervisor must be apprised of activities in each subarea. He must also help coordinate operations with other functional areas, particularly command, triage, and transport.

On-Scene Physicians

At some high-impact or long-term incidents, physicians may be used on scene to support EMS. Physicians may use their advanced medical knowledge and skills in several ways at an MCI. For example, they may be better able to make difficult triage decisions, perform advanced triage and treatment in the treatment area, or perform emergency surgery to extricate a patient as a last resort. Physicians also provide direct supervision and medical direction over paramedics in the treatment area, removing the need to operate under standing orders or radio contact. A contingency plan should be established outlining when and how physicians respond to and operate at an MCI.

Staging

Ambulances may be the most precious resource at a multiple-casualty incident. As a result, ambulances must be staged as they arrive to allow proper access to the scene and, equally important, egress with the patients. If ambulances arrive before they are needed to treat patients, they should be kept in a **staging area** that is supervised by a **staging officer**. This area may be a roadway, a parking lot,

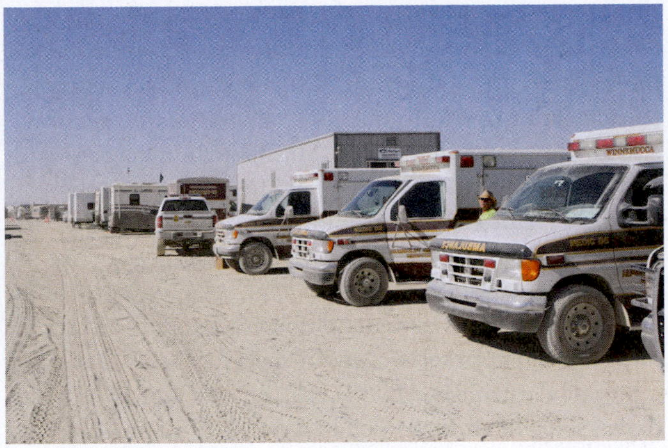

FIGURE 11-16 The staging area is an important component of any large MCI.

(*© Dr. Bryan E. Bledsoe*)

or some other site where the units can wait until they are deployed by command (Figure 11-16).

Depending on local protocols, drivers or crew members will be required to wait with the vehicles until they are needed for transport. A staging pool keeps personnel from "freelancing" and ensures their availability for quick deployment. It also prevents premature commitment of resources. If ambulances are required for immediate transport, the staging area can serve as a loading area for patients.

Transport Unit

The **transportation unit supervisor** coordinates operations with the staging officer and the treatment supervisor. His job is to get patients into the ambulances and routed to hospitals. If you are assigned to this role, you will need to be flexible in determining the order in which patients are packaged and loaded. You may, for example, elect to place two critical patients in one ambulance for transport to a trauma center. If you decide that the ambulance provider cannot adequately care for two critical patients, you may instead decide to transport one critical and one noncritical patient. You may also take into account the facilities at a given hospital and avoid overwhelming its resources with critical patients.

The routing of patients to hospitals is as important as getting them into the ambulances. Early in the incident, your communications center should contact local hospitals and determine how many patients in each triage category they can handle. You must take this information into account. You must also consider any specialties that a hospital may have, such as trauma centers, burn units, and neurologic teams. Keep in mind, too, that many patients may have left the scene before the arrival of EMS and transported themselves to the closest hospital. Depending on the scope and nature of the incident, you may have to factor in such self-transport as well.

As you might suspect from this discussion, a transportation supervisor needs to implement some type of tracking system or destination log. Ideally, the tracking sheet or log will include the following data:

- Triage tag number
- Triage priority
- Patient's age, gender, and major injuries
- Transporting unit
- Hospital destination
- Departure time
- Patient's name, if possible

The tracking sheet not only helps to organize activities at an MCI, but it also proves invaluable in reconstructing the incident at a later time. In addition, this record will help document on-scene patient care.

Extrication/Rescue Unit

Depending on your system, **extrication** or *rescue* may be a branch or a group. If this operation is considered an EMS function, it will be a group (sector) under the EMS branch. If it is a fire department function, it may be under the fire branch. If the rescue is extensive or long term, the operation may be separated into its own branch within the IMS.

In general, the extrication/rescue group removes patients from entanglements at the incident and arranges for them to be carried to treatment areas. The operation has many facets and may require specialized personnel and equipment. During extended operations, treatment personnel will need to work in this area and begin patient care prior to removal.

Depending on the circumstances, personnel operating in this area will need personal protective equipment, including helmets, eye protection, gloves, breathing apparatus, and/or protective clothing (Figure 11-17). Some rescue tools may also require specific support materials, such as gasoline, electricity, or compressed air. Extrication/rescue is a very dangerous area, and all efforts should be taken to ensure that operations are well supervised and safe.

Rehabilitation (Rehab) Unit

At extended operations, a special rehabilitation (rehab) area should be established to support on-scene responders. Arrangements should be made with logistics to ensure the necessary food, water, and medical monitoring supplies.

Ideally, rescuers should regularly rotate through a dedicated rehab area away from the incident. The site should provide thermal control and shelter from fumes, crowds, and the media. In this environment, rescuers can rest and hydrate themselves. Medical personnel operating in this area will take the vital signs of rescuers and watch for signs

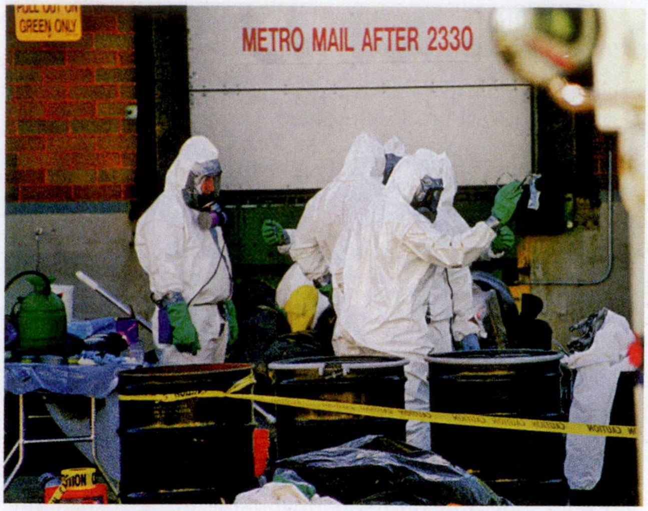

FIGURE 11-17 A hazardous materials team may be involved in the extrication and rescue phases of some multiple-casualty incidents. Here, a hazmat team prepares to enter the Brentwood mail facility on October 25, 2001, following an anthrax contamination.

(© AP Images/Ron Thomas)

of fatigue or incident stress. A predetermined threshold should be established so that rescuers with abnormal vitals are removed from the operation. This is especially important when working in extremely hot or cold conditions.

Provision should also be made for the availability of a **rapid intervention team**. If possible, an ambulance and crew should be dedicated to stand by outside the staging area. The incident commander can then contact the unit if a rescuer becomes ill or injured. Unfortunately, the demands of a large-scale MCI sometimes prevent implementation of this aspect of the IMS.

Communications

This chapter has already covered communications issues such as size-up, progress reports, frequency use, and more. However, it cannot be said too often: *Communication forms the cornerstone of the Incident Management System*. Therefore, it will be helpful to review some basic rules of communications within the system's EMS branch.

First, when communicating, think about what you are going to say before you say it. Does the message really need to be transmitted over the radio? Remember that the frequencies at an MCI will already be congested with messages. As a result, you should try to prevent as much unnecessary radio traffic as possible.

Second, key up your radio before transmitting. Wait 1 second after pressing the button to speak. This allows your radio to begin transmitting effectively and all other radios to begin listening before you begin your message. Keep in mind that missed messages mean missed chances at increased coordination and efficiency.

Third, acknowledge each message you receive with feedback to ensure that you understood it. For example, the message "Staging from Transport, please send two ambulances to pick up patients" should not be acknowledged with "Staging received." It should be answered with "Staging received two ambulances to pick up patients."

Other rules include points already covered in the chapter: the use of plain English instead of radio codes; the need for a common radio channel between command, groups (sectors), divisions, and units; face-to-face communications when appropriate; and respect for the lines of communication established by the IMS. In other words, report to the person you are supposed to report to at all times.

EMS Communications Officer

At large-scale incidents, the Incident Management System may provide for an **EMS communications officer**. This position may also be known as the *EMS COM* or the *MED COM*. This person works closely with the transportation unit supervisor to notify hospitals of incoming patients. A dedicated radio channel works best for this purpose, although use of cellular phones is common for this function. The EMS COM will not deliver complete patient reports, which would increase the communications traffic. Instead, he will transmit the basic information collected by the transportation unit supervisor, such as the number of Priority-1 or red patients en route to a hospital and the expected arrival time.

Alternative Means of Communication

Remember that your primary radio system may not always work at an MCI. Disasters can knock out radio towers and power. Frequencies can be overwhelmed. Telephone lines can be down. Radio batteries can fail. As a result, alternative means of communication should be included in every MCI preplan and should be practiced regularly. You might use cellular phones, mobile data terminals, alphanumeric pagers, fax machines, or other technology to overcome the failure of your primary radio system. When all else fails, runners can be used to hand-deliver messages around the incident scene. Although this method has obvious limitations, it may be your last resort—so know how to use it.

Disaster Management

Disasters can alter the operating procedures routinely used at high-impact events. For example, disasters can damage a region's infrastructure, preventing the operation of railroads, hospitals, radio systems, and so on. If a disaster occurs in your jurisdiction, you will be a victim as much as a responder, which is why outside assistance is often required. As a rule, **disaster management** occurs in four stages: mitigation, planning, response, and recovery.

Mitigation

Mitigation involves the prevention or limiting of disasters in the first place. For example, the public safety community tries to prevent people from building houses on floodplains or from putting up structures that are unable to withstand the impact of natural phenomena or terrorist attacks. In addition, most communities today have early-warning systems to alert people to weather emergencies, such as hurricanes and tornadoes, or to geological emergencies, such as volcanic eruptions or earthquakes.

Planning

As already indicated, planning is integral to the successful management of all high-impact emergencies. Every community, including your own, should take part in a hazard analysis and then rate these hazards according to their likelihood. For more on this analysis, see the section on preplanning later in this chapter.

Depending on your hazard analysis, devise relocation plans and/or evacuation procedures, as needed. When possible, every effort should be made to keep people in their natural social groupings. That is, provide home-based relocation instead of removing people to hospitals and clinics when they are not injured. If you must evacuate people, use whatever means you have to spread the message frequently and with urgency. Alert people to the nature of the disaster, its estimated time of impact, and description of its expected severity. Advise people of safe routes out of the area and the appropriate destinations for people who must leave an area.

Critical to any successful disaster plan will be provision for an efficient communications system in case the primary system fails. Decide, for example, where a central communications center might be established for people needing help. Set up guidelines on the use of radios by all EMS personnel. Make arrangements for portable radios and recorders as necessary.

Response

In a disaster, there is a great disparity between the casualties and resources. The event overwhelms the natural order and causes a great loss of property and/or life. As a result, a disaster almost always requires outside assistance and alternative operating plans. In general, you will follow the guidelines set up by the Incident Management System.

Recovery

Recovery involves the return of your department, your jurisdiction, and your community to normal as soon as possible. Actions taken will vary with the nature of the disaster and/or the disaster plan under which you operate. You may be involved with the reunion of families, follow-up care, and support of the personnel charged with handling potential hazards such as collapsed buildings or highways.

Meeting The Challenge of Multiple-Casualty Incidents

As implied in the preceding sections, you will never be more challenged in your EMS career than when you respond to an MCI. The routine actions that you do every day will suddenly become more difficult or, in some cases, impossible because of the stress or complexities of the incident. For this reason, you should anticipate various problems and work to overcome them.

Common Problems

Things can, do, and most assuredly will go wrong at MCIs and disasters. One way to avert or minimize complications is to anticipate them. As the saying goes, "Forewarned is forearmed." Studies of past incidents have revealed the following common problems, any one of which can hinder the success of a rescue operation:

- Lack of recognizable EMS command in the field
- Failure to provide adequate widespread notification of an event
- Failure to provide proper triage
- Lack of rapid initial stabilization of patients
- Failure to move, collect, and organize patients rapidly into a treatment area
- Overly time-consuming patient care
- Premature transportation of patients
- Improper or inefficient use of in-field personnel
- Improper distribution of patients to medical facilities
- Failure to establish an accurate patient-tracking system
- Inability to communicate with on-scene units, regional EMS agencies, or other personnel
- Lack of command vests for all IMS officers or supervisors
- Lack of adequate training and/or practice of rescuers at an MCI
- Lack of drills among regional agencies involved in the IMS
- Lack of proper community assessment, preplanning, and contingency plans

Preplanning, Drills, and Critiques

As we have mentioned several times, planning for an MCI or disaster makes response much smoother. Anticipate any problems that may occur and work toward removing them. Anything that can be planned in advance should be planned in advance.

The first step involves a complete assessment of the potential hazards, both natural and man-made, that could occur in your area. If you live in Kansas, for example, you might not worry about hurricanes, but tornadoes are a very real possibility. Sites of potential incidents in almost any community include chemical or nuclear plants, factories or mines, schools, jails, sporting arenas, entertainment centers, railroads, and airports.

Once you have completed the assessment, your agency should develop a plan that outlines the SOPs and protocols for potential incidents. You will not, of course, be able to plan for every possible scenario. If you develop 100 preplans, for example, you can expect to be summoned to scenario 101 or 102—that is, the unscripted event. For this reason, you must develop contingency plans for worst-case scenarios. For example, how would you communicate with ambulances if something or someone knocked out the dispatch center? What would you do if the local hospital suddenly became unusable because of chemical contamination?

After you have completed a preplan, test it. Start small. Tabletop drills, for example, are a good place to begin. Once you have worked out the wrinkles, distribute the plan to everyone in your department, the surrounding departments, local police, fire departments, hospitals—in short, to anyone who could be involved in the IMS in your area. Use the plan to ensure that the necessary mutual aid agreements are in place and that the appropriate personnel within the IMS know about these agreements.

Then make sure that all personnel who could show up at an MCI have received proper training in use of the IMS. As you have learned, the first responders on the scene will often determine the course of an event. Run or take part in drills so that you can gain practice in MCI operations and large-scale use of the IMS. Again, start small. Use local drills within your department to help personnel become familiar with the system. Then, aim for large-scale drills that involve outside agencies.

Finally, never say "It will never happen here." Experience has proven time and again that multiple-casualty incidents and disasters can occur almost anywhere and at any time. Make it part of your professional training to be ready to act as an incident commander, the person charged with establishing and organizing the IMS (Figure 11-18).

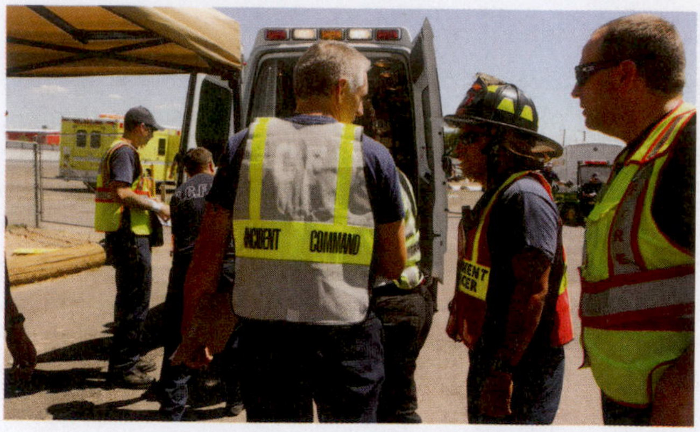

FIGURE 11-18 Planning for a local MCI should always include review of past similar MCI events. Make it part of your professional training to be ready to act as an incident commander.

Disaster Mental Health Services

The emotional well-being of both rescuers and victims is an important concern in any MCI. In the past, critical incident stress management (CISM) was recommended for use in emergency services. However, recent evidence has clearly shown that CISM and critical incident stress debriefing do not appear to mitigate the effects of traumatic stress and, in fact, may interfere with the normal grieving and healing process.[8,9]

However, an important role remains for competent mental health personnel in any MCI. Mental health personnel should be available on scene to provide psychological first aid for those affected by the event, including emergency personnel.[10] This requires no special training or certification and provides no psychological intervention but rather involves just meeting basic human needs. It includes:

- Listening
- Conveying compassion
- Assessing needs
- Ensuring that basic physical needs are met
- Not forcing personnel to talk
- Providing or mobilizing company from family or significant others
- Encouraging, but not forcing, social support
- Protecting from additional harm

Competent mental health personnel can also begin to screen both rescuers and victims for abnormal signs and symptoms associated with traumatic stress. Often, these symptoms take up to two months to develop. Because of this, mental health personnel should remain available and work with emergency personnel to identify anyone who may not be recovering normally from the event. Persons so affected may be referred for additional counseling or other mental health care.

Summary

Every paramedic should be thoroughly familiar with IMS procedures and should follow these procedures at every multiple-patient, multiple-unit response, from the smallest incident to the largest. Keep in mind the saying "We play as we practice." If you do, you will be prepared for the MCI or disaster that puts the emergency medical system to its biggest tests.

You Make the Call

At 5:15 A.M. on a dark and dreary Wednesday morning, the Hall County Sheriff's Office dispatch center receives a single call from a cellular phone reporting smoke coming from the back side of the Lone Pines Motel. The caller reports that he sees thick smoke in the area and smells something burning. The dispatcher immediately dispatches the Hall County Fire and Sheriff's Departments and your EMS agency. Hall County EMS responds with one ALS ambulance, one BLS ambulance, and the on-duty field supervisor in his ALS chase car (Figure 11-19).

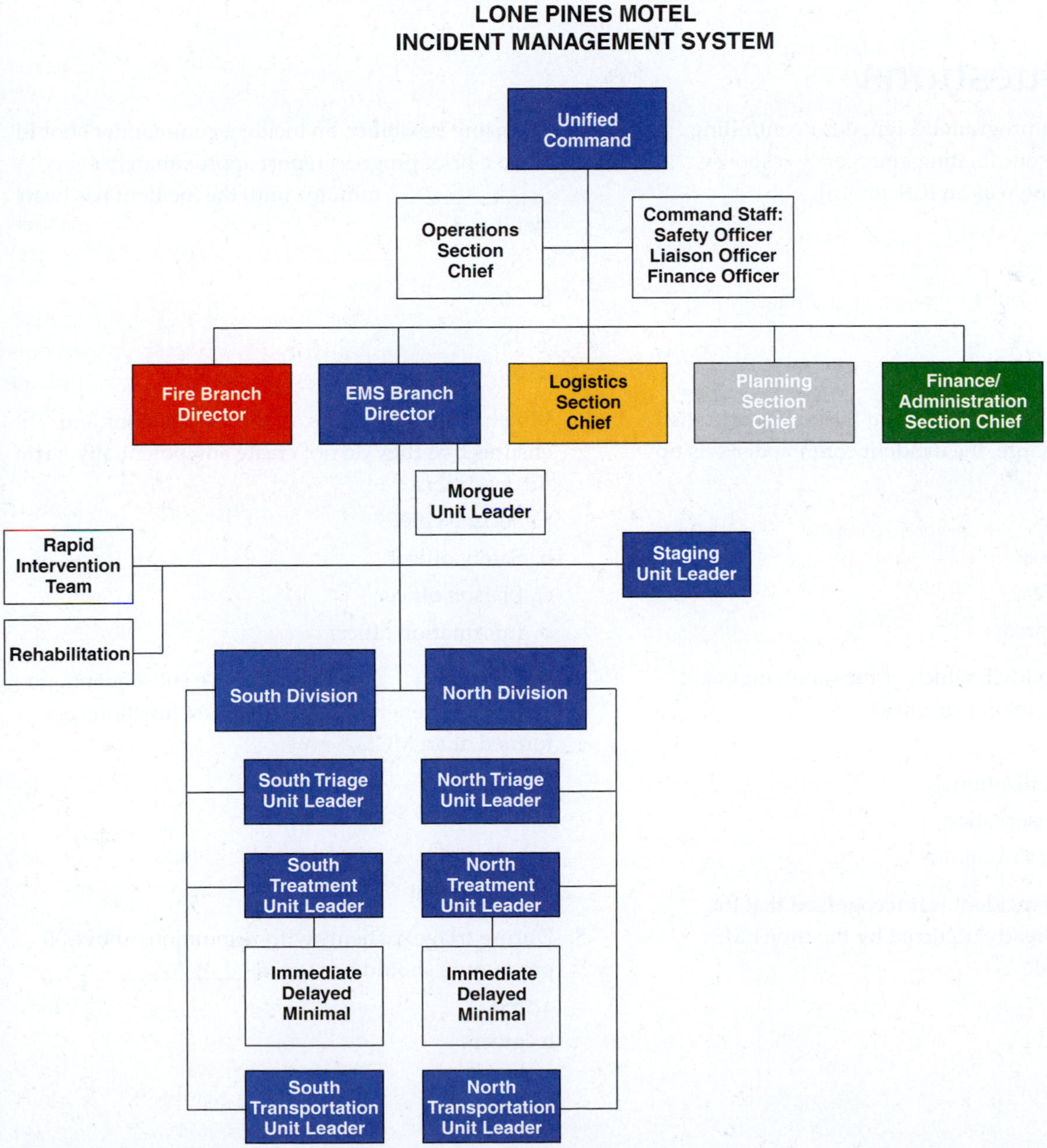

FIGURE 11-19 Sample command structure for a multiple-casualty incident at a motel.

You arrive in the ALS ambulance. You do a windshield survey and observe heavy fire and smoke coming from the rear portion of the building; several motel guests are now leaving their rooms. The night manager runs over and says that there are at least 20 people in those rooms in that part of the motel.

1. What two roles in the Incident Management System will you and your partner fill, as you are first on scene?
2. How would you size up the incident?
3. What additional resources would you anticipate, and what instructions would you provide for them?
4. How would you use the Incident Management System to organize this incident?
5. What would your initial radio report sound like in this incident?

See Suggested Responses at the back of this book.

Review Questions

1. A management program designed for controlling, directing, and coordinating emergency response resources is known as an ICS, or a(n) ____________
   a. MCI plan.
   b. IMS plan.
   c. ISC plan.
   d. PAR plan.
2. When the Incident Management System is expanded or the scene is large, the incident commander sets up a ____________
   a. control tower.
   b. command post.
   c. treatment area.
   d. operational area.
3. In managing an MCI, which of the following is *not* one of the three main priorities?
   a. Life safety
   b. Incident stabilization
   c. Property conservation
   d. Cost outlay evaluation
4. In what type of incident is it recognized that the injuries have already occurred by the time EMS arrives on scene?
   a. Open
   b. Uncontained
   c. Closed
   d. Controlled
5. To ensure flexibility, an incident commander should radio a brief progress report approximately every ____________ minutes until the incident has been stabilized.
   a. 5
   b. 10
   c. 15
   d. 20
6. Which person monitors all on-scene actions and ensures that they do not create any potentially harmful conditions?
   a. Section chief
   b. Safety officer
   c. Liaison officer
   d. Information officer
7. Because ____________ will drive subsequent operations, it is generally one of the first functions performed at an MCI.
   a. triage
   b. survey
   c. priority
   d. assessment
8. During triage, patients with respirations above 30 per minute should be tagged ____________
   a. red.
   b. green.
   c. black.
   d. yellow.

9. Which stage of a disaster management plan involves the return of your department, your jurisdiction, and your community to normal as soon as possible?
   a. Planning
   b. Response
   c. Recovery
   d. Mitigation

10. When command at a large-scale disaster event is transferred to another officer, it is done ________.
    a. face to face.
    b. via telephone.
    c. over the radio.
    d. in written documentation.

See Answers to Review Questions at the end of this book.

References

1. Department of Homeland Security. Homeland Security Presidential Directive 5: Management of Domestic Incidents. (Available at http://www.fas.org/irp/offdocs/nspd/hspd-5.html.)
2. Kahn, C. A., C. H. Schultz, K. T. Miller, and C. L. Anderson. "Does START Triage Work? An Outcomes Assessment after a Disaster." *Ann Emerg Med* 54 (2008): 424–430.
3. Hong, R., P. R. Sierzenski, M. Bollinger, C. C. Durie, and R. E. O'Connor. "Does the Simple Triage and Rapid Treatment Method Appropriately Triage Patients Based upon Injury Severity Score?" *Am J Disaster Med* 3 (2008): 265–271.
4. Gebhart, M. E. and R. Pence. "START Triage: Does It Work?" *Disaster Manag Response* 5 (2007): 68–73.
5. Deluhery, M. R., B. Lerner, R. G. Pirallo, and R. B. Schwartz. "Paramedic Accuracy Using SALT Triage after a Brief Initial Training." *Prehosp Emerg Care* 15(4) (2011): 526–532.
6. Lerner, E. B., R. B. Schwartz, P. L. Coule, et al. "Mass Casualty Triage: An Evaluation of the Data and Development of a Proposed National Guideline." *Disaster Med Public Health Prep* 2 Suppl 1 (2008): S25–S34.
7. Romig, L. E. "Pediatric Triage. A System to JumpSTART Your Triage of Young Patients at MCIs." *JEMS* 27 (2002): 52–58.
8. Bledsoe, B. E. "Critical Incident Stress Management (CISM): Benefit or Risk for Emergency Services?" *Prehosp Emerg Care* 7 (2003): 272–279.
9. MacNab, A. J., J. A. Russell, J. P. Lowe, and F. Gagnon. "Critical Incident Stress Intervention after Loss of an Air Ambulance: Two-Year Follow-Up." *Prehosp Disaster Med* 14 (1999): 8–12.
10. Everly, G. S., Jr., D. J. Barnett, N. L. Sperry, and J. M. Links. "The Use of Psychological First Aid (PFA) Training among Nurses to Enhance Population Resiliency." *Int J Emerg Ment Health* 12 (2010): 2131.

Further Readings

Molino, L. N., Sr. *Emergency Incident Management Systems: Fundamentals and Applications*. Hoboken, NJ: John Wiley and Sons, 2006.

National Incident Management System (NIMS). Washington, DC: U.S. Department of Homeland Security, 2004. NIMS information also available from the Department of Homeland Security website: http://www.dhs.gov (keyword: NIMS).

NFPA 1500. *Standard on Fire Department Occupational Safety and Health*. 2013 ed. Quincy, MA: National Fire Protection Association.

NFPA 1561. *Standard on Fire Department Incident Management System*. 2014 ed. Quincy, MA: National Fire Protection Association.

NFPA 1600. *Recommended Practices for Disaster Management*. 2013 ed. Quincy, MA: National Fire Protection Association.

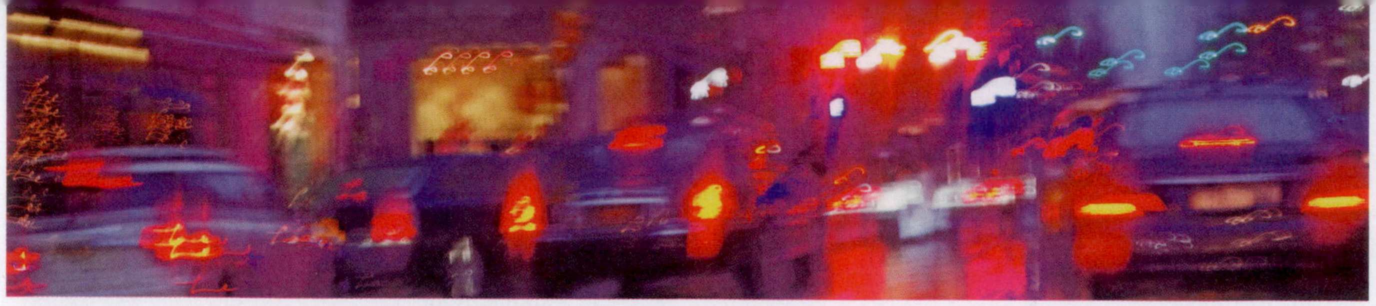

Chapter 12
Rescue Awareness and Operations

Bryan Bledsoe, DO, FACEP, FAAEM, EMT-P

STANDARD

EMS Operations (Vehicle Extrication)

COMPETENCY

Applies knowledge of operational roles and responsibilities to ensure patient, public, and personnel safety.

Learning Objectives

Terminal Performance Objective: After reading this chapter, you should be able to effectively perform the expected functions of EMS personnel in a rescue situation.

Enabling Objectives: To accomplish the terminal performance objective, you should be able to:

1. Define key terms introduced in this chapter.
2. Describe the concept of rescue awareness training with respect to the role of paramedics in rescue situations.
3. Identify the protective equipment needed by rescue and EMS personnel for a variety of rescue responses.
4. Identify equipment and safety processes used to protect patients in rescue situations.
5. Identify and describe the goals and tasks for each of the seven phases of a rescue situation.
6. Describe the principles and practices related to surface water and moving water rescues.
7. Describe the principles and practices related to hazardous atmosphere rescues.
8. Describe the principles and practices related to highway operations and vehicle rescues.
9. Describe the principles and practices related to hazardous terrain rescues.

KEY TERMS

active rescue zone, p. 332
disentanglement, p. 328
eddies, p. 337
extrication, p. 331
heat escape lessening position (HELP), p. 334
recirculating currents, p. 335
scrambling, p. 347
scree, p. 347
short haul, p. 350
strainers, p. 335

Case Study

A call comes into Fire Unit 1204, a volunteer-operated paramedic ambulance, to assist an injured person in a rural state park approximately 15 miles from the station. You hear the call over your radio and respond promptly, along with another volunteer.

Because of the distance and the winding roadways leading to the park, it takes nearly 30 minutes to arrive on scene. At the park entrance, one of the rangers informs you that a rock climber fell while trying to rappel down a popular cliff to meet his climbing partner on a rock ledge. Using a four-wheel-drive vehicle, the ranger takes you to the trail leading to the patient. Because the portable radio will not reach dispatch from the park, your partner stays with the ambulance.

From a vantage point along the trail, you spot the patient through binoculars. You see a young man lying on a rock ledge, about 55 feet below the trail. The climber's partner waves frantically to catch your attention, but seems unharmed. The cliff above the ledge is nearly vertical, with a smooth rock face. You quickly determine the need for a high-angle rescue team and possibly a helicopter for rescue and medical evacuation.

You relay the size-up information to the ambulance. Your partner, in turn, calls dispatch and requests the necessary resources. Dispatch arranges for two members of a regional high-angle rescue team to fly with the helicopter, which has been placed on stand-by.

On arrival, rangers lead the team to the emergency site. The two specially trained paramedics quickly confer with you, size up the situation, and ensure scene and personal safety. They then prepare their equipment for descent and access to the patient.

When the first rescuer rappels to the ledge, the uninjured climber blurts out: "I don't know what happened. He's such a good climber. Did you see all those leaves and pebbles near the anchor? I think he must have slipped while setting up his rappel. He's breathing but hasn't really moved since landing. A hiker saw the fall and called the ranger station with her cell phone—but that was so long ago. Please help—he's my best friend!"

To avoid having two patients, the rescuer directs the uninjured climber to "tie in" at a safe spot on the ledge. Because of the significant mechanism of injury, she performs a primary assessment on the patient, followed by a rapid secondary assessment. Her assessment reveals an unresponsive patient with multiple fractures. Nonetheless, his blood pressure and pulse appear stable at this time.

Because of the heavy forest canopy, rescuers decide not to do a short haul with the helicopter. While the other high-angle rescuer rigs the ropes and rescue system, the paramedic immobilizes the patient and establishes an IV of normal saline solution. Because she anticipates a prolonged removal time, the paramedic collects some of the patient history from the uninjured climber and begins the detailed physical exam. She starts a second IV, administers fentanyl, cleans and dresses all wounds, and splints all fractures.

It takes approximately 25 minutes for the team to rig the rescue and haul the patient off the ledge in a Stokes basket stretcher. Although badly shaken, the uninjured climber is hoisted to the top and turned over to your care. Meanwhile, the high-angle team carries the patient to the helicopter, which is waiting in a clearing about 200 yards down the trail. He is then flown to the nearest trauma unit for treatment. About 1 hour later, a violent thunderstorm hits the area. Without use of the high-angle team, the patient might still be lying unprotected on the ledge.

Introduction

EMS personnel usually have no trouble reaching their patients—that is, unless they are pinned beneath a vehicle, trapped in a collapsed building, or injured climbing a rock face or crawling into a cave. When people get injured or stranded in such situations, often someone must first rescue the patients before emergency medical care can even begin.

So what does *rescue* mean? According to the dictionary, it is "the act of delivering from danger or imprisonment." In the case of EMS, rescue means extricating and/or disentangling the victims who will become your patients. Without rescue, there are no patients.

Role of The Paramedic

Rescue is a patient-driven event, and EMS is a patient-driven profession. However, not all EMS crews have the training to perform rescues. In most cases, it is simply not practical to train every paramedic in the detailed knowledge or operational skills necessary for each rescue specialty (Figure 12-1). It is possible, though, to instruct paramedics in the concept of rescue and to train them to what is known as an "awareness level." Awareness training imparts enough knowledge about rescue operations to EMS personnel that they can recognize hazards and realize the need for additional expertise at the scene. Failing to train paramedics in rescue awareness will eventually end in the injury or death of EMS personnel, patients, or both.

Rescue involves a combination of medical and mechanical skills, with the correct amount of each applied at the appropriate time. Think of the medics who serve in the military. All armies throughout the world train and deploy medical people into combat. Even if the medics do not fire a weapon, they have enough military and medical training to treat patients in a combat situation. It's the same with the paramedics who serve on high-angle teams, SCUBA teams, and other specialized rescue units. If a rescue unit does not have medical training, your unit provides the balance.

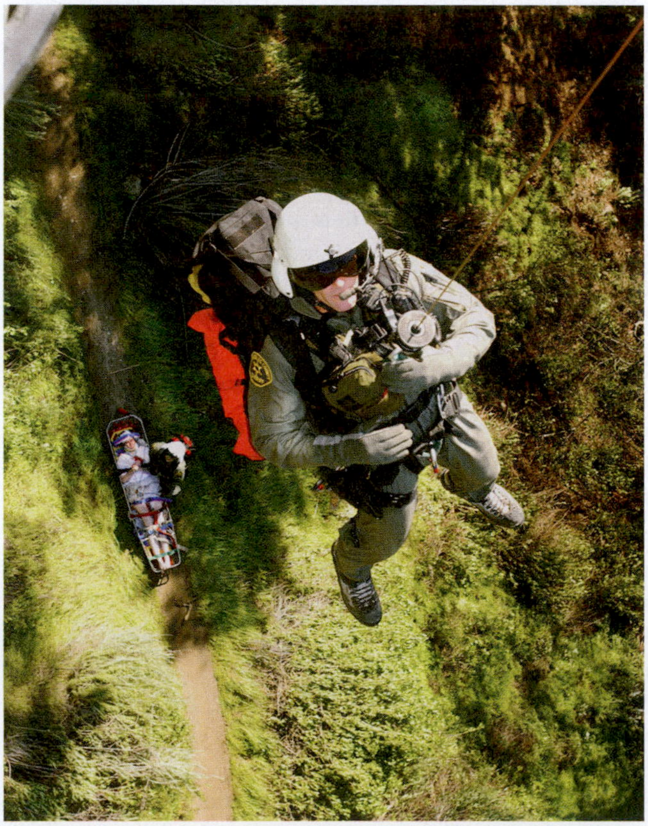

FIGURE 12-1 Rescue is a dangerous activity and safety is the number-one priority. It is impossible for an individual paramedic to be highly trained in all types of rescue. Instead, specialized rescue teams should be used.

(© Jeff Forster)

In any rescue situation, treatment begins at the site of the incident. If the patient can be accessed in any way, treatment may, in fact, start before the patient is actually released from entrapment. Once medical care begins, it continues throughout the incident. The trick is to balance the medical and mechanical rescue skills to ensure that the patient obtains effective and timely extraction. Teams must work together to provide a well-coordinated effort to meet the patient's medical and physical needs.

The role of EMS in a rescue operation varies from area to area. Some localities, for example, may require additional training beyond the awareness level. In general, however, all paramedics should have the proper training and personal protective equipment (PPE) to allow them to access the patient, provide assessment, and establish incident command.

As first responders, paramedics should understand the hazards associated with various environments, such as extreme heat or cold, potentially toxic atmospheres, and unstable structures. They should also be able to recognize when it is safe and unsafe to access the patient or attempt a rescue. If you deem an environment safe and if you have the training to effect a rescue, you should at least participate in the rescue under the guidance of individuals with additional expertise. You should also understand the rescue process, so you can decide when various treatments are indicated or contraindicated. In the climbing accident in the case study, for example, you would direct all parties not to move the patient until he was immobilized.

Because the field of rescue entails so many specialties, a single chapter cannot provide a step-by-step list of procedures and equipment for all the various scenarios you may encounter. Although practice scenarios can be found in related course materials, this chapter focuses on considerations that apply to most rescue situations. It discusses rescuer PPE and safety, presents the seven general phases of a rescue operation, and provides an "awareness level" of rescue operations in the following environments:

- ***Surface water***—such as "low head" dams, flat water, moving water
- ***Hazardous atmospheres***—such as confined spaces, trenches, hazmat incidents
- ***Highway operations***—such as unstable vehicles, hazardous cargoes, volatile fuels
- ***Hazardous terrains***—such as high-angle cliffs, off-road wilderness areas

Protective Equipment

The use of personal and patient safety equipment is paramount in any rescue situation. To prepare for a rescue response, you must develop a PPE cache. Without the appropriate protective gear, you will jeopardize both your own safety and the safety of the patient. Some of the equipment listed in the following sections has application in many rescue situations. Other pieces of gear are appropriate to specific environments or conditions.

Rescuer Protection

In all rescue environments, EMS personnel should wear highly visible clothing so they can be spotted easily. Ideally, PPE should fit the situation, but gear can be adapted, if necessary. For example, your PPE may not completely prevent exposure to infectious disease. Nonetheless, it minimizes the risk of infection (Figure 12-2). In fact, most PPE has not been specifically designed for EMS use. Instead, it has been borrowed from other fields, such as firefighting, mountaineering, caving, occupational safety, and more.

The use of adapted gear has resulted from the lack of a national uniform reporting system to identify risk-related exposures for EMS personnel. Future risk management and PPE design should be driven by such data. As a *minimum,* you should have the following equipment available:

- ***Helmets.*** The best helmets have a four-point, nonelastic suspension system (Figure 12-3). Most of the four-point suspension helmets are designed to withstand a greater impact than the two-point system found in hard hats worn at construction sites. Avoid helmets with nonremovable "duck bills" in the back—this will compromise your ability to wear the helmet in tight spaces. A compact firefighting helmet that meets National Fire Protection Association standards is adequate for most vehicle and structural applications. Climbing helmets work better for confined space and technical rescues, while padded rafting or kayaking helmets are more appropriate for water rescues.

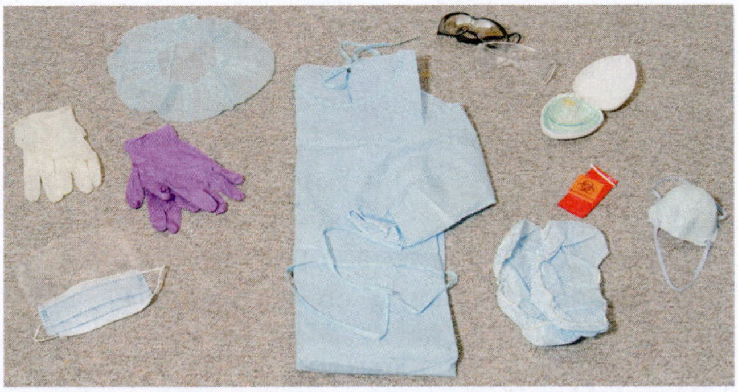

FIGURE 12-2 Your personal protective equipment helps to minimize the risk of exposure to infectious diseases. For more specialized operations, such as water rescues, you need more specialized equipment.

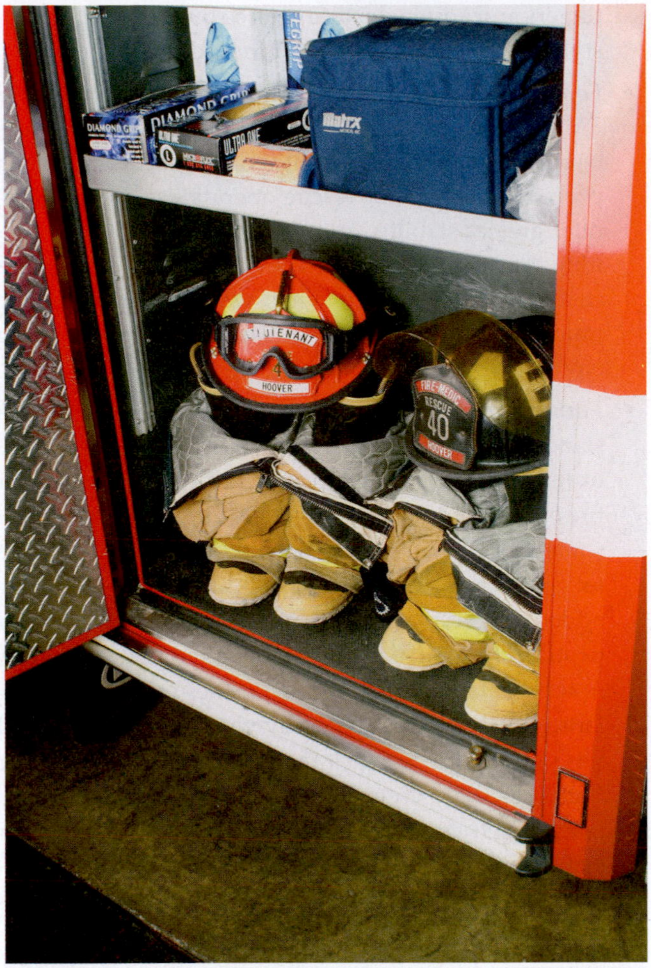

FIGURE 12-3 The quantity of safety and rescue equipment that can be carried on a standard ambulance is limited. However, helmets should be among the minimum types of rescue gear aboard each unit.

- ***Eye protection.*** Two essential pieces of eye gear are goggles, which should be vented to prevent fogging, and industrial safety glasses. These should be approved by the American National Standards Institute (ANSI). Do not rely on the face shields found in fire helmets. They usually provide inadequate eye protection.
- ***Hearing protection.*** From a purely technical standpoint, high-quality earmuffs provide the best hearing protection. However, you must take into account other factors such as practicality, convenience, availability, and environmental considerations. In high-noise areas, for example, you might use the multi-baffled rubber earplugs used by the military or the spongelike disposable earplugs.
- ***Respiratory protection.*** Surgical masks or commercial dust masks prove adequate for most occasions. These should be carried routinely on all EMS units.
- ***Gloves.*** Leather gloves usually protect against cuts and punctures. They allow free movement of the

fingers and ample dexterity. As a rule, heavy, gauntlet-style gloves are too awkward for most rescue work.

- ***Foot protection.*** As a rule, the best general boots for EMS work are high-top, steel-toed, and/or shank boots with a coarse lug sole to provide traction and prevent slipping. For rescue operations, lace-up boots offer greater stability and better ankle support by limiting the range of motion. They also do not come off as easily as pull-on boots when walking through deep mud. Insulation may be useful in some colder working environments.
- ***Flame/flash protection.*** Every service should have a standard operating procedure (SOP) calling for the use of flame/flash protection whenever the potential for fire exists. Turnout gear, coveralls, or jumpsuits all offer some arm and leg protection and help prevent damage to your uniform (Figure 12-4). They also have the added advantage of being quick and easy to don. For protection against the sharp, jagged metal or glass found at many motor vehicle crashes or structural collapses, turnout gear generally works best. For limited flash protection, use gear made from Nomex®, PBI®, or flame-retardant cotton. For high visibility, pick bright colors such as orange or lime and reflective trim or symbols. Some services, for example, have an SOP calling for highly visible gear and/or orange safety vests to be worn during all highway operations—both day and night. Insulated gear or jumpsuits are helpful in cold environments, but they can also increase heat stress during heavy work or in situations where high ambient temperatures prevail.

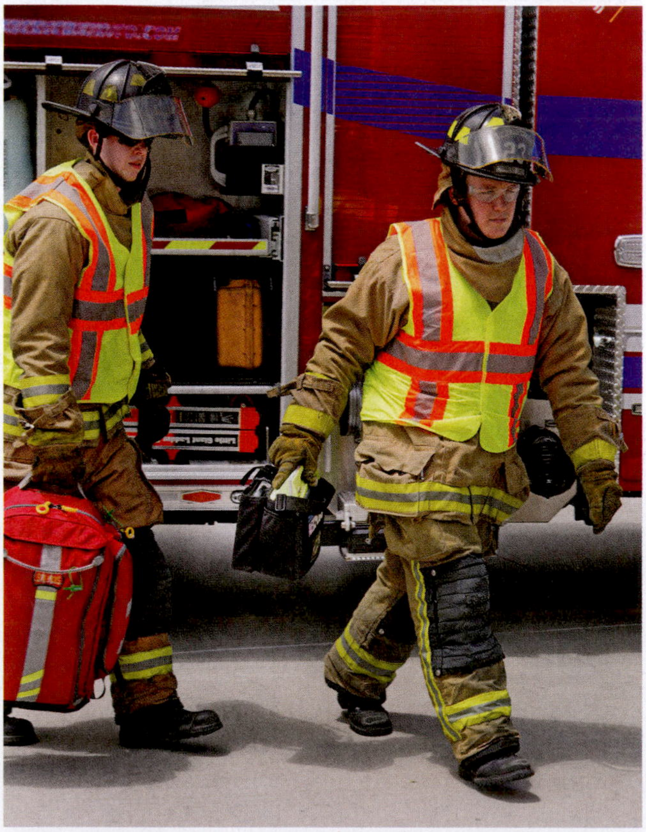

FIGURE 12-4 Full protective gear, including turnout gear, eye protection, helmet, and gloves.

CONTENT REVIEW

➤ Checklist for Backcountry Survival Pack
- PPE for inclement weather
- Provisions for drinking water
- Snacks for a few hours
- Temporary shelter
- Butane lighter
- Redundant light sources

- ***Personal flotation devices (PFDs).*** If your service includes areas where water emergencies can result, your unit should carry PFDs that meet the U.S. Coast Guard standards for flotation. They should be worn whenever operating on or around water. The Type III PFD is preferred for rescue work. You should also attach a knife, strobe light, and whistle to the PFD in such a way that they are easily accessible.
- ***Lighting.*** Depending on the type and location of the rescue, you might also consider portable lighting. Many rescuers carry at least a flashlight or, better yet, a headlamp that can be attached to a helmet for hands-free operation. Consider the long-burning headlamps commonly worn by mountaineers and found through catalogs, the Internet, or climbing/camping stores.
- ***Hazmat suits or self-contained breathing apparatus (SCBA).*** These items should only be made available to personnel who have been trained to use them. Most services or regions have special hazmat units to provide the highly specialized support required at rescue situations involving toxic substances. (For a discussion of hazmat training and equipment, see the "Hazardous Materials" chapter.)
- ***Extended, remote, or wilderness protection.*** If your unit provides service to a remote or wilderness area, you might need to hike into—or even be air transported into—a rugged environment. In such cases, you would be advised to have a backcountry survival pack as part of your gear. This backpack should be preloaded with PPE for inclement weather (cold, rain, snow, wind), provisions for personal drinking water (iodine tablets/water filter), snacks for a few hours (energy gels or bars), temporary shelter (tent/tarp/bivouac ["bivy"] sack), a butane lighter, and some redundancy in lighting in case of a light source failure.

Patient Protection

Many of the considerations for rescuer safety also apply to patients, with several significant differences. A patient protective equipment cache should include at least the following items:

- ***Helmets.*** Patients usually do not require the same heavy-duty helmets as rescuers. As a result, the less expensive, construction-style hard hats often provide adequate protection against minor hazards. However, if you anticipate greater danger, as in climbing or caving rescues, outfit patients with the same high-grade helmets as rescuers would use in the same or similar environments.
- ***Eye protection.*** Vented goggles, held in place by elastic bands, are ideal. They are not as easily dislodged as safety glasses. You might also use workshop face shields.
- ***Hearing and respiratory protection.*** Apply the same considerations for hearing and respiratory protection as you would for yourself. Earplugs are usually adequate.
- ***Protective blankets.*** You should have a variety of protective blankets to shield patients from debris, fire, or weather. Inexpensive vinyl tarps do a good job of protecting patients from water, weather, and most debris. Aluminized rescue blankets protect from fire, heat, or glass dust. Commercially available wool blankets provide excellent insulation from the cold. Plastic shielding (the kind used by landscapers) and plastic trash bags of many sizes and weights are also very useful. One 55-gallon-drum liner is large enough to cover a single patient. It can serve as a disposable blanket, poncho, vapor barrier, or, in a wilderness situation, bivy sack.
- ***Protective shielding.*** Circumstances may call for protective equipment that is more substantial than blankets or plastic sheets. All rescue teams should be trained to use backboards and other commonly found equipment as shields to protect patients from fire, weather, falling rock or debris, glass, or other sharp-edged objects. Shields specifically designed for a Stokes basket should be available. Keep in mind, though, that a device that shields a patient from debris or the elements may also limit rescuers' access to the patient. The more securely you package a patient, the more difficult it will be for you to monitor him. As patient care becomes more complicated, changing patient conditions may be overlooked.

Safety Procedures

As you already know, safety—your own and that of your crew–is your first priority. In rescue situations, however, a number of factors prod you to take action: your own desire to access the patient for treatment, the urging of people to "do something," the patient's cries for help, the presence of media, frustration at rescuers' lack of medical experience, and more. One mistake, though, can spell disaster for you, your crew, and/or the entrapped victim. One way to curb "heroics" is by establishing rescue SOPs, determining crew assignments, and, above all else, preplanning scenarios well in advance of actual rescues.

Rescue SOPs

Standard operating procedures are the nuts and bolts of effective EMS practice. At rescue situations, all teams should have written safety procedures familiar to everyone. Contents should include sections on all types of anticipated rescues. Each section should specify required safety equipment, required or prohibited actions, and any rescue-specific modifications in assignments. SOPs should include a statement requiring that a safety officer be present and an explanation of that person's relationship to incident command. Ideally, the safety officer should be someone with the knowledge and authority to intervene in unsafe situations. This person makes the "go/no go" decision in the operation. (For more on the role of safety officers, see the chapter "Multiple Casualty Incidents and Incident Management.")

Crew Assignments

In addition to SOPs, an EMS unit must anticipate crew assignments and special needs *before* the rescue operation. This task can be done through personnel screening, careful preplanning, and regular practice of any dangerous rescue techniques that members of your unit may be trained to perform (Figure 12-5).

Search-and-rescue planners often use personnel screening to determine the participants in the rescue process. Programs exist to identify the physical capabilities of crew members. Findings of these programs could have a significant impact on personnel assignments. In addition, psychological testing is recommended. It may even be desirable to screen for specific traits, such as phobias. For example, a rescuer's inordinate fear of heights or small spaces should be taken into account when assigning duties.

Preplanning

As stressed in the chapter "Multiple Casualty Incidents and Incident Management," one of the most critical factors in promoting safety and operational success is preplanning. Preplanning starts with the identification of potential rescue locations, structures, or activities within your area. Effective preplanning then evaluates the specific training and equipment needed to manage each of these events. The preplan also generates ideas on efficient use of existing resources and anticipates the need for additional equipment, rescuers, and/or expertise.

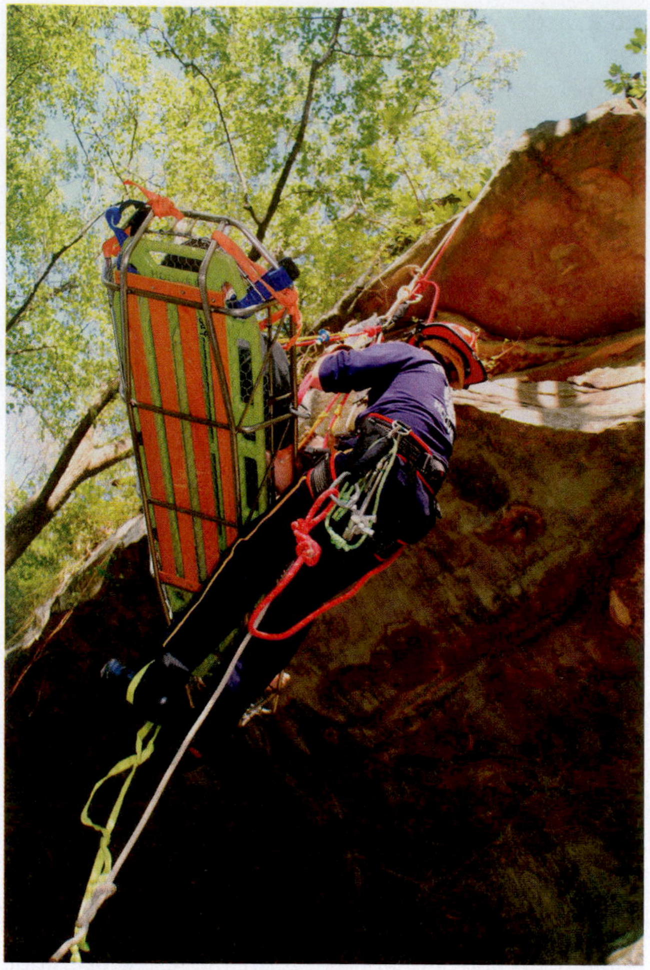

FIGURE 12-5 Dangerous rescue techniques, such as vertical rescue, should be practiced frequently to ensure the utmost safety during actual rescue situations.

Because of the intensity and length of many rescue operations, provisions must be made for the maintenance and rotation of rescue personnel. Plans should be made for "stand-by" or staging sites that offer protection from the weather. Sites should be away from the immediate operations area and secure from bystanders and the media. Personnel should be rotated at controlled intervals. Predetermined policies should be set regarding food and hydration of crews. On-scene diets should be high in complex carbohydrates and low in sugars and fats. Fluid replacement should consist of diluted (at least 50 percent) electrolyte solutions, such as those found in sports drinks. The classic coffee-and-donuts regimen should be avoided altogether.

The preplanning should be the basis of a broader regional emergency rescue plan, to be tested and modified in practice exercises. When possible, other specialized rescue agencies, such as high-angle teams, should take part in the exercises. These "test run" scenarios will give you and other members of your unit ample opportunity to utilize the Incident Command System (ICS) as it applies to rescue situations.

Rescue Operations

CONTENT REVIEW

➤ Phases of a Rescue Operation
- Arrival and size-up
- Hazard control
- Patient access
- Medical treatment
- Disentanglement
- Patient packaging
- Removal/transport

As already mentioned, there are several types of rescue operations, each of which includes technically difficult procedures, very specialized equipment, or both. *They should be attempted only by personnel with special training and experience in these areas.* Some of these special rescue operations are examined later in the chapter. First, however, you need to be aware of the general approach to most rescue situations.

As in any other EMS incident, rescue operations go through phases. Although specific procedures vary from area to area and from rescue to rescue, most calls will go through seven general phases: arrival and size-up, hazard control, patient access, medical treatment, **disentanglement**, patient packaging, and removal/transport.

Phase 1: Arrival and Size-Up

Size-up begins with the dispatcher's call and subsequent arrival at the scene (Figure 12-6). Although the dispatcher's message may indicate a rescue situation, you must still understand the environment and potential risks. On arrival, you or another paramedic must quickly establish medical command and appoint a triage officer. You must also conduct a rapid scene size-up, determine the number of patients, and notify dispatch of the magnitude of the event. Now is the time to implement the ICS, any mutual-aid agreements, and the procedures for contacting off-duty personnel or backup advanced life support (ALS) units.

Prompt recognition of a rescue situation and identification of the specific type of rescue are essential. You may be summoned to a structural collapse, vehicle rollover, or climbing accident. Each of these situations holds out the potential for entrapment and the need for specialized crews and equipment. Often, you must make a quick risk-versus-benefit analysis based on the conditions found on arrival. Be careful not to overestimate your capability to handle a rescue situation. As indicated, individual acts of courage may be called for, but safety comes first. If in doubt, err on the side of safety.

In calling for backup, follow this precaution: "Don't undersell overkill." Remember that it is always easier to send back a rescue crew than to rectify a personal tragedy caused by too few rescuers or hasty heroics. Also keep in mind the realistic time needed to access and evacuate an entrapped patient. Make use of the ICS to shave off valuable response minutes in what may be a life-threatening situation.

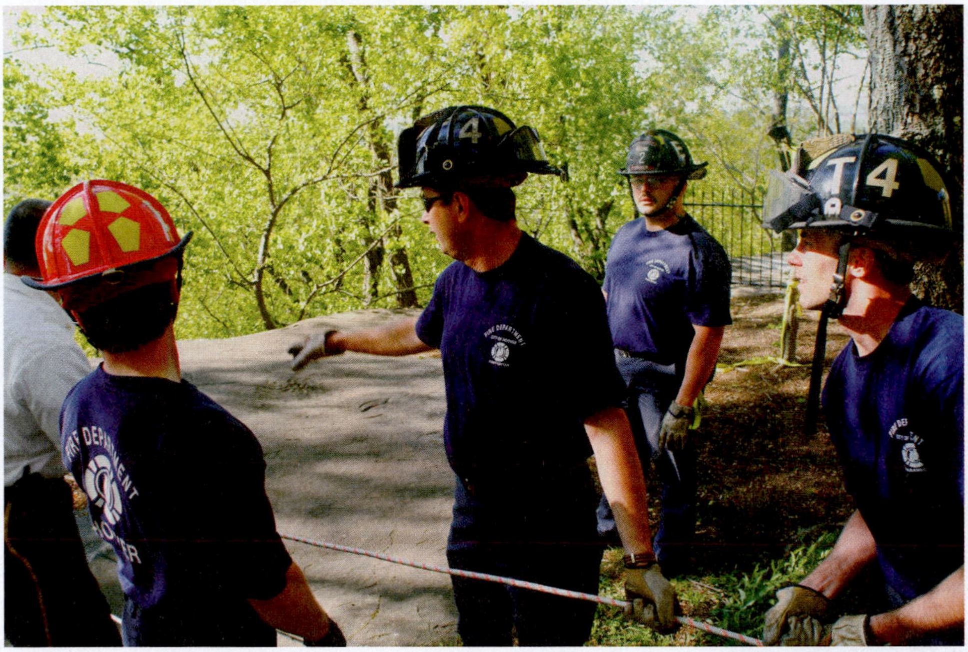

FIGURE 12-6 The first phase of a rescue operation is arrival and scene size-up. If the scene assessment reveals any hazards, efforts must be taken to control them, the second step of a rescue operation.

The very environment in which you stand can be risk filled. Look around to determine the possibility of lightning, avalanches, rock slides, cave-ins, and so on. Manage and minimize the risks from uncontrollable hazards as soon as possible to avoid other injuries. Ensure that all personnel, for example, wear appropriate PPE. Never forget the dangers of traffic. EMS providers have been killed at highway crash sites by drunks attracted to the bright lights, striking crew members in nonreflective gear. The following are some other potential hazards that you may be confronted with. As you skim this list, keep in mind that these are only a sampling of the conditions you may encounter.

- Poisonous or caustic substances
- Biological agents or germ-infected materials
- Swiftly moving currents, floating debris, or water contaminated with toxic agents
- Confined spaces such as vessels, trenches, mines, or caves
- Extreme heights or icy rock faces, especially in mountainous situations
- Possible psychological instability, as is often experienced in hostage crises, urban violence, mass hysteria, or individual emotional trauma on either the part of the patient or the crew (Recall the need for preassessment of crew members.)

Phase 2: Hazard Control

On-scene hazards must be identified with speed and clarity (Figure 12-7). You must often deal with these hazards before even attempting to reach the patient. To do otherwise would place you and other personnel at risk. Control as many of the hazards as possible, but do not attempt to manage any condition beyond your training or skills. Some situations, for example, involve chemical spills, radiation, gas leaks, explosives, or other dangerous substances. You will need to employ a hazmat team and confine your actions to a safe area. (For more on setting up zones at a hazmat scene, see the "Hazardous Materials" chapter.) Electric wires hold a "double threat" for fire and shock.

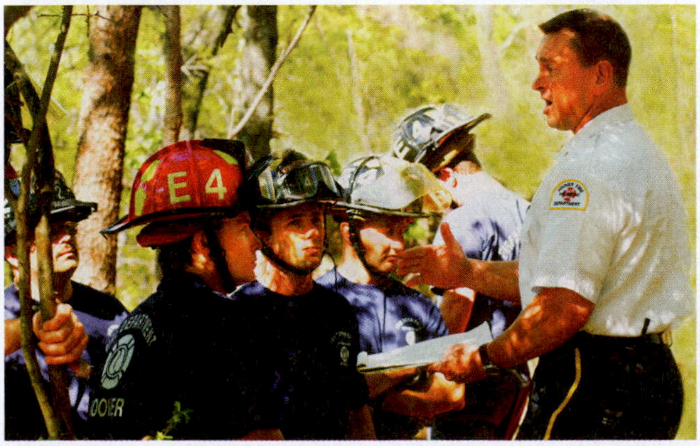

FIGURE 12-7 The second phase of a rescue operation is hazard control. Hazards must be quickly identified and dealt with.

Phase 3: Patient Access

After controlling hazards, you will then attempt to gain access to the patient or patients (Figure 12-8). Begin by formulating a plan. Determine the best method to gain access and deploy the necessary personnel. Make sure that you take steps to stabilize the physical location of the patient. For example, look for threats of structural collapse, cave-ins, or vehicle rollovers.

Access triggers the technical beginning of the rescue. While gaining access, you must use appropriate safety equipment and procedures. This is the point when you and/or the incident commander and safety officer must honestly evaluate the training and skills needed to access the patient. Untrained, poorly equipped, or inexperienced rescue personnel must not put their safety and the safety of others at risk by attempting foolhardy, heroic rescues.

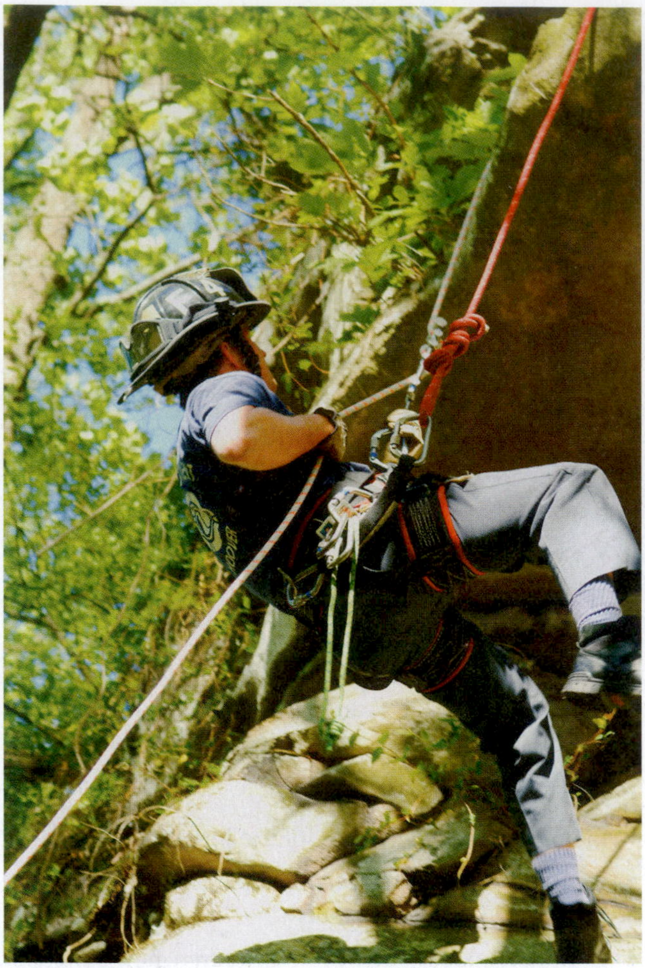

FIGURE 12-8 The third phase of a rescue operation is gaining access to the patient. In specialized rescues, such as vertical rescue, this can be a long process.

During the access phase, key medical, technical, and command personnel must confer with the safety officer on the strategy they will use to accomplish the rescue. To ensure that everyone understands and supports the rescue plan, a formal briefing should be held for rescue personnel before the operation begins. Even with well-trained personnel and adequate equipment, rescue efforts can be poorly executed because team members do not understand the "big picture" or they do not know what is expected of each member of the team.

Phase 4: Medical Treatment

After devising a rescue plan, medical personnel can begin to make patient contact. Remember: No personnel should enter an area to provide patient care unless they are physically fit, are protected from hazards, and have the technical skills to reach, manage, and remove patients safely. The interests of both rescuer and patient may be served by a first responder with expertise in the type of rescue required. However, if a first responder does not have the required fitness or skills, he may end up needing to be rescued because of some hasty, ill-advised effort to treat the patient.

Legal Considerations

Rescue Calls, Routine Calls, and Safety. A major concern of rescue is the safety of the patient and the rescuers. Rescue operations, especially when the incident management system is in place, seem to cause rescue personnel to be more alert with regard to safety issues. However, it is important to remember that the single biggest risk for EMS personnel is the routine ambulance call. Responding with lights and sirens places emergency personnel in peril. An unrestrained paramedic in the back of an ambulance caring for a patient is at extreme risk for injury in the event of a crash. Thus, it is important always to wear safety belts and harnesses any time the ambulance is in operation. Also, a significant risk for EMS personnel is traffic near an emergency scene. Every year EMTs and paramedics are killed when struck by vehicles while attempting to access or care for patients. Safety is a fundamental aspect of rescue. It also is a fundamental aspect of EMS and should be practiced at all times.

In general, a paramedic has three responsibilities during this phase of the rescue operation:

- Initiation of patient assessment and care as soon as possible
- Maintenance of patient care procedures during disentanglement
- Accompaniment of the patient during removal and transport

Again, whether or not you actually fulfill each of these responsibilities depends on the medical expertise of the special rescue team. Recall, for example, the opening case study, in which a trained high-angle paramedic accessed *and* treated the patient.

If you are treating the patient, take these actions if the conditions allow. Quickly conduct a primary assessment (mental status, ABCs, and C-spine status) on each patient (Figure 12-9). The next critical steps include rapid

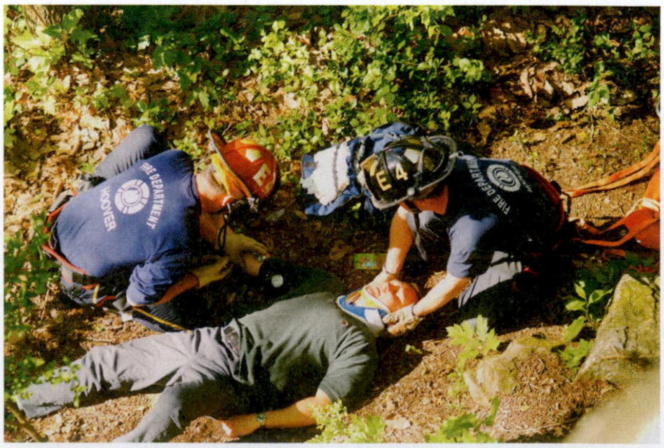

FIGURE 12-9 The fourth phase in a rescue operation is patient treatment. Assessment and care may need to be modified, depending on the on-scene environment and any special hazards.

CONTENT REVIEW

➤ Goals of Rescue Assessment
- Identify and care for existing patient problems.
- Anticipate changing patient conditions and determine in advance the assistance and equipment needed.

secondary assessment for the patient with a significant mechanism of injury, detailed physical exam, and medically oriented recommendations to the evacuation team.

Because a long time may elapse before transport, a patient's condition may change dramatically during disentanglement and removal. As a result, you should perform patient assessment with two goals in mind. First, identify and care for existing patient problems. Second, anticipate changing patient conditions, and determine the assistance and equipment needed to cope with those changes.

Continually evaluate risks to both rescuers and the patient. In many situations, the best overall patient care requires rapid stabilization and immediate removal. A final positive patient outcome may depend on initial sacrifice of definitive patient care so that the patient and rescuers can be removed from imminent danger. Examples of such situations might include:

- Injured, stranded high-rise window cleaners; workers on water, radio, or TV towers; high-rise construction workers
- Workers or bystanders involved in a trench cave-in
- Persons stranded in swift-running, rising water
- Patients entrapped in vehicles with an associated fire
- Patients overcome by life-threatening atmospheres
- Victims entrapped with unstable and/or volatile hazardous materials

In such cases, rapid transport of a nonstabilized patient to a safer location may be justified by the risk of injury to the rescuers and exposure of the patient to even greater complications. Rapid movement might be required even though the transport will aggravate existing patient injuries. Generally, management for the entrapped patient has the same foundation as all emergency care. Steps include:

- Primary assessment of the MS-ABCs
- Management of life-threatening airway, breathing, and circulation problems
- Immobilization of the spine
- Splinting of major fractures
- Packaging with consideration to patient injuries, **extrication** requirements, and environmental conditions
- Ongoing reassessment during the transport phase

Specifics of patient management during a rescue often follow the same or similar protocols to those used "on the street." However, some specifics may be, or should be, significantly different. Differences result mainly from the lengthy time periods often required to access, disentangle, and/or evacuate the patient. EMS personnel are trained in rapid stabilization and transport, particularly with trauma patients. However, during a rescue mission, the desire to achieve speedy transport may be impossible to fulfill. As a result, you must be able to "shift gears" mentally to an extended care situation. (For some background on time-related changes in treatment, see the discussion of distance in the chapter "Rural EMS.")

In addition to extended field time, you must be prepared to provide more in-depth psychological support for rescue patients than might otherwise be required. This is especially true in situations in which a patient has already been entrapped for a considerable amount of time. Establish a solid rapport with the patient, striking up a constant and reassuring conversation. In quieting the fears of rescue patients, keep in mind the following tips:

- Learn and use the patient's name.
- Be sure that the patient knows your name and knows that you will not abandon him.
- Be sure that other team members know and use the patient's correct name. The term "it" should never be substituted for the patient's name in any prehospital setting.
- Avoid negative or fearful comments regarding the operation, the causes of the operation, or the patient's condition within earshot of the patient.
- Explain all delays to the patient and identify the steps that will be taken to remedy the situation.
- Ask special rescue teams to explain any technical aspects of the operation that could frighten the patient or affect the patient's condition. Translate these operations into clear, simple terms for the patient.
- Do not lie to the patient. If something may hurt during rapid movement, acknowledge it. If the patient suspects an unstable environment, acknowledge that too. However, be sure to explain what will be done to mitigate the situation (i.e., the pain or the unstable environment).
- Above all else, stay calm and act every bit the professional. If you do not know the answer to a question, find somebody who does. Remember: Rescues are driven by patient needs.

Phase 5: Disentanglement

Disentanglement involves the actual release from the cause of entrapment, such as the dashboard of a wrecked automobile, a concrete slab from a structural collapse, or the blocked entry to a cave. This phase may be the most technical and

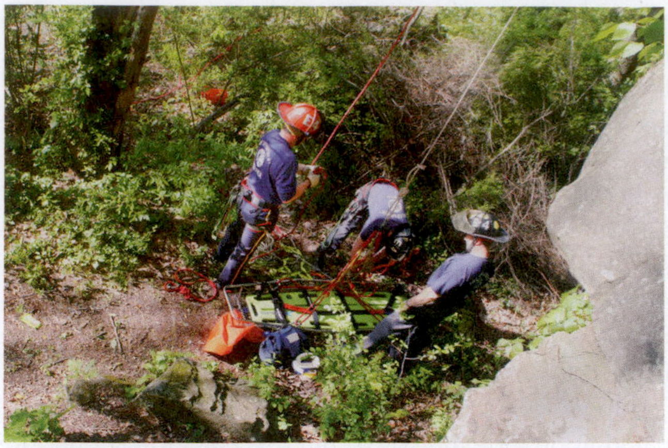

FIGURE 12-10 The fifth phase in a rescue operation is disentanglement. It can be prolonged, as in the case of auto entrapment.

time-consuming portion of the rescue (Figure 12-10). If assigned to patient care during this phase of the rescue, you have three responsibilities:

- Personal and professional confidence in the technical expertise and gear needed to function effectively in the **active rescue zone**, sometimes referred to as the "hot zone" or "inner circle"
- Readiness to provide prolonged patient care, that is, medical support of technical efforts
- Ability to call for and/or use special rescue resources

If you or another member of the rescue team cannot fulfill these requirements, reassess available rescue personnel and call for backup. Disentanglement is not a task for persons who are claustrophobic—extrication may involve crawling into a tight space. Disentanglement is also not a task for the squeamish—in some cases, an amputation may be required.

Methods used to disentangle the patient must be constantly analyzed on a risk-to-benefit basis. You and/or other members of the rescue team must balance the patient's medical needs with such concerns as the time it will take to perform treatment, the safety of the environment, and so on. If a patient has a severely crushed extremity and it will take an inordinate amount of time to release the extremity, the patient may, in fact, bleed to death without an amputation. This is only one of the hard treatment decisions that may be faced during the disentanglement phase of the operation.

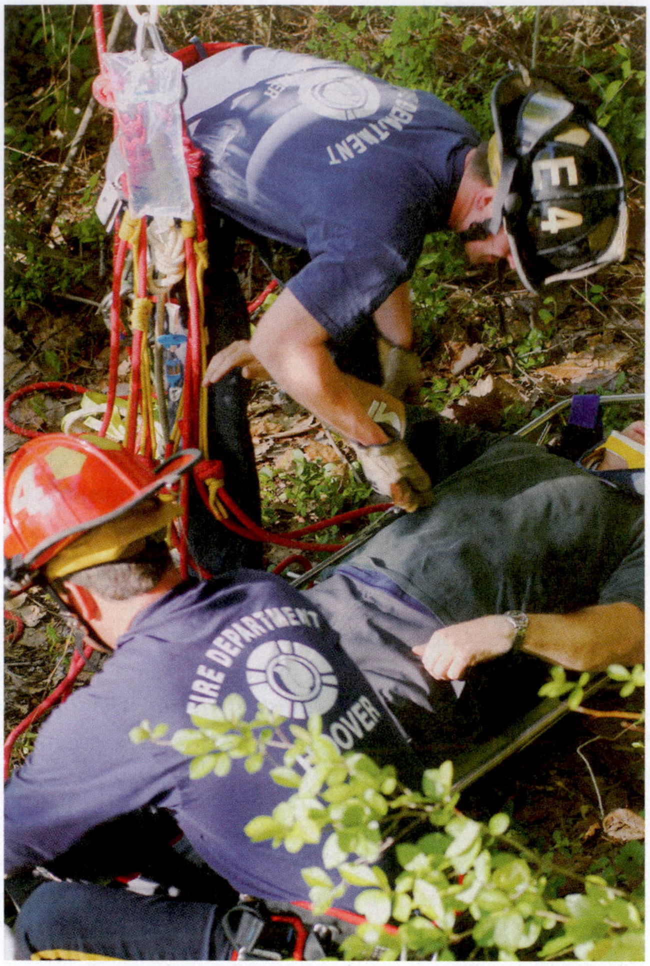

FIGURE 12-11 The sixth phase in a rescue operation is packaging of the patient.

Phase 6: Patient Packaging

After disentanglement, a patient must be appropriately packaged to ensure that all medical needs are addressed (Figure 12-11). You must consider such things as the means of egress—for example, a litter carry through the woods versus walking a patient out. You must also factor time based on the patient's medical conditions—for instance, rapid extrication techniques versus application of a Kendrick extrication device (KED). Some forms of patient packaging can be more complex than others, depending on the specialized rescue techniques required to extricate the patient—for example, being lifted out of a hole in a Stokes basket by a ladder truck, being vertically hauled through a manhole in a Sked stretcher, and so on. In situations in which the patient may be vertical or suspended in a Stokes basket, it is paramount that the rescuer know how to properly package the patient to prevent additional injury.

Phase 7: Removal/Transport

Removal of the patient may be one of the most difficult tasks to accomplish (Figure 12-12a) or it may be as easy as placing the person on a stretcher and wheeling the stretcher to a nearby ambulance. Activities involved in the removal of a patient will require the coordinated effort of all personnel. Transportation to a medical facility should be

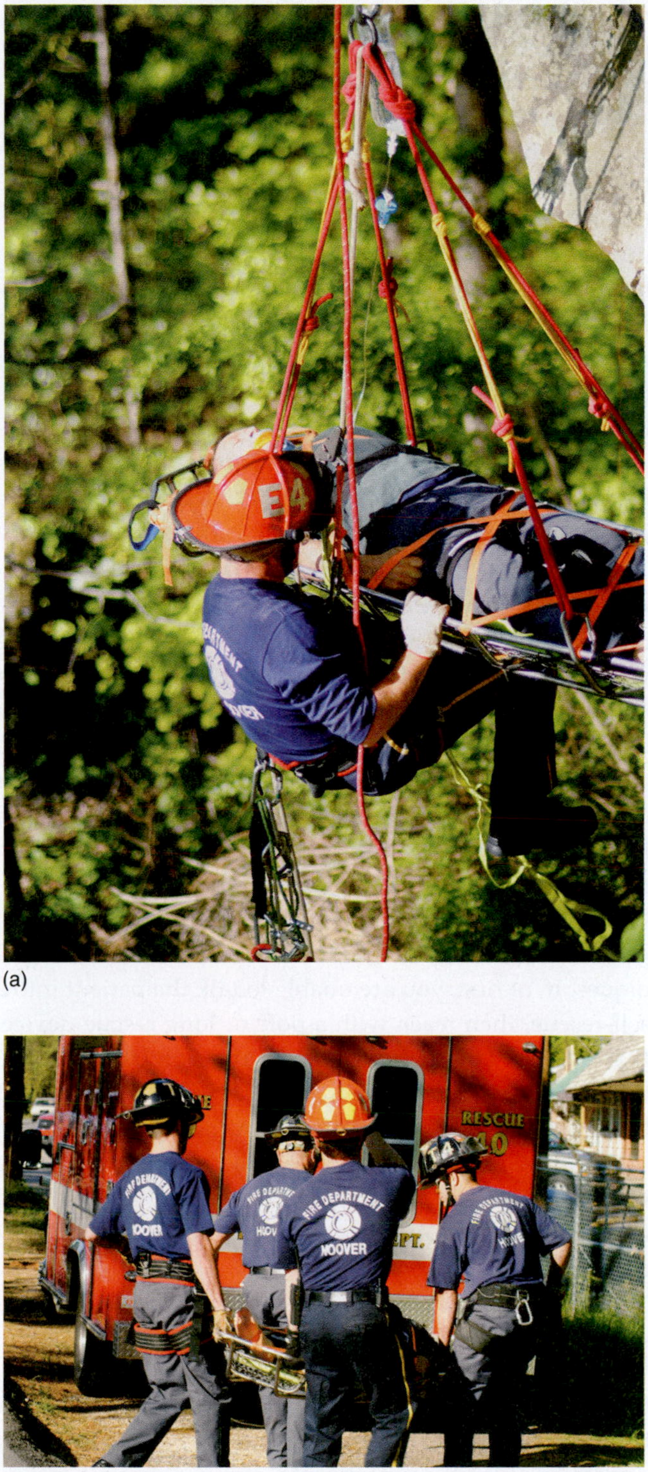

(a)

(b)

FIGURE 12-12 The seventh and final phase in a rescue operation is (a) removal and (b) transport of the patient. This can be by helicopter or by ground ambulance, depending on the situation and the condition of the patient.

planned well in advance, especially if you anticipate any delays. Decisions regarding patient transport—whether by ground vehicle (Figure 12-12b), by aircraft, or by physical carry-out—should be coordinated based on advice from medical direction. En route to the hospital, perform the reassessment, repeating vitals every 5 minutes for an unstable patient and every 15 minutes for a stable patient. Update the patient's condition and administer additional therapy per medical direction.

Surface Water Rescues

As previously mentioned, there are a number of different categories of rescue operations in which you may apply the principles and practices described thus far in the chapter. Water emergencies are among the most common. Because people are attracted to water in such great numbers and for such a wide variety of activities, accidents can take many different forms.

Most water rescues are resolved without the involvement of EMS personnel—for example, bystanders jump into a pool to pull out a struggling swimmer or other boaters rescue someone whose canoe has overturned. However, some water emergencies require that the rescuers have special training and equipment. In such cases, the temperature and dynamics of flat or moving water place both the victim and the rescuer at high risk of entrapment. Although all the possible scenarios for water rescue training cannot be supplied in a single section of a chapter, the following are some general concepts and methods to raise your "water rescue awareness."

General Background

Water rescues may involve many kinds of water bodies: pools, rivers, streams, lakes, canals, flooded gravel pits, or even the ocean. Some communities also have drainage systems that remain dry until flash floods turn them into raging rivers.

Most people who get injured or drown in these bodies of water do not intend to get into trouble. But one or more factors conspire to create an emergency: The weather changes, swimmers underestimate the water's power, nonswimmers neglect to wear a PFD and fall in, people develop a muscle stitch or cramp while in the water, submerged debris knocks waders off their feet, boats collide, and more.

Nearly all incidents in and around water are preventable. It is important for you to become familiar with safe aquatic practices. First and foremost, know how to swim and make swimming part of your physical exercise. Second, remember that even the strongest swimmer can get into trouble. Therefore, always carry PFDs aboard your unit and always wear a PFD whenever you are around water or ice (Figure 12-13). (Make sure your crew does the same.) Third, you might consider taking a basic water rescue course.

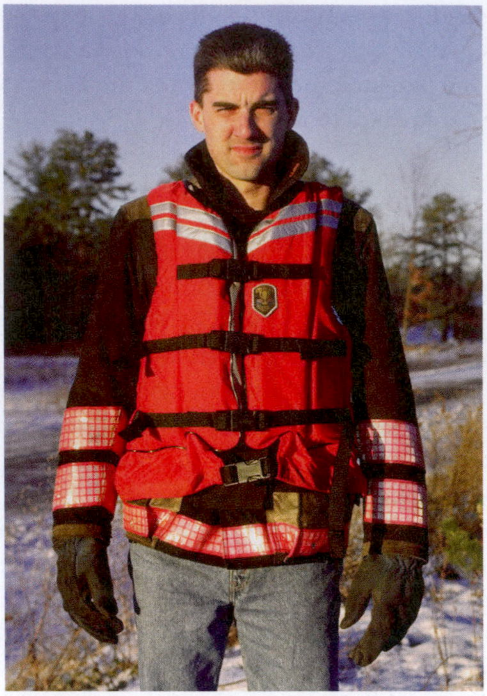

FIGURE 12-13 A personal flotation device (PFD) is mandatory equipment for any water-related rescue.

Water Temperature

Because the human body temperature is normally 98.6°F (37°C), almost any body of water is colder and will cause heat loss. Water temperature in smaller bodies of water varies widely with the seasons and the amount of runoff. Even on warm days, though, water temperature can be quite cold in most places. As a result, water temperature and heat loss figure in the demise of most victims and ill-equipped rescuers.

As implied, immersion can rapidly lead to hypothermia, a condition discussed in the chapter "Environmental Trauma." As a rule, people cannot maintain body heat in water that is less than 92°F (33°C). The colder the water, the faster the loss of heat. In fact, water causes heat loss 25 times faster than the air. Immersion in 35°F (1.6°C) water for 15 to 20 minutes is likely to kill a person.[1,2] Factors contributing to the demise of a hypothermic patient include:

- Incapacitation and an inability to self-rescue
- Inability to follow simple directions
- Inability to grasp a line or flotation device
- Laryngospasm (caused by sudden immersion) and greater likelihood of drowning

A number of actions can delay the onset of hypothermia in water rescues. The use of PFDs slows heat loss and reduces the energy required for flotation. If people suddenly become submerged, they can also assume the **heat escape lessening position (HELP)**. This position involves floating with the head out of water and the body in a fetal tuck. Researchers estimate that someone who has practiced with HELP can reduce heat loss by almost 60 percent, as compared to the heat expended when treading water. If a group of victims find themselves in the water, researchers also suggest huddling together. This technique not only prevents heat loss, but also provides a better target (more visibility) for members of a rescue team.

CONTENT REVIEW

➤ Actions to Delay Hypothermia
- Use of PFDs
- Use of HELP
- Huddling together

Basic Rescue Techniques

Basic rescue techniques vary with the dynamics of the water; rescue in moving water will differ from rescue in nonmoving (flat) water. If your unit responds to frozen bodies of water, you may also add techniques for ice rescue and include the proper cold-water-entry dry suits as part of your PPE cache (Figure 12-14). Also keep in mind that a PFD is useless if it is not worn. Therefore, all EMS personnel should put one on, even for shore-based rescues.

The water rescue model is reach–throw–row–go. All paramedics should be trained in reach-and-throw techniques. If, at first, you are unable to talk the patient into a self-rescue, then reach with a pole or long rescue device. If this is not effective or if the victim is too far out, try throwing a flotation device. All paramedics should become proficient with a water-throw bag for shore-based operations. Remember: Boat-based techniques require specialized rescue training. Water entry ("go") is used only as the last resort—and is an action best left to specialized water rescuers.

Moving Water

By far the most dangerous water rescues involve water that is moving. Competency at handling the power and dynamics of swift-water rescues comes only with extensive training and experience. The force of moving water can be very deceptive. The hydraulics of moving water change with a number of variables, including water depth, velocity, obstructions to flow, changing tides, and more. Only specially trained rescuers can readily recognize these factors.

To train for swift-water entry, rescuers must develop a proficiency in many specialized skills. In preparation for technical rope rescues, they must master the skills required for high-angle rope rescues. They must also

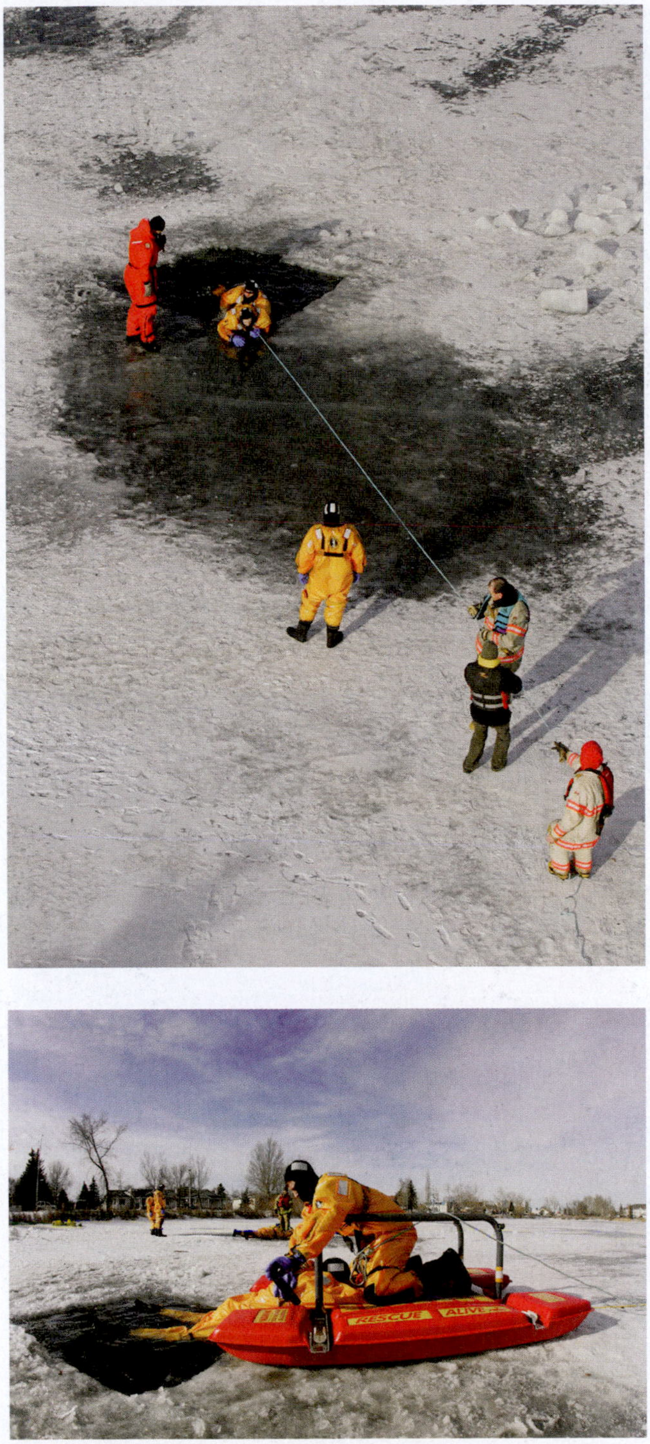

FIGURE 12-14 Safe ice rescue requires proper equipment and protective clothing.

(© Both Photos: Kevin Link/Science Source)

become well practiced in such skills as crossing moving bodies of water, defensive swimming, use of throw bags and boogy boards, shore-based swimming, boat-based rescue techniques, management of water-specific emergencies, and the capability to package the patient with water-related injuries.

Four swift-water rescue scenarios present a special challenge and danger to rescuers. They are recirculating currents ("drowning machines"), strainers, foot/extremity pins, and dams or hydroelectric intakes.

Recirculating Currents

Recirculating currents result from water flowing over a uniform obstruction such as a large rock or low head dam. The movement of currents can literally create what is known as a "drowning machine" (Figure 12-15).

On first appearance, recirculating currents can look very tame. Anglers, for example, often fish on the downstream portion of a low head dam, casting their lines into the recirculating waters. This is a good place to catch fish because they can often be seen just below the dam. But think about it. If fish, with their natural ability to swim, get stuck in the recirculating currents, imagine what would happen to humans if they got too close to the dam. Once caught in the recirculating currents, people find it very difficult to escape. The resulting rescue can be extremely hazardous, even for specially trained rescuers.

Strainers

When moving water flows through obstructions such as downed trees, grating, or wire mesh, an unequal force is created on the two sides of the so-called **strainers** (Figure 12-16). Currents can literally force a patient up against a strainer, making it difficult to remove him because of the power of the current. In some cases, the current might be flowing into a drainage pipe under the surface, which is in turn covered by a rebar (metal) grate. Victims can get sucked into the grate and then pinned against it.

This, too, can be a hazardous rescue. If you get stuck floating downstream and see the potential of getting pinned against a strainer, attempt to swim over the object. Whatever you do, do not put your feet on the bottom of the river—your feet could get stuck or, even worse, you could get swept off your feet and slammed into the obstruction.

Foot/Extremity Pins

For the sake of safety, keep this point in mind: It is always unsafe to walk in fast-moving water over knee depth because of the danger of entrapping a foot or extremity. When this occurs, the weight and force of the water can knock you below the surface of the water. To remove the foot or extremity, it must be extracted the same way it went in. Water currents often make this extremely difficult. Again, this is a hazardous rescue because of the need to work below the surface in already dangerous water conditions.

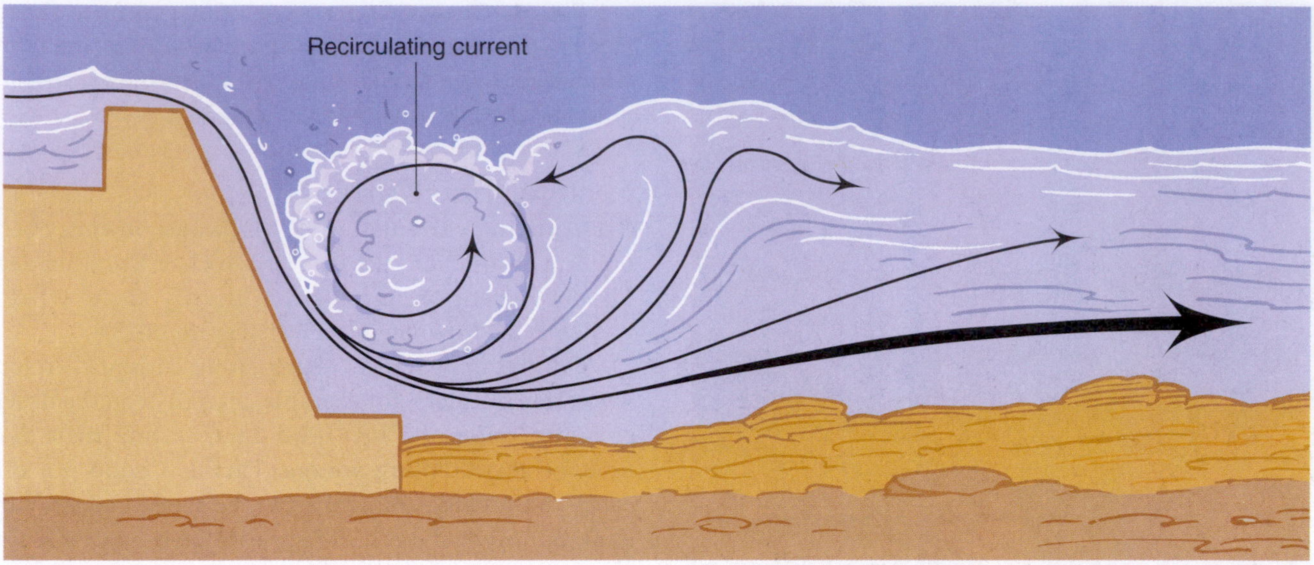

FIGURE 12-15 When water flows over a large uniform object, it can create a hydraulic trap or hole with a recirculating current that moves against the river's flow and can trap people.

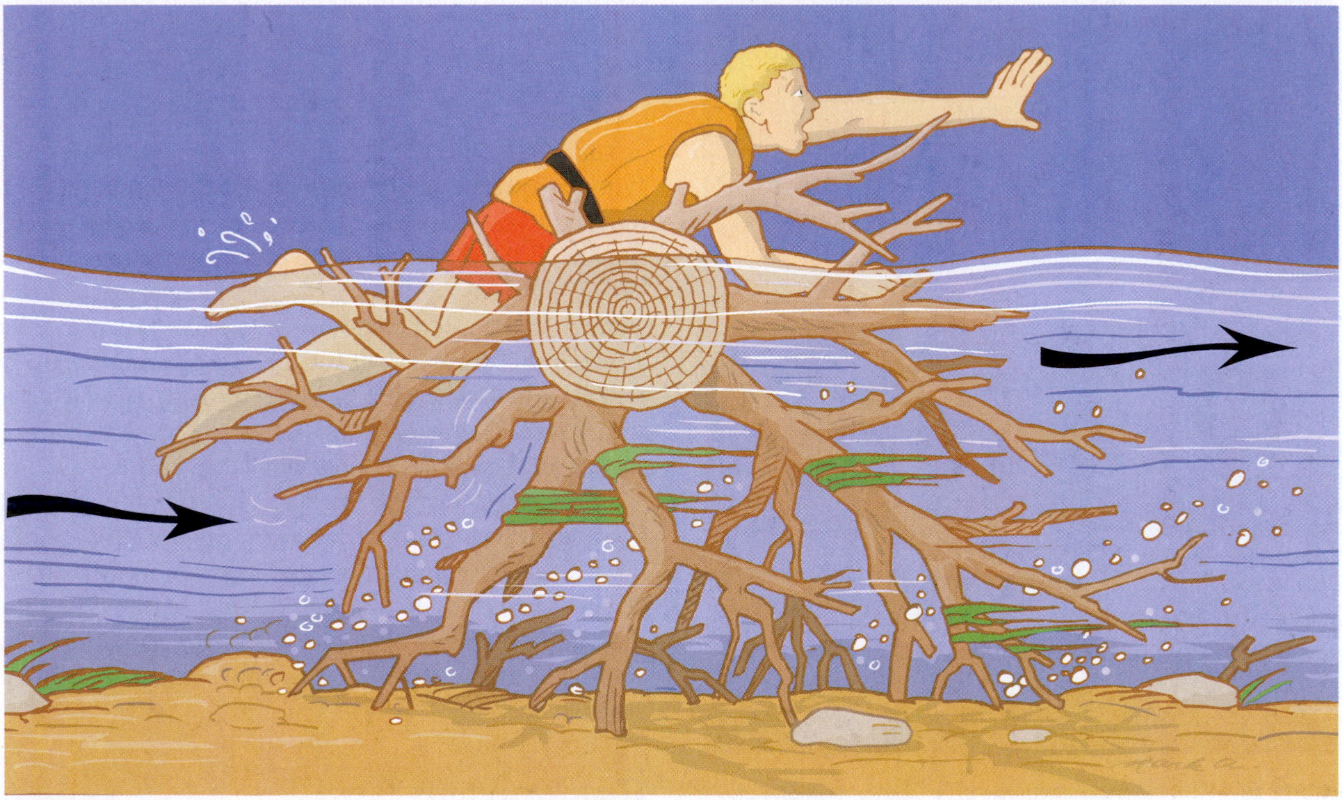

FIGURE 12-16 Strainers are objects that allow water to flow through them but that will trap other objects—and people.

Dams/Hydroelectric Intakes

Yet another dangerous situation involves dams and hydroelectric intakes, such as those often found along rivers. The height of the dam is no indication of the degree of hazard. As already indicated, low head dams can create powerful drowning machines. As a result, assume that all dams have the ability to form recirculating currents. Hydroelectric intakes, however, serve as dangerous strainers with all the accompanying hazards.

Self-Rescue Techniques

Some water survival techniques, such as wearing PFDs and the use of HELP, have already been mentioned.

However, if you suddenly fall in swift-running water (or flat for that matter), keep these suggestions in mind:

- Cover your mouth and nose during entry.
- Protect your head and, if possible, keep your face out of the water.
- Do not attempt to stand up in moving water.
- Float on your back, with your feet pointed downstream.
- Steer with your feet, and point your head toward the nearest shore at a 45-degree angle or continue to float downstream until you come to an area where the water slows enough for you to swim to the edge.
- If the water turns a bend, remember that the outside of the curve moves faster than the inside of the curve.
- Look for large objects, such as rocks, that can block the water and cause recirculating currents or strainers.
- Learn to identify **eddies**—water that flows around especially large objects and, for a time, flows upstream around the downside of the obstruction. These back currents move more slowly and can actually sweep you toward the edge—and safety.
- Above all else, take precautions not to fall into the water in the first place. Remember: Reach–throw–row–go, with "go" being the absolutely last resort.

Flat Water

The greatest problem with flat water is that it looks so calm. However, a large proportion of drowning or near-drowning incidents take place in flat or slow-moving water (Figure 12-17). Some of the factors in these deaths were mentioned earlier. In a significant number of cases, alcohol plays a role in the incident. Nearly 50 percent of boating fatalities, for example, result from alcohol intoxication or impairment. As a result, many states have enacted tough laws to restrict the operation of boats while under the influence of alcohol, which impairs the ability to think, reason, and survive in an alcohol-related water incident.[3]

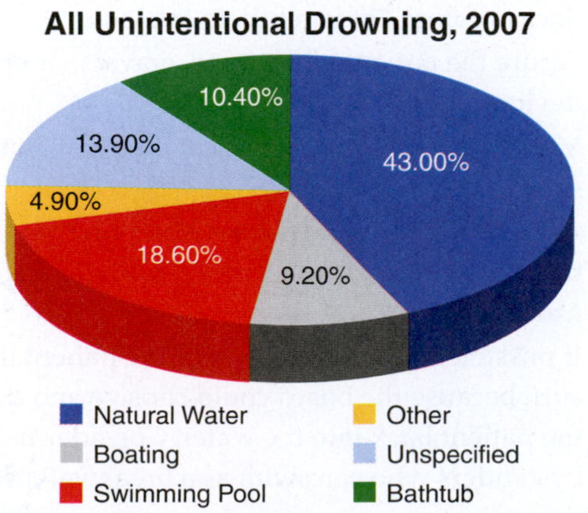

FIGURE 12-17 Unintentional drowning. From "Drowning Risks in Natural Water Settings," Centers for Disease Control and Prevention, http://www.cdc.gov/Features/dsDrowningRisks/.

CONTENT REVIEW

➤ Factors Affecting Survival
- Age
- Posture
- Lung volume
- Water temperature
- Use of PFDs

Factors Affecting Survival

A number of factors help determine the demise or survival of a patient. A person's "survivability profile" is affected by age, posture, lung volume, water temperature, and more. Two especially important factors include the presence of PFDs and what is known as the "cold-protective response."

Personal Flotation Devices

Many recreational water users associate "life preservers" with rough water or people who cannot swim. However, PFDs should be essential items for all water-related activities. One study, for example, linked nearly 89 percent of all boating fatalities to the lack of a PFD. This fact is a reminder of why you should don a PFD whenever you approach water.

Every system should have a strict SOP mandating the use of PFDs for all EMS personnel. Even services in arid regions can be involved in water rescues. They can be called to swimming pool incidents or river-rafting accidents. In some places, especially in the Southwest, they can respond to flash flooding in canyons that can trap or kill hikers or "canyoneers." The same flash flooding can overload drainage systems, creating hazardous conditions for the public and rescuers alike.

Cold-Protective Response

Brain cells deprived of oxygen will normally begin to die in as little as 4 to 8 minutes. Keeping the head above water, as in the HELP and self-rescue techniques discussed earlier, ensures that the person can breathe and keep the brain supplied with oxygen. Additionally, although cold water can cause death from hypothermia, cold water can also trigger a protective response known as the "mammalian diving reflex." This is how it works: When the face of a human, or any mammal, is plunged into cold water less than 68°F (20°C), the parasympathetic nervous system is stimulated. The heart rate rapidly decreases to a bradycardic rhythm. Meanwhile, blood pressure drops and vasoconstriction occurs throughout the body. Blood is shunted from less vital organs to the heart and brain, temporarily delivering life-sustaining oxygen. As a general rule, the colder the water, the more oxygen is diverted.

Two factors, then, can significantly delay death when a person is in cold water: the length of time the person is able to keep his head above water and the mammalian diving reflex once the person's face becomes submerged. Some patients have been resuscitated after 45 minutes underwater. (The record is 66 minutes for a patient rescued in Salt Lake, Utah, on June 10, 1989.) As a rule, the reflex is more pronounced in children than in adults.

Location of Submerged Victims

Because of protective physiologic responses, rescuers must make every effort to locate submerged victims. Interview witnesses to establish a relative location. Ask each witness, for example, to locate an object across the water to form a line. Repeat this process with each witness. Use the point of convergence among lines to target the most accurate "last seen" location. Start searching from this point and fan out in larger and larger circles, forming a radius equal to the depth of the water.

Rescue versus Body Recovery

A number of conditions determine when a rescue turns into a body recovery. Some factors are length of time submerged, any known or suspected trauma, age and physical condition of the victim, water temperature and environmental conditions, and estimated time for rescue or removal.

Once a patient is recovered, you should attempt resuscitation on any hypothermic and/or pulseless, non-breathing patient who has been submerged in cold water. (Some experts advise providing resuscitation to every drowning patient, regardless of water temperature, even those who have been in the water for some time.) A patient must be rewarmed before an accurate assessment can be made. Remember: Water-rescue patients are "never dead until they are warm and dead." (For more on drowning and near-drowning, see the chapter "Environmental Trauma.")

In-Water Patient Stabilization

In flat water where you are able to safely stand, it is important that you know how to perform in-water stabilization (Figure 12-18). Cervical spine injuries are associated with trauma (e.g., diving) rather than simple submersion.[4] In general, the procedure mirrors the application of a long board, with the following modifications:

- ***Phase One: In-Water Spinal Stabilization***
  1. Apply the head-splint technique. (There are other techniques, but they do not work as well because of the use of PFDs by the rescuers.)
  2. Approach the patient from the side.
  3. Move the patient's arms over the head.
  4. Hold the patient's head in place by using the patient's arms as a "splint."
  5. If the patient was found in a face-down position, perform steps 1 through 4, then rotate the patient toward the rescuer in a face-up position.
  6. Ensure an open airway.
  7. Maintain this position until a cervical collar is applied.
- ***Phase Two: Cervical Collar Application (If Indicated)***
  1. A second rescuer determines proper collar size.
  2. This second rescuer then holds the open collar under the victim's neck.
  3. The primary rescuer maintains stabilization and a patent airway.
  4. The second rescuer brings the collar up to the back of the patient's neck and the primary rescuer allows the second rescuer to bring the collar around the patient's neck while the primary rescuer maintains the airway.
  5. The second rescuer secures the fastener on the collar while the primary rescuer maintains the airway.
  6. The second rescuer secures the patient's hands at the waist of the patient.
- ***Phase Three: Backboarding and Extrication from the Water***
  1. Secure the necessary personnel—two rescuers in the water and additional rescuers at the water's edge—and the correct equipment. Rescuers are strongly urged to use a floating backboard for water rescue.
  2. Submerge the board under the patient's waist.
  3. Never lift the patient to the board. Instead, allow the board to float up to the victim. (If the board does not float, lift it gently to the victim.)
  4. Secure the patient with straps, cravats, or other devices.
  5. Move the patient to an extrication point along the shore or boat.
  6. Always extricate the patient head first, so the body weight does not compress possible spinal trauma.
  7. If possible, avoid extrication of the patient through surf, because the board could capsize and dump the patient back into the water. Consider using bystanders who can swim as a breakwall behind the patient.
  8. Maintain airway management during extrication.

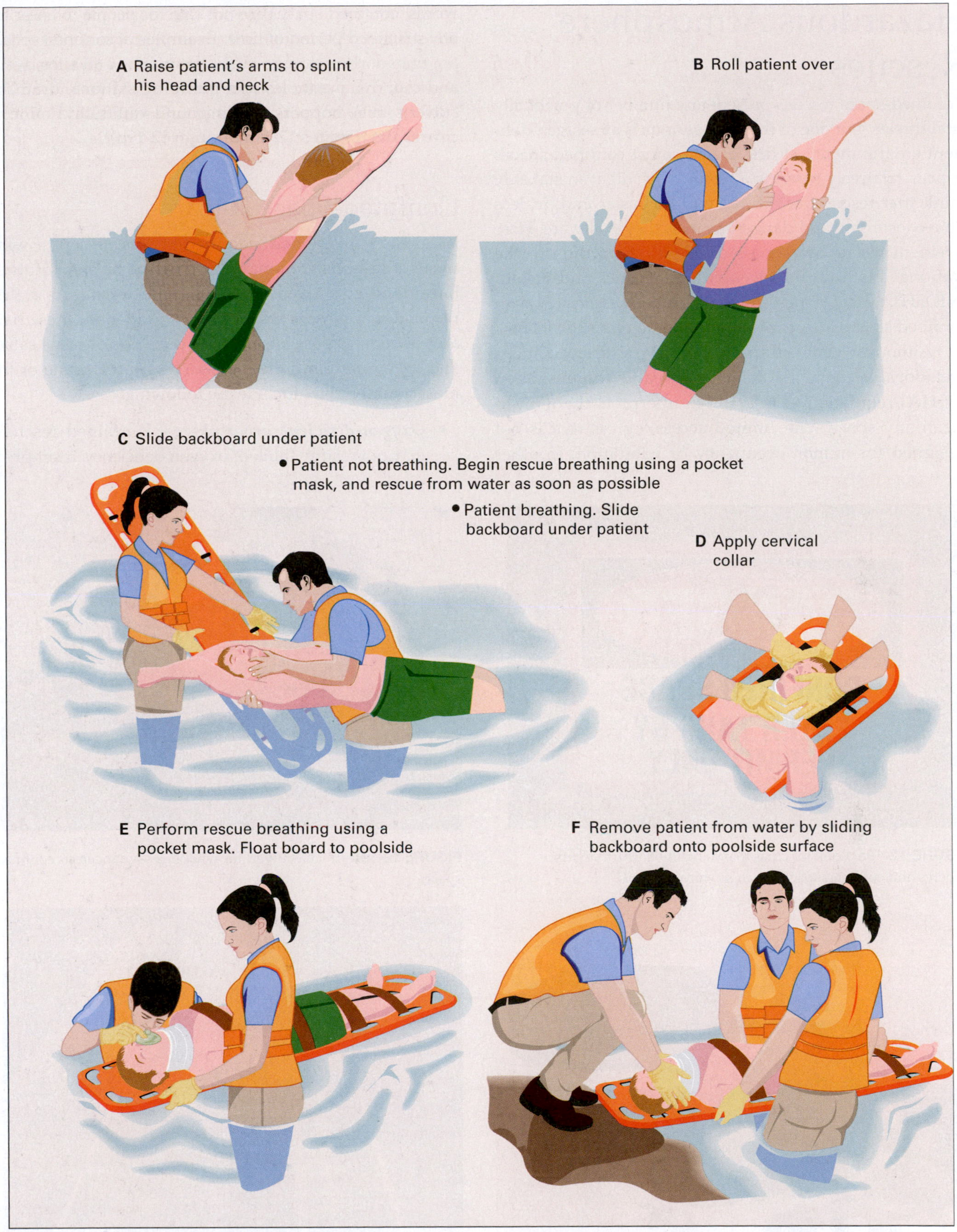

FIGURE 12-18 Water rescue, possible spinal injury.

Hazardous Atmosphere Rescues

Confined-space rescues present any number of potentially fatal threats, but one of the most serious is an oxygen-deficient environment. At first glance, most confined spaces appear relatively safe. As a result, you might mistakenly think that rescue procedures will be easier and/or less time-consuming and dangerous than they really are. Here is where rescue awareness comes in. According to the National Institute for Occupational Safety and Health (NIOSH), nearly 60 percent of all fatalities associated with confined spaces are people attempting to rescue a victim.

Although "confined space" can have a variety of interpretations, Occupational Safety and Health Administration (OSHA) regulation CFR 1910.146 interprets the term to mean any space with limited access/egress that is not designed for human occupancy or habitation. In other words, confined spaces are not safe for people to enter for any sustained period of time. Examples of confined spaces are transport or storage tanks, grain bins and silos, wells and cisterns, manholes and pumping stations, drainage culverts, pits, hoppers, underground vaults, and mine or cave shafts (Figures 12-19a through 12-19d).

Confined-Space Hazards

As already mentioned, confined spaces present a wide range of hazards. You may confront one or more of these hazards in any given confined-space rescue. As a first responder, it is your responsibility to identify these hazards as soon as possible, both for purposes of scene safety and for summoning the necessary support. Some of the most common risks include the following:

- ***Oxygen-deficient atmospheres.*** Untrained rescuers may not readily think of oxygen deficiency. It simply is

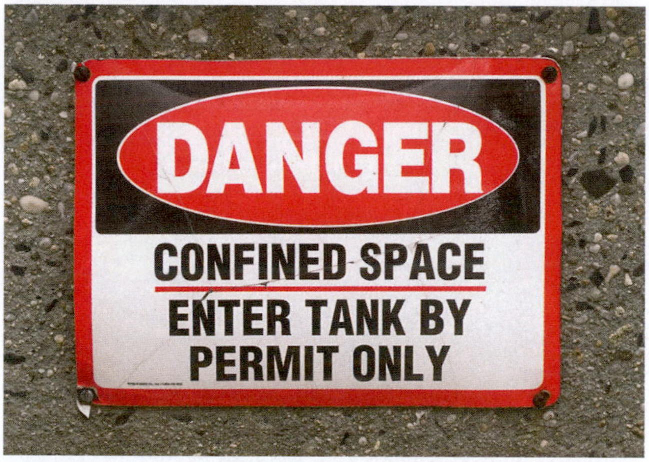

FIGURE 12-19a Look for clues to potentially hazardous atmospheres and confined spaces, such as warning signs.

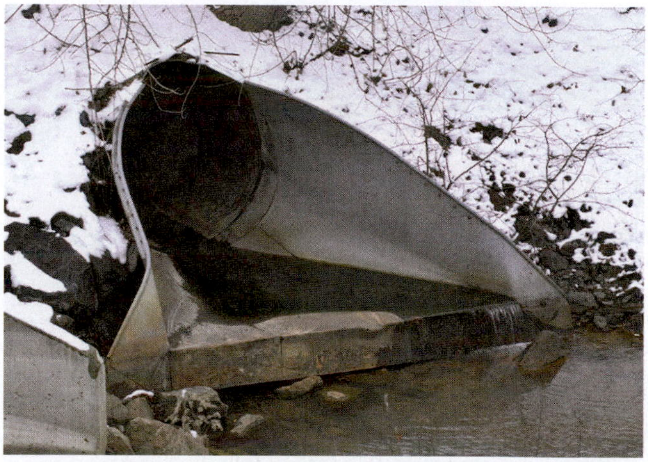

FIGURE 12-19b Treat a culvert for what it is—a dangerous confined space.

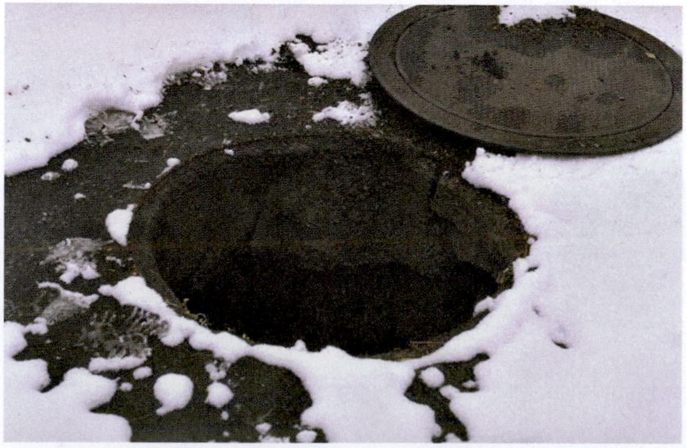

FIGURE 12-19c Manholes provide access to underground utility vaults. The vault may have a limited or hazardous atmosphere and may offer the potential for entrapment.

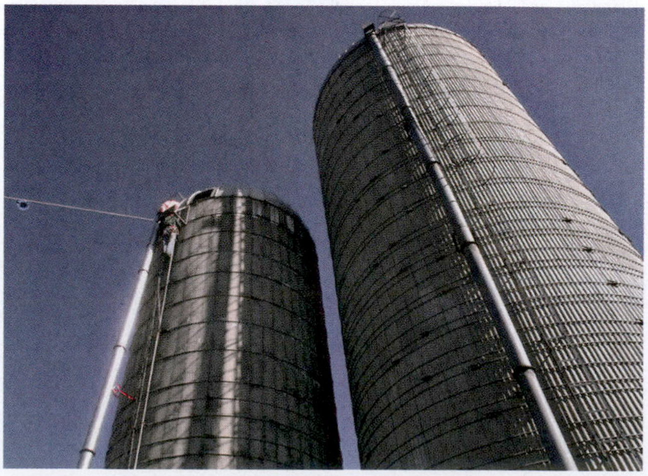

FIGURE 12-19d Rescuers should never be permitted to enter confined spaces, such as silos, unless they have training, equipment, and experience in this environment.

(© Michal Heron)

not a "visible" threat. Special entry teams know otherwise. Before going into a confined space, they monitor the atmosphere to determine oxygen concentration, levels of hydrogen sulfide, explosive limits, flammable atmosphere, or toxic contaminants. They are also aware that increases in oxygen content for any reasons—such as a gust of wind—can give atmospheric monitoring meters a false reading. The bottom line is this: Confined spaces often mean hazardous atmospheres.

- ***Toxic or explosive chemicals.*** Many chemicals found in confined spaces can be toxic, especially if inhaled (Figure 12-20). Some of the poisonous fumes contain gases that displace oxygen in the red blood cells. Other chemicals are highly explosive. Dangerous chemical gases commonly found in confined spaces include hydrogen sulfide (H_2S), carbon dioxide (CO_2), carbon monoxide (CO), exceptionally low or high oxygen concentrations, chlorine (Cl_2), ammonia (NH_3), and nitrogen dioxide (NO_2).
- ***Engulfment.*** Some confined spaces contain physical substances—grain, coal, sand, and so on—that can literally bury a patient or a rescuer who falls into the space. Dust from these materials can also create a highly explosive atmosphere.

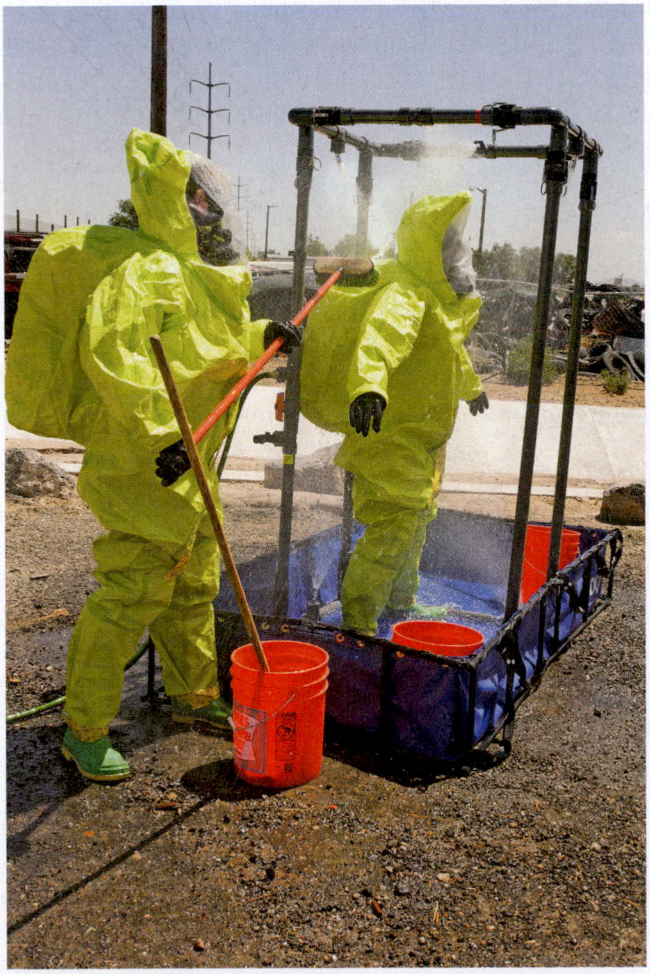

FIGURE 12-20 Rescuers exposed to toxic or hazardous materials will need to go through decontamination.

- ***Machinery entrapment.*** Confined spaces come with all sorts of machinery or equipment that can entrap a person. Augers or screws can also entrap a victim.
- ***Electricity.*** Confined spaces often contain motors or materials management equipment powered by electricity. In addition to the risk of shock or electrocution, these machines may contain stored energy. To ensure safe entry, rescue crews will have to take a number of steps. First, it may be necessary to blank out the flow of all power into the site. Second, stored energy should be dissipated, and all machinery should be shut down following lock-out/tag-out procedures. (After you shut off the equipment, lock off the switch and place a tag on the switch stating why it is shut off to prevent inadvertently tripping the switch.) Third, the space may need to be ventilated to ensure against oxygen deficiency or explosive dust particles. Remember: It takes only one spark to trigger an explosion.
- ***Structural concerns.*** Structure supports and shapes further complicate confined-space rescues. Some confined spaces have I-beams that can cause injury due to limited light and height. Other confined spaces have noncylindrical shapes that present difficult extrication problems. Confined spaces can be shaped in the form of Ls, Ts, Xs, and any combination thereof. Because of limited access, rescuers may find it difficult or even impossible to use standard self-contained breathing apparatus. They may have to resort to supplied air breathing apparatus (i.e., oxygen lines). They may also need to be lowered into the space with a full-body harness or other system to make retrieval easier in case something goes wrong.

Confined-Space Protections in the Workplace

Fortunately, state and federal laws require most industries to develop a confined-space rescue program. This means that employers must provide a training program for all employees who work in or around confined spaces. These employees may be called on to perform on-site rescues and may indeed be an important part of the emergency response.

OSHA also requires a permit process before workers may enter a confined space such as a trench. In addition, most industries must fulfill strict requirements such as ongoing atmospheric monitoring, posted warnings, and work-site permits with detailed data on hazard management. The area must be made safe and workers must don PPE. Retrieval devices must also be in place whenever workers enter the spaces. Nonpermitted sites are the most likely locations for emergencies because of the oxygen deficiencies that result from inadequate atmospheric monitoring.

The types of confined-space emergencies most commonly encountered in the workplace include falls, medical emergencies (often hazmat related), oxygen deficiencies or asphyxia, explosions, and entrapment. You should never allow rescuers into a confined space unless they have the training, equipment, and experience specific to the particular environment involved. You will almost always summon outside specialized agencies for support.

Cave-Ins and Structural Collapses

As earthquakes in California have proven, it can be very dramatic to watch rescues from cave-ins or structural collapses. It does not take an earthquake to produce this type of confined-space emergency, however. Collapsed trenches or cave-ins can occur in almost any community. In fact, most trench collapses occur in trenches less than 12 feet deep and 6 feet wide, particularly in trenches that do not comply with OSHA regulations (Figure 12-21).

To understand the medical magnitude of a collapsed trench, consider these facts. A typical cubic foot of soil weighs 100 pounds. As a result, just 2 feet of soil on top of a worker's chest or back, which could have a surface area of 4 to 5 square feet, would weigh between 800 and 1,000 pounds. People are literally buried alive. Unless uncovered quickly, they suffer death by asphyxiation.

Reasons for Collapses/Cave-Ins

Trenches collapse or cave-in for a number of reasons. The most common reasons include:

- Contractors disregard safety regulations, either out of negligence or out of efforts to save money. (Federal law requires either shoring or a trench box for excavations deeper than 5 feet. Anything less is an invitation to trouble.)
- The lip of one or both sides of the trench caves in.
- The wall shears away or falls in entirely.
- The "spoil pile," or dirt removed from the hole, is placed too close to the edge of the trench.
- Water seepage, ground vibrations, intersecting trenches, or previously disturbed soil weaken the structural integrity.

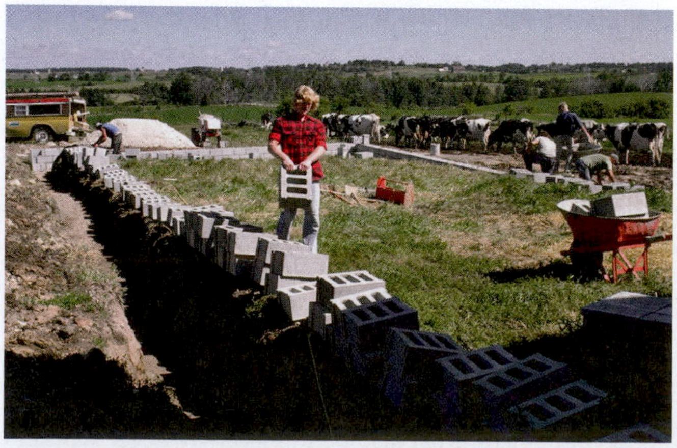

FIGURE 12-21 If trenches do not comply with OSHA regulations, the possibility of collapse is increased.

(© Michal Heron)

Rescue from Trenches/Cave-Ins

If a collapse has caused burial, a secondary collapse is likely. Therefore, your initial actions should be geared toward safety. Secure the scene, establish command, secure a perimeter, and immediately summon a team specializing in trench rescue. While waiting for the team to arrive, do not allow entry in the area surrounding the trench or cave-in. Safe access can take place only when proper shoring is in place.

Highway Operations and Vehicle Rescues

As you already know, the most common rescue situations encountered by EMS personnel involve motor vehicle collisions. These incidents generally go through the phases covered at the start of this chapter. However, certain modifications must be made to meet the special hazards associated with traffic control and the extrication of patients from wrecked vehicles.

Hazards in Highway Operations

To prepare for highway rescues, you must size up the scene, identify all hazards, and ensure scene safety—that is, control any potentially dangerous situations. In the case of highway operations, this means reducing traffic-related hazards and identifying hazards related to the vehicle crash itself.

Traffic Hazards

Traffic flow is the largest single hazard associated with EMS highway operations. You may have to respond to incidents on roads with limited access and to incidents on highways with unlimited access. In either situation, you will need to work closely with police to avoid unnecessary congestion, as well as other injuries. Remember that traffic backups impede the flow both to and from the scene.

An even bigger personal danger results from the risk of vehicles hitting EMS apparatus or personnel. Studies have shown that drivers who are tired, drunk, or drugged actually drive right into the emergency lights. Spectators can worsen the situation by getting out of their cars to watch or even "help."

At this point in your career, you probably already know some of the things you can do to reduce traffic hazards. Here are a few tried and tested techniques:

- ***Staging.*** Staging is always critical at any multiple-casualty incident, but it takes on added importance on limited-access roads or highways. Always consider staging emergency vehicles away from the scene, then have command bring the vehicles in whenever there is an appropriate place and/or assignment for the crews. The staging area should be within a minute or two of the scene, ideally in a large parking lot or less congested area. Some situations simply cannot accommodate the entire response at once.
- ***Positioning of apparatus.*** When apparatus does arrive, ensure that it causes the minimum reduction of traffic flow. As much as possible, apparatus should be positioned to protect the scene. The ambulance loading area should *not* be directly exposed to traffic. Also, *do not* rely solely on ambulance lights to warn traffic away. These lights are often obstructed when medics open the doors for loading.
- ***Emergency lighting.*** Use only a minimum of warning lights to alert traffic of a hazard and to define the actual size of your vehicle. Too many lights can confuse or blind drivers, causing additional collisions. Experts strongly advise that you turn off all headlights when parked at the scene and rely instead on amber scene lighting.
- ***Redirection of traffic.*** Be sure that traffic cones and flares are placed early in the incident. If the police are not already on scene, this is your responsibility. As a first responder, you must redirect traffic away from the collision and away from all emergency workers. In other words, you need to create a safety zone. Make sure that you do not place lighted flares too near any sources of fuel or brush; otherwise, you risk an explosion or fire. Once you light the flares, allow them to burn out. *Do not* try to extinguish them. Attempting to pick up a flare can cause a very severe thermal burn.
- ***High visibility.*** As already mentioned, all rescuers should be dressed in highly visible clothing. Because many EMS, police, and fire agencies wear dark-colored uniforms, you should don a brightly colored turnout coat or vest with reflective tape. You can apply the tape at the scene.

Other Hazards

Other hazards besides traffic control exist at highway operations. In some communities, paramedics receive training to manage these hazards. In other communities, they receive "awareness training" and learn to summon specialized rescue personnel. Regardless of the procedure in your service area, you must be able to recognize all nontraffic hazards (Figure 12-22). Otherwise, you risk injuring yourself, your crew, the patient, or even passing motorists. Some of these nontraffic hazards include:

- ***Fire and fuel.*** Fuel spilled at the scene increases the chances of fire. Be very careful whenever you smell or see pools of liquid at a collision. Keep in mind that bystanders who are smoking can cause a bigger problem than the original crash if they flick lighted ashes into a fuel leak. *Do not* drive your emergency vehicle over a fuel spill or—worse yet—park on one. Remember that all automobiles manufactured since the 1970s have catalytic converters. They run at a temperature of around 1,200°F—hot enough to heat fuel to the point of ignition. Be especially careful when a vehicle has gone off the road into dry grass or brush. The debris can be just as dangerous as spilled fuel, especially when brought into contact with a blazing hot catalytic converter.
- ***Alternative fuel systems.*** Be equally cautious of vehicles powered by alternative fuel systems. High-pressure tanks, especially if filled with natural gas, are extremely volatile. Even vehicles powered by electricity can be dangerous. The storage cells possess the energy to spark, flash, and more.
- ***Hybrid and electric vehicles.*** Hybrid and electric vehicles pose a particular danger for rescuers. These vehicles have high-voltage systems that can be a risk for rescuers unfamiliar with the vehicles.
- ***Sharp objects.*** Automobile collisions mean lots of sharp objects, including glass, metal, plastic, and fiberglass. Be sure to wear appropriate protective gear, such as heavy leather gloves and eyewear.
- ***Electric power.*** Contact with downed power lines or underground electrical feeds can be lethal. If a vehicle

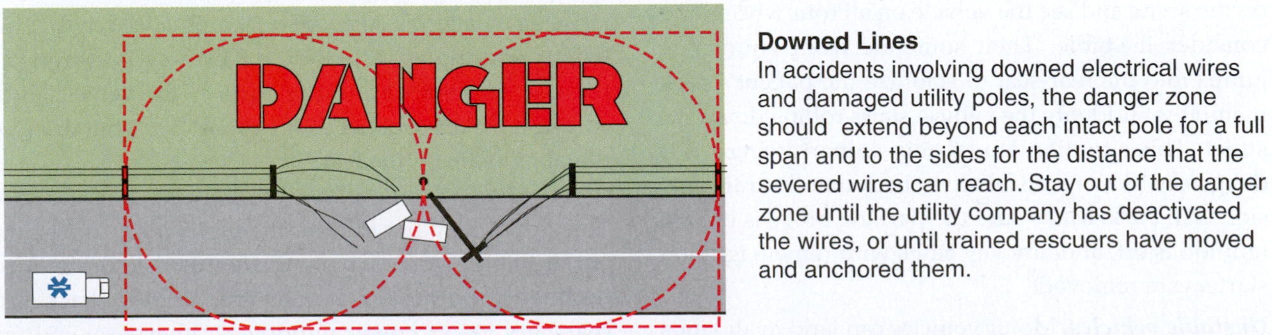

FIGURE 12-22 Establish a danger zone in motor vehicle collisions involving electrical hazards.

is in contact with electrical lines, consider it to be "charged" and call the power company immediately. In most newer communities, electrical lines run underground. However, a vehicle can still run into a transformer or an electrical feed box. As a result, make sure you look under the car and all around it during your scene size-up. *Do not* touch a vehicle until you have ruled out all electrical hazards.

- ***Energy-absorbing bumpers.*** The bumpers on many vehicles come with pistons and are designed to withstand a slow-speed collision. The intent is to limit front- or rear-end damage. Sometimes, however, these bumpers become "loaded" in the crushed position and do not immediately bounce back out. When exposed to fire or even just tapped by rescue workers, the pistons can suddenly unload their stored energy. Some bumpers have been thrown a hundred feet from the vehicle when they unload. As a result, you must examine bumpers for loading. If you discover a loaded bumper, stay away from it unless you are specially trained to deal with this hazard.
- ***Supplemental restraint systems (SRSs)/air bags.*** Air bags also have the potential to release stored energy. If they have not deployed during the collision, they may do so during the middle of an extrication. As a result, these devices must be deactivated prior to disentanglement. Auto manufacturers can provide information about power removal or power dissipation for their particular brand of SRS. Also, keep in mind that many new model vehicles come equipped with side impact bags.
- ***Hazardous cargoes.*** An incredible amount of hazardous material travels across the highways of North America. You will learn much more about the role of EMS in highway crashes involving hazmat in the "Hazardous Materials" chapter. For your personal safety, suspect hazmat at any scene involving commercial vehicles.
- ***Rolling vehicles.*** As you already know, you must size up the position of a vehicle whenever you arrive at the scene of a collision. Do not overlook the subtle situations that can occur at any collision. You might arrive on the scene and see the vehicle on all four wheels and consider it stable. Then someone from your crew jumps into the rear seat to stabilize the patient's neck manually. Suddenly the vehicle starts rolling down the street. This situation is not only embarrassing—it is dangerous! As a result, always check that the transmission is in park. Make sure the parking brake is on, the ignition is off, and any key rings with remote ignition starters are removed.
- ***Unstable vehicles.*** Motor vehicles can land in all kinds of unstable positions. They can roll onto a side or the roof. They can stop on an incline or unstable terrain. They can be suspended over a cliff or river. They can come to rest on a patch of ice or an on-site spill or leak. In such situations, you need to request the necessary stabilization crews or equipment. You should also know how to apply proper techniques for temporary stabilization, using ropes, chocks, or a come-along. Under no circumstances should you allow rescuers to access the patient until the vehicle is stabilized.

Auto Anatomy

Motor vehicle collisions present EMS personnel with the most common access and/or extrication problems. As a result, you must know some basic information about automobile construction or "anatomy." Obviously, vehicles can differ greatly, both in terms of manufacture and design. However, most recent automobiles have certain features in common that can guide you in simple access situations.

Basic Construction

Vehicles can have either a unibody or a frame construction. Most automobiles today have a unibody design, whereas older vehicles and lightweight trucks have a frame construction. For unibody vehicles to maintain their integrity, the roof posts, floor, firewall, truck support, and windshield must all remain intact.

Both types of construction have roofs and roof supports. The support posts are lettered from front to back. The first post, which supports the roof at the windshield, is called the "A" post. The next post is the "B" post. The third post, found in sedans or station wagons, is the "C" post. Station wagons have an additional rear post, known as the "D" post.

If you remove the plastic molding on the posts, the remaining steel can be easily cut with a hacksaw. Application of power steering fluid helps reduce the heat produced by cutting. In the case of a unibody design, remember that cutting a post will interrupt the vehicle's construction.

Firewall and Engine Compartment

The firewall separates the engine compartment from the occupant compartment. Frequently, the firewall can collapse on a patient's legs during a high-speed, head-on collision. Sometimes, a patient's feet may go through the firewall. Movement at other parts of the vehicle, such as cutting a rocker panel or roof support post, can place additional pressure on the feet.

The engine compartment usually contains the battery. This can cause a fire hazard; therefore, many rescue teams cut the battery cables to eliminate this risk. Before disconnecting the power, it is a good idea to move back electric seats and lower power windows. Otherwise, you might needlessly complicate the extrication.

Glass

Vehicles have two types of glass: safety glass and tempered glass. Safety glass is made from three layers of fused materials: glass–plastic laminate–glass. It is found in windshields and designed to stay intact when shattered or broken. However, safety glass can still produce glass dust or fracture into long shards. These materials can easily get into a patient's eyes, nose, or mouth and/or create cuts. As a result, be sure to cover a patient whenever you remove this type of glass.

Tempered glass has a high tensile strength. However, it does not stay intact when shattered or broken. It fractures into many small beads of glass, all of which can cause injuries and cuts.

Doors

The doors of most newer vehicles contain a reinforcing bar to protect the occupant in side-impact collisions. They also have a case-hardened steel "Nader" pin. Named for consumer advocate Ralph Nader, these pins help keep the doors from blowing open and ejecting the occupants. If the Nader pin has been engaged, it will be difficult to pry open the door. You must first disengage the latch or use hydraulic jaws.

Before attempting to assist a patient through a door, you should be trained in proper extrication techniques. In general, you should follow these steps:

- Try all four doors first—a door is usually the easiest means of access.
- Otherwise, gain access through the window farthest away from the patient(s).
- Alternatively, use simple hand tools to peel back the outer sheet of metal on the door, exposing the lock mechanism. Unlock the lock and pry the cams from around the Nader pin. Then pry out the door.

These steps can be highly useful in situations in which the patient must be promptly removed from the vehicle or the vehicle rescue team is delayed for some reason. Before removing a patient, keep in mind the earlier points about deactivating or dissipating front and/or side air bags.

Hybrid Vehicles

Hybrid automobiles, also called hybrid electric vehicles (HEVs), are becoming increasingly popular. HEVs contain both an electric motor and an internal combustion motor (Figure 12-23). A large array of batteries powers the electric motor, whereas the internal combustion motor is powered by gasoline or diesel fuel. This combination allows significantly increased fuel efficiency and decreases the release of pollutants.

The electrical system of HEVs contains a high-voltage and a 12-volt battery. The high-voltage component poses a particular risk for rescue personnel. The easiest way to inactivate the high-voltage component is to simply turn off the vehicle and remove the key from the ignition. This prevents electric current from flowing into the cables from the motor or high-voltage battery, and turns off power to the air bags and the seat belt pretensioners. To ensure rescuer safety, it is recommended that the 12-volt battery also be disconnected to further isolate the electrical system.

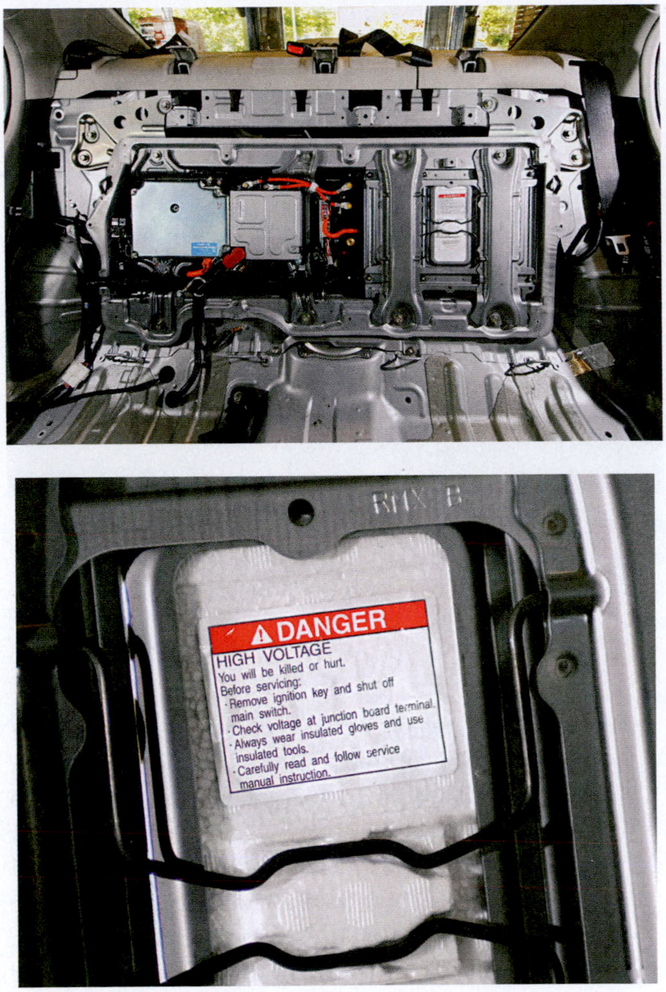

FIGURE 12-23 Modern hybrid electrical vehicle (HEV). These vehicles have a high-voltage electrical system that poses a particular hazard to rescuers.

Because battery locations vary by vehicle type, rescuers should be familiar with the popular HEV types on the market.

Rescue Strategies

In managing highway operations or vehicle rescues, you should use the following general strategies:

- ***Initial scene size-up.*** Establish command, call for appropriate backup, then locate and triage the patients. Triage may be delayed until hazards are controlled.
- ***Control hazards.*** This topic has already been covered. But always remember this point: Traffic can be your worst enemy at a collision.

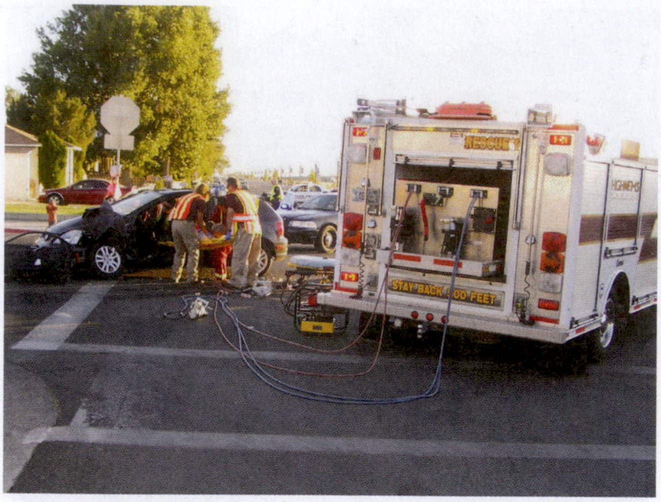

FIGURE 12-24 Modern extrication equipment is essential for a fast, efficient rescue. Paramedic skill in using these devices will depend on local protocols and the location of extrication units.

(© Pat Songer)

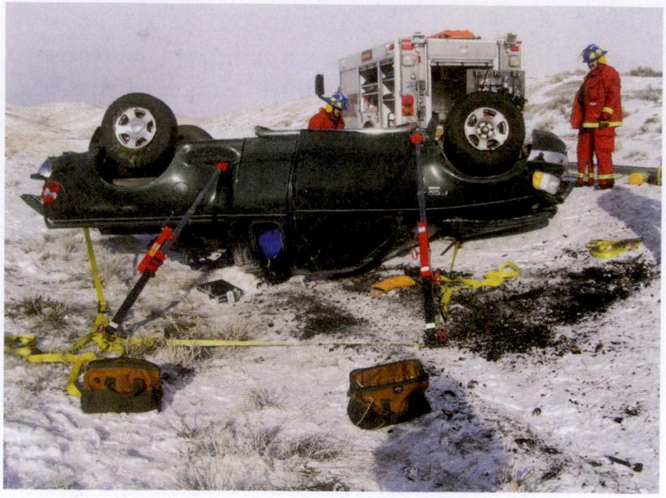

FIGURE 12-25 Vehicle stabilization equipment must be used to protect rescuers during extrication operations.

(© Pat Songer)

- ***Assess the degree of entrapment and fastest means of extrication.*** Try all doors. If they cannot be opened, decide whether it is advisable and/or necessary to break glass. Although you may not have the training or responsibility to use extrication equipment, you should observe its use so you know what technical skills are available should you need them (Figure 12-24). Be aware of the considerations and techniques for door removal, roof removal, dashboard or firewall rollup, and construction of a new door.
- ***Establish circles of operation.*** Set up two circles of operation early in the incident. The inner circle is the area where the actual rescue takes place. Limit the number of workers in this area to team members operating rescue tools and/or charged with actual patient care. If two different units must work in the inner circle (e.g., a fire department extrication crew and an EMS crew), you will need to maintain a good working balance between the crews to avoid "over-rescuing." The outer circle is where staging takes place. Hold all additional equipment and personnel in this area until they are assigned a duty.
- ***Treatment, packaging, removal.*** As a rule, the role of EMS personnel in vehicle stabilization and removal is that of patient care provider. Once specialized rescue personnel assure you that the vehicle is stable and the scene is safe to enter, you may approach the patient, initiate assessment, and administer emergency care. Patient care always precedes removal from the vehicle unless delay would endanger the life of the patient, EMS personnel, or other rescuers. Again, work with rescuers in any way possible to minimize risk, both to the patient and to on-scene personnel. You should be well practiced in the application of long spine boards for rapid removal of the patient through the doors or vertical extrication through removed roofs.

Rescue Skills Practice

Depending on local protocols, you should practice or observe the use of the rescue skills and equipment needed for initial vehicle stabilization (Figure 12-25). Some of the common tools used for vehicle stabilization can be found in Table 12-1.

You should also make a point of practicing and/or observing the various disentanglement or extrication skills commonly used with vehicle rescues, many of which have already been mentioned. Know how to gain access using hand tools through nondeformed doors, deformed doors, safety and tempered glass, trunks, and floors. Become familiar with the use of heavy hydraulic equipment employed by special rescue teams in your area and take part in practice scenarios to build agency cooperation. Again, preplan and prepare so that you are ready when this all-too-common type of rescue occurs.

Hazardous Terrain Rescues

In recent years, outdoor activities—mountain climbing, rock climbing, ice climbing, mountain biking, cross-country skiing, snowboarding, and hiking—have drawn more and more people into rugged areas. Inevitably, accidents happen, and they happen in places that can be difficult to reach. You do not have to live in the wilderness to take part in a hazardous terrain rescue. For example, a mountain biker can get injured along the trails that run along many power lines or a rock climber can get injured on an

Table 12-1 Vehicle Stabilization Equipment

Type	Description and Use
Air bag	Synthetic bag, available in various shapes and sizes, that, when inflated, has great lifting capability
Come-along	Ratcheting cable device used to pull in a straight direction
Cribbing	4-X 4-inch or 2-X 4-inch blocks of hardwood cut to approximately 18-inch-long sections
Hydraulic cutter	Hydraulic power tool used to cut metal
Hydraulic ram	Hydraulic power tool used to push or pull in a straight direction
Hydraulic spreader	Hydraulic power tool used to open, spread, or separate items such as vehicle doors
Jack	Manual device used much as a ram would be used
Step chock	Set of several 2-X 6-inch blocks of hardwood cut to varying lengths and secured together to form "steps"
Wedge	4-X 4-inch piece of cribbing tapered to an edge on one end
Winch	Powered cable reel, usually electrically or hydraulically driven and mounted to a truck, which is used for pulling

CONTENT REVIEW

➤ Types of Hazardous Terrain
- Steep slope or "low-angle" terrain
- Vertical or "high-angle" terrain
- Flat terrain with obstructions

outcropping in a relatively populated area. Some climbers even scale the sides of buildings!

As a paramedic, you must know how to take part in rugged terrain rescues. At a minimum, you should know how to perform litter evacuations without causing additional injury to patients. Even more important, you should develop a "rescue awareness" so that you know when to call specialized teams and how to work with those teams once they arrive on scene.

Types of Hazardous Terrain

In general, there are three types of hazardous terrain: steep slope or "low-angle" terrain, vertical or "high-angle" terrain, and flat terrain with obstructions. Low-angle terrains typically can be accessed by walking or **scrambling**—climbing over boulders or rocks using both hands and feet. Footing can be difficult, and it may be hazardous to carry a litter, even with multiple people. As a result, low-angle teams use ropes to counteract gravity and/or may set a rope to act as a hand line. Any error can result in a fall or tumble. Depending on the presence of boulders, brush, downed trees, and so on, injuries can be quite serious.

High-angle terrain usually involves a cliff, gorge, side of a building, or terrain so steep that hands must be used when scaling it. Crews depend on rope and/or aerial apparatus for access and litter movement. Errors are likely to cause serious, life-threatening injuries. In many cases, falls can be fatal.

Flat terrain with obstructions includes trails, paths, or creek beds. Obstructions can take many forms such as downed trees, rocks, slippery leaves or pine needles, and **scree**—the loose pebbles or rock debris that can form on the slopes or bases of mountains.

Although this is the least hazardous type of rugged terrain, it is still possible to slip while carrying a patient, causing injury.

Patient Access in Hazardous Terrain

Unless you have been trained in high-angle or low-angle rescue, patient access and removal should be left to specialized teams. Even if you have the skills to perform the rescue, you will, in all likelihood, need additional resources to provide the necessary balance of technical and medical support for the patient.

High-Angle Rescues

High-angle, or vertical, rescuers must constantly contend with the effects of gravity. Any organization that could be assigned a vertical technical rescue must have extensive initial training, additional advanced training, frequently supervised practice sessions, and top-of-the-line equipment (Figure 12-26a). Each member of a high-angle team must have complete competency in knot tying, use of ladders and/or ropes to ascend and descend a steep face, ability to rig a hauling system, and the skills for packaging a patient for evacuation by litter and rope. Some of the specialized terms that you will hear high-angle rescuers use include:

- *Aid*—using means other than hands, feet, and body to get up a vertical face, such as in "aided ascent"
- *Anchor*—technique for securing rescuers to a vertical face; an anchor may be rope or a combination of rope and other special hardware or "gear"
- *Belay*—procedure for safeguarding a climber's progress by controlling a rope attached to an anchor (The

person controlling the rope is sometimes also called the belay.)

- *Rappel*—to descend by sliding down a fixed double rope, using the correct anchor, harness, and gear

Low-Angle Rescues

Many EMS systems have trained their paramedics in the skills of low-angle rescue or "off-the-road" rescue. Like high-angle rescues, crews require rope, harnesses, hardware, and the necessary safety systems (Figure 12-26b). A rescue is considered a low-angle rescue up to 40°, except if the face is overly smooth. Then a high-angle team will be better able to handle the more technical access and evacuation.

Each member of a low-angle crew must know how to assemble a hasty harness tied from 2-inch tubular webbing (or don a climbing harness), rappel and ascend by rope, package a patient in a litter, and rig a simple hauling system to assist the litter team up the embankment. Teams must also know how to set up a hasty rope slide to assist with balance and footing on rough terrain. Although low-angle rescues involve less technical skill than high-angle rescues, they still require ongoing practice and proper equipment.

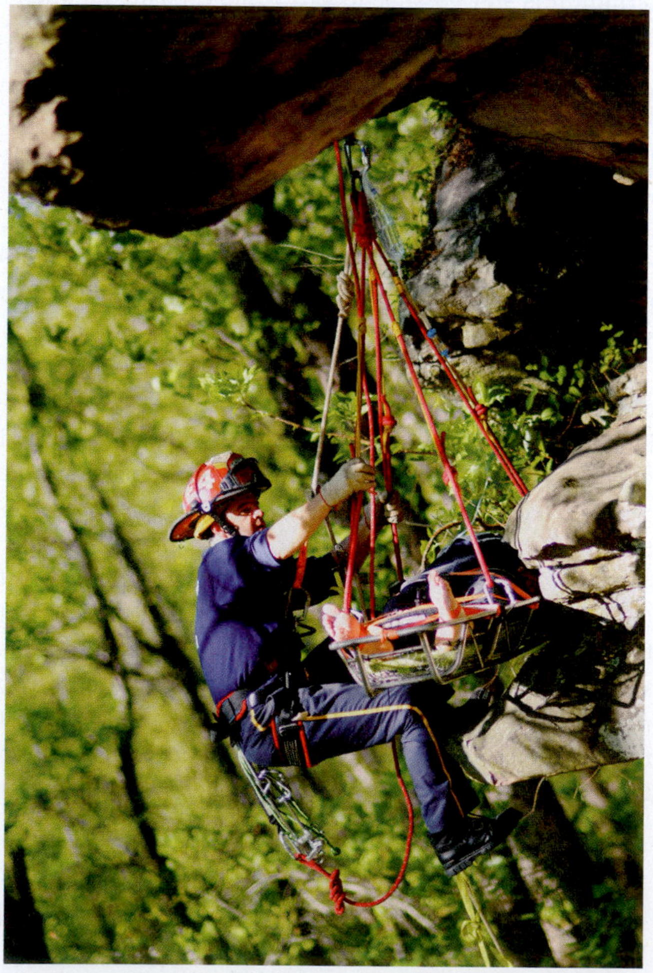

FIGURE 12-26a High-angle rescue is dangerous and difficult. It should be deferred to persons trained and experienced in high-angle rescue techniques.

Patient Packaging for Rough Terrain

Packaging a patient is a critical aspect of any hazardous terrain rescue. The Stokes basket stretcher is the standard litter for rough terrain evacuation (Figures 12-27a and 12-27b). It provides a rigid frame for patient protection and is easy to carry with an adequate number of personnel.

Stokes baskets come in wire and tubular, as well as plastic, styles. The older "military-style" wire mesh Stokes basket will not accept a backboard. Newer models, however, offer several advantages:

- Generally, greater strength
- Less expense per unit
- Better air/water flow through the basket
- Better flotation, an important concern in water rescues

Plastic basket stretchers are usually weaker than their wire mesh counterparts. They are often rated for only 300 to 600 pounds. However, they tend to offer better patient protection. In general, Stokes baskets with plastic bottoms and steel frames are best. These versatile units can also be slid in snow when necessary.

Most Stokes baskets, regardless of their style, are not equipped with adequate restraints. As a result, they will require additional strapping or lacing for rough terrain evacuation and/or extrication. A plastic litter shield can be used to protect the patient from dust and objects that may fall on the person's face. When moving across flat terrain, lace the patient into the Stokes basket to limit movement. When using a Stokes basket for high-angle or low-angle evacuation, take the following additional steps:

- Apply a harness to the patient.
- Apply leg stirrups to the patient.

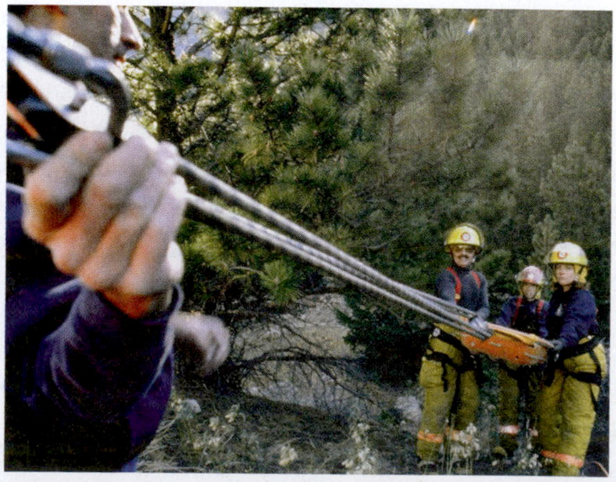

FIGURE 12-26b Low-angle situations are not the same as high-angle situations. Therefore, many EMS agencies have trained their paramedics in the skills of low-angle rescue.

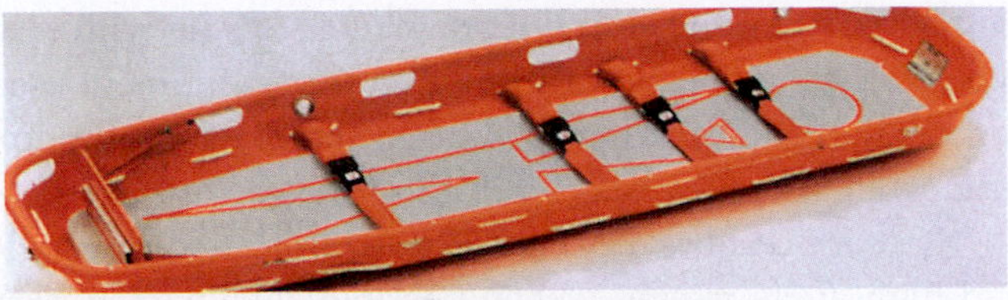

FIGURE 12-27a A basket stretcher.

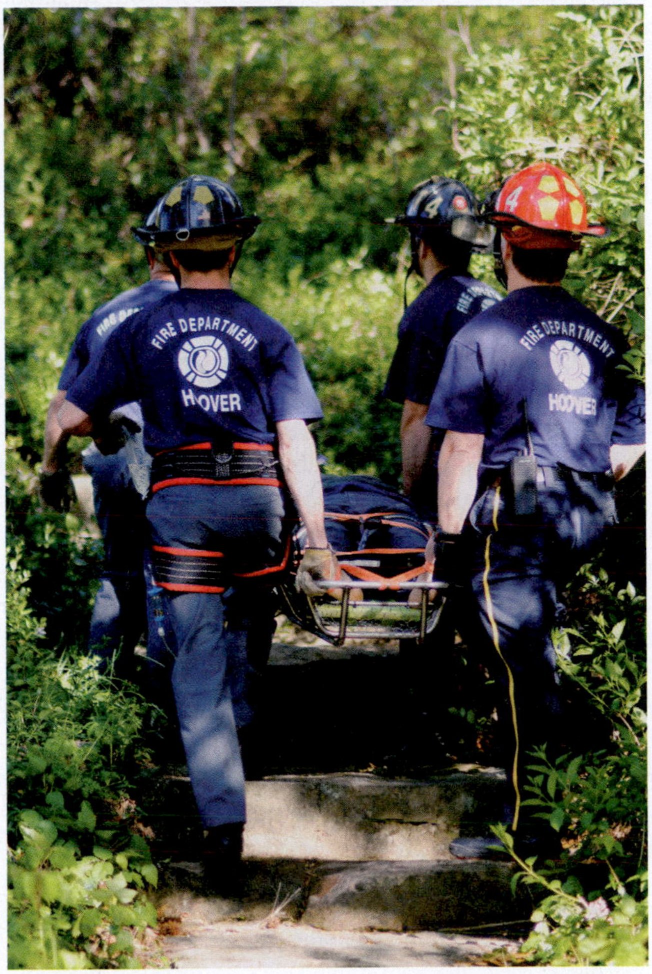

FIGURE 12-27b A basket stretcher is often used to carry patients over rough terrain.

- Secure the patient to a litter to prevent movement.
- Tie the tail of one litter line to the patient's harness.
- Use a helmet or litter shield to protect the patient.
- Administer fluids (IV or orally).
- Allow accessibility for taking blood pressure, performing suction, and assessing distal perfusion.
- Ensure adequate padding—a crucial consideration.
- Consider use of a patient heating/cooling system, especially for prolonged evacuations.
- Provide for an airway clearing system via a gravity "tip line," if necessary.

Patient Removal from Hazardous Terrain

When removing the patient from hazardous terrain, a non-technical/nonrope evacuation is usually faster. In other words, when possible, walk the patient out. Remember: Carrying a patient on a litter over flat ground can be a strenuous task, even under ideal conditions. As the terrain becomes rougher, the litter carry becomes more demanding.

Flat, Rough Terrain

When removing a patient in a litter from flat, rough terrain, make sure you have enough litter carriers to "leapfrog" ahead of each other to save time and to rotate rescuers. An adequate number of litter bearers would be two—or, better yet, three—teams of six. Litter bearers on each carry should be approximately the same height.

Several devices exist to ease the difficulty of a litter carry. For example, litter bearers can run webbing straps over the litter rails, across their shoulders, and into their free hands. This will help distribute the weight across the bearers' backs. Another helpful device is the litter wheel. It attaches to the bottom of a Stokes basket frame and takes most of the weight of the litter. Bearers must keep the litter balanced and control its motion. As you might suspect, the litter wheel works best over flatter terrain.

Low-Angle/High-Angle Evacuation

As already mentioned, low-angle and high-angle evacuations require specialized knowledge and skills. Before beginning patient removal, rescuers must ensure that all anchors are secure. They must check their own safety equipment and recheck patient packaging. They must also have the necessary lowering and hauling systems in place, again doing the recommended safety checks.

Materials, especially ropes, should never be used if there is any question of their safety. If you see a frayed rope or any stressed or damaged equipment, do not hesitate to point it out to the rescuers in a polite, but professional manner. Also, because hauling sometimes requires many "helpers," you may be asked to assist. Make sure you understand all directions given by the rescuers. Evacuation is a team effort.

Some high-angle units, especially fire departments, make use of aerial apparatus such as tower-ladders or bucket trucks to assist in the removal of a patient in a Stokes basket. These units are usually employed in structural environments, but can be adapted to hazardous terrain if there is room for a truck.

When using aerial apparatus, it is necessary to provide a litter belay during movement to a bucket. Litters, of course, must then be attached correctly to the bucket. Use of aerial ladders can be difficult because upper sections are usually not wide enough to slot the litter. The litter must always be properly belayed if being slid down the ladder. Finally, ladders or other aerial apparatus should *not* be used as a crane to move a litter. They are neither designed nor rated for this work. Serious stress can cause accidents, resulting in patient death.

Use of Helicopters

Helicopters can be useful in hazardous terrain rescues, especially when hospitals lie at a distant location (see the "Air Medical Operations" chapter). You must understand the capabilities of local helicopter systems and know who provides helicopter rescue in your region. Be aware of the difference in mission, crew training, and capabilities of helicopters that do air medical care versus helicopters that do rescue. You should be familiar with the advantages, disadvantages, and local restrictions for each of the following practices or techniques *before* you summon a helicopter from the field:

- Boarding and deboarding practices
- Restrictions on carrying noncrew members
- Use of cable winches for rescues
- Weight restrictions
- Restrictions on hovering rescues
- Use of **short hauls** or sling loads of equipment and/or personnel, as opposed to the more dangerous rappel-based rescues

Packaging/Evacuation Practice

Depending on local protocols, you should practice the packaging and evacuation techniques expected of EMS personnel in your region (Figure 12-28). You should familiarize yourself with the specific types of basket stretchers and litters available to your unit and the proper packaging, immobilization, and restraint techniques for use with each type. You should also practice with other equipment used for rough-terrain rescues, including the Sked and appropriate half-spine devices.

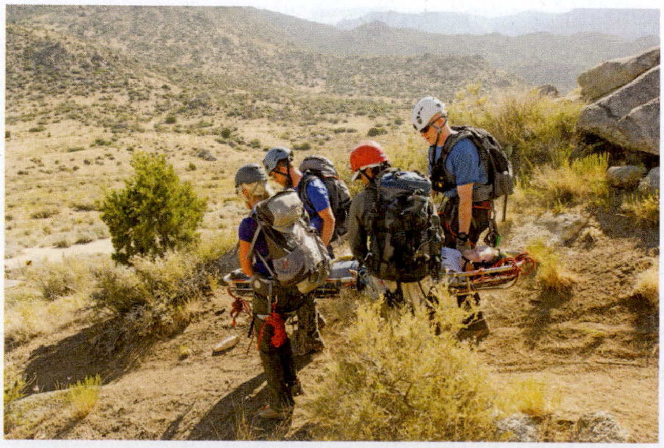

FIGURE 12-28 Patient removal over rough terrain requires adequate planning and personnel.

Practice or observe the skills required for low-angle and high-angle rescues. When possible, take part in exercises with the rescue units that you would summon to perform these evacuations. By fully understanding the capabilities of the rescue response teams in your area, you will circumvent any "turf" issues. You will also know how to work together whenever a multijurisdictional event occurs.

Extended Care Assessment and Environmental Issues

As you learned in the "Environmental Trauma" chapter, environmental emergencies can present their own special challenges. For rescue operations, at least some personnel should have formal training in managing patients whose injuries have been aggravated by prolonged lack of treatment, often under extreme conditions. If SOPs do not already exist, procedures adopted from wilderness medical research will prove useful. Position papers written by the Wilderness Medical Society or the National Association for Search and Rescue can serve as guidelines for protocols.

Regardless of the source, you will discover that many protocols for extended care vary substantially from standard EMS procedures. If your agency anticipates involvement in some of the rescue situations described in this chapter, you should consider protocols that at least address the following areas:

- Long-term hydration management
- Repositioning of dislocations
- Cleansing and care of wounds
- Removal of impaled objects
- Nonpharmacological pain management—using proper splinting, distracting the patient by talking or asking questions, scratching or creating sensory stimuli when doing painful procedures
- Pharmacological pain management—using pharmacological agents with isolated trauma, such as amputation or fracture, or with multiple trauma, such as crushing or pinning of more than an extremity
- Assessment and care of head and spinal injuries
- Management of hypothermia or hyperthermia
- Termination of CPR
- Treatment of crush injuries and compartment syndromes (For a review of these injuries, see the trauma chapters.)

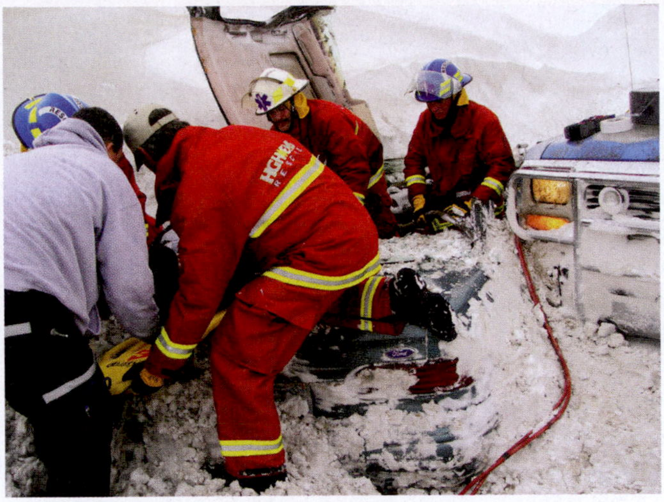

FIGURE 12-29 Rescue operations can involve multiple risks including environmental hazards, road hazards, and entrapment, as seen here.

(© Pat Songer)

A number of environmental issues can affect your assessment during a rescue situation (Figure 12-29). Some of the most important issues include the following:

- ***Weather/temperature extremes.*** Extreme weather or temperature conditions increase the risk of patient hypo/hyperthermia. These conditions also make it difficult or impossible to expose the patient completely for full assessment and treatment. As a result, your physical examination may be compromised. Use of tarps, blankets, or plastic sheeting may help in some cases, but your assessment will usually be limited at best.
- ***Limited patient access.*** Parts of the patient may not be accessible for examination because they are pinned beneath debris or stuck in a confined space. Cramped space and low lighting conditions also make assessment difficult. For this reason, it is important that you carry a headlamp with extended battery packs.
- ***Difficulty transporting street equipment.*** Hazardous terrain often makes it difficult to transport typical street equipment to the patient. Tackle boxes and heavy equipment may be inappropriate to take into a confined space or the backwoods, or down a hasty rappel. As a result, equipment usually must be downsized. Often you will use a backpack to keep your hands free for carrying. Essential equipment for the initial assessment and management include:
    - *Airway*—oral and nasal airways, manual suction, intubation equipment
    - *Breathing*—thoracic decompression equipment, small oxygen tank/regulator, masks/cannulas, pocket mask/BVM
    - *Circulation*—bandages/dressings, triangular bandages, occlusive dressings, IV administration equipment, and BP cuff and stethoscope
    - *Disability*—extrication collars
    - *Expose*—scissors
    - *Miscellaneous*—headlamp/flashlight, space blanket, padded aluminum splint (SAM® splint), PPE (leather gloves, latex gloves, eye shields)
- ***Cumbersome PPE.*** Necessary, but cumbersome, PPE can restrict rescuer mobility. In certain instances, some of the PPE might be removed to perform care steps. For example, the heavy outer gloves worn in extremely cold conditions might be taken off during administration of an IV. However, all PPE should be reapplied as soon as possible.
- ***Patient exposure.*** Patients should be quickly covered to ensure thermal protection. During the extrication, place hard protection, such as a spine board, and take steps to prevent patient contact with sharp objects or debris. For example, use an aluminized blanket to prevent glass shards from contacting the patient.
- ***Use of ALS skills.*** Good basic life support skills are mandatory in hazardous terrains, but limit ALS skills to those that are really essential. More wires and tubing complicate the extrication process. Continuous oxygenation and definitive airway control and volume may be essential. However, rescuers cannot carry lots of oxygen tanks into rugged terrains. As a result, you may have to use your tank at a slower flow rate so it will last a longer period of time.
- ***Patient monitoring.*** Hazardous terrain can alter your use of monitoring equipment. In high-noise areas, for example, you may have to take BP by palpation or use a compact pulse oximetry unit. An ECG monitor can be cumbersome during extrication and will be more difficult to use than in a street situation.
- ***Improvisation.*** Improvisation is common in rescue situations. To minimize the amount of equipment carried over hazardous terrain, you may want to consider such techniques as tying upper extremity fractures to the torso or tying lower extremity fractures to the uninjured leg. Lightweight SAM splints can be very useful in the backwoods and should be part of your downsized medical gear. Whatever you do, continue talking to the patient and explain exactly what is happening. Answer any questions, particularly if you are improvising. The patient is already frightened by the entrapment. Do not worsen the situation by making the patient feel even more out of control.

Summary

All rescue operations can be divided into seven functional stages: arrival and size-up, hazard control, patient access, medical treatment, disentanglement, patient packaging, and removal/transport. Whenever you function in any one of these phases, you must be properly outfitted with protective equipment. You must also have training specific to the assigned rescue.

In any rescue, you must access the scene quickly so assessment and management can begin. Situational threats to the rescuer and/or patient should be identified and remedied as thoroughly as conditions permit. Patients should be reassessed throughout the rescue and repackaged as extrication and removal progress.

During the operational phases of the rescue, you must provide direct patient care and work with technical teams to ensure optimal patient management. Any paramedic assigned to rescue duties should have training in the care of patients who may require prolonged management. Such training results from the increased time to locate, access, remove, and/or transport a rescue patient.

Either you or a paramedic on your crew must accompany the patient throughout the transportation phase. This person should constantly monitor any changes in condition, while coordinating patient transport to an appropriate medical facility. If a specialized rescue team includes a trained paramedic, this person may fulfill these functions.

You Make the Call

You and your partner are working on Medic Ambulance 642, covering the north portion of town. You receive a call for a motor vehicle collision on Interstate 94. Upon arrival, you quickly determine that the collision involves more than the average complications. Apparently, the vehicle swerved off the road and rolled down an embankment. Traffic is already backed up for about half a mile. Several motorists have gotten out of their cars.

When you look over the embankment, you discover that two bystanders have climbed down the hill and are standing near the overturned automobile. They yell up: "There's just one guy inside. He's breathing, so we know he's alive. But we can't get any response out of him. Do you want us to do something?" While you are directing the bystanders to stand clear of the car, "rubbernecking" in the other lane causes a low-speed collision right on the highway.

1. What are your immediate considerations as you size up the scene?
2. Why would you consider this a rescue operation?
3. What additional resources would you request?

See Suggested Responses at the back of this book.

Review Questions

1. The safest helmets incorporate a ______________ suspension system within them.
   a. two-point, elastic
   b. two-point, nonelastic
   c. four-point, elastic
   d. four-point, nonelastic

2. Although specific procedures in rescue operations vary from area to area and from rescue to rescue, most calls will go through how many general phases?
   a. Four
   b. Five
   c. Seven
   d. Ten

3. During a rescue, what triggers the technical beginning of the rescue?
   a. Access
   b. Arrival
   c. Size-up
   d. Hazard control
4. Which phase may be the most technical and time-consuming portion of a rescue operation?
   a. Hazard control
   b. Patient access
   c. Disentanglement
   d. Patient packaging
5. Decisions regarding patient transport should be coordinated based on advice from ____________
   a. the safety officer.
   b. medical direction.
   c. the liaison officer.
   d. the communications officer.
6. As they pertain to rescue operations, examples of confined spaces include all of the following *except* ____________
   a. open water.
   b. drainage culverts.
   c. wells and cisterns.
   d. grain bins and silos.
7. The types of confined-space emergencies most commonly encountered in the workplace are ____________
   a. falls.
   b. explosions.
   c. entrapment.
   d. all of the above.
8. What part of an automobile is usually the easiest means of access during an MVC?
   a. Door
   b. Window
   c. Trunk
   d. Windshield
9. As a rule, the primary role of EMS personnel in vehicle stabilization and removal is that of ____________
   a. extrication.
   b. scene control.
   c. patient care provider.
   d. communications officer.
10. A technique for securing rescuers to a vertical face is called a(n) ____________
    a. aid.
    b. belay.
    c. anchor.
    d. rappel.

See Answers to Review Questions at the end of this book.

References

1. Ducharme, M. S. and D. S. Lounsbury. "Self-Rescue Swimming in Cold Water: The Latest Advice." *Appl Physiol Butr Metab* 32 (2007): 799–807.
2. Giesbrecht, G. G. "Prehospital Treatment of Hypothermia." *Wilderness Environ Med* 12 (2001): 24–31.
3. Driscoll, T. R., J. A. Harrison, and M. Steenkamp. "Review of the Role of Alcohol in Drowning Associated with Recreational Aquatic Activity." *Inj Prev* 10 (2004): 107–113.
4. Watson, R. S., P. Cummings, L. Quan, S. Bratton, and N. S. Weiss. "Cervical Spine Injuries among Submersion Victims." *J Trauma* 51 (2001): 658–662.

Further Readings

Auerbach, P. S. *Wilderness Medicine.* 6th ed. St. Louis, MO: Mosby–Year Book, 2011.

Martinette, C. V., Jr. *Trench Rescue.* 2nd ed. Sudbury, MA: Jones and Bartlett Publishers, 2007.

Tilton, B. and F. Hubbell. *Medicine for the Backcountry.* 3rd ed. Guilford, CT: Globe Pequot, 2000.

Vines, T. *High-Angle Rescue Techniques.* 3rd ed. St. Louis: Mosby, 2004.

Wilkerson, J. A. *Medicine for Mountaineering* and *Other Wilderness Activities.* 6th ed. Seattle: The Mountaineers, 2010.

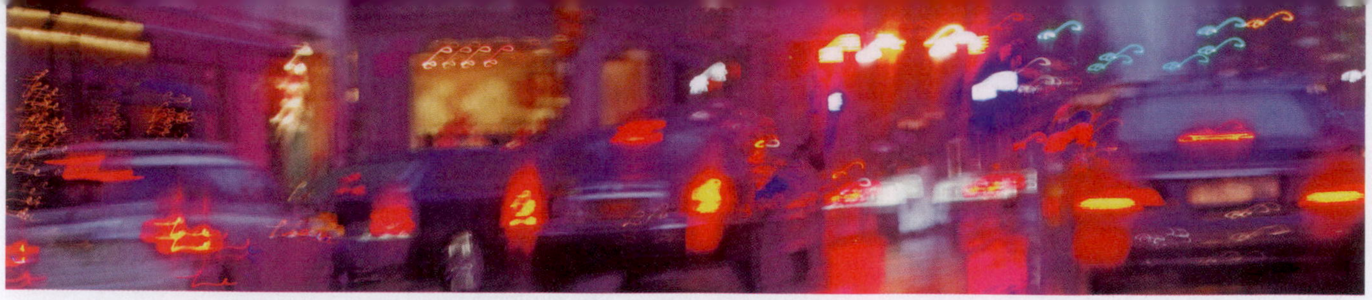

Chapter 13
Hazardous Materials

Bryan Bledsoe, DO, FACEP, FAAEM, EMT-P

STANDARD
EMS Operations (Hazardous Materials)

COMPETENCY
Applies knowledge of operational roles and responsibilities to ensure patient, public, and personnel safety.

Learning Objectives

Terminal Performance Objective: After reading this chapter, you should be able to effectively perform the expected functions of EMS personnel in a hazardous materials incident.

Enabling Objectives: To accomplish the terminal performance objective, you should be able to:

1. Define key terms introduced in this chapter.
2. Relate the paramedic's training in response to toxicological emergencies, multiple-casualty incidents, and terrorism to the response to hazardous materials.
3. Identify the federal agencies that provide regulations and standards related to hazmat emergencies, and describe the levels of training for hazmat responders.
4. Identify the EMS provider's role in initial hazmat incident size-up.
5. Given a variety of scenarios involving hazardous material release, describe resources available to help identify the substance involved and what actions to take.
6. Describe the various control zones established at a hazardous materials incident.
7. Discuss the types of contamination, routes of exposure, and actions to protect yourself and other responders from exposure at the scene of a hazardous materials incident.
8. Describe the levels of hazardous materials protective equipment available and approaches to decontaminating patients exposed to a variety of hazardous materials.
9. Given a variety of hazardous materials scenarios, discuss safe and effective patient care.
10. Describe the role of EMS personnel in monitoring and rehabilitating those responding to a hazardous materials incident.

KEY TERMS

acetylcholinesterase (AChE), p. 368
acute effects, p. 367
air-purifying respirator (APR), p. 373
biotransformation, p. 367
CAMEO®, p. 362
CHEMTEL, p. 362
CHEMTREC, p. 362
cold zone, p. 364
cytochrome oxidase, p. 368
delayed effects, p. 367
hazardous materials (hazmat), p. 356
hot zone, p. 364
local effects, p. 367
safety data sheet (SDS), p. 362
primary contamination, p. 365
secondary contamination, p. 365
semi-decontaminated patient, p. 371
shipping papers, p. 362
synergism, p. 367
systemic effects, p. 367
UN number, p. 360
warm zone, p. 364
warning placard, p. 358
weapons of mass destruction (WMD), p. 359

Case Study

The radio dispatches your unit to a chemical burn incident at the Acme Chicken Processing Plant. You jump aboard the ambulance and travel to the address given by the dispatcher. On arrival, you observe about 50 workers standing in the parking lot. A security guard approaches the ambulance and points toward the loading dock. He tells you, "A couple of people were sprayed with refrigerant when the hose broke open. Some of them got burned."

You proceed to the loading dock and find six patients. All of them are experiencing shortness of breath. Several have burns, including one patient with obvious facial injuries. Bystanders have already begun flushing his eyes with water. The plant supervisor tells you that the refrigerant was anhydrous ammonia. You relay the initial scene size-up to the dispatch center. Then you request additional ambulances, a supervisor, the fire department, and a local hazmat team.

As the first on-scene unit, you initiate the Incident Command System. You assume the role of incident commander while your partner acts as triage officer. She quickly tags three patients red and three patients yellow. She reports one patient with some facial burns and possible eye injuries. Two other patients have chemical burns on their backs and extremities and are suffering respiratory distress. The remaining three patients have no burns but are having difficulty breathing.

You instruct the patients to immediately remove all their clothing for decontamination. By this time, additional units have already begun to arrive. The fire chief requests a quick report and then initiates gross decontamination measures with large amounts of water. Meanwhile, you relocate all personnel to avoid contact with the runoff dilution.

You assign the patient with facial burns and eye injuries to a crew from one of the ALS ambulances. They complete decontamination and begin treatment. Other crews decontaminate and treat the remaining patients in the order established by triage. All patients receive oxygen. Paramedics establish intravenous lines and administer albuterol by small-volume nebulizer to the patients who are wheezing. Crews also apply dressings to the burn patients as necessary.

By now the supervisor has arrived, and you complete a face-to-face transfer of command. The supervisor oversees hazmat operations and notifies hospitals of incoming patients. The hazmat team dons the necessary equipment and provides paper garments for the patients. Because decontamination is not very demanding, transport begins quickly. Your ambulance remains on scene as a dedicated unit for the hazmat team.

You assess two hazmat crew members before they enter the plant. In analyzing the damage, the hazmat team determines that the anhydrous ammonia must be cleaned up by a contractor. However, if no one enters the building, the chemical poses no immediate hazard to the workers, the public, or the environment.

You now perform a post-entry evaluation of the hazmat team. You find that they have not suffered significant heat stress during their entry. The supervisor then terminates the incident and orders the plant closed until the contractor completes the cleanup operation.

Introduction

Hazardous materials (hazmat) are all around us. Companies in the United States manufacture more than 50 billion tons of hazardous materials a year. Some 4 billion tons of hazardous materials are shipped throughout the United States by truck, pipeline, railroad, and tankers (Figure 13-1).[1] They can exist as solids, liquids, or gases. They can irritate, burn, poison, corrode, or asphyxiate.

You learned about some hazardous materials in the chapters "Toxicology and Substance Abuse," "Multiple Casualty Incidents and Incident Management," "Rescue Awareness and Operations" and will learn more in the chapters "Rural EMS" and "Responding to Terrorist Acts." This chapter deals with the hazardous materials spilled or released as a result of an accident, equipment failure, human error, or an intentional violation of the laws and regulations that govern their manufacture, use, and disposal.

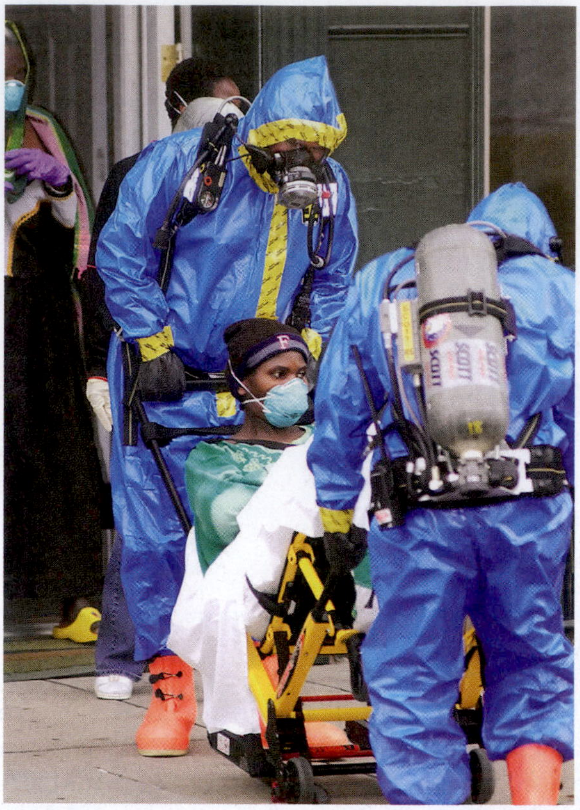

FIGURE 13-1 A hazardous materials emergency can involve countless substances and occur in many situations. Warning placards on a truck should immediately alert you to the possible need of a hazmat team.
(© AP Images/Herald-Mail, Erick Gibson)

Patho Pearls

Hazmat and Terrorism. The dangers of hazardous materials have been well documented. However, the rapid escalation of terrorism in the world has made the likelihood of having to respond to a hazardous materials event even greater—and the danger surrounding those events has escalated. Dangers that were once thought of as rare (anthrax) or eradicated (smallpox) now pose a true and present danger for all. The fall of the Soviet Union and black-market profiteering in weapons of mass destruction has possibly made very dangerous substances available to those who desire to harm us and our way of life. Because of these and other factors, it is important that all EMS personnel be familiar with the various weapons of mass destruction, including biological, chemical, and radiologic agents (as discussed in the chapter "Responding to Terrorist Acts"). It is also important for all EMS personnel to understand their roles in a response to a hazmat situation and to ensure that they have the appropriate protective equipment and/or antidotes before approaching a possible hazmat scene.

For purposes of this chapter, keep in mind the definition of a hazardous material offered by the U.S. Department of Transportation (DOT). A hazardous material can be regarded as "any substance which may pose an unreasonable risk to health and safety of operating or emergency personnel, the public, and/or the environment if not properly controlled during handling, storage, manufacture, processing, packaging, use, disposal, or transportation."

Role of the Paramedic

Hazardous materials incidents, or hazmat incidents, present some of the most challenging situations that you will face as a paramedic. As mentioned, a hazmat event can involve all kinds of substances: corrosive chemicals, pulmonary irritants, pesticides, chemical asphyxiants, hydrocarbon solvents, and radioactive wastes. The exposure to hazardous materials may be limited to just a few victims, or it may cause widespread destruction and loss of many lives. However, as the opening case study shows, even a small-scale incident is almost always a multijurisdictional event. For this reason, EMS agencies should train all their personnel how to respond to hazmat incidents and how to interact with other agencies that might be summoned to the scene.[2]

Traditionally, paramedics do not perform defensive (containment) and offensive (control) functions at a hazardous materials response. Even so, paramedics are still an integral part of a community's hazmat response system. As you will learn in this chapter, EMS personnel fulfill a variety of tasks at a hazmat incident. As first responders, they may size up the incident, assess the toxicologic risk, and activate the Incident Command System (ICS) needed to handle the event. They will also be called on to evaluate decontamination

CONTENT REVIEW

➤ Role of EMS Hazmat First Responders
- Size up incident
- Assess toxicologic risk
- Activate the ICS
- Establish command

CONTENT REVIEW

- Hazmat Requirements/Standards
  - OSHA publication CFR 1910.120
  - EPA regulation 40 CFR 311
  - NFPA standard 473

methods, to treat and transport exposed patients, and to perform medical monitoring of hazmat teams that enter the area.[3]

Requirements and Standards

Two federal agencies, the Occupational Safety and Health Administration (OSHA) and the Environmental Protection Agency (EPA), have set forth a number of regulations and standards for dealing with hazmat emergencies. The most important of these are found in OSHA publication CFR 1910.120, *Hazardous Waste Operations and Emergency Response Standard* (2004). This standard provides specific response procedures, including use of an incident management system, use of personal protective equipment (PPE), use of a safety officer, and special training requirements. The EPA has published a mirror regulation, 40 CFR 311, that applies to those agencies that fall outside OSHA's jurisdiction.

In addition, the National Fire Protection Association (NFPA) has published NFPA 473, *Standard Competencies for EMS Personnel Responding to Hazardous Materials Incidents.* This standard, along with two other NFPA standards for hazmat response, deals with the training standards for EMS personnel assigned to hazmat incidents.

Levels of Training

The documents just mentioned set forth three levels of training appropriate to EMS response at hazmat incidents: Awareness Level, EMS Level 1, and EMS Level 2. The Awareness Level applies to responders who may arrive first at a scene and discover a toxic substance. Training focuses on recognition of hazmat incidents, basic hazmat identification techniques, and individual protection from involvement in the incident. All EMS personnel, as well as police officers and firefighters, need to be trained to the Awareness Level.

EMS Level 1 training, or the "operations level," is required for those who may perform patient care in the cold zone on patients who do *not* present a significant risk of secondary contamination. This training focuses on hazard assessment, patient assessment, and patient care for previously decontaminated patients.

EMS Level 2 training, or the "technician level," is required for those who may perform patient care in the warm zone on patients who still present a significant risk of secondary contamination. This training focuses on personal protection, decontamination procedures, and treatment for patients who are beginning or undergoing decontamination.

The level of training required for each individual depends on that person's role in the hazmat response system. All systems require some individuals to be trained in both the EMS Level 1 and Level 2 standards. In this way, patient care can begin during decontamination and continue after the patient has been cleaned of contaminants.

Incident Size-Up

Sizing up a hazardous materials incident is a very difficult task. You often receive inaccurate or incomplete information; in addition, events tend to develop very quickly during each phase of the incident. As already indicated, you can also expect a number of agencies to be involved in the response. As a result, you should be skilled in the use of the ICS discussed in the chapter "Multiple Casualty Incidents and Incident Management" and practice it regularly with the other agencies that typically respond to a hazmat call.

ICS and Hazmat Emergencies

Priorities for a hazmat incident are the same as those for any other major incident: life safety, incident stabilization, and property conservation. However, you should be prepared for the special circumstances surrounding most hazmat emergencies. Some incidents, for example, will require immediate evacuation of patients from a contaminated area. Other incidents will have ambulatory contaminated patients who seek out EMS personnel as soon as you arrive on scene. In performing early hazmat interventions, you face the challenge of avoiding exposure to the hazardous material yourself. As a result, never compromise scene safety during the early phase of a hazmat operation. Otherwise, you risk becoming a contaminated patient. (The subject of "self-rescued" patients is discussed later in the chapter.)

In setting priorities, you must also quickly determine whether the hazmat emergency is an open incident or a closed incident. That is, does the event have the potential for generating more patients? As you learned in the chapter "Multiple Casualty Incidents and Incident Management," the answer to this question will determine the resources that you request, how you stage them, and the way in which you deploy personnel. In reaching your decision, remember that some chemicals have delayed effects. Triage must be ongoing, because patient conditions can change rapidly.

Finally, in employing the ICS at a hazmat incident, you must take into account certain special conditions when choreographing the scene. The most preferable site for deploying resources will be uphill and upwind. This will help prevent contamination from ground-based liquids, high-vapor-density gases, runoff water, and vapor clouds.

The basic ICS at a hazmat incident will require a command post, a staging area, and a decontamination corridor. Depending on the event, the incident commander may also establish separate areas, such as treatment areas and personnel staging areas, to prevent unnecessary exposure to contamination. A backup plan for areas of operations must be determined early in the event. For example, what would you do if the wind direction suddenly shifted and a cloud of chlorine gas headed toward your staging area?

Incident Awareness

One of the most critical aspects of any hazmat response is the simple awareness that a dangerous substance may be present. Virtually every emergency site—residential, business, or highway—possesses the potential for hazardous materials. For example, most households keep ammonia and liquid bleach in the kitchen or laundry room. When combined, these substances can produce a toxic gas. Homes with kerosene heaters or blocked flues can be filled with carbon monoxide. Do not take any chances. Always keep the possibility of dangerous substances in mind whenever you approach the scene of an emergency. If you suspect the presence of hazardous materials, use binoculars to inspect the scene from a distance (Figure 13-2).

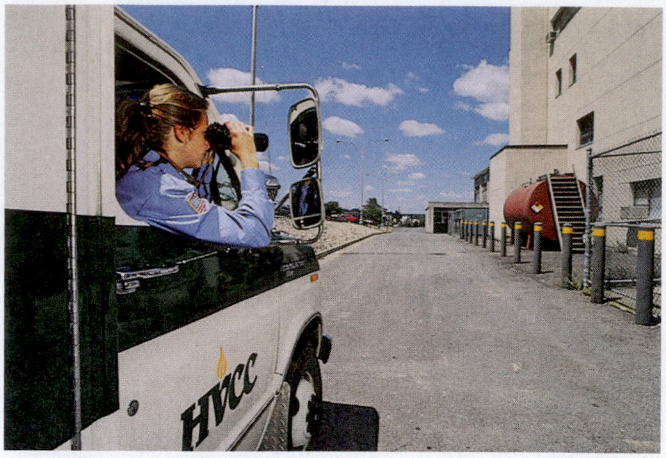

FIGURE 13-2 Don't take any chances. Use binoculars to make a visual inspection of a potentially hazardous situation—such as a suspicious storage tank—from a safe distance.

Transportation

Any transportation accident—automobile, truck, or railroad—should raise a suspicion of the presence of hazardous materials (Figure 13-3). Maintain a high degree of hazmat awareness whenever you are summoned to collisions involving commercial vehicles, pest control vehicles, tanker trucks, tractor-trailers, or cars powered by alternative fuels. Do not rule out the presence of hazardous materials just because you do not see a **warning placard**. Hospitals and laboratories, for example, routinely and

Establishing the Danger Zone

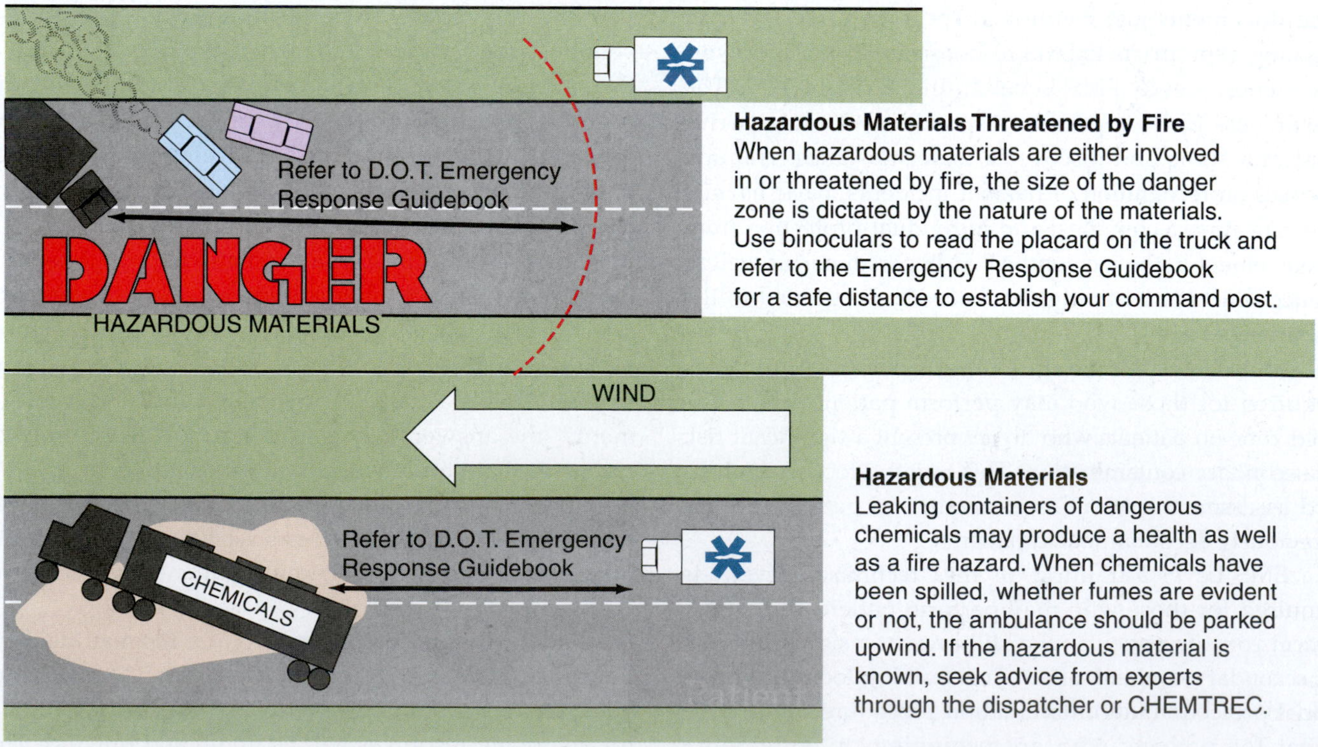

FIGURE 13-3 Transportation incidents involving hazardous materials.

legally transport medical radioactive isotopes in unmarked passenger cars. You could look into the back seat of a crashed automobile and see a container with a label indicating radioactive contents.

Railroad accidents merit special attention for two reasons. First, railroad cars can carry large quantities of hazardous materials. The largest tanker truck, for example, has about a 14,000-gallon capacity, whereas a railroad tank car can carry up to 34,000 gallons. Second, several tank cars may be hitched together on a freight train. Obviously, there is a greater chance for a major incident if one or more of these tanks are ruptured in an accident. Fortunately, railroads run along fixed lines, which means you can preplan your response in case a railroad accident occurs within your jurisdiction.

Fixed Facilities

Hazmat incidents can also take place at fixed facilities where dangerous substances are produced or stored. Chemical plants and all manufacturing operations have tanks, storage vessels, and pipelines used to transport products and/or wastes. Additional fixed sites with possible hazardous materials include warehouses, hardware or agricultural stores, water treatment centers, and loading docks. If you work in a rural area, keep in mind the number of places where you can find hazardous materials on a farm or ranch: silos, barns, greenhouses, and more. (For information on rural hazmat emergencies, see the chapter "Rural EMS.")

Finally, remember that many communities have some kind of fixed pipelines, especially in urban settings. These pipelines can be damaged by acts of nature (earthquakes), by construction crews, or, if aboveground, by vehicle crashes. A rupture or leak in a gas or oil pipeline can spell disaster, especially if ignited.

Terrorism

Unfortunately, a new type of hazmat incident has emerged in the form of terrorism. Terrorists may use any variety of chemical, biological, or nuclear devices to strike at government or high-profile targets. These **weapons of mass destruction (WMD)** can be manufactured from materials as simple as those found on most farms, as was the case in the bombing of the Alfred P. Murrah Federal Building in Oklahoma City (see the chapter "Responding to Terrorist Acts"). The perpetrators can come from within the United States or from abroad.

The most frightening aspect of terrorism is the lack of predictability about when or where an attack might take place. Lacking a clear verbal or written threat, it can happen almost anywhere. However, terrorists usually select their targets by activity, particularly government or industrial, and by the number of people present. Potential targets include public buildings, multinational headquarters, shopping centers, workplaces, and sites of assembly such as arenas, stadiums, transportation centers, or places of worship. All these locations should be identified in any mass casualty or disaster plan for your community.

CONTENT REVIEW

➤ Potential Terrorist Targets
- Public buildings
- Multinational headquarters
- Shopping centers
- Workplaces
- Sites of assembly

In responding to a suspected terrorist incident, look for potential clues. Patients in a closed environment, such as a subway or an office building, will exhibit similar symptoms if they have been exposed to a chemical or biological weapon of mass destruction. In the case of an explosion, remember that a secondary device may exist. Take every precaution not to fall victim to a terrorist attack yourself. Make full use of the ICS and all specialized agencies able to respond to the scene of suspected terrorism.

For more on this topic, see the chapter "Responding to Terrorist Acts."

Recognition of Hazards

To aid in the visual recognition of hazardous materials, two simple systems have been developed. The DOT has implemented placards to identify dangerous substances in transit, and the NFPA has devised a system for fixed facilities.

Placard Classifications

Although many vehicles are required by law to carry placards (Figure 13-4), the absence of a placard does not mean the absence of a hazmat threat. Regulations depend on the type of substance and/or the amount of substance in transit.

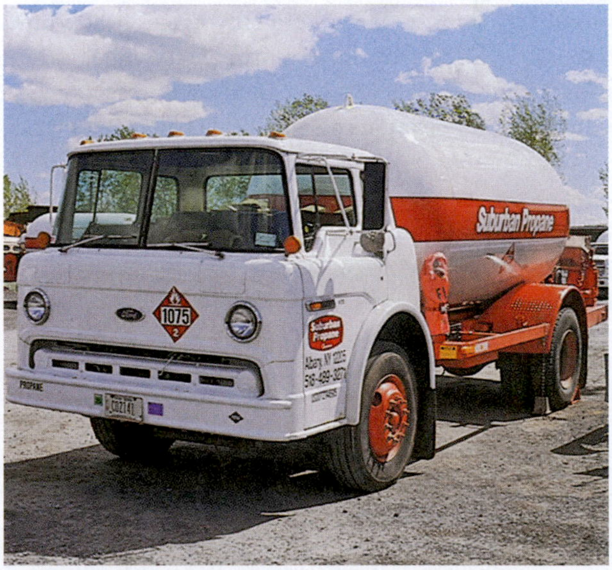

FIGURE 13-4 Vehicles carrying hazardous materials are required to display placards indicating the nature of their contents. Even if you have studied these placards earlier in your EMS career, you should regularly review the symbols, color codes, and hazard class numbers so that you can identify dangerous materials.

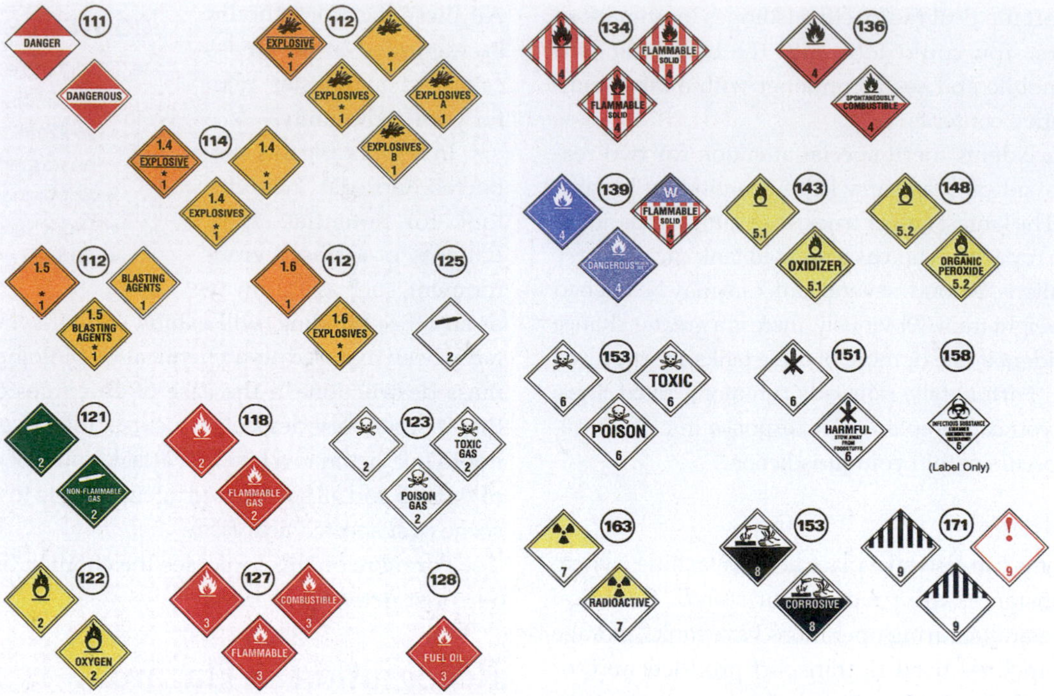

FIGURE 13-5 Sample labels and warning placards required by the DOT for all packages, storage containers, and vehicles containing hazardous materials.

(U.S. Department of Transportation)

Placards are easily spotted because of their diamond shape (Figure 13-5). Each placard indicates hazmat classifications through use of a color code and hazard class number. Some placards also carry a **UN number**—a four-digit number specific to the actual chemical. For quick reference, keep in mind the general classifications listed in Table 13-1.

In addition to numbers and colors, placards also use symbols to indicate hazard types. For example, a flame symbol indicates a flammable substance, a ball-on-fire symbol indicates an oxidizer, a propeller symbol indicates a radioactive substance, and a skull-and-crossbones symbol indicates a poisonous substance. When combined with numbers and colors, these symbols help you to recognize the specific nature of the hazardous material. For instance, a red placard with the number 2 and a flame symbol means that the vehicle is carrying a flammable gas. Over time, you will become more familiar with these and other important symbols such as a "W" with a line through it, which means "reacts with water."

In using the placard system, keep in mind several shortcomings. Although some substances are required to show a placard in any quantity, others need to be placarded only if they are transported in large quantities. This means that a truck may be carrying hazardous materials, but because the amount falls below the quantity required for placarding, no placard is shown. Also, the "Dangerous" placard means that there are two or more substances onboard, between 1,000 and 5,000 pounds total weight. However, the generic placard tells you nothing about the hazardous nature of the materials. Finally, people can remove placards or fail to apply them in the first place. In this case, you have no immediate indication at all of a dangerous hazmat situation.

Table 13-1 Hazard Classes and Placard Colors

Hazard Class	Hazard Type	Color Code
1	Explosives	Orange
2	Gases	Red or green
3	Liquids	Red
4	Solids	Red and white
5	Oxidizers and organic peroxides	Yellow
6	Poisonous and etiologic agents	White
7	Radioactive materials	Yellow and white
8	Corrosives	Black and white
9	Miscellaneous	Black and white

NFPA 704 System

The NFPA 704 System identifies hazardous materials at fixed facilities. Like the DOT placards, the system uses diamond-shaped figures, which are placed on tanks and storage vessels. The diamond is divided into four sections and color coded (Figures 13-6a and 13-6b). The top segment is red and indicates the flammability of the substance. The left segment is blue and indicates the health hazard. The

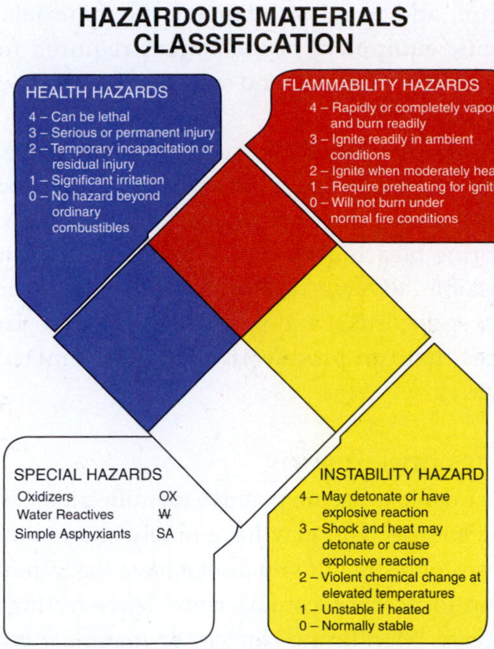

FIGURE 13-6a NFPA 704 hazardous materials classification.

(Reprinted with permission from NFPA 704-2012, System for the Identification of the Hazards of Materials for Emergency Response, Copyright © 2011, National Fire Protection Association. This reprinted material is not the complete and official position of the NFPA on the referenced subject, which is represented solely by the standard in its entirety. The classification of any particular material within this system is the sole responsibility of the user and not the NFPA. The NFPA bears no responsibility for any determinations of any values for any particular material classified or represented using this system.)

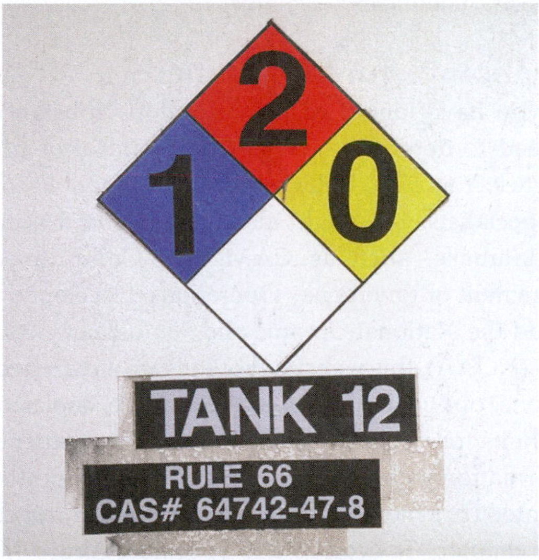

FIGURE 13-6b NFPA 704 labeling on a tank.

right segment is yellow and indicates the product's instability. The bottom segment is white and indicates special information. The hazards listed may include water reactivity, oxidizing properties, or simple asphyxiant.

Flammability, health hazard, and reactivity are measured on a scale of 0 to 4. A designation of 0 indicates no hazard, whereas a designation of 4 indicates extreme hazard. The degrees of hazard are summarized in the figures. The NFPA 704 standard should be referred to for specific criteria used to rate the materials.

> **CONTENT REVIEW**
>
> ➤ Hazmat References
> - *Emergency Response Guidebook* (ERG)
> - Shipping papers
> - Safety data sheets
> - Monitors/chemical tests
> - Databases (CAMEO)
> - Hazmat telephone hotlines (CHEMTREC; CHEMTEL)
> - Poison control centers
> - Toxicologists
> - Reference books

Identification of Substances

Once you have determined that an incident involves hazardous materials, you must next try to identify the particular substance. This is the crux, or most difficult aspect, of dealing with a hazmat incident. You will often lack adequate on-scene information to make a positive identification, or you will get conflicting preliminary information. For this reason, you must be familiar with the resources that can assist you in identification of a hazardous material and become skilled at using each of them.

To prevent dangerous interpretations, try to locate two or more concurring reference sources. Do not take action until you find this information—otherwise, you risk making mistakes and providing incorrect patient treatment.

Emergency Response Guidebook

You have already read about UN numbers, the four-digit numbers specific to actual chemicals. Some placards will include the UN number as well as the hazard class information. For example, you may see a tanker truck with a red (3) placard with the number 1203 in the middle. Based on what you already know, you can determine that the incident involves a flammable liquid. To identify the specific flammable liquid, you will need the *Emergency Response Guidebook* (ERG) (Figure 13-7).

The ERG, published by the U.S. Department of Transportation, Transport Canada, and the Secretary of Communications and Transportation of Mexico, should be carried on every emergency vehicle. It lists more than a thousand hazardous materials, along with placards, UN numbers, and chemical names. It also cross-references each identification number to specific emergency procedures related to the chemical. The ERG includes, for example, a list of evacuation distances for the most hazardous substances. It is revised frequently, and the most up-to-date version should be readily available to all crew members. Newest updates are available on the Internet from the DOT.

When using the ERG, keep in mind two shortcomings. First, the reference provides only basic generic information on medical treatment. One recommendation, for instance, involves calling EMS. Obviously, this is not very helpful for EMS personnel. Second, more than one chemical often

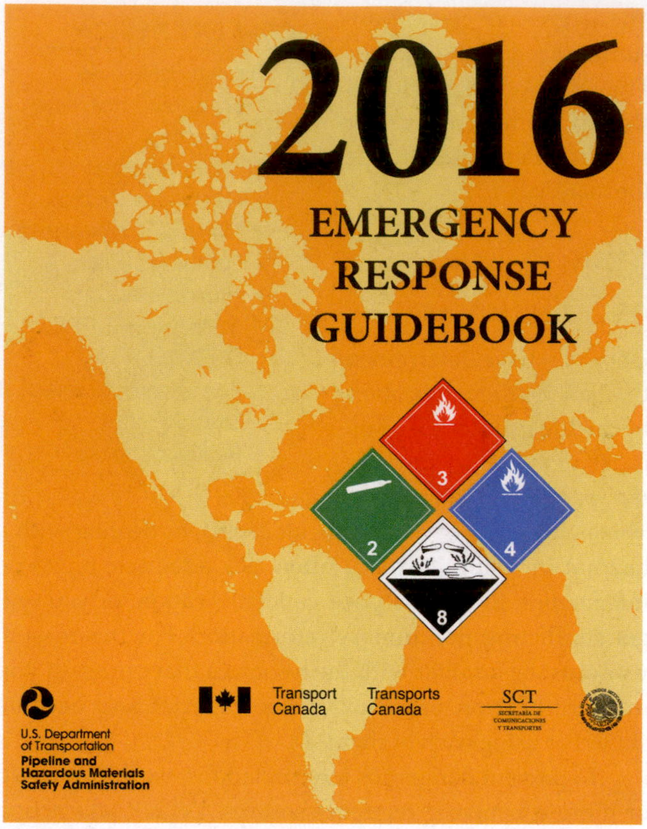

FIGURE 13-7 Carry a copy of the *Emergency Response Guidebook* in your vehicle at all times.

have the same UN number. For example, UN 1203 may be diesel fuel, gasohol, gasoline, motor fuels, or motor spirits. The difference between a gasoline leak and a diesel fuel leak, for instance, is dramatic, highlighting the need to use other methods of positive identification.

Shipping Papers

The most accurate information about a transported substance can be found in the **shipping papers**, or bill of lading. Trucks, boats, airplanes, and trains routinely carry these documents. Ideally, they should list the specific substances and quantities carried. However, drivers, pilots, or engineers may not take these papers when they exit the vehicle or craft, and you may find the scene too unstable to retrieve the documents yourself. In some cases, the papers may be incomplete or inadequate, requiring you to consult additional sources of identification.

Safety Data Sheets

In the case of fixed facilities, employers are required by law to post **safety data sheets (SDSs)**—formerly called *material safety data sheets (MSDSs)*. These sheets contain detailed information about all potentially hazardous substances found on site. The sheets typically list the names and characteristics of the materials; what types of health, fire, and reactivity dangers the materials pose; any specific equipment or techniques required for safe handling of the materials; and suggested emergency first aid treatment.

Even simple chemicals, such as window cleaners, should have SDSs posted in an easily accessible location. Figure 13-8 shows the SDS posted for a familiar chemical—chlorine bleach. Among other information, it indicates possible adverse reactions in cases of accidental exposure, spills, leaks, and so on. Note, too, the range of substances that can produce toxic fumes if mixed with the bleach.

Monitors and Testing

If you are unable to secure positive identification using the preceding sources, you may have to rely on monitors and other means of testing. If you do not have the training and equipment to do the reconnaissance, leave testing to the hazmat team. Monitoring devices or materials typically include:

- ***Air and gas monitors***—typically determine the percentage of oxygen in the air and measure the presence of explosive gases, carbon monoxide, and toxic gases such as hydrogen sulfide
- ***Litmus paper***—measures the approximate pH of a liquid, indicating whether it is an acid or a base
- ***Colorimetric tubes***—suction the air and search for specific chemicals

Other Sources of Information

Once you have identified the hazardous substance, you will need to determine its specific chemical or physical properties. You can consult textbooks, handbooks, or technical specialists. You might also make use of a computerized database, such as **CAMEO**®—Computer-Aided Management of Emergency Operations. Developed by the EPA and the National Oceanic and Atmospheric Administration (NOAA), this website provides answers to technical questions, opportunities for skills practice, copies of software, links for networking, and more. Yet another source of information includes your local or regional poison control center. (For more on the use of poison control centers, see the chapter "Toxicology and Substance Abuse.")

Two other sources of information are **CHEMTREC**—the Chemical Transportation Emergency Center—and **CHEMTEL**. Established by the American Chemistry Council (formerly the Manufacturing Chemists Association), CHEMTREC maintains a 24-hour, toll-free hotline. It provides information on the chemical properties of a substance and explains how the material should be handled. If necessary, CHEMTREC will even contact shippers and manufacturers to find out more detailed information about the incident and provide field assistance. In the United

THE Clorox Company
7200 Johnson Drive
Pleasanton, California 94566
Tel. (415) 847-6100

Safety Data Sheets

Health	2+
Flammability	0
Reactivity	1
Personal Protection	B

I – CHEMICAL IDENTIFICATION

Name regular Clorox Bleach	CAS No. N/A
Description clear, light yellow liquid with chlorine odor	RTECs No. N/A

Other Designations	Manufacturer	Emergency Procedure
EPA Reg. No. 5813-1 Sodium hypochlorite solution Liquid chlorine bleach Clorox Liquid Bleach	The Clorox Company 1221 Broadway Oakland, CA 94612	• Notify your supervisor • Call your local poison control center OR • Rocky Mountain Poison Center (303)573-1014

II – HEALTH HAZARD DATA

• Causes severe but temporary eye injury. May irritate skin. May cause nausea and vomiting if ingested. Exposure to vapor or mist may irritate nose, throat and lungs. The following medical conditions may be aggravated by exposure to high concentrations of vapor or mist: heart conditions or chronic respiratory problems such as asthma, chronic bronchitis or obstructive lung disease. Under normal consumer use conditions the likelihood of any adverse health effects are low. FIRST AID: EYE CONTACT: Immediately flush eyes with plenty of water. If irritation persists, see a doctor. SKIN CONTACT: Remove contaminated clothing. Wash area with water. INGESTION: Drink a glassful of water and call a physician. INHALATION: If breathing problems develop remove to fresh air.

III – HAZARDOUS INGREDIENTS

Ingredients	Concentration	Worker Exposure Limit
Sodium hypochlorite CAS# 7681-52-9	5.25%	not established

None of the ingredients in this product are on the IARC, NTP or OSHA carcinogen list. Occasional clinical reports suggest a low potential for sensitization upon exaggerated exposure to sodium hypochlorite if skin damage (e.g., irritation) occurs during exposure. Routine clinical tests conducted on intact skin with Clorox Liquid Bleach found no sensitization in the test subjects.

IV – SPECIAL PROTECTION INFORMATION

Hygienic Practices: Wear safety glasses. With repeated or prolonged use, wear gloves.

Engineering Controls: Use general ventilation to minimize exposure to vapor or mist.

Work Practices: Avoid eye and skin contact and inhalation of vapor or mist.

V – SPECIAL PRECAUTIONS

Keep out of reach of children. Do not get in eyes or on skin. Wash thoroughly with soap and water after handling. Do not mix with other household chemicals such as toilet bowl cleaners, rust removers, vinegar, acid or ammonia containing products. Store in a cool, dry place. Do not reuse empty container; rinse container and put in trash container.

VI – SPILL OR LEAK PROCEDURES

Small quantities of less than 5 gallons may be flushed down drain. For larger quantities wipe up with an absorbent material or mop and dispose of in accordance with local, state and federal regulations. Dilute with water to minimize oxidizing effect on spilled surface.

VII – REACTIVITY DATA

Stable under normal use and storage conditions. Strong oxidizing agent. Reacts with other household chemicals such as toilet bowl cleaners, rust removers, vinegar, acids or ammonia containing products to produce hazardous gases, such as chlorine and other chlorinated species. Prolonged contact with metal may cause pitting or discoloration.

VIII – FIRE AND EXPLOSION DATA

Not flammable or explosive. In a fire, cool containers to prevent rupture and release of sodium chlorate.

IX – PHYSICAL DATA

Boiling point.................................212°F/100°C (decomposes)
Specific Gravity (H_2O = 1).............1.085
Solubility in Water.........................complete
pH...11.4

FIGURE 13-8 An example of a safety data sheet (SDS).

States and Canada, the toll-free number for CHEMTREC is 800-424-9300. For collect calls and calls from other points of origin, contact 703-527-3887. CHEMTREC can also refer you to the proper agencies for emergencies involving radioactive materials.

CHEMTEL, Inc. maintains another 24-hour, toll-free emergency response communications center for the United States and Canada. In addition to providing support for chemical emergencies, CHEMTEL also supplies the names of state and federal authorities that deal with radioactive incidents. For toll-free calls, dial 800-255-3924. For collect calls and calls from other points of origin, contact 813-248-0585.[4]

The contact numbers given here are printed on the back cover of the ERG.

Hazardous Materials Zones

As already mentioned, your main priority at a hazmat incident is safety. First, you protect your own safety and the safety of your crew. Then you attend to the safety of the patient(s) and the public. To ensure that expert help arrives, request it right away—just as you would under the ICS. Establish command and hold it until relieved by somebody higher in the chain of command.

While waiting for additional support, keep a bad situation from becoming worse by evacuating people from the area around the incident. Do not risk anyone's safety by allowing "heroic" rescues. The result can be only an increased number of contaminated patients. Prepare for the arrival of additional resources by setting up the control zones shown in Figure 13-9. They are:

- ***Hot (red) zone:*** The **hot zone**, also known as the *exclusionary zone*, is the site of contamination. Prevent anyone from entering this area unless they have the appropriate high-level PPE. Hold any patients who escape from this zone in the next zone, where decontamination and/or treatment will be performed.
- ***Warm (yellow) zone:*** The **warm zone**, also called the *contamination reduction zone*, lies immediately adjacent to the hot zone. It forms a "buffer zone" in which a decontamination corridor is established for patients and EMS personnel leaving the hot zone. The corridor has both a "hot" and a "cold" end.
- ***Cold (green) zone:*** The **cold zone**, or *safe zone*, is the area where the incident operation takes place. It includes the command post, medical monitoring and rehabilitation, treatment areas, and apparatus staging. The cold zone must be free of any contamination. No people or equipment from the hot zone should enter until they have undergone the necessary decontamination. You and your crew should remain inside this zone unless you have the necessary training, equipment, and support to enter other areas.

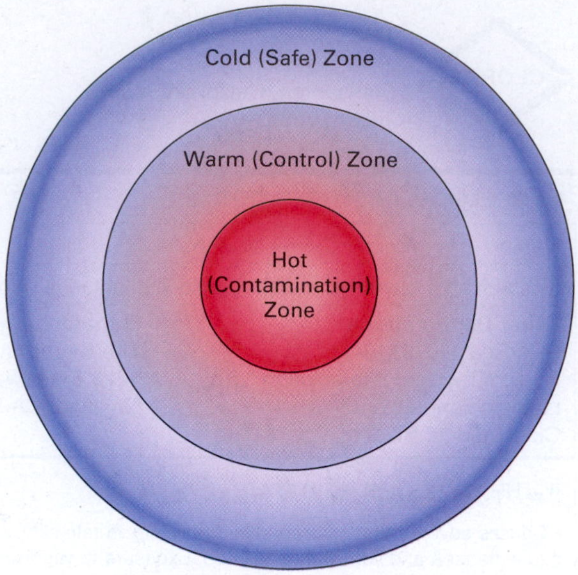

Hot (Contamination) Zone

- Contamination is actually present.
- Personnel must wear appropriate protective gear.
- Number of rescuers limited to those absolutely necessary.
- Bystanders never allowed.

Warm (Control) Zone

- Area surrounding the contamination zone.
- Vital to preventing spread of contamination.
- Personnel must wear appropriate protective gear.
- Lifesaving emergency care is performed.

Cold (Safe) Zone

- Normal triage, stabilization, and treatment are performed.
- Rescuers must shed contaminated gear before entering the cold zone.

FIGURE 13-9 The three zones typically established at a hazmat incident.

Specialized Terminology

To prevent conflicts between the personnel or departments working at a hazmat incident, everyone should use the same terminology. This helps to eliminate dangerous misunderstandings during operations and treatment.

Terms for Medical Hazmat Operations

The following are the general terms that you can expect to encounter during a medical hazmat operation. They apply to situations involving chemical and/or radioactive materials.

- ***Boiling point***—temperature at which a liquid becomes a gas.
- ***Flammable/explosive limits***—range (upper and lower) of vapor concentration in the air at which an ignition will initiate combustion. The lower explosive limit (LEL) is the lowest concentration of chemical that will burn in

the air. Below the LEL, there is not enough chemical to support combustion. The upper explosive limit (UEL) is the highest concentration of chemical that will burn in the air. Above the UEL, there is too much chemical and not enough oxygen to support combustion.

- ***Flash point***—lowest temperature at which a liquid will give off enough vapors to ignite.
- ***Ignition temperature***—lowest temperature at which a liquid will give off enough vapors to support combustion; slightly higher than the flash point.
- ***Specific gravity***—the weight of a volume of liquid compared with an equal volume of water. Chemicals with a specific gravity greater than 1 will sink in water, whereas chemicals with a specific gravity less than 1 will float on water.
- ***Vapor density***—the weight of a vapor or gas compared with the weight of an equal volume of air. Chemicals with a vapor density greater than 1 will fall to the lowest point possible, whereas chemicals with a vapor density less than 1 will rise.
- ***Vapor pressure***—pressure of a vapor against the inside walls of a container. As temperatures increase, so do vapor pressures.
- ***Water solubility***—ability of a chemical to dissolve into solution in water.
- ***Alpha radiation***—neutrons and protons released by the nucleus of a radioactive substance (Figure 13-10). These are very weak particles and will travel only a few inches in the air. Alpha particles are stopped by paper, clothing, or intact skin. They are hazardous if inhaled or ingested.
- ***Beta radiation***—electrons released with great energy by a radioactive substance. Beta particles have more energy than alpha particles and will travel 6 to 10 feet in the air. Beta particles will penetrate a few millimeters of skin.
- ***Gamma radiation***—high-energy photons, such as X-rays. Gamma rays have the ability to penetrate most substances and to damage any cells within the body. Heavy shielding is needed for protection against gamma rays. Because gamma rays are electromagnetic (rather than particles), no decontamination is required. (For more information on the hazards and protection strategies of the three types of radiation, see the chapters "Toxicology and Substance Abuse" and "Environmental Trauma.")

Toxicologic Terms

It is equally important to learn the terminology related to the toxic effects of hazardous materials. Here are the most important toxicologic terms used in the field:

- ***Threshold limit value/time weighted average (TLV/TWA)***—maximum concentration of a substance in the air that a person can be exposed to for 8 hours each day, 40 hours per week, without suffering any adverse health effects. The lower the TLV/TWA, the more toxic the substance. The *permissible exposure limit (PEL)* is a similar measure of toxicity.
- ***Threshold limit value/short-term exposure limit (TLV/STEL)***—maximum concentration of a substance that a person can be exposed to for 15 minutes (time weighted); not to be exceeded or repeated more than four times daily with 60-minute rests between each of the four exposures.
- ***Threshold limit value/ceiling level (TLV-CL)***—maximum concentration of a substance that should never be exceeded, even for a moment.
- ***Lethal concentration/lethal doses (LCt/LD)***—concentration (in air) or dose (if ingested, injected, or absorbed) that results in the death of 50 percent of the test subjects. Also referred to as the LCt50 or LD50.
- ***Parts per million/parts per billion (ppm/ppb)***—representation of the concentration of a substance in the air or a solution, with parts of the substance expressed per million or billion parts of the air or solution.
- ***Immediately dangerous to life and health (IDLH)***—level of concentration of a substance that causes an immediate threat to life. It may also cause delayed or irreversible effects or interfere with a person's ability to remove himself from the contaminated area.

Contamination and Toxicology Review

You have already covered some of the following material in the chapter "Toxicology and Substance Abuse." These points serve as a review, highlighting topics of particular relevance to hazmat situations. Keep this material in mind whenever you come onto any scene in which you suspect the presence of dangerous substances.

Types of Contamination

Whenever people or equipment come into contact with a potentially toxic substance, they are considered to be contaminated. The contamination may be either primary or secondary.

Primary contamination occurs when someone or something is directly exposed to a hazardous substance. At this point, the contamination is limited, that is, the exposure has not yet harmed others.

Secondary contamination takes place when a contaminated person or object comes in contact with an uncontaminated person or object—that is, the contamination is

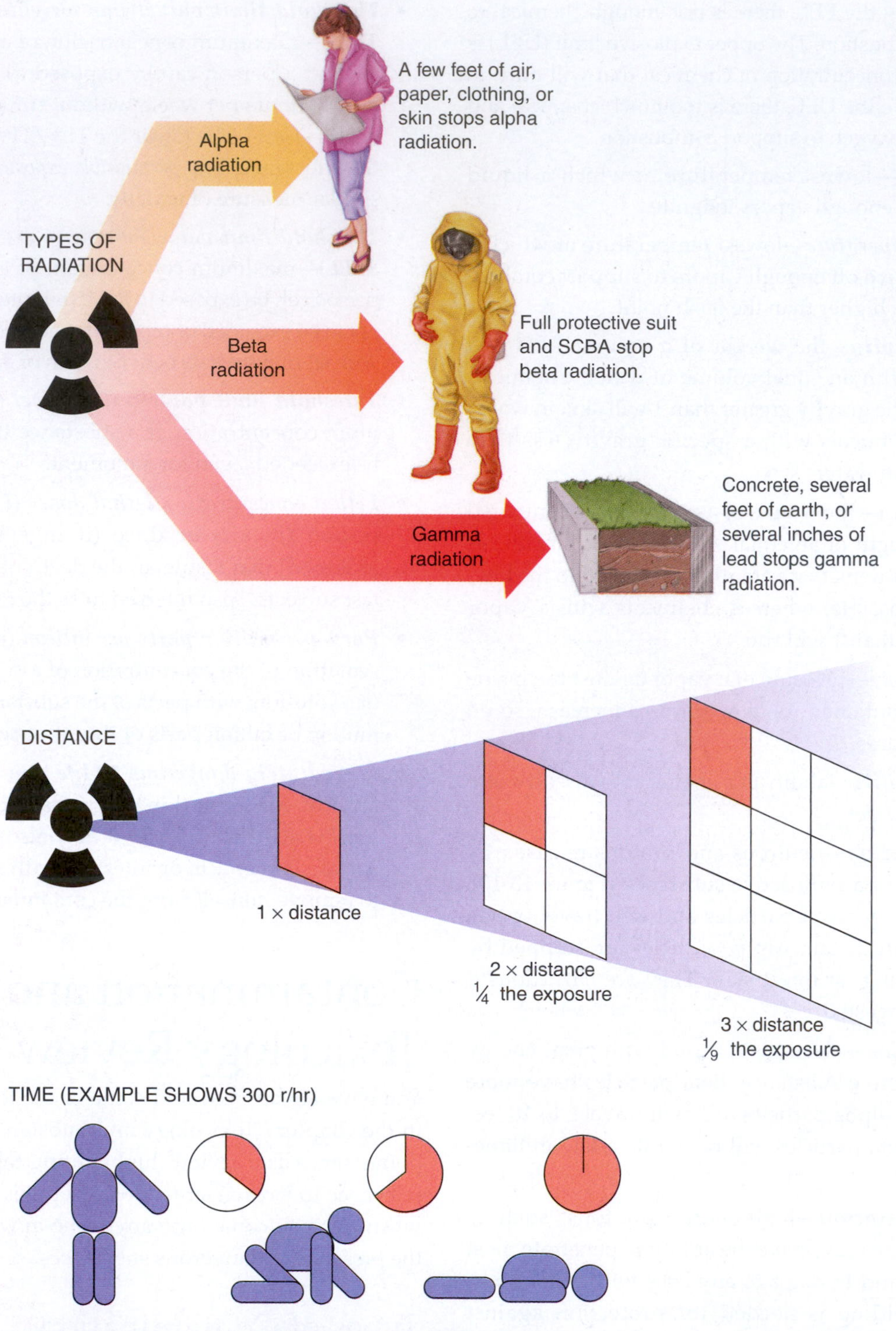

FIGURE 13-10 Alpha, beta, and gamma rays have different powers of penetration.

transferred. If you touch a contaminated patient, for example, you can become a contaminated care provider. Although gas exposure rarely results in secondary contamination, liquid and particulate matter are much more likely to be transferred.

To understand the difference between primary and secondary contamination, consider this example. A chemical pipeline ruptures and sprays several people with a hazardous substance. This is primary contamination. One of these patients walks out of the area and calls an ambulance. On arrival, this same patient climbs into the back of the ambulance, exposing the paramedics and the ambulance to the contaminant. This is secondary contamination. As a member of the EMS crew, you must make every effort not to become part of the incident through such secondary contamination.[5]

CONTENT REVIEW

- Common Routes of Hazmat Exposure
  - Respiratory inhalation
  - Topical absorption
  - Parenteral injection
  - Gastrointestinal ingestion

Routes of Exposure

As you know from the chapter "Toxicology and Substance Abuse," a person can be exposed to a hazardous substance in four ways. The most common method is respiratory inhalation. Gases, liquids, and particulate solids can all be inhaled through the nose or mouth. Once substances enter the bronchial tree, they can be absorbed quickly, especially in oxygen-deficient atmospheres. The substance then enters the central circulation system and is distributed throughout the body. As a result, inhaled substances often trigger a rapid onset of symptoms.

Toxic substances may also be introduced into the body through the skin, either by topical absorption or parenteral injection. Any toxic substance placed topically on intact skin and transferred into the person's circulation is considered a medical threat. In the case of injections, poisons directly enter the body via a laceration, a burn, or a puncture.

In hazmat situations, the least common route of exposure is through gastrointestinal ingestion, but it does happen. In occupations involving hazardous materials, people can be exposed to poisons by eating, drinking, or smoking around deadly substances. Foodstuffs can be exposed to a chemical and then eaten. People can forget to wash their hands and introduce the substance into their mouths.

Cycles and Actions of Poisons

Absorption—the rate at which a substance is delivered into the bloodstream—varies with the type and dosage of the poison. In general, the higher the dose, the greater the effect the substance will have on the body. Because of the wide variety of toxic substances, you will need to rely on the resources mentioned earlier to determine a given substance's actions, distribution to target organs, likely areas of deposit, and so on.

Basically, a poison's actions may be acute or delayed. **Acute effects** include signs and symptoms that manifest themselves immediately or shortly after exposure. **Delayed effects** may not become apparent for hours, days, weeks, months, or even years. If a person is exposed to chlorine gas, for example, he immediately develops shortness of breath—an acute effect. If a person is exposed to a carcinogen, on the other hand, it may take many years before a malignancy develops—a delayed effect. Some substances, such as mustard gas (a military blister agent), cause immediate damage, but victims do not develop symptoms for many hours.

Once a substance is introduced into the body, it is distributed to target organs. Effects from a chemical may be local or systemic. **Local effects** involve areas around the immediate site and should be evaluated based on standard criteria such as the rule of nines, which was described in the chapter "Burns." You can usually expect some skin irritation (topical) or perhaps acute bronchospasm (respiratory). An acid sprayed on the skin, for example, creates immediate skin damage at the point of contact.

Systemic effects occur throughout the body. They can affect the cardiovascular, neurologic, hepatic, and/or renal systems. For example, although hydrofluoric acid may cause local skin burns on contact, it can also trigger hypocalcemia and arrhythmias. As a result, exposure to this substance can be potentially fatal.

The organs most commonly associated with toxic substances are the liver and the kidneys. The liver metabolizes most substances by chemically altering them through a process known as **biotransformation**. The kidneys can usually excrete the substances through the urine. However, both the liver and kidneys may be adversely affected by chemicals as are other organ systems. In such situations, the body may not be able to eliminate the toxic substances, creating a life-threatening situation.

When treating patients exposed to toxic substances, keep in mind that two substances or drugs may work together to produce an effect that neither of them can produce on their own. This effect, known as **synergism**, is part of the standard pharmacological approach to medicine. Before administering any medication, be sure to consult with medical direction or the poison control center on possible synergistic effects or treatments.

Treatment of Common Exposures

As noted several times, patients can be exposed to an incredibly large number of chemicals. Their treatment ranges from supportive care to specific antidotes. After ensuring your own safety, you should see that all patients receive the necessary supportive measures: airway support and suctioning, respiratory support, supplemental oxygen, circulatory support, and intravenous access. Before administering specific pharmacological treatment, at least two sources should agree on the medication. In addition, you should confer with medical direction, as previously mentioned.

The following subsections cover several of the most common classifications of chemicals to which patients may be exposed. A brief overview of effects and treatment procedures is provided for each circumstance. Keep in mind that this is a generic discussion

CONTENT REVIEW

- Hazmat Chemical Classifications
  - Corrosives—acids and bases
  - Pulmonary irritants—fumes from chlorine and ammonia
  - Pesticides—carbamates and organophosphates
  - Chemical asphyxiants—carbon monoxide and cyanides
  - Hydrocarbon solvents—xylene and methylene chloride

and is not intended to replace the specific identification resources already described.

Corrosives

Corrosives—acids and alkalis (bases)—can be found in many everyday materials. Most drain cleaners, for example, contain the alkali sodium hydroxide. Depending on the concentration, these substances can damage skin and other tissues. Corrosives can be inhaled, ingested, absorbed, or injected. Primary effects include severe skin burns, respiratory burns, and/or edema. Some corrosives may also have systemic effects.

When decontaminating a patient exposed to solid corrosives, brush off dry particles. In the case of liquid corrosives, flush the exposed area with large quantities of water. Tincture of green soap may help in decontamination. Irrigate eye injuries with water, possibly using a topical ophthalmic anesthetic such as tetracaine to reduce eye discomfort. In patients with pulmonary edema, consider the administration of furosemide (Lasix) or albuterol. If the patient has ingested a corrosive, *do not* induce vomiting. If the patient can swallow and is not drooling, you may direct the person to drink 5 mL/kg water up to 200 mL. As with other injuries, maintain and support the ABCs: airway, breathing, and circulation.

Pulmonary Irritants

Many different substances can be pulmonary irritants, including the fumes from chlorine and ammonia. When inhaled, chlorine mixes with respiratory secretions to produce hydrochloric acid. Ammonia mixes with respiratory secretions to produce ammonium hydroxide, an alkali. In addition to tissue damage, these chemicals can cause pulmonary edema. The substances can also injure intact skin. Liquid ammonia, for example, will cause cold burns.

Primary respiratory exposure cannot be decontaminated. However, you should remove the patient's clothing to prevent any trapped gas from being contained near the body. You should also flush any exposed skin with large quantities of water. Irrigate eye injuries with water, possibly using tetracaine to reduce eye discomfort. Treat pulmonary edema with furosemide, if indicated. Again, treatment includes maintaining and supporting the ABCs.

Pesticides

Toxic pesticides or insecticides include primarily carbamates and organophosphates. Patients may come in contact with these chemicals through any of the four routes of exposure: inhalation, absorption, ingestion, or injection. The substances can act to block **acetylcholinesterase (AChE)**, an enzyme that stops the action of acetylcholine, a neurotransmitter. The result is overstimulation of the muscarinic receptors and the SLUDGE syndrome: Salivation, Lacrimation, Urination, Diarrhea, Gastrointestinal distress, and Emesis. Stimulation of the nicotinic receptor may also trigger involuntary contraction of the muscles and pinpoint pupils.

These chemicals will continue to be absorbed as long as they remain on the skin. As a result, decontamination with large amounts of water and tincture of green soap is essential. Remove all clothing and jewelry to prevent the chemical from being trapped against the skin. Maintain and support the ABCs. Secretions in the airway may need to be suctioned.

The primary treatment for significant exposure to pesticides is atropinization. The dose should be increased until the SLUDGE symptoms start to resolve. For carbamates, pralidoxime is *not* recommended. If an adult patient presents with seizures, administer 5 to 10 mg of diazepam. Do *not* induce vomiting if the patient has ingested the chemical.

Chemical Asphyxiants

The most common chemical asphyxiants include carbon monoxide (CO) and cyanides such as bitter almond oil, hydrocyanic acid, potassium cyanide, wild cherry syrup, prussic acid, and nitroprusside. Keep in mind that both CO and cyanides are by-products of combustion, so patients who present with smoke inhalation may need to be assessed for these substances as well. Most patients are exposed to CO and cyanides through inhalation. However, keep in mind that cyanides can also be ingested, absorbed, or injected.

These two chemicals have different actions once inhaled. Carbon monoxide has a very high affinity for hemoglobin—approximately 200 times greater than oxygen. As a result, it displaces oxygen in the red blood cells. Cyanides, however, inhibit the action of **cytochrome oxidase**. This enzyme complex, found in cellular mitochondria, enables oxygen to create the adenosine triphosphate (ATP) required for all muscle energy. Primary effects of CO exposure include changes in mental status and other signs of hypoxia such as chest pain, loss of consciousness, or seizures. Primary effects of cyanides include rapid onset of unconsciousness, seizures, and cardiopulmonary arrest.

Decontamination of patients exposed to CO and cyanide asphyxiants is usually unnecessary. However, these patients must be removed from the toxic environment without exposing rescuers to inhalation. Take off the patient's clothing to prevent entrapment of any toxic gases, while maintaining airway, breathing, and circulatory support. Definitive treatment for CO inhalation is oxygenation. In some cases, it may be provided through hyperbaric therapy, which increases the displacement of carbon monoxide from hemoglobin molecules by oxygen.

Definitive treatment for cyanide exposure can be provided by one of two cyanide antidotes. The older system, generally referred to as a cyanide antidote kit (also called a Pasadena, Lilly, or Taylor kit) contains three medications:

CONTENT REVIEW

- ➤ Use of Cyanide Kit
  - Administer ampule of amyl nitrite for 15 seconds.
  - Repeat at 1-minute intervals until sodium nitrite is ready.
  - Administer infusion of sodium nitrite, 300 mg IV push over 5 minutes.
  - Follow with infusion of sodium thiosulfate, 12.5 g IV push over 5 minutes.
  - Repeat at half original doses, if necessary.

amyl nitrite, sodium nitrite, and sodium thiosulfate. If this kit is used, first administer amyl nitrite. This short-acting vasodilator has the ability to convert hemoglobin to methemoglobin, which forms a nontoxic complex with cyanide ions. Wrap an ampule in gauze or cloth and crush it between your fingers. Then place it in front of a spontaneously breathing patient for 15 seconds. Repeat at 1-minute intervals until an infusion of sodium nitrite is ready. Keep in mind that amyl nitrite is volatile and highly flammable when mixed with air or oxygen. Next, administer the sodium nitrite, 300 mg IV push over 5 minutes. (Sodium nitrite also produces methemoglobin.) Quickly follow the sodium nitrite with an infusion of sodium thiosulfate, 12.5 g IV push over 5 minutes. The sodium thiosulfate converts the cyanide/methemoglobin complexes into thiocyanate, which can be excreted by the kidneys. If the signs and symptoms reappear, the process should be repeated at half the original doses.

A safer and less toxic antidote is now available (Figure 13-11). This antidote, called hydroxocobalamin, is commercially available and packaged as Cyano-Kit™. Hydroxocobalamin is a precursor to cyanocobalamin (vitamin B_{12}). When hydroxocobalamin is administered, it binds cyanide from cytochrome oxidase and forms cyanocobalamin. Excess cyanocobalamin is excreted from the body via the kidneys.[6]

Hydrocarbon Solvents

Many different chemicals can act as solvents, including xylene and methylene chloride. Usually found in liquid form, they give off easily inhaled vapors. Primary effects include arrhythmias, pulmonary edema, and respiratory failure. Delayed effects include damage to the central nervous system and the renal system. Exposure to these chemicals may be intentional, such as among drug abusers seeking the central nervous system effects (euphoria) produced by the fumes. If the patient ingests the chemical and vomits, aspiration may lead to pulmonary edema.

Treatment varies with the route of exposure. In cases of topical contact, decontaminate the exposed area with large quantities of warm water and tincture of green soap. If the patient has ingested the solvent, *do not* induce vomiting. If the adult patient presents with seizures, administer 5 to 10 mg of diazepam. In the case of inhalation, maintain and support the ABCs.

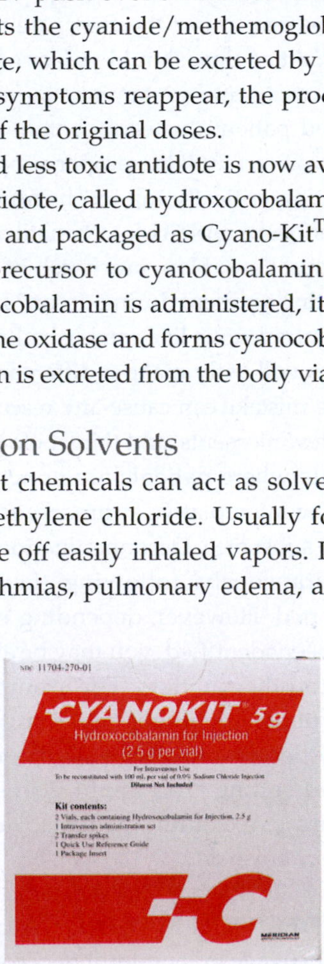

FIGURE 13-11 The Cyano-Kit.
(© Dr. Bryan E. Bledsoe)

Approaches to Decontamination

Decontamination, as you have read, attempts to reduce or remove hazardous substances from people and/or equipment to prevent adverse health effects. Decontamination can be accomplished by physical or chemical means. Physical decontamination involves the removal of chemicals by separating them from the person or equipment, whereas chemical decontamination focuses on changing the hazardous substance into something less harmful.

Decontamination (decon) procedures serve several purposes. First, decon reduces the dosage of the material to which patients are exposed. Second, it reduces the risk of secondary contamination of rescuers, on-scene personnel, bystanders, hospital personnel, the families of rescuers, and the general public.

Methods of Decontamination

The four methods of decontamination are dilution, absorption, neutralization, and isolation/disposal. The method used depends on the type of hazardous substance and the route of exposure. In many instances, rescuers will use two or more of these methods during the decontamination process.

Dilution

Dilution involves the application of large quantities of water to the contaminated person or item. Water is considered the universal decon solution, especially for reducing topical absorption. It may be aided by use of a soap, such as tincture of green soap. Mixing hazardous substances with water significantly reduces their concentration, hopefully to a level at which they are no longer dangerous. Be aware that a small number of chemicals should never be mixed with water.

CONTENT REVIEW

- ➤ Methods of Decontamination
  - Dilution
  - Absorption (blotting)
  - Neutralization
  - Isolation/disposal

Absorption

Absorption entails the use of pads or towels to "blot" up the hazardous material. The process is usually applied after washing with water—that is, as a means of drying the patient. Absorption further reduces the contamination levels but is not usually a primary method of decon. Absorption is more commonly used during environmental cleanup.

Neutralization

Neutralization occurs when one substance reduces or eliminates the toxicity of another substance, such as adding an acid to a base. Although this is a third method of patient decontamination, it is almost never used by EMS personnel. In a field setting, it is difficult to identify the exact hazardous substance and the proper neutralizing agent. In addition, neutralization often produces an exothermic reaction, or release of large quantities of heat. The heat can be just as damaging as, or even more damaging than, the original chemical. Lavage usually dilutes and removes the chemical faster and is more practical given the typical on-scene equipment.

Isolation/Disposal

Isolation and/or disposal involves separating the patient or equipment from the hazardous substance. Isolation begins by establishing zones at the incident to prevent any further contamination or exposure. Next, hazmat teams remove patients from the hot zone to the warm zone. Last, any items that might contain or trap a hazardous substance should be removed, including a patient's clothing and jewelry. All contaminated items should be properly disposed of or stored.

Decontamination Decision Making

In performing decontamination, always recall the priorities of incident management: life safety, incident stabilization, and property conservation. These priorities should guide your decision making throughout the incident. For example, you should try to prevent any water runoff used for decontamination from damaging the environment. However, environmental considerations form a major concern only when there are no life threats—that is, when patients are stable and not expected to deteriorate during the decon process. If life threats exist, the patients come first; environmental considerations come last.

Modes of Operation

In general, EMS personnel engage in one of two modes of operation at hazmat incidents that generate patients: "fast-break" decision making or long-term decision making. Fast-break decision making occurs at incidents that call for immediate action to prevent rescuer contamination and/or to handle obvious life threats. Long-term decision making takes place at extended events in which hazmat teams retrieve patients, identify the hazardous substance, and determine methods of decontamination and treatment.

FAST-BREAK DECISION MAKING At hazmat incidents where patients are conscious, contaminated victims will often self-rescue. They will walk from the primary incident site to the EMS units. In such cases, you must make fast-break decisions to prevent rescuer contamination. Keep in mind that it may take time for a hazmat team to arrive and set up operations. In the interim, the conscious, contaminated patients may try to leave the scene entirely. As a result, all EMS units must be prepared for gross decontamination. Basic personal protective equipment should be onboard and all personnel should be familiar with the two-step decontamination procedures covered later in this chapter.

Implement this mode of decision making at all incidents with critical patients and unknown or life-threatening materials. Fire apparatus often respond very quickly and carry large quantities of water that can be used for decon. Remove patient clothing, treat life-threatening problems, and wash with water. Although it is preferable to use warm water to prevent hypothermia, this option is not always available. Please remember the first rule of EMS: *Do not become a patient!* At no time should you or other crew members expose yourselves to contaminants—even to rescue a critically injured patient. Instead, contain and isolate the patient as best you can until the proper support arrives.

When treating critically injured hazmat patients, it is important to perform a rapid risk-to-benefit assessment. Ask yourself these questions: How much risk of exposure will I incur by intubating a patient during decon? Does the patient really need an intravenous line established right now? Few ALS procedures will truly make a difference if performed rapidly, but one mistake can cause any rescuer to become a patient. Take a few moments, and think before you act.

At incidents where patients are noncritical, rescuers can take a more contemplative approach, especially if they can identify the substance. Decontamination and treatment proceed simultaneously, following the general steps already mentioned. However, depending on whether the substance has been identified, you may be able to give special attention to other matters. For example, you might contain water runoff. You might better protect patient privacy by grossly decontaminating ambulatory patients in a more controlled setting. You might also spend time on patient monitoring, reclothing patients, isolating or containing patients, and so on.

LONG-TERM DECISION MAKING At more extended events, you will engage in long-term decision making. This mode of operation most often occurs when patients remain in the hot zone and have not self-rescued. Traditionally,

CONTENT REVIEW

➤ Most Common Decontamination Solvents
- Water
- Tincture of green soap
- Isopropyl alcohol
- Vegetable oil

CONTENT REVIEW

➤ Two-Step Decon
- Removal of clothing and personal effects
- Gross decontamination (two times)

EMS personnel have not been trained or equipped to enter the hot zone to retrieve these patients. Instead, a hazmat team is summoned promptly, and the EMS crew awaits the team's arrival. The team will not make its entry until you or members of your crew perform the necessary medical monitoring and establish a decontamination corridor. It often takes 60 minutes or more for actual team deployment.

This mode of operation provides a number of advantages: a better opportunity for thorough decontamination, better PPE, less chance of secondary decontamination, greater consideration of the environment, and more detailed research of the actual hazardous substance. Obviously, long-term decision making presents less opportunity for error and is preferable to fast-break decision making. Unfortunately, self-rescued patients often force a decision about the mode of operation the minute you arrive on the scene. Be prepared for fast-break operations whenever you suspect a potential hazmat incident.

Field Decontamination

As mentioned, the decontamination method and type of PPE depend on the substance involved. If in doubt, assume the worst-case scenario. When dealing with unknowns, do not attempt to neutralize. Brush dry particles off the patient before the application of water to prevent possible chemical reactions. Next, wash with great quantities of water—the universal decon agent—using tincture of green soap if possible. Isopropyl alcohol is an effective agent for some isocyanates, and vegetable oil can be used to decon water-reactive substances.

Two-Step Process

Use the two-step decon process for gross decontamination of patients who cannot wait for a more comprehensive decon process, usually patients at a fast-break incident.

- **Step 1:** Rescuers remove or instruct patients to remove all clothing, including shoes, socks, and jewelry. (Remember to have some method of accounting for personal effects *before* hazmat incidents occur.)
- **Step 2:** Rescuers wash and rinse the patients with soap and water, making sure that they do not stay in contact with the runoff. Repeat the process, allowing the fluid to drain away each time. It is important to pay special attention to difficult contamination areas such as the scalp and hair, ears, nostrils, axillae, fingernails, navel, genitals, groin, buttocks, behind the knees, between the toes, and toenails.

Eight-Step Process

The eight-step process takes place in a complete decontamination corridor and is much more thorough. To leave the hot zone, the hazmat rescuers follow these steps:

- **Step 1:** Rescuers enter the decon area at the hot end of the corridor and mechanically remove contaminants from the victims.
- **Step 2:** Rescuers drop equipment in a tool-drop area and remove outer gloves.
- **Step 3:** Decon personnel shower and scrub all victims and rescuers, using gross decontamination. As surface decontamination is removed, the dilution is conducted into a contained area. Victims may be moved ahead to Step 6 or Step 7.
- **Step 4:** Rescuers remove and isolate their self-contained breathing apparatus (SCBA). If reentry is necessary, the team dons new SCBA from a noncontaminated side.
- **Step 5:** Rescuers remove all protective clothing. Articles are isolated, labeled for disposal, and placed on the contaminated side.
- **Step 6:** Rescuers remove all personal clothing. Victims who have not had their clothing removed have it taken off here. All items are isolated in plastic bags and labeled for later disposal or storage.
- **Step 7:** Rescuers and victims receive a full-body washing, using soft scrub brushes or sponges, water, and mild soap or detergent. Cleaning tools are bagged for later disposal.
- **Step 8:** Patients receive rapid assessment and stabilization before being transported to hospitals for further care. EMS crews medically monitor rescuers, complete exposure records, and transport rescuers to hospitals as needed.

These procedures are not set in stone. Small variations may exist from system to system. You should become familiar with the specific procedures in the jurisdiction where you practice.

Transportation Considerations

Remember that no patient who undergoes field decontamination is truly decontaminated. Field-decontaminated patients, sometimes called **semi-decontaminated patients**, may still need to undergo a more invasive decon process at a medical facility. Depending on the type of exposure, wounds may need debridement, hair or nails may need to be trimmed or removed, and so on. However, it is always better to deliver a grossly decontaminated living patient to the hospital than a perfectly decontaminated corpse. Just make sure that field-decontaminated patients are transported to facilities capable of performing more thorough decon procedures.

When transporting field-decontaminated patients, always recall that they may still have some contamination in or on them. For example, a patient may have ingested a chemical, which can be expelled if the patient coughs or vomits. As a result, use as much disposable equipment as possible. Keep in mind that any airborne hazard not only can incapacitate the crew in the back of the ambulance but can affect the driver as well. Although it is not practical to line the ambulance in plastic, you can isolate the patient using a stretcher decon pool. The pool can help contain any potentially contaminated body fluids. Plastic can also be used to cover the pool, adding yet another protective barrier.

Hazmat Protection Equipment

As you know, the personal protective equipment used at a hazmat incident is specifically designed to prevent or limit rescuer injuries (Figures 13-12a through 13-12d). Hard hats, for example, protect rescuers against impacts to the head. There are basically four levels of hazmat protective equipment, ranging from Level A (the highest level) to Level D (the minimum level).

- *Level A*—provides the highest level of respiratory and splash protection. This hazmat suit offers a high degree of protection against chemical breakthrough and fully encapsulates the rescuer, even covering the SCBA. The sealed, impermeable suits are typically used by hazmat teams entering hot zones with an unknown substance and a significant potential for both respiratory and dermal hazards.
- *Level B*—offers full respiratory protection when there is a lower probability of dermal hazard. The Level B suit is nonencapsulating, but chemically resistant. Seams for zippers, gloves, boots, and mask interface are usually sealed with duct tape. The SCBA is worn outside the suit, allowing increased maneuverability

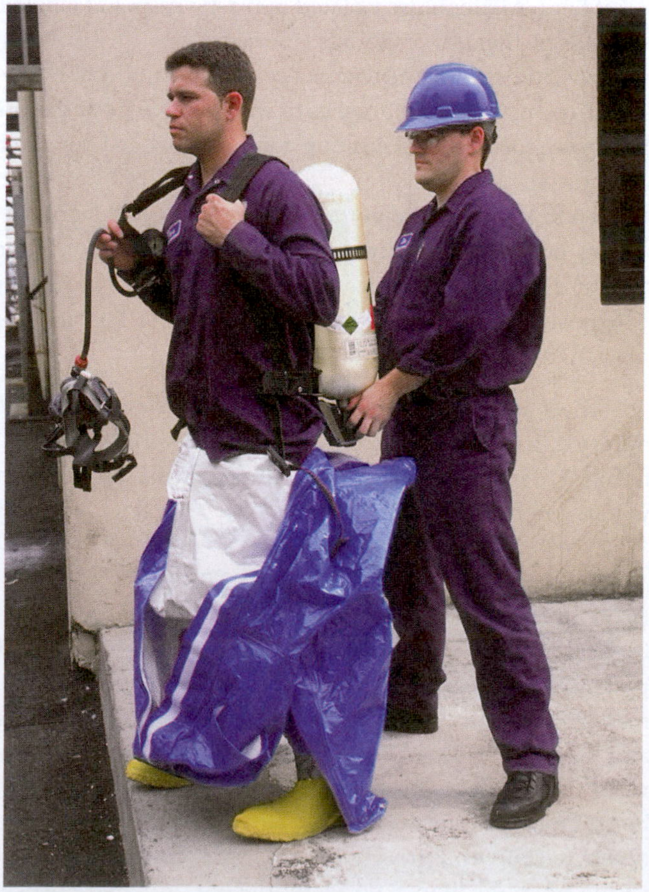

FIGURE 13-12a Assisting with an air tank.

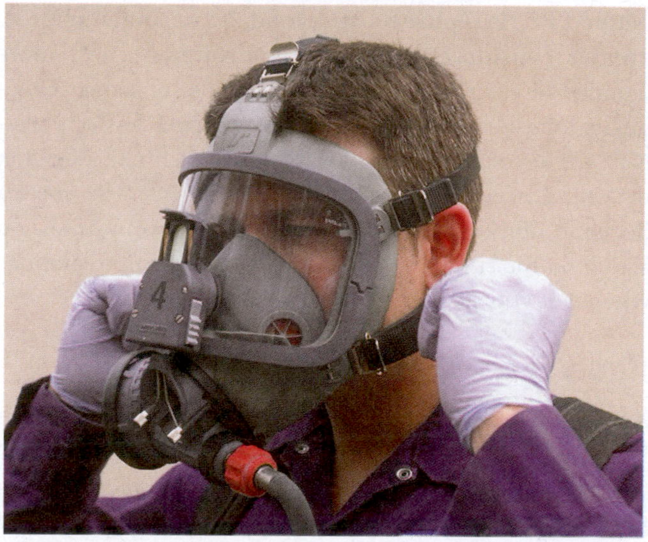

FIGURE 13-12b Putting on a mask.

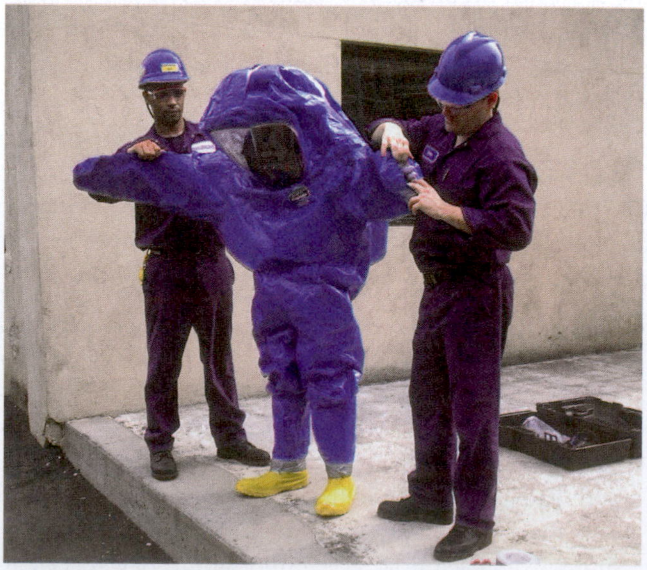

FIGURE 13-12c Assisting with a hood.

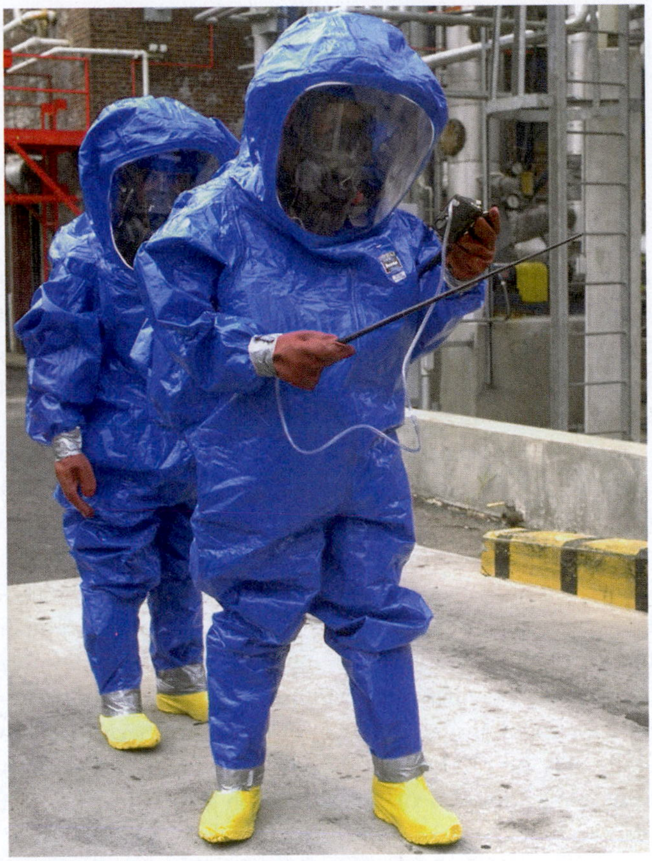

FIGURE 13-12d Hazmat team fully suited.

and greater ease in changing SCBA bottles. The decon team typically wears Level B protective equipment.

- *Level C*—includes a nonpermeable suit, boots, and gear for protecting eyes and hands. Instead of SCBA, Level C protective equipment uses an **air-purifying respirator (APR)**. The APR relies on filters to protect against a known contaminant in a normal environment. As a result, the canisters in the APR must be specifically selected and are not usually implemented in a hazmat emergency response. Level C clothing is usually worn during transport of patients with the potential for secondary contamination.
- *Level D*—consists of structural firefighter, or turnout, gear. Level D gear is usually not suitable for hazmat incidents.

The level of hazmat protective gear worn depends on the chemical or substance involved. Ideally, the chemical should be identified so a permeability chart can be consulted to determine the breakthrough time. No single material is suitable to all hazmat situations. Some materials are resistant to certain chemicals and nonresistant to others.

EMS personnel should not become involved in any hazmat situation without the proper PPE. All ambulances carry some level of PPE, even if not ideal. If the situation is emergent and the chemical unknown, use as much barrier protection as possible. Full turnout gear (Level D) or a Tyvek suit is better than no gear at all. High-efficiency particulate air (HEPA) filter masks and double or triple gloves offer good protection against some hazards. Keep in mind that latex gloves are not chemically resistant. Instead, use nitrile gloves, which have a high resistance to most chemicals. Also remember that leather boots will absorb chemicals permanently, so be sure to don rubber boots.

Medical Monitoring and Rehabilitation

As noted, one of the primary roles of EMS personnel at a hazmat incident is the medical monitoring of entry personnel. All hazmat team members should undergo regular annual physical examinations, with baseline vital signs placed on file.

Entry Readiness

Prior to entry, you or other EMS crew members will assess rescuers and document the following information on an incident flow sheet: blood pressure, pulse, respiratory rate, temperature, body weight, ECG, and mental/neurologic status. If you observe anything abnormal, do not allow the hazmat team member to attempt a rescue.

Hazmat team members will enter the hot zone only in groups of two, with two more members in PPE remaining outside the hot zone as a backup team. The PPE used at hazmat incidents can cause significant stress and dehydration. As a result, entry team personnel should prehydrate themselves with 8 to 16 ounces of water or sports drinks. Because sports drinks are more effective at half strength, dilute them with 50 percent water when possible.

Post-Exit Rehab

After the hazmat entry team exits the hot zone and completes decontamination, they should report back to EMS for post-entry monitoring (Figure 13-13). Measure and document the same parameters on the flow sheet. Rehydrate the team with more water or diluted sports drinks. You can use weight changes to estimate any fluid losses. Check with medical direction or protocols to determine fluid replacement by means of PO or IV. Entry team members should not be allowed to reenter the hot zone until they are alert, nontachycardic, normotensive, and within a reasonable percentage of their normal body weight.

CONTENT REVIEW

➤ Pre-Entry/Post-Exit Documentation
- Blood pressure
- Pulse
- Respiratory rate
- Temperature
- Body weight
- ECG
- Mental/neurologic status

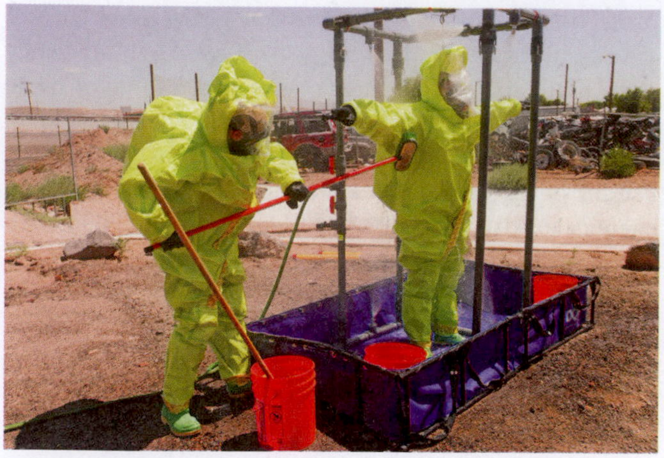

FIGURE 13-13 Rescuers involved in the decontamination process.

Heat Stress Factors

In evaluating heat stress, you will need to take many factors into account. Primary considerations include temperature and humidity. Prehydration, duration and degree of activity, and the team member's overall physical fitness will also have a bearing on your evaluation. Keep in mind that Level A suits protect a rescuer, but prevent cooling. A rescuer essentially works inside an encapsulated sauna. The same suit that seals out hazards also prevents heat loss by evaporation, conduction, convection, and radiation. Therefore, place heat stress at the top of your list of tasks for post-exit medical monitoring.

Importance of Practice

As a paramedic, you will play an important role at any hazmat incident. You may establish command, make the first incident decisions, and help protect all on-scene personnel, including the hazmat team. As a result, you should practice skills that you can expect to use in most EMS systems.

Here are some things you should routinely do. Put on and take off Level B hazmat protective equipment. Set up a rapid two-step decontamination process and an eight-step decontamination process, preferably with the help of the local hazmat team. With a crew member, identify a simulated chemical, determine the correct PPE, and establish the proper decontamination methods. Practice pre-entry and post-exit medical monitoring and documentation. Prepare a patient and ambulance for transport. Because these skills may be rarely used except in the busiest EMS systems, you should work closely with your local hazmat team to practice these skills on a regular basis.

Summary

Every member of an EMS team should be prepared to face the challenges of a hazmat incident. At all times, keep in mind the high potential for rescuer involvement in a hazmat incident, especially during the early phases. As with any EMS operation, the primary consideration is your own safety. No patient's life is worth your own. This is especially true at a fast-break incident in which you must resist heroic efforts that will place you in contact with ambulatory, self-rescued patients. You become useless at a hazmat incident if you become contaminated yourself.

You Make the Call

You are dispatched to a motor vehicle collision on an interstate highway. You arrive on scene and find that a car has rear-ended a tractor-trailer. Two people exit the cab of the truck and begin to walk toward the ambulance. Both have obvious respiratory distress. You note that the driver of the car appears to be unresponsive behind the steering wheel.

You do a quick windshield size-up for hazards and see a black-and-white placard on the rear of the truck. The placard bears a skull and crossbones and two numbers, 6 and 2783. You notice some liquid dripping from the rear door of the truck onto the hood of the car.

The occupants of the truck walk up to the side of the ambulance. You observe that they are drooling, tearing, and sweating profusely. One of them knocks on your window and says, "Please help us. We can't breathe."

1. What do you suspect has happened based on your quick scene size-up?
2. What are your initial priorities?

3. How will you identify the substance involved in the accident?
4. What additional resources would you request?
5. Is this a fast-break or a long-term incident? Explain.
6. What are your first actions?

See Suggested Responses at the back of this book.

Review Questions

1. Which standard, along with two other NFPA standards for hazmat response, deals with the training standards for EMS personnel assigned to hazmat incidents?
   a. CRF 1910.120
   b. 40 CFR 311
   c. NFPA 473
   d. ASTM 1147
2. Which of the following does *not* represent one of the three levels of training appropriate to EMS response at hazmat incidents?
   a. Awareness Level
   b. EMS Technician Level
   c. EMS Level 1
   d. EMS Level 2
3. The basic Incident Command System (ICS) at a hazmat incident will require which component(s)?
   a. Command post
   b. Staging area
   c. Decontamination corridor
   d. All of the above
4. Which organization has implemented a placard system to identify dangerous substances in transit?
   a. UN
   b. DOT
   c. NFPA
   d. NIOSH
5. Which source of information maintains a 24-hour, toll-free hotline; provides information on the chemical properties of a substance; and explains how the material should be handled?
   a. EPA
   b. NOAA
   c. CHEMTREC
   d. CAMEO
6. Within which zone does the incident operation take place, including the command post, medical monitoring and rehabilitation, treatment areas, and apparatus staging?
   a. Hot (red) zone
   b. Warm (yellow) zone
   c. Exclusionary (orange) zone
   d. Cold (green) zone
7. Which is the most common method by which a person can be exposed to a hazardous substance?
   a. Respiratory inhalation
   b. Topical absorption
   c. Parenteral injection
   d. Gastrointestinal ingestion
8. What is considered to be the universal decon solution, especially for reducing topical absorption?
   a. Water
   b. Oxygen
   c. Atropine
   d. Sodium nitrite
9. You may need to use "fast-break decision making" when dealing with what type of patient at a hazardous scene?
   a. A pediatric patient who was covered in gasoline from a car wreck
   b. A grossly contaminated but uninjured patient walking away from the scene of the incident
   c. A dead patient who is contaminated, and may contaminate others when he is moved
   d. Any patient who is found unresponsive at the scene of a hazardous spill
10. With time and supplies allowing, what should be used when assisting with the decontamination of a victim covered with a water-reactive substance?
    a. Isopropyl alcohol
    b. Water
    c. Vegetable oil
    d. Dehydronated water

See Answers to Review Questions at the end of this book.

References

1. U. S. Department of Transportation, Pipeline and Hazardous Materials Safety Administration. Definitions. (Available at http://www.phmsa.dot.gov/public/definitions.)
2. Keim, M. M. "The Public Health Impact of Industrial Disasters." *Am J Disaster Med* 6 (2011): 265–272.
3. Decker, R. J. "Acceptance and Utilization of the Incident Command System in the First Response and Allied Disciplines: An Ohio Study." *J Bus Contin Emer Plan* 5 (2011): 224–230.
4. Oberg, M., N. Palmen, and G. Johanson. "Discrepancy among Acute Guidelines for Emergency Response." *J Hazard Mater* 184 (2010): 439–447.
5. Scanlon, J. "Chemically Contaminated Casualties: Different Problems and Possible Solutions." *Am J Disaster Med* 5 (2010): 95–105.
6. Hall, A. H, J. Saiers, and F. Baud. "Which Cyanide Antidote?" *Crit Rev Toxicol* 39 (2009): 514–552.

Further Readings

De Lorenzo, R. A., and R. S. Porter. *Weapons of Mass Destruction: Emergency Care*. Upper Saddle River, NJ: Pearson/Prentice Hall, 2000.

Emergency Response Guidebook: A Guidebook for First Responders During the Initial Phase of a Dangerous Goods/Hazardous Materials Transportation. Washington, DC: U.S. Department of Transportation, 2008.

Leonard, J. E., and G. D. Robinson. *Managing Hazardous Materials*. Rockville, MD: Institute of Hazardous Materials Management, 2002.

Meyer, E. *Chemistry of Hazardous Materials*. 4th ed. Upper Saddle River, NJ: Pearson/Prentice Hall, 2005.

NFPA 473. *Standard Competencies for EMS Personnel Responding to Hazardous Materials Incidents*. 2013 ed. Quincy, MA: National Fire Protection Agency.

NFPA 704. *Standard for Identification of the Fire Hazards of Materials*. 2012 ed. Quincy, MA: National Fire Protection Agency.

Noll, G. G., M. S. Hildebrand, and J. G. Yvorra. *Hazardous Materials: Managing the Incident*. 3rd ed. Chester, MD: Red Hat Publishing, 2005.

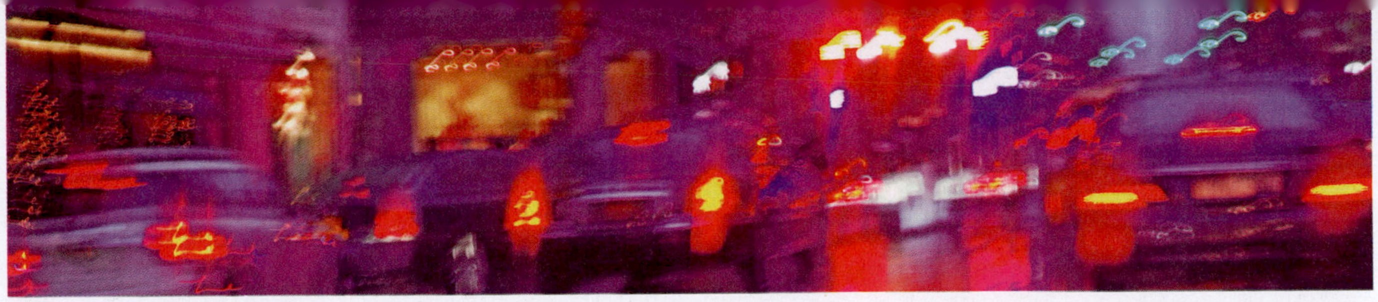

Chapter 14
Crime Scene Awareness

Bryan Bledsoe, DO, FACEP, FAAEM, EMT-P
Dale Carrison, DO, FACEP, FACOEP
Daniel Limmer, AS, EMT-P

STANDARD
Assessment (Scene Size-Up)

COMPETENCY
Integrates scene and patient assessment findings with knowledge of epidemiology and pathophysiology to form a field impression. This includes developing a list of differential diagnoses through clinical reasoning to modify the assessment and formulate a treatment plan.

Learning Objectives

Terminal Performance Objective: After reading this chapter, you should be able to integrate the special considerations involved in response to crime scenes and increased risk of violence into the overall approach to scene management and patient care.

Enabling Objectives: To accomplish the terminal performance objective, you should be able to:

1. Define key terms introduced in this chapter.
2. Describe the epidemiology and demographics of violence in the United States.
3. Describe the actions you should take to protect your safety when you are advised of danger before you reach the scene, to observe danger on arriving at the scene, and when danger arises during a call.
4. Identify steps to take to avoid dangers you may encounter when responding to calls on the roadside or highway, or responding to violent street events.
5. Describe the tactical options of retreat, concealment, cover, distraction, evasion, contact and cover, warning signals, and communication when situations call for their use.
6. Identify the advantages and limitations of using body armor.
7. Describe the role of tactical EMS.
8. Discuss the roles of EMS and how to integrate into and interact cooperatively with law enforcement to provide patient care while maintaining awareness of crime scene and evidence considerations.

KEY TERMS

blood spatter evidence, p. 390
body armor, p. 387
concealment, p. 385
CONTOMS, p. 388
cover, p. 386
EMT-Tacticals (EMT-Ts), p. 388
hate crimes, p. 382
particulate evidence, p. 390
special weapons and tactics (SWAT) team, p. 387
tactical emergency medical service (TEMS), p. 379

Case Study

At 10:30 P.M., your paramedic unit receives a call for an unknown problem at 4926 Magnolia Boulevard. The residence lies in a well-kept part of the city. As you turn onto Magnolia, you shut off the vehicle's emergency lights. Before arriving on scene, you request further information from dispatch. The dispatcher tells you that an older male requested an ambulance because "someone is sick and needs help, now!" He then quickly hung up without providing any further details, which makes you suspicious. Computer-aided dispatch shows no prior calls at the residence and no history of violence at the location.

Your partner stops the ambulance two houses away from the scene. You both observe the quiet single-family residence. Because you see no signs of danger, your partner moves the rig closer. Both you and your partner exit the vehicle and approach the residence with only the necessary equipment. The two of you take separate, unpredictable paths to the residence, keeping each other in sight. This provides a better view of the dwelling.

Your partner looks in the front window and observes an older man standing over a woman about the same age. She seems to be very ill. There are no signs of fighting, intoxication, or other unusual behavior.

You and your partner decide that it is safe to approach the door. You knock, and the man urges you to enter quickly. "My wife is so sick," he exclaims. "I don't know what to do. Please follow me.

You introduce yourself and immediately notice that the man has difficulty hearing you. He is older than you had suspected and is obviously distraught. The combination of factors explains why he may have failed to provide adequate information to dispatch.

You learn that the patient is experiencing chest discomfort and has been vomiting. You treat her according to ALS protocols and then transport both the patient and her husband to the hospital.

No violence on this call! Yet neither you nor your partner has any doubt about your cautious approach to the call. You have learned from experience that quiet calls can be just as worrisome as those made with loud voices. At least with loud voices, you have some reason to suspect trouble. Although you discovered a reasonable explanation for this suspicious call, you know all too well that your personal safety depends on your ability to detect potentially violent situations before you even step outside your ambulance.

Introduction

Violence can occur anywhere. Regardless of where you work as a paramedic—the inner city, the suburbs, or rural America—you can be affected by violence. The violence can take all forms, from interpersonal abuse in the home to gang activities in the street. The violence can also involve any number of weapons, ranging from fists to guns to explosives.

Although people of all ages and backgrounds commit acts of violence, the past two decades have seen a dramatic increase in violence among youth. According to the Division of Violence Prevention at the National Center for Injury Prevention and Control, arrest rates for homicide, rape, robbery, and aggravated assault are consistently higher for people ages 15 to 34 than for all other age groups. Even more alarming, an average of 16 youth (ages 10–24) homicides occur in the United States every day. Among 10- to 24-year-olds, homicide is the leading cause of death for African Americans and the second leading cause of death for Hispanics.[1]

Approximately one of six victims of violent crimes requires medical attention, often by emergency medical services. Several studies suggest that a substantial number of these victims fail to report the violence to the police. As a result, the emergency medical services may be a victim's only contact with professionals who can intervene to prevent further harm.

A more recent phenomenon is bullying. Bullying is a form of youth violence and can result in physical injury, social and emotional distress, and even death. Victimized youth are at increased risk for mental health problems such as depression and anxiety, psychosomatic complaints such as headaches, and poor school adjustment. Youths who bully others are at increased risk for substance use, academic problems, and violence later in adolescence and adulthood.

Despite the increased presence of violence, EMS providers find it almost impossible to predict exactly when and where a violent incident will occur. Nearly all calls that you or any other paramedic handle on a given day will progress without any threat of danger. In fact, you have a higher risk of being injured by oncoming traffic than by a violent act. Even so, you cannot let down your "crime scene awareness." Otherwise, you risk becoming a victim or hostage of a violent situation.

As this chapter shows, your most important safety tactic is an ability to identify potentially violent situations as soon as possible. Although you cannot predict violence hours in advance, you can remain alert to signs of danger. You can also become aware of local issues that hold a potential for violence, such as the presence of street gangs or a known area of drug activity.

Equally as important, you should familiarize yourself with standard operating procedures (SOPs) for handling violent situations and/or the specialized resources that you can call on for backup. Find out, for example, whether your unit has access to a **tactical emergency medical service (TEMS)**, which is a unit that provides on-site medical support to law enforcement.[2,3] If so, know how and when to access it. Above all else, remain alert to the signs of danger from the start of a call to the time you return your ambulance to service.

Approach to the Scene

Your safety strategy begins as soon as you are dispatched on a call. Even the most basic information can provide important tactical clues. Emergency medical dispatchers try to keep callers on the line to obtain as much information as possible. They remain alert to background noises such as fighting or intoxicated persons, so they can warn incoming units of these dangers. Modern computer-aided dispatch programs provide instant information on previous calls at a particular location and display "caution indicators" to notify dispatchers when a location has a history of violence.

Even in the age of computers, however, some of your best information can still come from your own experience and that of other crews. Your memory of previous calls can serve as an important indicator of trouble. For example, if a bar or club has a reputation for fights and you are summoned there, you will already have a high suspicion of danger before you arrive.

Possible Scenarios

There are three possible scenarios in which you might observe violence during an EMS call. The dispatcher may advise you of a potentially violent scene en route to the call. Obviously, you will be alert to danger from the start. In other cases, you may not spot danger until you arrive on the scene and begin your size-up and approach. In yet a third scenario, you may not face danger until the start of patient care or transport.

Advised of Danger en Route

When the dispatcher reports possible danger, do not approach the scene until it has been secured by law enforcement personnel. Remember that lights and sirens can draw a crowd and/or alert the perpetrator of a crime, so use them cautiously or not at all.

Never follow police units to the scene. To do so might place you at the center of violence. If you arrive first, keep the ambulance out of sight so the rig does not attract the attention of bystanders or any of the parties involved in the incident. While you wait for police to secure the scene, set up a staging area.

Management of the incident depends on interagency cooperation. Communicate with the police—you are in this together. Be sure you understand any differences in dispatch terminology. For example, a code 1 emergency for police units is a code 3 emergency for EMS units. Work with police to determine if and when you should approach the scene.

Keep in mind that violence can occur or resume even with the police present. Furthermore, depending on your uniform colors and the use of badges, people might mistake you for the police, especially if you exit from a vehicle with flashing lights and siren. They might expect you to intervene in a violent situation, or they might direct aggression toward you as an authority figure. If the scene cannot be made safe, retreat immediately (Figure 14-1).

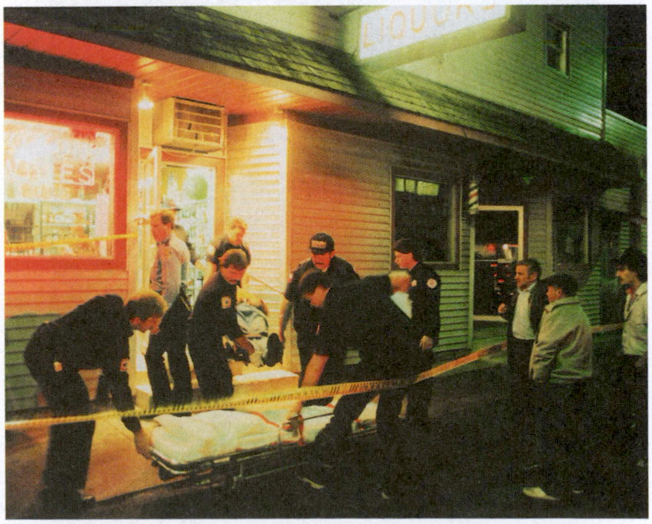

FIGURE 14-1 Never approach the scene until you have been advised that the scene is secure. Remember, even if a scene has been declared secure, violence may still erupt.

(© Craig Jackson/In the Dark Photography)

Observing Danger on Arrival

Even if dispatch has not alerted you to danger, you must still keep this possibility in mind once you arrive on scene. One of the main purposes of the scene size-up is to search for any possible hazards. This includes nonviolent dangers such as downed power lines, dangerous pets, unstable vehicles, or hazmat. As you look for these dangers, observe for other signs of trouble such as crowds gathering on the street, an unusual silence, or a darkened residence. Obviously, you will adopt a different approach for a confirmed medical emergency than for an "unknown problem, caller hang-up." Even so, do not exit the vehicle until you have ruled out all immediate hazards.

If you have any doubts about a call, park away from the scene. If you must park in view of the location, take an unconventional approach to the door (Figure 14-2). People will expect you to use the sidewalk. Therefore, approach from the side, on the lawn, or flush against the house. Avoid getting between a residence and the lighted ambulance so you do not "backlight" yourself. In addition, hold your flashlight to the side rather than in front of you (Figure 14-3). Armed assailants often fire at the light.

Before announcing your presence, listen and observe for signs of danger. If you can, look in windows for evidence of fighting, the presence of weapons, or the use of alcohol or drugs. Gradually make your way to the doorknob side of the door, or the side of the door opposite the hinges (Figure 14-4). Listen for any signs of danger, such as loud noises, items breaking, incoherent speech, or the lack of any sounds at all.

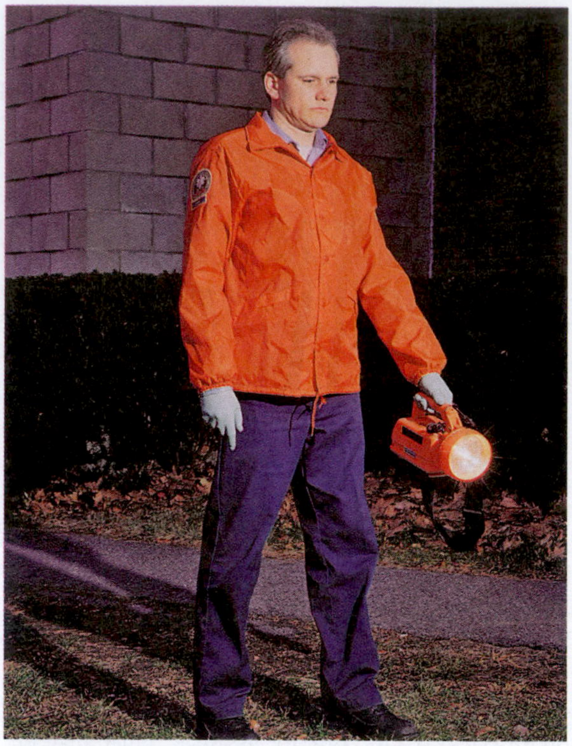

FIGURE 14-3 Hold a flashlight to the side of your body, not in front of it. Armed assailants usually aim at the light.

If you spot danger at any time during your approach, immediately stop and reevaluate the situation. Decide whether it is in the interest of your own safety to continue or to retreat until law enforcement officials can be

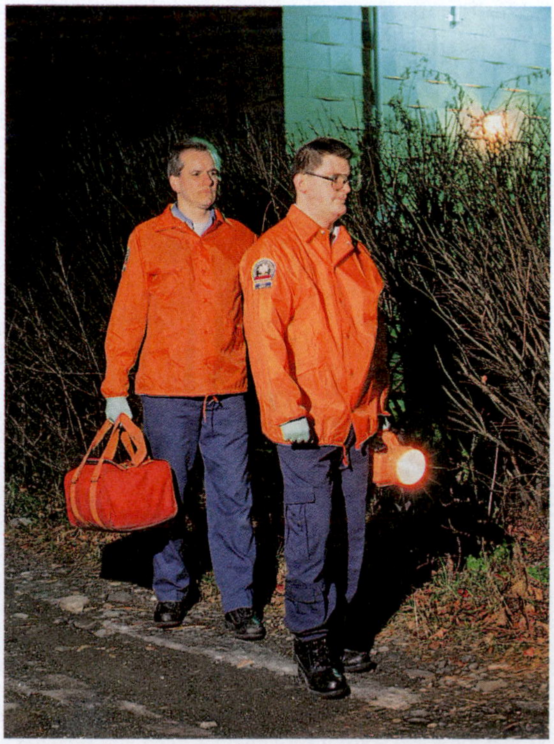

FIGURE 14-2 Approach potentially unstable scenes single file along an unconventional path.

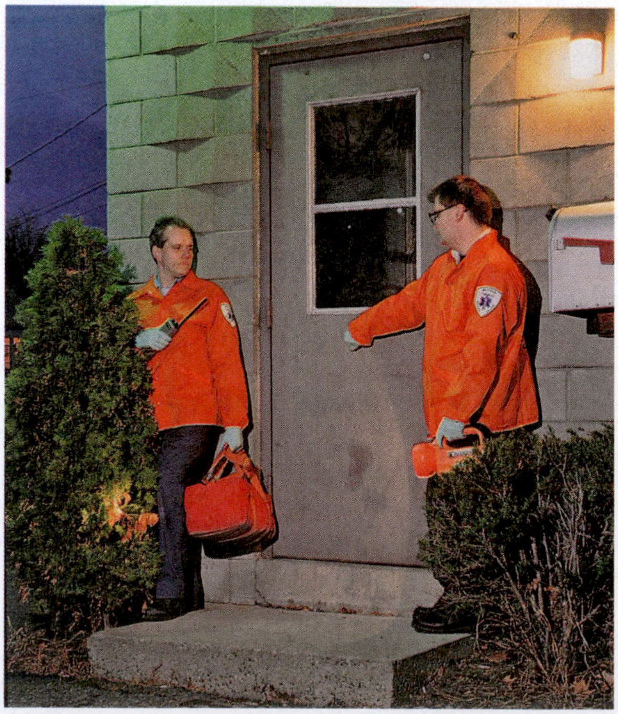

FIGURE 14-4 Stand to the side of the door when knocking. Do not stand directly in front of a door or window, making yourself an unwitting target.

summoned. Rather than risk becoming injured or killed, err on the side of safety.

Eruption of Danger During Care or Transport

Remain alert throughout a call, especially in areas with a history of violence. You may enter the scene and spot weapons or drugs. Additional combative people may arrive on scene. The patient or bystanders may become agitated or threatening. Even if treatment has begun, you must place your own safety first. You now have two tactical options: (1) quickly package the patient and leave the scene with the patient or (2) retreat without the patient.

Your choice of action depends on the level of danger. Abandonment is always a concern. However, in most cases, you can legally leave a patient behind when there is a *documented* danger. As discussed later in the chapter, keep accurate records of incidents involving violence. If you must defend yourself, use the minimum amount of force necessary. Immediately summon police and retreat as needed.

Regardless of the situation, always have a way out. Your failure to plan will undoubtedly lead to an emergency at some point in time. Make sure that SOPs include an escape plan. Then adhere to this plan so you do not become a victim of violence yourself.

Specific Dangerous Scenes

Most prehospital services were developed to meet the needs of individual patients in controlled situations. However, in recent years, EMS personnel trained for this limited role have been pressed increasingly into service in potentially hazardous situations. The result has been the employment of specialized resources with the tactical judgment and skills not normally taught in EMS programs. Your ability to survive a violent street encounter depends on recognition of threats and an understanding of some of the things that can be done to provide for rescuer and patient safety. The following sections describe some of the known dangers that you may face while on the street. (A discussion of tactical safety strategies appears later in the chapter.)

CONTENT REVIEW

➤ Potentially Dangerous Scenes
- Highway encounters
- Violent street incidents
- Drug-related crimes
- Clandestine drug labs
- Domestic violence

Highway Encounters

The preceding examples of known dangers have focused largely on residences. However, EMS units frequently report to roadside calls involving motor vehicle collisions, disabled vehicles, or sick and/or unresponsive people inside a car—for example, "man slumped over wheel" calls. The chapters "Ground Ambulance Operations" and "Rescue Awareness and Operations" have already indicated the dangers of highway operations and the steps that you should take to protect yourself. Additionally, keep in mind that highway operations also hold the risk of violence from occupants who may be intoxicated or drugged, fleeing from the police, or in possession of weapons. Some potential warning signs of danger include:

- Violent or abusive behavior
- An altered mental state
- Grabbing or hiding items inside the vehicle
- Arguing or fighting among passengers
- Lack of activity where activity is expected
- Physical signs of alcohol or drug abuse (e.g., liquor bottles, beer cans, or syringes)
- Open or unlatched trunks (a potential hiding spot for people or weapons)
- Differences among stories told by occupants

To make a safe approach to a vehicle at a roadside emergency, follow these steps:

- Park the ambulance in a position that provides safety from traffic.
- Notify dispatch of the situation, location, the vehicle make and model, and the state and number of the license plate.
- Use a one-person approach. The driver should remain in the ambulance, which is elevated and provides greater visibility.
- The driver should remain prepared to radio for immediate help and to back or drive away rapidly once the other medic returns.
- At night, use the ambulance lights to illuminate the vehicle. However, do not walk between the ambulance and the other vehicle. You will be backlighted, forming an easy target.
- Because police approach vehicles from the driver's side, you should approach from the passenger's side—an unexpected route.
- Use the A, B, and C door posts for cover.
- Observe the rear seat. Do not move forward of the C post unless you are sure there are no threats in the rear seat or foot wells.
- Retreat to the ambulance (or another strategic position of cover) at the first sign of danger.
- Make sure you have mapped out your intended retreat and escape with the ambulance driver.

Violent Street Incidents

You can encounter many different types of violence while working on the streets. You see examples on the news all the time. Incidents can range from random acts of violence against individual citizens to organized efforts at domestic or international terrorism. Some of the dangerous street situations that you may face at some point in your EMS career are discussed next.

Murder, Assault, and Robbery

Although the overall crime rate has dropped in recent years, millions of violent acts still occur annually. They take place at residences, at schools, and at commercial establishments. However, according to the U.S. Department of Justice, the most common location for violent crimes is on the streets—often within 5 miles of the victim's home. In order of occurrence, the most frequent crimes include simple assaults, aggravated assaults, rapes and sexual assaults, robberies, and homicides.

In one-quarter of the incidents of violent crime, offenders used or threatened the use of a weapon. Homicides are most commonly committed with handguns, but knives, blunt objects, and other types of guns or weapons may also be used. About one in five violent victimizations involves the use of alcohol.

Although motives vary, the late 1990s and early 2000s saw a rise in **hate crimes**—crimes committed against a person solely on the basis of the individual's actual or perceived race, color, national origin, ethnicity, gender, disability, or sexual orientation. A number of states or communities have passed legislation on the management of hate crimes, including the steps to be taken on scene. Determine whether these laws exist in your area, and establish protocols that your agency should follow. Crew assignments, for example, should be well thought out in advance of the response to a hate crime. You should also know the specific type of information that must be documented for later use by the courts.

In responding to the scene of any violent crime, keep these precautions in mind:

- Dangerous weapons may have been used in the crime.
- Perpetrators may still be on scene or could return to the scene.
- Patients may sometimes exhibit violence toward EMS, particularly if they risk criminal penalties as a result of the original incident.

Dangerous Crowds and Bystanders

As mentioned earlier, you must remain aware of crowd dynamics whenever you respond to a street incident. Crowds can quickly become large and volatile, especially in the case of a hate crime. Violence can be directed against anyone or anything in the path of an angry crowd. Your status as an EMS provider does not give you immunity against an out-of-control mob.

Whenever a crowd is present, look for these warning signs of impending danger:

- Shouts or increasingly loud voices
- Pushing or shoving
- Hostilities toward anyone on scene, including the perpetrator of a crime, the victim, and police
- Rapid increase in the crowd size
- Inability of law enforcement officials to control bystanders

To protect yourself, constantly monitor the crowd and retreat, if necessary. If possible, take the patient with you so you do not have to return later. Rapid transport may require limited or tactical assessment at the scene with more in-depth assessment done inside the safety of the ambulance. Be sure to document reasons for the quick assessment and transport.

Street Gangs

Gangs include groups of people who band together for a variety of reasons: fraternization, self-protection, creation of a surrogate family, or, most frequently, the pursuit of criminal enterprises. Street gangs can be found in big cities, suburban towns, and lately in rural America. No EMS unit is totally immune from gang activity. In fact, some organized gangs have purposely branched out into smaller towns in an effort to escape surveillance and expand their illicit businesses.

Youth gangs account for a disproportionate amount of youth violence across the nation. Gang activity is associated with high levels of delinquency, illegal drug use, physical violence, and possession of weapons. Young people from all demographic backgrounds report some knowledge of gangs or gang activity.

Some of the largest and best-known gangs include the Crips, Bloods, Almighty Latin King Nation (Latin Kings), Hell's Angels, Outlaws, Pagans, MS-13, and Banditos. Local variations of these and other gangs can be found throughout the country. In some places, gangs have used firebombs, Molotov cocktails, and, on a limited basis, military explosives (hand grenades) as weapons of revenge and intimidation. Links have been drawn between street gangs and the sale of drugs, which in turn finance gang activities.

Commonly observed gang characteristics include the following:

- *Appearance*—Gang members frequently wear unique clothing specific to the group. Because the clothing is often a particular color or hue, it is referred to as the gang's "colors." Wearing a color, even a bandana, can signify gang membership. Within the gang itself, members sometimes wear different articles to signify rank.

- *Graffiti*—Gangs have definite territories, or "turfs." Members often mark their turf with graffiti broadcasting the gang's logo, warning away intruders, bragging about crimes, insulting rival gangs, or taunting police.
- *Tattoos*—Many gang members wear tattoos or other body markings to identify their gang affiliation. Some gangs even require these tattoos. The tattoos will be in the gang's colors and often contain the gang's motto or logo.
- *Hand signals/language*—Gangs commonly create their own methods of communication. They give gang-related meanings to everyday words or create codes. Hand signs provide quick identification among gang members, warn of approaching law enforcement, or show disrespect to other gangs. Gang members often perform signals so quickly that an uninformed outsider may not spot them, much less understand them.

EMS units venturing into gang territory must be extremely cautious because of the potential for violence. Danger is increased if your uniform looks similar to the uniform worn by police. Gangs with a history of arrest may in fact make every effort to prevent you from transporting one of their members to a hospital or any other place beyond the reach of the gang. Do not force the issue if your safety is at stake.

Drug-Related Crimes

The sale of drugs goes hand in hand with violence (Figure 14-5). Hundreds of people die each year in drug deals gone bad. In addition, drug dealers protect their drug stashes and shooting galleries with booby traps, weapons, and abused dogs that are likely to attack. The combination of high cash flow, addiction, and automatic weapons threatens anyone who unwittingly walks onto the scene of a drug deal or threatens to uncover an illicit drug operation.

A number of signs can alert you to the involvement of drugs at an EMS call:

- Prior history of drugs in the neighborhood of the call
- Clinical evidence that the patient has used drugs of some kind
- Drug-related comments by bystanders
- Drug paraphernalia visible at the scene, such as the following:
  - Tiny zip-top bags or vials
  - Sandwich bags with the corners torn off (indicating drug packaging) or untied corners of sandwich bags (indicating drug use)
  - Syringes or needles
  - Glass tubes, pipes, or homemade devices for smoking drugs
  - Chemical odors or residues

Whenever you observe any of the preceding items, assume the use or presence of drugs at the scene. Even if the patient is not involved, others at the scene may still pose a danger. Keep in mind that not all patients who use drugs will be seeking to harm you. Some may, in fact, be looking for help. Evaluate each situation carefully. Above all else, remember to retreat and/or request police backup at the earliest sign of danger.

Clandestine Drug Laboratories

Drug dealers often set up "laboratories" to manufacture controlled substances or to otherwise refine or convert a controlled substance to another more profitable or usable

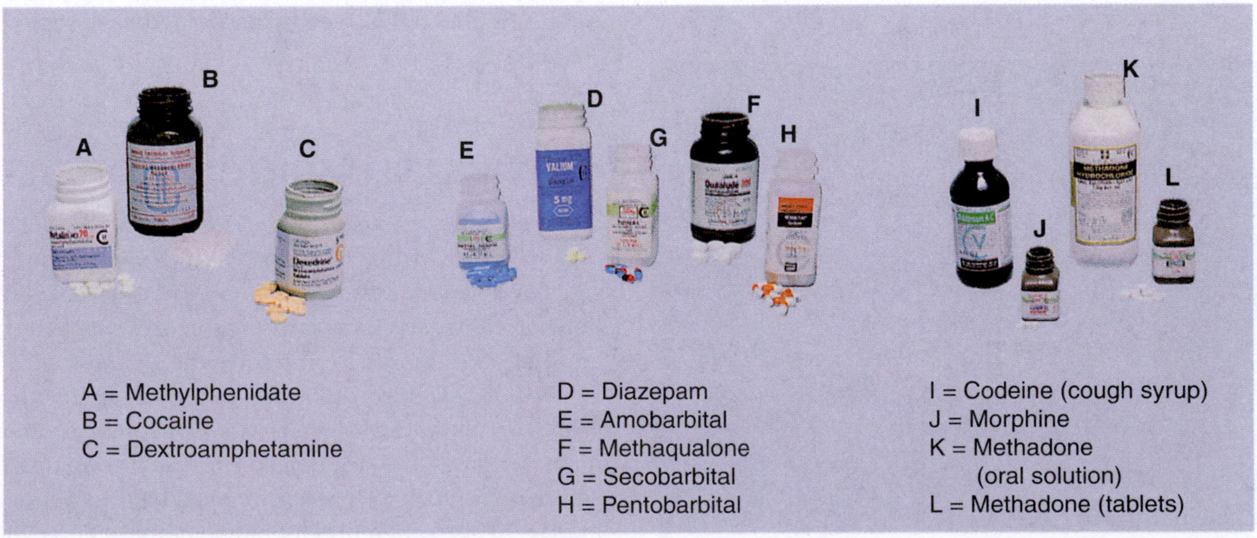

FIGURE 14-5 Substances abused and sold come in all forms. Some of the most commonly prescribed substances sold or used on the streets are shown here. Persons who abuse or deal in drugs may exhibit violent behavior.

form, such as tablets. One of the most common types of substances manufactured in drug laboratories is methamphetamine, also known by street names such as "meth," "crank," "speed," or "crystal." Other drugs include LSD and "crack."

Clandestine drug laboratories, or "clan labs," have three requirements: privacy, utilities, and equipment such as glassware, chemical containers, and heating mantles or burners (Figure 14-6). Most clan labs are uncovered by neighbors who report suspicious odors, deliveries, or activities.

Drug raids on clan labs have a way of turning into hazmat operations. All too often, the labs contain toxic fumes and volatile chemicals. The people on scene complicate matters by fighting or shooting at the rescuers who come to extricate them from the toxic environment. As they retreat, drug dealers may also trigger booby traps or wait for police or EMS personnel to trigger them. If you ever come upon a clan lab, take these actions:

- Leave the area immediately.
- Do not touch anything.
- Never stop any chemical reactions already in progress.
- Do not smoke or bring any source of flame near the lab.
- Notify the police.
- Initiate IMS and hazmat procedures.
- Consider evacuation of the area.

Remember that laboratories can be found anywhere—on farms, in trailers, in city apartments, and elsewhere. They may be mobile, roaming from place to place in a camper or truck. Or they may be disassembled and stored in almost any variety of locations. The job of raiding clan labs belongs to specialized personnel—not EMS crews.

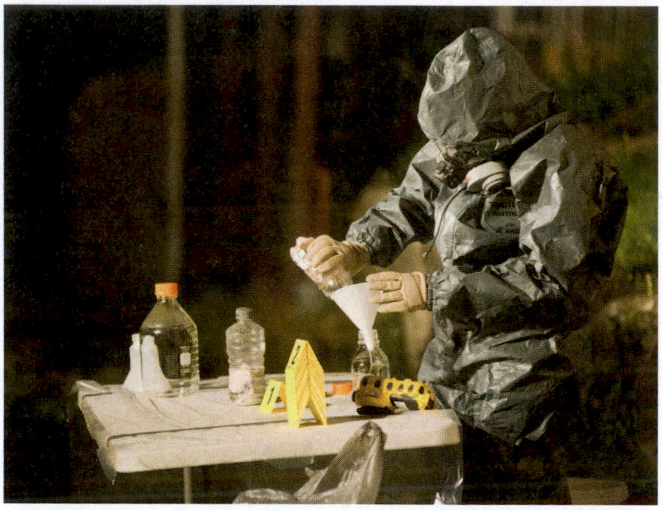

FIGURE 14-6a Clandestine labs, particularly methamphetamine ("meth") labs, pose a risk for rescuers. Many of the solvents and reagents are toxic and highly explosive.

(© AP Photo/The News-Item, Larry Deklinski)

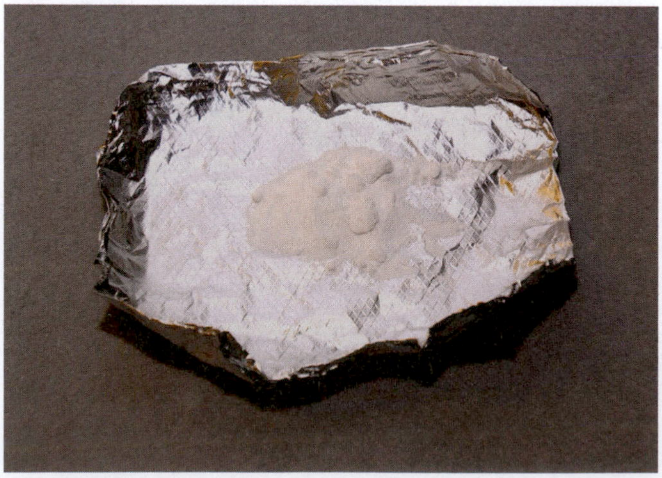

FIGURE 14-6b Powdered meth.

(Photo courtesy of US Drug Enforcement Administration)

Domestic Violence

Domestic violence involves people who live together in an intimate relationship. The violence may be physical, emotional, sexual, verbal, or economic. It may be directed against a spouse or partner, or it may involve children and/or older relatives who live at the residence.

At a scene involving domestic violence, the abuser may also turn on you or other members of your crew. Calls involving domestic violence are among those with the highest risk of injury or death for police officers and other responders.

Always retreat when a scene becomes unsafe. Retreating is a matter of personal safety, not cowardice, in violent situations. Bear in mind that an injured paramedic may be unable to care for the ill or injured patient. For more on the indications of domestic violence and the appropriate actions of EMS crews, see the chapter "Abuse, Neglect, and Assault."

Tactical Considerations

As mentioned on several occasions, your best tactical response to violence is observation. Know the warning signs and stay out of danger in the first place. If the dispatcher alerts you to hazards, resort to staging until the appropriate authorities can resolve the situation.

Nevertheless, you still may find yourself in situations with a potential for danger—a suspicious call that you must check out, the eruption of violence during treatment, and so on. In such instances, you must have a "game plan" in place. This section presents some of the actions you can take to protect your own safety while attempting to provide tactical patient care.

CONTENT REVIEW

- ➤ Safety Tactics
  - Retreat
  - Cover and concealment
  - Distraction and evasion
  - Contact and cover
  - Warning signals and communication

Safety Tactics

Dangerous situations mean extreme stress. As a result, your response to danger will be most effective if you practice tactical options frequently. Even on routine calls, think about safety, contact and cover, escape routes, and other strategies that can help you make a better decision when you are faced with actual danger. To borrow a phrase from professional sports, "You will play the game the way you practice." If you have rehearsed the responses to danger before you actually need them, you will be more likely to use them successfully. The following sections describe some proven methods for EMS safety in dangerous situations.

Retreat

The prudent strategy is to retreat whenever you spot indicators of violence or potential physical confrontations, particularly with fleeing criminals or people with emotional disturbances (Figure 14-7). Retreat in a calm, but decisive, manner. Be aware that the danger is now at your back and integrate cover into your retreat.

Ideally you will retreat to the ambulance so that you can summon help. However, if a dangerous obstacle, such as a crowd, blocks access to your rig, retreat by foot or by whatever means possible. Nothing in the ambulance is worth your life.

In deciding how far to retreat, your primary goal is to protect yourself from any potential danger. You must be out of the immediate line of sight. You must also seek cover from gunfire. Finally, you must allow enough distance to react if a person or crowd attempts to move toward you again. You need time and space to respond to changing situations.

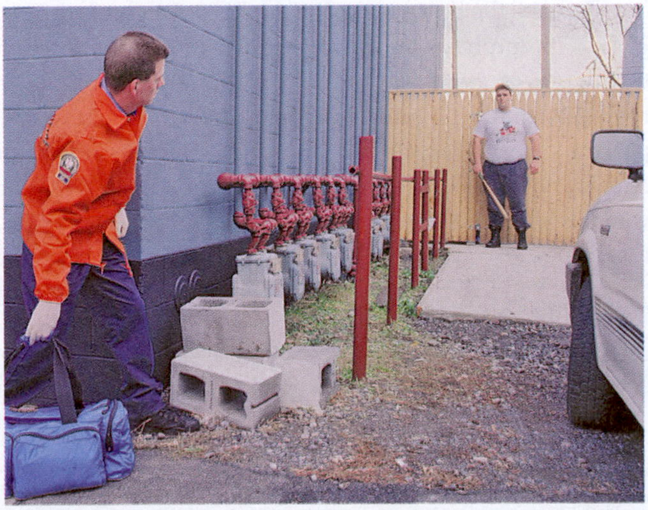

FIGURE 14-7 A patient's stance and position can indicate a potential for violence. If you suspect such a situation, put your own personal safety first. Retreat and request police backup.

As soon as possible, notify other responding units and agencies of the danger. Activate appropriate codes, SOPs, and/or interagency agreements, particularly with law enforcement departments. Be sure to document your observations of danger and your specific responses. Include information such as the following:

- Actions taken while on scene
- Reasons you retreated
- Time at which you left and/or returned to the scene
- Personnel or agencies contacted

Also keep in mind that retreat does not mean the end of a call. As already mentioned, you should seek to stage at a safe area until police secure the scene and you can respond once again. Staging, along with thorough documentation, will reduce liability and provide evidence to refute charges of abandonment.

Cover and Concealment

When faced with danger, two of your most immediate and practical strategies are cover and concealment (Figures 14-8a and 14-8b). **Concealment** hides your body, as when you

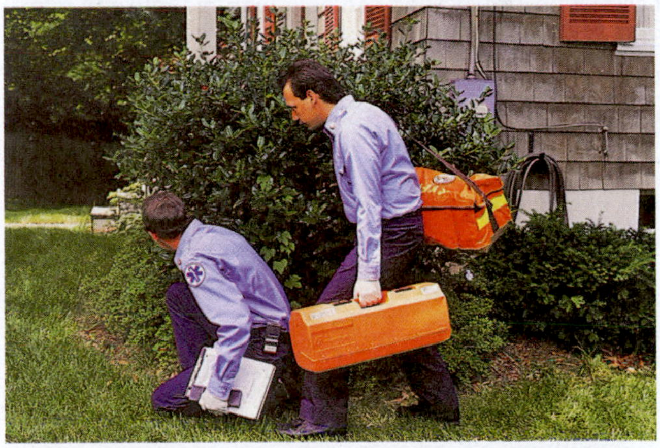

FIGURE 14-8a Concealing yourself means placing your body behind an object that can hide you from view.

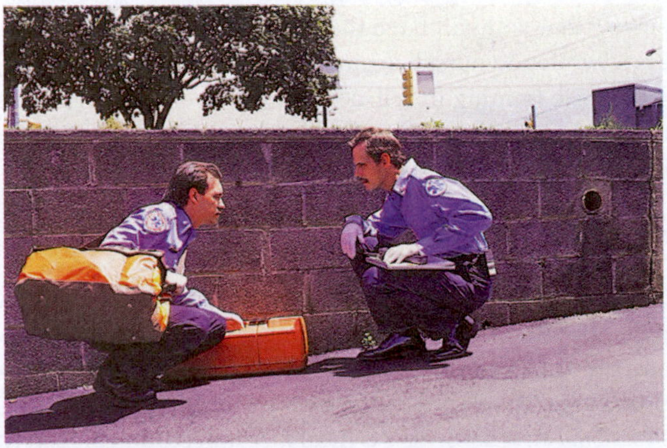

FIGURE 14-8b Taking cover means finding a position that both hides you and protects your body from projectiles.

crouch behind bushes, wallboards, or vehicle doors. However, most common objects do not stop bullets. During armed encounters, seek **cover** by hiding your body behind solid and impenetrable objects such as brick walls, rocks, large trees or telephone poles, and the engine blocks of vehicles.

For cover and concealment to work, they must be used properly. In applying these safety tactics, keep in mind the following general rules:

- As you approach any scene, remain aware of the surroundings and any potential sources of protection in case you must retreat or are "pinned down."
- Choose your cover carefully. You may have only one chance to pick your protection. Select the item that hides your body adequately, while shielding you against ballistics.
- Once you have made your choice of cover, conceal as much of your body as possible. Be conscious of any reflective clothing that you may be wearing. Armed assailants can use it as a target, especially at night.
- Constantly look to improve your protection and location.

Distraction and Evasion

Distraction and evasion can be integrated into any retreat. Some specific techniques to avoid physical violence include:

- Throwing equipment to trip, slow, or distract an aggressor
- Wedging a stretcher in a doorway to block an attacker
- Using an unconventional path while retreating
- Anticipating the moves of the aggressor and taking countermoves
- Overturning objects in the path of the attacker
- Using preplanned tactics with your partner to confuse or "throw off" an aggressor

The key to the success of these safety tactics is your own physical well-being. Regular exercise and good health ensure that you will have the strength to outrun or, if necessary, defend yourself against an attacker. Some units provide basic training in self-defense or have protocols on its use. Make sure you take advantage of this training and/or know the protocols related to the application of force.

Situational Awareness

Concentrating on the care of patients, particularly complex patients, requires that you focus on the patient. However, a narrow focus can be dangerous if you forget your surroundings. Awareness of your surroundings—known as *situational awareness*—is a critical factor in paramedic safety. It is a skill you can learn that will be a valuable safety tool for you, your crew, and your patients.

First, you need to learn to scan the scene while providing patient care—to continually evaluate for environmental dangers, unknown persons entering the scene, the return of the person that caused the injury, and similar dangerous situations. Your ability to be aware of the overall environment may be the key to knowing when to move the patient to a different location for treatment, when to load and go, or even when to stop care and retreat.

Additionally, you and your crew can improve safety by learning and practicing contact-and-cover skills and the skills of reading and communicating warning signals, as described in the next two sections.

Contact and Cover

The concept of contact and cover comes from a police procedure developed in San Diego, California, where several officers were injured or killed while interviewing suspects. Studies of the incidents revealed that the officers focused directly on the suspect, reducing their ability to observe the "big picture." This left them exposed to threats of physical violence and/or encounters with edged weapons or firearms.

To solve this problem, the San Diego Police Department adopted an interview approach in which one officer "contacts" the suspect while another officer stands 90 degrees to the side. By standing at a different angle, the second officer can provide "cover" to the officer dealing with the suspect.

When adapted to EMS practice, the procedure assigns the roles shown in Table 14-1. As with any tactic adopted from another discipline, contact and cover has obvious advantages and drawbacks. The tactic is ideal for street encounters with intoxicated persons or subjects acting in a suspicious manner. An obvious drawback is that two medics working on a cardiac arrest will not be able to designate one person to act solely as a "cover" medic.

Perhaps the best application of this police procedure to EMS is its emphasis on the importance of observation and teamwork. A crew that works well together will assign roles—formally or informally—to guarantee safety and patient care. In its most basic form, contact and cover means that you will watch your partner's back while he watches yours.

Table 14-1 Contact and Cover

Contact Provider	Cover Provider
Initiates and provides direct patient care.	Observes the scene for danger while the contact provider cares for the patient.
Performs patient assessment.	Generally avoids patient care duties that would prevent observation of the scene.
Handles most interpersonal scene contact.	In small crews, may perform limited functions such as handling equipment.

Warning Signals and Communication

Communication forms a vital part of EMS regardless of the situation. In the case of street survival, it is an invaluable safety tool. Every team or crew should develop methods of alerting other providers to danger without alerting the aggressor. Devise prearranged verbal and nonverbal clues and then practice them.

Be sure to involve dispatch in the process. Choose signals that will indicate a variety of circumstances while sounding harmless to an attacker. This can be a lifesaving technique in situations when you find yourself, the crew, and/or the patient held hostage. Your so-called routine radio reports can spell out the nature of the trouble and summon help from a **special weapons and tactics (SWAT) team**, a trained police unit equipped to handle hostage holders or other difficult law enforcement situations.

Tactical Patient Care

The increased involvement of care providers in violent situations has raised discussion and debate over the tactical training and protection offered to the EMS community. Interagency planning is essential, especially for clarifying the duties and roles of EMS and law enforcement agencies at crime scenes, riots, or terrorist events. Other aspects of tactical patient care include the use of body armor by EMS providers and the training of special tactical EMS personnel.

Body Armor

Several years ago, few EMS providers would have considered wearing **body armor**, or bulletproof vests, while on duty. However, today more and more providers are taking "tactical patient care" seriously. To protect EMS personnel against danger, an increasing number of EMS agencies have chosen to supply body armor or to provide a sum of cash toward its purchase. Body armor manufacturers have responded by designing and marketing vests specifically for the EMS community.

Unlike conventional armor, body armor is soft. A series of fibers such as Kevlar™ are woven tightly together to form the vest. The tight weave and strength of the material offer protection from many handgun bullets, most knives, and blunt trauma. The number of layers of fiber determine the rating or "stopping power" of a vest. Most body armor is rated from level 1 (least protective) to level 3 (most protective). Specialty vests with steel inserts and other materials are available for use by the military or by SWAT teams.

Some critics of body armor claim that wearers may feel a false sense of security. They point out that body armor offers reduced protection when wet. They also note that it provides little or no protection against high-velocity bullets, such as those fired by a rifle, or from thin or dual-edged weapons. An ice pick, for example, can penetrate between the fibers of most vests.

Supporters of body armor feel that it should be viewed just like any other PPE offered to rescuers. They point to the new threats faced by emergency responders, such as paramilitary groups, international terrorists, drug-related violence, and the widespread possession of handguns.

Whether you purchase or wear body armor is a personal decision (Figure 14-9). However, for it to be effective, you must follow several guidelines:

- Keep in mind the limitations of body armor. Never do anything you would not do without it.
- Remember that body armor does not cover the whole body. You can still get seriously injured or killed.
- Even though body armor can prevent many types of penetration, you can still experience severe cavitation.
- For body armor to work, it must be worn. The temptation not to wear it, especially in hot temperatures, can render even the best body armor useless.

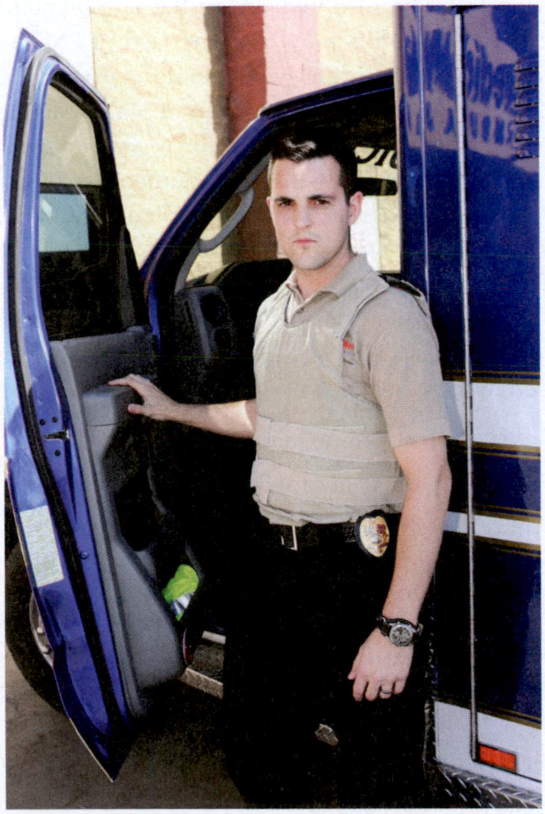

FIGURE 14-9 Body armor has been shown to save lives in the military and police setting. As a result, an increasing number of EMS providers have started wearing body armor (bulletproof vests) while on duty.

(© Dr. Bryan E. Bledsoe)

Tactical EMS

As already mentioned, the provision of care in violent or tactically "hot" zones, such as sniper situations, often necessitates risks far beyond those found on most EMS calls. Medical personnel assigned to such incidents require special training and authorization. Like hazmat teams, they must don special equipment, function with compact gear, and, in most cases, work as medical adjuncts to the police or military.

The patient care offered by TEMS differs from routine EMS care in several ways:

- A major priority is extraction of the patient from the hot zone.
- Care may be modified to meet tactical considerations.
- Trauma patients are encountered more frequently than medical patients.
- Treatment and transport interventions must almost always be coordinated with an incident commander.
- Patients must be moved to tactically cold zones for complete assessment, care, and transport.
- Metal clipboards, chemical agents, and other tools may be used as defensive weapons.

Local protocols, standing orders, and issues of medical direction must be resolved before the employment of a TEMS unit. The units may be composed of EMTs, paramedics, and/or physicians who operate as part of a tactical law enforcement team. Certification of SWAT-Medics and **EMT-Tacticals (EMT-Ts)** is offered by several organizations, including the **CONTOMS** (Counter-Narcotics Tactical Operations) program and the National Tactical Officers Association (NTOA).

The training required of EMT-Ts or SWAT-Medics involves strenuous physical activity, under a variety of conditions. In a CONTOMS program, medics may be exposed to scenarios or skills such as the following:

- Raids on clandestine drug laboratories
- Emergency medical care in barricade situations
- Wounding effects of weapons and booby traps
- Special medical gear for tactical operations
- Use of CS (a component of tear gas), CN (mace), capsaicin (pepper spray), CR (more powerful than CS, so incapacitating it has been nicknamed "firegas"), or other riot-control agents
- Blank-firing weapons
- Helicopter operations
- Pyrotechnics (smoke and distraction devices)
- Operation under extreme conditions, darkness, and psychological stress
- Firefighting and hazmat operations

In summoning or working with a TEMS unit, follow the same general approaches and procedures as with other units and teams. If you have not had exposure to such a unit, find out more about EMT-Ts or SWAT-Medics from local law enforcement officials or from sites sponsored by CONTOMS or NTOA on the Internet.

EMS at Crime Scenes

A crime scene can be defined as a location where any part of a criminal act has occurred and where evidence relating to a crime may be found. The goal of performing EMS at a crime scene is to provide high-quality patient care while preserving evidence. *Never* jeopardize patient care for the sake of evidence. However, do not perform patient care with disregard of the criminal investigation that will follow.

EMS and Police Operations

Often, emergencies arise in which police and EMS personnel respond to the same crisis. Both are there for specific purposes. The EMS crew has arrived on scene to treat patients and save lives. Law enforcement officers have come to protect the public and to solve a crime. These two primary goals sometimes create tension between the two teams. For example, police and paramedics often work under different time constraints. As a paramedic, you have a limited time at the scene. The police, on the other hand, spend much more time at the location of a crime. In some major cases, police can remain at the scene for days or weeks as they methodically look for evidence (Figure 14-10).

The key to cooperation between EMS and law enforcement personnel is communication. You should become aware of the nature and significance of physical evidence at a crime scene and, if possible, keep that evidence intact.

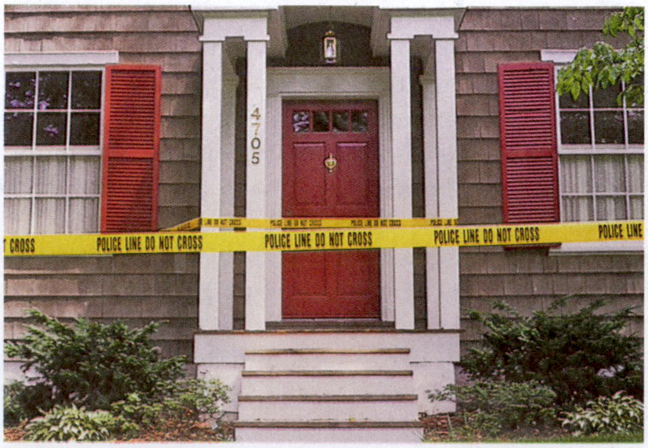

FIGURE 14-10 Police can remain at the scene of a crime for days, methodically searching for evidence. An EMS crew has a limited time at the scene. During that time, they must protect themselves, treat the patient, *and* preserve potential evidence, if at all possible.

Police, on the other hand, should be aware that the first and foremost responsibility of a paramedic is to save the life of the victim. However, police and paramedics can usually reach a common ground. By preserving evidence, you can help the police lock up a criminal before the person hurts, injures, or kills someone else. Remember: EMS personnel and law enforcement are really on the same side. Talk to each other.

Preserving Evidence

To prevent future violent injuries, be aware that anything on and around the patient may be evidence. You never know when a seemingly unimportant item may, in fact, be crucial evidence that could help solve a crime. Whenever in doubt, save or treat an object as evidence.

If you are the first person at the scene of a crime, be aware that anything you touch, walk on, pick up, cut, wipe off, or move could be evidence. Developing an awareness of evidence will even affect the way you treat patients. You will need to observe the patient carefully and to disturb as little direct evidence as possible. For example, if clothing must be removed, never cut through a gunshot or knife wound. Instead, try to cut as far away from the wound as possible. Instead of placing the cut cloth or garment in a plastic bag, put it in a brown paper bag so condensation does not build up and destroy body fluid evidence.

In addition, when examining a patient, remember that you may be at risk. The victim may have a concealed weapon, such as a knife or gun. Or the person who committed the crime may be intent on finishing it and reappear to attack the patient. As a result, your first responsibility is to protect yourself. If you have any suspicions at all about the patient or the safety of the scene, wait for the police to frisk the patient and/or secure the scene.

Legal Considerations

Preserving Evidence at a Crime Scene. Modern science has made solving crimes easier. The advent of forensic science and DNA technology has greatly increased the ability of authorities to link a person to a crime scene.

EMS personnel are often the first to arrive at the scene of a crime—sometimes ahead of law enforcement personnel. Although the paramedic's primary responsibilities are scene safety and care of the patient, it is important to be cognizant of crime scene evidence and make every effort to avoid contaminating or disturbing it. For example, when cutting away the clothing of a gunshot or stabbing victim, take care not to cut through the gunshot or stab entrance wound. Furthermore, never handle any weapons found at the scene. If you arrive at a scene and find your victim dead, your responsibility should turn to protecting the scene and any evidence until law enforcement personnel arrive and release you from the scene.

It is important for EMS and law enforcement personnel to work together. Although our jobs are different, we share a common dedication to justice, and protection of crime scene evidence is just one way to accomplish this.

CONTENT REVIEW

- ➤ Types of Evidence
  - Prints—fingerprints, footprints, tire prints
  - Blood and blood spatter
  - Body fluids
  - Particulate evidence
  - On-scene EMS observations

Types of Evidence

Gathering evidence is a specialized and time-consuming job. Although it is unrealistic to train EMS personnel in the details of police work, it is not unrealistic to ask them to develop an awareness of the general types of evidence that they may expect to encounter at a crime scene. Some of the main categories of evidence are prints, blood and body fluids, particulate evidence, and your own observations at the scene.

PRINTS Prints include fingerprints, footprints, and tire prints. Of the three, fingerprints can be the most valuable source of evidence. No two people have identical fingerprints—the distinctive patterns left on a surface by the natural oils and moisture that form on a person's fingertips. The patterns can be compared with the millions of fingerprints already on file or compared to the fingerprints of a suspect charged with the crime.

As a paramedic, you have two concerns when it comes to fingerprints. First, try not to disturb any fingerprint evidence that may be present. Second, do not leave behind your own fingerprints at a crime scene.

The only way to preserve fingerprints is simply not to touch anything. Of course, this is impossible when treating a patient. However, you can and should minimize what you touch. If you must touch or move an item, remember to tell the police that you did so.

Because of Standard Precautions, you will be wearing disposable gloves as a part of infection control. These gloves prevent you from leaving your own fingerprints—but they will not prevent you from smudging existing prints. Again, touch as little as possible. In addition, bring in only the necessary equipment. The more equipment you have, the more evidence you can potentially disturb, including fingerprints.

Scan the approach to the scene and the scene itself for footprints or tire prints. These prints have value because they give the police an idea of what a perpetrator was wearing (e.g., sneakers vs. work boots) or the type of tread on a vehicle's tires. These patterns may be later matched to the footwear or vehicle used by an alleged perpetrator.

BLOOD AND BODY FLUIDS Blood and body fluids also give police a lot of information about a crime. For example, if the victim scratched or injured the perpetrator, blood samples might be found under the fingernails, on clothing, on hands, or elsewhere. By ABO blood typing these samples, the field of suspects can be narrowed down.

Identification of DNA (deoxyribonucleic acid) has been called "genetic fingerprinting." Matching the DNA found in blood samples or other body fluids to the DNA of a suspect is nearly 100 percent accurate. There is only one chance in several million that the DNA could be from someone else. The high cost of DNA testing prevents its widespread use. However, when performed, medical technologists need only a small sample to ascertain the genetic code of the person from which it came.

The way in which blood is splattered or dropped at the scene provides yet other clues for police. This so-called **blood spatter evidence** can indicate the type of weapon used, the position of the attacker in relation to the victim, and the direction or force used in the attack.

Preserving blood evidence can be performed in the following ways:

- Avoid mixing samples of blood whenever possible. Cross-contamination of blood will render blood evidence useless.
- Avoid tracking blood on your shoes. You will leave your own footprints, and you risk contaminating other blood evidence.
- If you must cut bloody clothing from a victim, place each piece in a separate brown paper bag. If the garment is wet, gently roll it in the paper bag to layer it. Place the entire contents in a second paper bag and then in a plastic bag for body fluid protection.
- Do not throw clothes stained with blood or other body fluids in a single pile or in a puddle of blood.
- Do not clean up or smudge blood spatter left at a scene.
- If you leave behind blood from a venipuncture, notify police.
- Because blood can be a biohazard, ask police whether the scene should be secured for evidence collection.

PARTICULATE EVIDENCE **Particulate evidence**, also known as *microscopic* or *trace evidence*, refers to evidence that cannot be readily seen by the human eye, such as hairs or carpet and clothing fibers. Particulate evidence can help identify the actual crime scene, such as in cases when a body has been moved, or the DNA of the perpetrator. Minimal handling of a victim's clothes by EMS personnel may help to preserve this evidence.

ON-SCENE OBSERVATIONS Everything that you and other members of the EMS crew see and hear can serve as evidence. Your observations of the scene will become part of the police record—and, ultimately, part of the court record. Be sure to look for and record the following information:

- Conditions at the scene (e.g., absence or presence of lights, locked or unlocked doors, open or closed curtains)
- Position of the patient/victim
- Injuries suffered by the patient/victim
- Statements of persons at the scene
- Statements by the patient/victim
- Dying declarations
- Suspicious persons at, or fleeing from, the scene
- Presence and/or location of any weapons

If the victim is deceased by the time you arrive, any staff not immediately needed on the scene should leave to minimize the risk of disturbing evidence. If a gun is seen or found on the deceased victim, do not touch or move it unless it must be secured for the safety of others. Pick it up only as a last resort, and touch it only by the side grips or handles. The grips are coarse and will not generally leave good fingerprints. *Never* put anything into the barrel of the gun to lift or move it. The barrel of a gun can house the majority of the evidence used by the police: traces of gunpowder, rifling patterns, and even flesh or blood from the victim.

Documenting Evidence

Record only the facts at the scene of a crime, and record them accurately. Otherwise, they might be thrown out of court as evidence. Use quotation marks to indicate the words of bystanders and any remarks made by the patient. Avoid opinions not relevant to patient care. If the patient has died, do not offer any judgments that might contradict later findings by the medical examiner. For example, a knife wound is not a knife wound until it is proven that a knife caused the laceration. Instead, describe the shape and anatomic location of the puncture or cut.

Also keep in mind the protocols, local laws, and ethical considerations in reporting certain crimes such as child abuse, rape, geriatric abuse, and domestic violence. (For more on reporting these kinds of crimes, see the chapter "Abuse, Neglect, and Assault.") Finally, follow local policies and regulations regarding confidentiality surrounding any criminal case. Any offhand remarks that you make might later become testimony in a courtroom along with other documents that you prepare at the scene.

Summary

Your first priority at any crime scene is your own safety. To protect your life and the lives of others, you need to develop a "crime scene awareness." Whenever you survey the scene of any call, keep in mind some of the telltale signs of potential violence, such as a suspiciously darkened house or a lack of activity. Do not needlessly expose yourself to dangers better left to professional emergency medical personnel such as SWAT-Medics or EMT-Ts. When you do treat the victim(s) at a crime scene, keep in mind that police and EMS personnel must work together to preserve the evidence that may lead to conviction of the perpetrator. Touch only items or objects that pertain directly to patient care.

You Make the Call

Your ambulance receives a call about a 65-year-old man with chest pain. You arrive at the scene and scan for dangers. Detecting no visible hazards, you enter the patient's home and begin assessment. The patient describes the pain as crushing and points to the center of his chest. You observe labored breathing and begin care. You direct your partner to administer oxygen, while you look for a peripheral IV site.

While treatment progresses, the patient's son bursts through the door. He appears intoxicated and is obviously agitated at the presence of an ambulance. The patient whispers, "My son isn't quite right when he's drinking. You better be careful."

While you introduce yourself to the son, your partner slips away to radio the police. The dispatcher advises her that it could be a few minutes before the police can arrive on scene. Meanwhile, you tell the son why it is important that you start an IV. The son yells, "You're no doctor. Get away from my father. He needs to get to a hospital, not stay here in the living room. Get out of here before I throw you out."

1. What is your evaluation of this situation from a safety perspective?
2. What are your options?

See Suggested Responses at the back of this book.

Review Questions

1. The most common place where violent crime takes place is in ____________
   a. a bar.
   b. the home.
   c. the street.
   d. a school.
2. Crimes committed against a person solely on the basis of the individual's actual or perceived race, color, national origin, ethnicity, gender, disability, or sexual orientation are termed ____________
   a. social crimes.
   b. hate crimes.
   c. interpersonal crimes.
   d. prejudice crimes.
3. Which of the following are warning signs of impending danger whenever a crowd is present?
   a. Pushing or shoving
   b. Rapid increase in crowd size
   c. Inability of law enforcement officials to control bystanders
   d. All of the above
4. The contact-and-cover tactic is ideal to use to when ____________
   a. escaping from imminent danger.
   b. interviewing a potentially violent patient on the street.
   c. signaling incoming departments of potential danger.
   d. retreating and then returning to the scene at a later time.

5. "A trained police unit equipped to handle hostage holders or other difficult law enforcement situations" describes a ______________ team.
   a. TEMS
   b. EMT-T
   c. SWAT
   d. HAZMAT
6. How should you hold your flashlight when approaching a dark house at a potential crime scene?
   a. Behind you
   b. Over your head
   c. To your side
   d. In front of you
7. At a crime scene, you should preserve evidence containing body fluids by placing it in what type of container?
   a. Sterile container
   b. Sealed plastic bag
   c. Brown paper bag
   d. Airtight container
8. Which of the following is an appropriate way to avoid crime scene evidence contaminations?
   a. Clean up blood spatter.
   b. Wear gloves while on scene.
   c. Place small articles of clothing in a plastic bag.
   d. Fold blood-stained clothes and place them in a single pile.

See Answers to Review Questions at the end of this book.

References

1. Centers for Disease Control and Prevention. Violence Prevention. (Available at http://www.cdc.gov/violenceprevention/.)
2. Tang, N. and G. D. Kelen. "Role of Tactical EMS in Support of Public Safety and the Public Health Response to a Hostile Mass Casualty Event." *Disaster Med Public Health Prep* 1(1Suppl) (2007): S55–S56.
3. Rinnert, K. J. and W. L. Hall, 2nd. "Tactical Emergency Medical Support." *Emerg Med Clin North Am* 20 (2002): 929–952.

Further Readings

DeLorenzo, R A. and R. S. Porter. *Weapons of Mass Destruction: Emergency Care.* Upper Saddle River, NJ: Pearson/Prentice Hall, 2000.

Eliopilos, L. N. *Death Investigator's Handbook: A Field Guide to Crime Scene Processing, Forensic Evaluation, and Investigation Techniques.* Expanded and updated edition. Boulder, CO: Paladin Press, 2003.

Schwartz, R. D., J. G. McManus, and R. E. Swienton. *Tactical Emergency Medicine.* Philadelphia: Lippincott Williams and Wilkins, 2007.

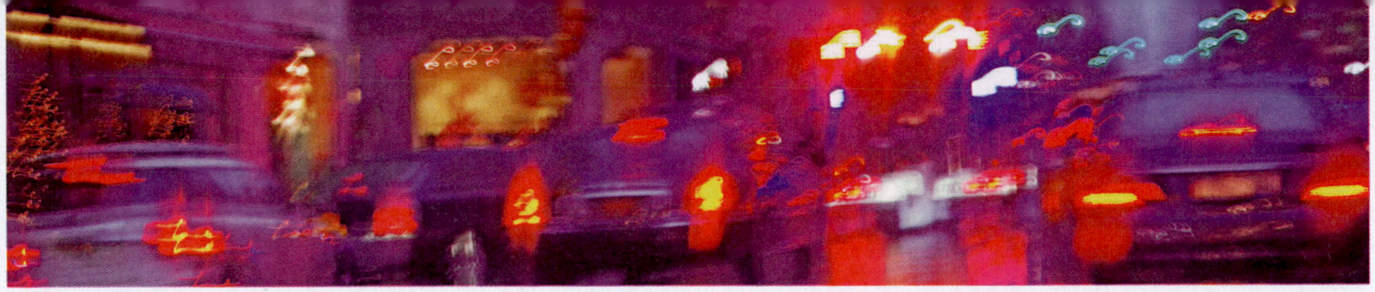

Chapter 15
Rural EMS

Bryan Bledsoe, DO, FACEP, FAAEM, EMT-P

Deborah J. McCoy-Freeman, BS, RN, NREMT-P

STANDARDS

Assessment (Scene Size-Up); EMS Operations (Air Medical)

COMPETENCY

Integrates scene and patient assessment findings with knowledge of epidemiology and pathophysiology to form a field impression. This includes developing a list of differential diagnoses through clinical reasoning to modify the assessment and formulate a treatment plan.

Applies knowledge of operational roles and responsibilities to ensure patient, public, and personnel safety.

Learning Objectives

Terminal Performance Objective: After reading this chapter, you should be able to effectively perform the expected functions of EMS personnel in a rural setting.

Enabling Objectives: To accomplish the terminal performance objective, you should be able to:

1. Define key terms introduced in this chapter.
2. Describe the demographics, health status, and health access issues of rural populations.
3. List and describe the special challenges faced by rural EMS systems.
4. Identify solutions to solving special challenges faced by rural EMS systems.
5. Given a variety of scenarios, integrate the special challenges and considerations of rural EMS into patient care decision making.
6. Recognize mechanisms of injury and particular hazards involved in agricultural emergencies.
7. Anticipate injuries associated with various recreational activities and discuss strategies to help mitigate these injuries in a rural environment.

KEY TERMS

air bags, p. 401
compartment syndrome, p. 401
cribbing, p. 401
crush points, p. 404
lock-out/tag-out, p. 400
pinch points, p. 402
prompt care facilities, p. 398
rust out, p. 396
shear points, p. 404
silo gas, p. 400
wrap points, p. 402

Case Study

It's a warm sunny afternoon in July when a call comes in to your paramedic unit for "a man down in a farmyard." The communications officer has dispatched the local volunteer basic life support (BLS) squad. However, because the call involves an unresponsive patient, the dispatcher has also requested backup from the nearest paramedic unit. Your unit, which is stationed more than 29 miles away, receives the call.

It takes the local volunteer squad 5 minutes to assemble and get an ambulance en route to the farm, which lies at the edge of the squad's district. Your unit—a full-time paid agency—is off the floor in less than 1 minute. Because both units must travel quite a distance, they race against the clock to reach the scene safely.

The BLS squad arrives at the farm just a few minutes ahead of your unit. Crew members meet the patient's wife at the door of the house. She says, "Please hurry. Follow me. I'll show you where my husband is." The squad leader informs the wife that crew members will proceed as soon as they ensure that the scene is safe. By this time, the man's wife is frantic. She yells, "You've got to help my husband right now!"

At this point, your unit arrives on the scene and you assist the squad leader in calmly obtaining information. As the woman gestures toward a silo, you notice a man lying at its base. About a foot away from the patient, you see a ladder propped up against the silo. A rope runs up the ladder to the top of the silo.

When the squad leader asks the woman what may have happened, she says, "My husband was going to clean the silo today. Everything seemed OK, until I heard him yelling. When I looked out the window, my husband was having trouble climbing down the ladder. As he got near the ground, he seemed to keel over and fall."

The squad leader then finds out whether the woman's husband was using any hazardous materials and whether she has had any ill effects from being near the silo. She responds "no" to both questions. You and the squad leader agree that the scene is probably safe and relay this information to the dispatch center.

As you move toward the base of the silo, you note no apparent trauma to the victim. You ask the woman, "How far do you think your husband fell?" The patient's wife now says that he did not actually fall to the ground, but slumped forward to his current face-down position. Her comment corroborates your initial observation.

Because the patient is unresponsive, you assume control of the situation. You and your partner carefully logroll the patient to assess the airway. You note that the man is breathing, but his respirations are less than 8 per minute. He is diaphoretic, ashen, and unconscious. His pulse is slow and weak.

The downtime is now 40 minutes. Because the patient must be ventilated, your partner assists breathing with a bag-valve-mask (BVM) unit. Meanwhile, you place a monitor on the patient and note a bradycardia. You establish an IV, using aseptic techniques, while your partner obtains vitals. She reports blood pressure 60 by palpation and a pulse of 40 bpm.

The patient is now receiving ventilations at 14 bpm, using capnography as a guide. You order the airway secured with a number 8.0-mm ET tube. Using a landline, you report the situation to medical direction. The medical director orders 0.5 mg of atropine IV push (IVP). Because this is a rural setting, you realize that the ambulance may experience communication blackouts. As a result, you must anticipate any problems that may arise en route to the hospital. In case the atropine does not help, you request orders for transcutaneous pacing (TCP) and/or additional doses of atropine according to advanced cardiac life support (ACLS) protocols.

After receiving approval from medical direction, you administer the prescribed atropine and load the patient into the ambulance. The total time of treatment prior to transport is 11 minutes. En route, you apply the TCP and achieve mechanical capture at 60 milliamperes (ma) on the rate of 70 bpm. The patient responds well to the treatment and is taken to a local hospital 33 miles away. At the hospital, he receives a temporary pacemaker. The patient is then transferred to the regional cardiac center for an internal pacemaker. The actions of the BLS and paramedic crews in this rural emergency have made the difference between life and death.

Introduction

Recent census data indicate that more than 53 million people in the United States live in rural areas. In fact, some states have rural populations of nearly 50 percent or more. In the West, states with large rural populations include Alaska, Montana, North Dakota, and South Dakota. In the South, they include Arkansas, Kentucky, Mississippi, North Carolina, South Carolina, and West Virginia. In the Northeast, they include Maine, New Hampshire, and Vermont.

People choose to live in rural areas for a variety of reasons. Their families have always lived there. They work at occupations such as farming, ranching, or mining. They like the solitude, open space, or recreational activities found in rural areas. Regardless of the reason, most rural dwellers face a similar problem: lack of easy access to the health care facilities found in most urban and suburban areas.

In the rural setting, resources such as full-service hospitals, fire departments, and EMS units are often as thinly distributed as the population. Specialty teams may be nonexistent. One of the challenges for rural EMS providers is to ensure that their patients receive the same high-quality care as people living elsewhere in the nation.[1] The following sections outline some of the obstacles and decisions typically faced by rural EMS providers.

Patho Pearls

Quality Considerations in Rural EMS. It has been said that the farther a person is from a hospital, the more sophisticated the prehospital care should be. This is an ideal situation in an ideal world—yet is rarely true. Many rural EMS providers routinely make emergent patient transports of an hour or longer. In some parts of this great land, especially in the frontier regions, air medical transport is not even available, thus forcing paramedics to transport critically ill or injured patients for hours before they reach any level of health care facility. The paradox is this: Although the level of prehospital care in rural areas should be high, the less frequent call volumes prevent this from occurring. Furthermore, it is much more difficult to get the required education in a rural setting, and skills decay is a particular problem. However, through outreach programs and skills retention programs, these problems can be overcome.

Rural paramedics must have and develop skills that will allow them to care for patients for a prolonged period of time. These skills include definitive airway management, fluid replacement therapy (possibly with hemoglobin-based oxygen-carrying solutions), selected fracture and dislocation reduction, and other aspects of prolonged patient care. Nasogastric tube and Foley catheter placements are often helpful during prolonged patient transports. Likewise, the ability to provide adequate analgesia, second-line antidysrhythmic agents, and, in certain cases, fibrinolytic therapy can often mean the difference between life and death.

Rural EMS has been neglected for a long time. Now, through several initiatives, attention has once again turned to rural EMS and the plight of the rural EMT and paramedic and their patients.

Practicing Rural EMS

In general, the U.S. government defines rural areas in terms of their sparse populations and distances from cities, towns, or villages. In relation to health care, rural areas can also be characterized by their higher percentage of people over age 65 and their lower physician-to-patient ratios.[2] Whereas one in five people in the United States lives in rural settings, only about one in ten doctors chooses to practice in these locations.

It has been found that rural residents experience a disproportionate number of serious injuries and chronic health conditions. Because of the greater distances to health care facilities, rural residents suffer a higher level of mortality associated with trauma and medical emergencies. In many cases, an EMS unit may provide the definitive care. In meeting the challenge of practicing rural EMS, paramedics and other health care personnel need to be aware of the special problems facing them.

Special Problems

As already indicated in this text, the cost of medical care and the rise of health maintenance organizations have expanded the roles and responsibilities of EMS personnel in the 21st century. The need for nonemergent transports, especially in rural areas, has increased. The shortage of specialized doctors and well-equipped hospitals in rural areas has become an even more critical problem. In the years ahead, a growing number of patients may have to be transported to urban areas to receive the care unavailable to them in rural facilities.

In the case of natural disasters, such as tornadoes, floods, or hurricanes, the situation is equally serious. In such instances, EMS personnel may be the *only* available medical support until state or federal agencies can be transported into the area.

Regardless of the circumstances surrounding a call, rural EMS crews face a number of obstacles and challenges not found in most urban areas. If you currently work for a rural EMS unit, you may already be aware of some of these situations from firsthand experience. As a paramedic, you will assume an expanded leadership role in directing other EMS personnel on how best to handle or overcome the following special problems.

Distance and Time

Rural EMS often relies on volunteer services. In responding to calls, volunteers must first travel varying distances to a squad building. Once aboard the ambulance, they then

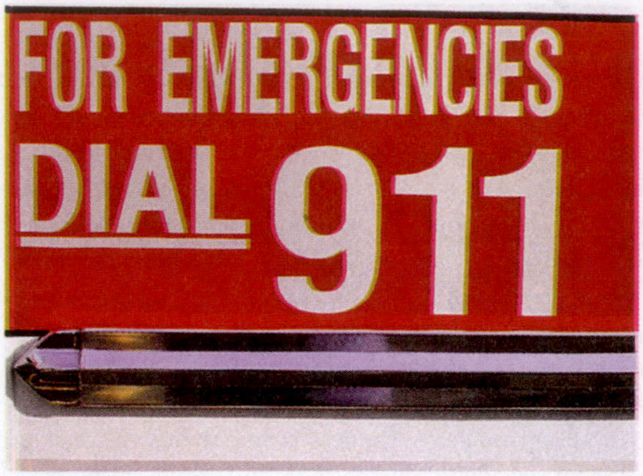

FIGURE 15-1 A universal access number, such as 911, is essential for rapid public access to the EMS system. However, many rural areas lack such a number, hampering communications and increasing response times.

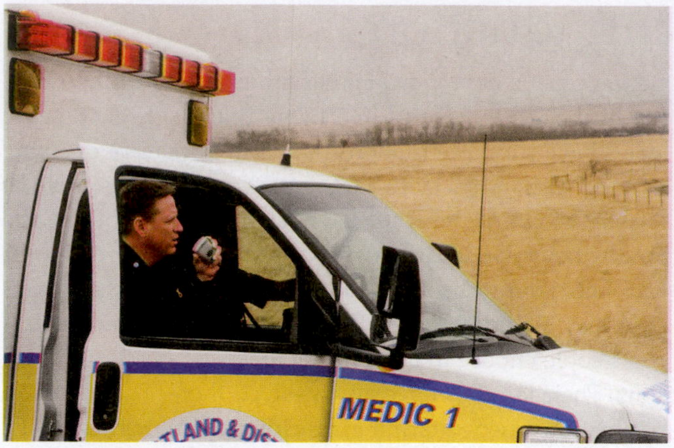

FIGURE 15-2 A rural paramedic must anticipate radio dead spots and request orders to treat any possible medical conditions that may arise during transport.

travel the distance to the patient and later the distance to the hospital. As a result, every decision that a paramedic makes in a rural setting needs to be made with the thought of distance in mind. (The "distance factor," one of the most critical aspects of rural EMS, is discussed in more detail later in this chapter.)

Communication Difficulties

In rural areas, poor or old communication equipment often hampers public access to EMS. A rural area, for example, may not have universal access to 911 (Figure 15-1). Lack of 911 service will delay response time or, in many cases, lead people to turn telephone operators into dispatchers.

Rural EMS crews can also be hampered by inadequate communications. Antiquated "fire phones" or "crash bars" might notify them of an emergency call, but crew members may have no way of communicating with each other en route to the service vehicle. Crews may also lack information from dispatch until they arrive at the squad building or are onboard the ambulance.

While traveling on the ambulance, rural EMS providers may experience dead spots where they cannot transmit (Figure 15-2). Frequencies can also be overloaded with static from highway departments and school buses. This impairs a paramedic's ability to communicate with other ambulance crews or with medical direction. As a result, rural paramedics must often think ahead, asking for orders in anticipation of medical conditions that might develop while traveling within a dead spot.

Enrollment Shortages

Because many rural EMS providers work on a volunteer basis, units or squads can experience enrollment shortages. Volunteers must respond to calls from their jobs or homes. The greater distances and time involved in many rural EMS calls can take volunteers from their work or families for lengthy periods. This situation can affect their ability to earn a living or to raise their children. As a result, they often serve for only short stretches or resign entirely.[3]

Training and Practice

Access to training and continuing education is not readily available in many rural areas. In addition, the cost and amount of time required for certification as a paramedic has increased. For the volunteer, this means increased personal expense and time away from home. The net effect can be EMS providers with a less advanced level of training than their paid urban counterparts.

This situation can be further complicated by the low volume of EMS calls in some rural areas. EMS providers simply do not have the opportunity to practice their skills on a consistent basis. Members of rescue squads may experience what has become known as **rust out**, or an inability to keep abreast of new technologies and standards. The networking opportunities or volume of calls simply do not exist.[4]

Inadequate Medical Support

As might be expected, rural areas sometimes have difficulty obtaining EMS medical direction. Local physicians may lack the training in EMS operations or feel that EMS operations should not be part of their job.

Rural areas also may not have the budgets to buy new equipment and ambulances. In addition, air medical transport may not always be readily available because of many factors, such as distance, lack of landing areas, cost, or too few helicopters for a large area.

Finally, hospitals and rural EMS agencies may not always implement protocols or standards for prehospital providers. Roles may not be clearly defined, or hospitals may have varying protocols. A rural paramedic faced with the decision to transport a patient to two different hospitals may have to deal with two different sets of protocols for prehospital care. That means that volunteers must seek out and familiarize themselves with these protocols often on their own.

Creative Problem Solving

To overcome the obstacles involved in the practice of rural EMS, agencies have turned to creative problem solving. The following sections outline some of the possible solutions available to rural EMS providers.

Improved Communications

In recent years, some rural counties have been fortunate enough to receive grants to modernize or supplement their communications equipment. In other areas, rural counties have joined together to share in the cost of implementing 911 systems. As 911 systems enter rural areas, dispatchers gain valuable education in medical priority dispatch and medical-assist dispatch. Dispatchers with specialized training can provide lifesaving instructions while rural crews are en route to emergencies.

Radio dead spots and crowded frequencies can be handled by requesting additional frequencies and/or by upgrading radio equipment. One possible solution is more powerful base station radios and towers. A group effort in the form of a 911 user advisory board or consortium of agencies can help reduce or eliminate the problem of radio traffic overcrowding. Such advisory boards or consortiums can also provide a forum for discussion of common communication concerns and other issues.

A technological innovation that promises to improve communications in rural areas is the cell or mobile phone. Through the use of cell phones, rural paramedics can communicate with emergency department physicians or their medical directors. Another innovation currently under consideration is the designation of cells for EMS use only.

Recruitment and Certification

One of the most important ways being used to improve rural EMS centers is the effort to increase the number of trained paramedics in rural areas. Recognizing the problem of distance, units with paramedics onboard can intercept basic life support (BLS) crews that require advanced life support measures for their patients. Paramedic units can thus help ensure the highest level of service in rural counties.

The issues of recruitment and certification of paramedics in rural areas can be addressed through flexible training sessions and ongoing education. Agencies can pool their resources with neighboring squads to offer education to all their members.

To increase interest in volunteer EMS, rural agencies can use "explorer" and "ride-along" programs, when appropriate. Paramedics can serve as "recruiters" by taking the lead

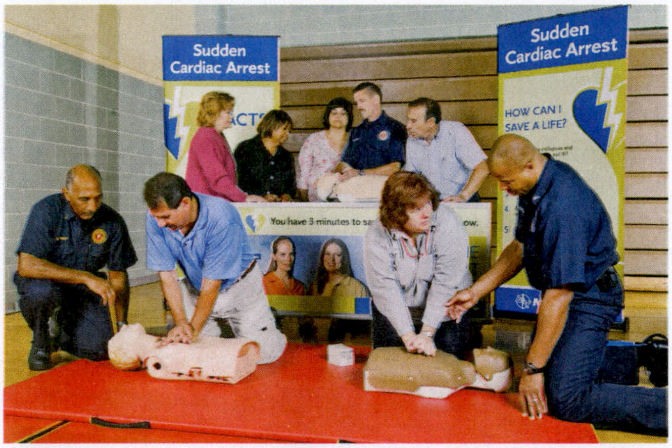

FIGURE 15-3 Public education is a critical part of fulfilling enrollment shortages in rural areas. As a paramedic, you should involve yourself in the training of techniques used by first responders such as CPR.

in training rural residents as CPR drivers or first responders (Figure 15-3). The goal is to involve them in ambulance service or quick response units as soon as possible. Once part of the EMS system, these volunteers can be encouraged to advance to the EMT and paramedic levels of training.

Some of the most important training advancements for rural areas have come through the use of computers and the Internet. Using the Internet, of course, means accessing valid sources of information. However, once these sources are identified, EMS personnel can use "distance learning" to develop an awareness of new standards and procedures. The Internet also provides rural squads with a cost-effective way to interface with other agencies. Networking over the Internet can be an excellent way to promote creative problem solving or to share new ideas.

Even without benefit of the Internet, agencies or units can purchase interactive CD-ROMs and EMS computer simulation programs. These programs allow crew members to maintain a high level of knowledge and skills. They also help EMT-Basics or EMT-Intermediates to train as paramedics (Figure 15-4).[5]

Improved Medical Support

The National Association of EMS Physicians provides numerous educational opportunities for physicians interested in learning more about the supervision and oversight of EMS operations. Conferences held by this organization offer courses in EMS medical direction. Although many doctors choose to practice in urban areas, some highly trained physicians live in rural areas. If you live in a rural area, you or an officer in your agency might approach such physicians and determine their willingness to serve as emergency medical directors. If it is impossible to find a medical director among local physicians, you may need to search at the nearest urban hospital.

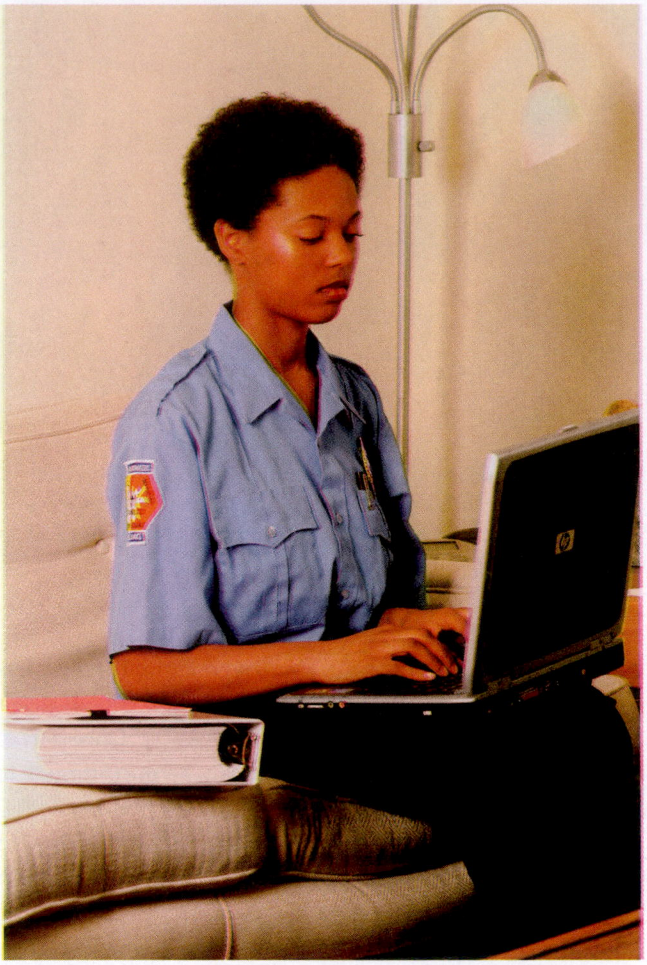

FIGURE 15-4 As a rural paramedic, your education should never end. You can overcome lack of access to classroom instruction through use of the Internet or computerized programs and simulations. You have a responsibility to provide patients with the same high-level care as your urban counterparts.

Regardless of where a paramedic lives, positive relationships with a hospital depend on good communications. A paramedic should spend time at the hospitals that serve his district and, when possible, request to sit in on relevant in-service training sessions provided for the hospital staff.

Ingenuity and Increased Responsibilities

Rural EMS requires ingenuity. For most rural agencies, it is a constant struggle to retain members, supplement budgets, update equipment, provide quality education programs, and network with other health care facilities. As a rural paramedic, you will be involved in most, if not all, of these aspects of rural EMS.

As a rural paramedic, you can expect your role to grow as counties attempt to fill the "health care gap" between rural and urban areas. You may find yourself involved in hospital outreach programs such as **prompt care facilities**, or agencies that provide limited care and nonemergent medical treatment. In such cases, you may work under the direction of a physician or a physician's assistant (PA) and administer immunizations, handle wound care, and provide emergent transport as necessary.

Governments in some rural areas are also considering the involvement of paramedics in the public health system when not responding to emergency calls. Whatever the future may hold, you will be challenged as a rural paramedic to raise the standard of prehospital care offered to the rural residents who make up nearly one-quarter of the nation's population.

Typical Rural EMS Situations and Decisions

Rural paramedics must be highly skilled and highly practiced to compensate for the extended run times and more complicated logistics found in many rural settings. The following sections discuss some of the unique factors a rural paramedic must consider. The scenarios that appear at the end of each section challenge you to consider some of the complex decisions faced by paramedics working in rural areas. In reviewing this material keep in mind one key point: Increased time and distance mean an increased chance of shock.

The Distance Factor

In rural settings, it is often necessary to travel great distances. As a result, you may spend far more time with the patient on board the ambulance than at the scene itself. With this in mind, actions taken by a rural paramedic during transport can have a definitive impact on the patient's outcome. During transport, for example, you could treat a CHF patient with nitrates, CPAP, and an ACE inhibitor. By the time you reach the hospital, the patient may be completely out of crisis. For this reason, you must keep accurate and complete documentation during any lengthy transport.

Another factor to consider during transport is the availability of emergency staff at the local hospital. In most urban areas, hospitals stay active all night. They have full-time emergency departments with around-the-clock staffing able to handle complicated procedures 24 hours a day, 7 days a week. Some rural hospitals, however, may have only a part-time emergency department with only one or two doctors on staff. In such cases, you may have to call the hospital from the patient's home to arrange for the necessary personnel to be in the building when you arrive. You may also have to make a judgment call on whether or not to transport a critically injured patient to a more distant full-time trauma center. In the case of cardiac problems, the availability of fibrinolytic therapy or PCI might be the deciding factor.

In rural EMS, every decision depends on the situation. Because paramedics live in a world of advanced cardiac life support and trauma life support, you may have access to advanced equipment that is unavailable at your local hospital. A rural hospital under budget constraints, for example, may be unable to purchase equipment such as 12-lead ECG monitors and similar technology. In such instances, you might decide with approval of medical direction to use your equipment at the local hospital or to transport the patient to a definitive treatment center at a more distant location.

In treating seriously ill or injured patients, keep in mind that you may see all phases of a patient's death before reaching a distant medical facility. Consider a motor vehicle collision patient with a serious head trauma. At first, your patient may be alert, conscious, and oriented. The patient then becomes agitated and aggressive. He may begin to have memory lapses and become more confused. You notice dilated pupils. If the transport is long enough, the patient will go into a decorticate posture, then a decerebrate posture. You face this situation knowing that there is little or nothing you can do to change the patient outcome because of the unavoidable transport time.

Given scenarios such as the one just described, rural paramedics must know when and how to use air transport. (For more on air transport, see the chapter "Air Medical Operations.")

To assess the effect of distance on the decisions made in many rural emergencies, consider Rural Scenario 1 and the questions that appear at the end of it.

Agricultural Emergencies

Agriculture provides one of the major sources of income in the rural setting. Emergencies related to farming or ranching can range from equipment-related injuries to pesticide poisoning to any number of medical problems exacerbated by agricultural labor.[6] When faced with an agricultural emergency, keep in mind the considerations discussed in the following sections.

Safety

As in any emergency situation, you must place crew safety first. Interpret the situation described by the dispatcher and think of all the scenarios that could be connected with

Rural Scenario 1

You are a rural volunteer paramedic. It's a foggy night, and you are en route to conduct training at an outlying quick response unit (QRU). On your radio, you hear dispatch sending this same QRU to a car-versus-train collision 10 miles ahead of you.

In approximately 10 minutes, you arrive at a very foggy scene with many flashing lights. You determine that the QRU and its fire department have already arrived. You also see a vehicle in the ditch near a railroad crossing. The first responder unit recognizes you as a paramedic and asks for your assistance. Crew members direct you to a 35-year-old man trapped behind the wheel of his vehicle.

On assessment, you find the patient alert and oriented but very anxious. Your physical exam shows blunt chest trauma, decreased breath sounds on the left, a rigid painful abdomen, and several lacerations and abrasions on the head and arms. You record the following vital signs: HR 160; RR 32 and shallow; BP 90/60 mmHg.

Fire department personnel inform you that it will take approximately 20 minutes to extricate the patient. A volunteer BLS ambulance will be on scene in 15 minutes. The closest hospital is a 20-bed Level IV trauma facility located 30 miles east. The nearest Level II trauma center, with an advanced life support (ALS) ambulance service, is 75 miles east and south of the scene.

1. On arrival on scene, you notice that the first responders with the QRU were not attempting to stabilize the cervical spine. They also were not using recommended Standard Precautions. How and when would you correct this situation?

   (After taking control of the scene, you correct any deficiencies that you might note right away. You would tell the first responders to stabilize the head and neck using manual stabilization and don the necessary gear.)

2. To which of the two trauma facilities would you transport this patient? Why?

   (Because the patient is in decompensated shock with a possible pneumothorax and abdominal bleeding, the need for surgery is imminent. As a result, you should transport the patient to the Level II trauma center.)

3. What resources would you call on to help ensure that this patient receives the highest level of care?

   (Because of the mechanism of injury and distance to the appropriate hospital, you would request air transport as well as dispatch of the closest ALS unit. This will ensure that you receive the correct equipment on scene. Keep in mind that the foggy weather may make it impossible for the helicopter to land or necessitate intercept at a safer landing zone.)

4. Having no ALS equipment with you, are there any liability issues that might dictate your actions at the scene and during transport? Explain.

   (You have a duty to act in this situation. As a result, there will be no liability solely for the fact that you do not have gear. Remember that you are always a paramedic and, in this case, your knowledge is as important as your equipment. This does not, however, cover any harm that you may cause to the patient in your treatment. Because you provided treatment on this patient, you must fully document all your actions.)

this situation. In agricultural emergencies, many possibilities for injury exist. Potential dangers include livestock, chemicals, fuel tanks, fumes in storage bins and silos, and heavy or outdated farm equipment.

FARM MACHINERY If you live in an agricultural area, you must familiarize yourself with the range of equipment used on farms or ranches (Figures 15-5a to 15-5c). Farm equipment can be very different from a car, in which a simple turn of the key shuts off the vehicle.

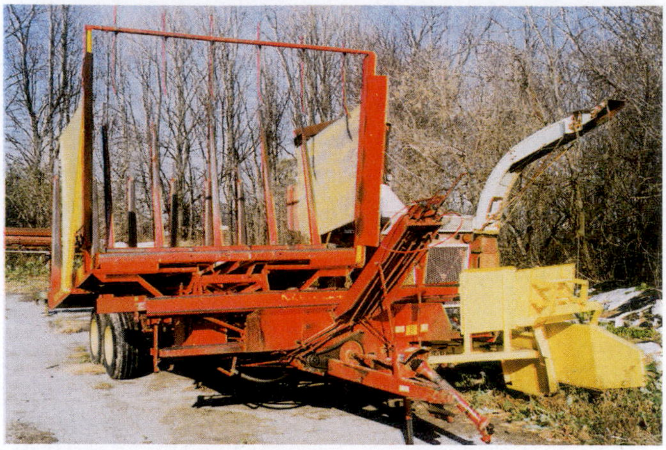

FIGURE 15-5a Hay bale stacker.

(© Mark Foster)

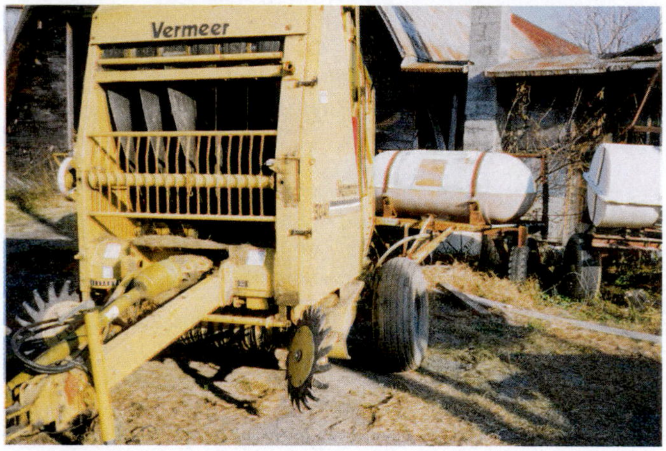

FIGURE 15-5b Round hay baler.

(© Mark Foster)

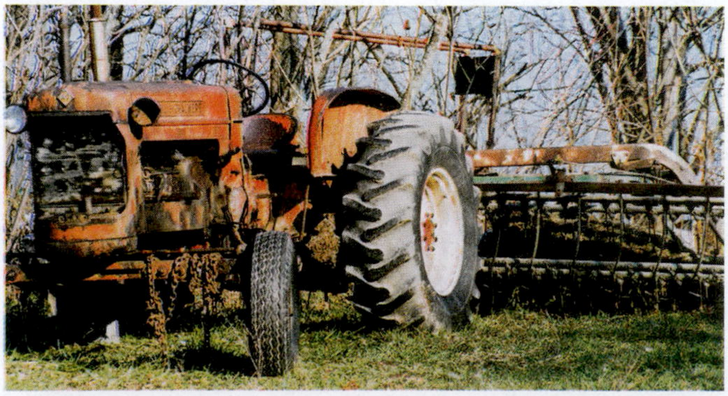

FIGURE 15-5c Tractor and hay rake, typical of the old equipment found on many rural farms.

(© Mark Foster)

To prevent on-scene injuries, you need to make sure that farm equipment is both stable and locked down. Keep in mind that many types of farm equipment have fuel line shut-offs or power-kill switches. For this reason, it is important that you place personnel familiar with the equipment in charge of shutting off and locking down all machinery. Keep in mind the safety principle of **lock-out/tag-out**. After you shut off the equipment, you lock off the switch and place a tag on the switch stating why it is shut off. This prevents accidental retripping of switches.

Remember, too, that the possibility for injury exists even after the equipment has been turned off. Engines fueled by gasoline, diesel, or propane hold the potential for explosion. Equipment that is not properly stabilized or chained can still roll or turn over. When lifting equipment, the center of gravity can shift, increasing the pressure on the patient or causing injury to crew members.

HAZARDOUS MATERIALS Hazardous materials can be found in many places on a farm or ranch (Figures 15-6 and 15-7). They exist in greenhouses, bins used to store pesticides, the equipment used to spray or dust crops, and the manure storage pits on large livestock facilities. For this reason, a self-contained breathing apparatus (SCBA) should be standard equipment on every rural EMS unit.

Be especially wary of rescues involving grain tanks and silos. Over time, grain and silage will ferment if stored long enough. During fermentation, crops release high levels of CO_2, **silo gas** (oxides of nitrogen, or NO_2), and methane.[7] In rescues involving silos, you face the added risk of high angles, confined spaces, and the possibility of entombment under grain or silage. In such cases, determine whether any other agencies might be needed at the scene. Keep in mind the distance factor; don't arrive at the scene to find out you lack the correct apparatus or support for the call. (For more on management of hazardous materials, see the "Hazardous Materials" chapter. For more on confined-space rescues, see the "Rescue Awareness and Operations" chapter.)

Potential for Trauma

Many farmers or ranchers work seven days a week, from sunrise to sunset. They endure extremes of heat, cold, and all kinds of weather conditions. They may spend a large part of the day in remote areas, far from telephones and help if injured.

The risk of serious agricultural accidents and injuries is increased by the equipment and machines routinely used by farmers. In some cases, farmers rely on old or outdated equipment because they cannot afford to replace it. They often wear little or no protective gear and may attempt to repair dangerous equipment themselves. All

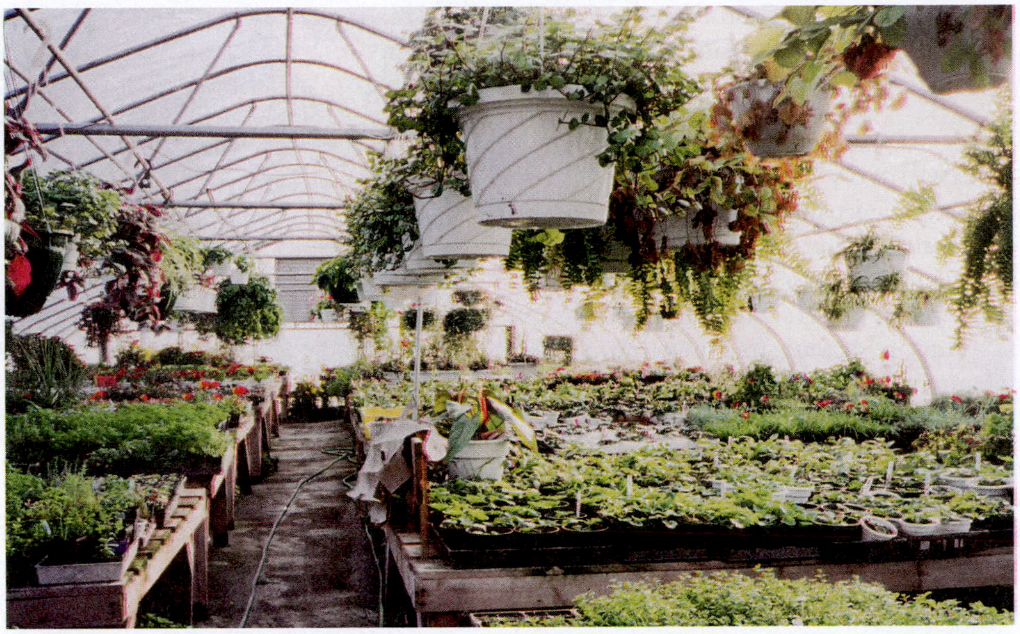

FIGURE 15-6 Greenhouses hold many hidden dangers, such as pesticides, insecticides, and fertilizers. Remember that fertilizers contain nitrites. When mixed with diesel fuel, as in the Oklahoma federal building bombing, they can form powerful explosives.

(© Mark Foster)

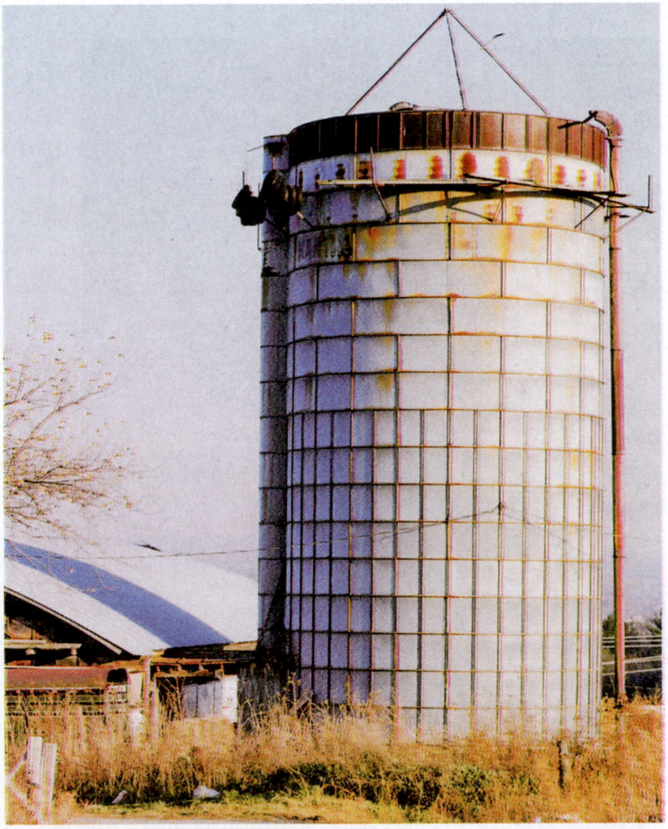

FIGURE 15-7 This old silo looks harmless, but it possesses the potential for entombment in a confined space and exposure to toxic silo gas.

(© Mark Foster)

these situations expose farm workers to equipment-related trauma. Depending on the type of machinery, the mechanism of injury could be crushing, twisting, tearing, penetrating, or a combination of mechanisms.

Equipment-related trauma is complicated by a number of factors related to agriculture. First, a wound may become contaminated by pesticides or manure. Second, a patient may become easily trapped or entangled under heavy equipment, making extrication both difficult and time consuming. Standard extrication devices that are used efficiently for automobiles may be unable to handle the weight of heavy farm equipment. In some cases, extrication equipment may be unavailable and crews will need to improvise using other farm equipment.

Lengthy extrications can worsen the patient's condition. You might use **air bags** (inflatable high-pressure pillows that, when inflated, can lift up to 20 tons) or **cribbing** (wooden slats used to shore up equipment) to relieve some of the equipment's weight. However, if extrication goes on too long, a patient may suffer from **compartment syndrome** or similar problems (e.g., rhabdomyolysis, renal failure). This occurs when circulation to a portion of the body is cut off. Over a period of time (usually hours), toxins develop in the blood, and when circulation is restored the patient goes into shock. This is a serious complication that can be fatal unless proper treatment is given in a timely manner. (For more on the treatment of shock, see the chapters "Hemorrhage and Shock,"and "Orthopedic

Trauma." For more on extrication and delayed treatment and transport, see the chapter "Rescue Awareness and Operations.")

Mechanisms of Injury

Suspect many different mechanisms of injury in accidents involving agricultural equipment. For example, most farm machinery have spinning parts, such as fans, power take-off (PTO) shafts, augers, pulleys, and wheels. These can cause sprains, strains, avulsions, fractures, and possible amputations. Common mechanisms of injury include the following:

- *Wrap points:* **Wrap points** are points at which an appendage can get caught and significantly twisted (Figure 15-8). As noted earlier, spinning parts such as fans, PTO shafts, augers, pulleys, and wheels can catch and twist arms, hands, legs, and feet.
- *Pinch points:* **Pinch points** occur when two objects come together and catch a portion of the patient's body between them. This could be anything from a plow blade falling on somebody's foot to catching a hand in a log splitter (Procedure 15-1).

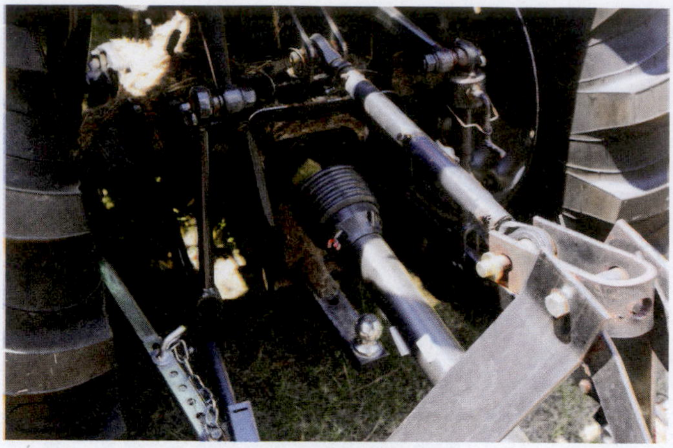

FIGURE 15-8 A tractor's PTO is a prime example of a possible mechanism for a wrap point injury.

(© Dr. Bryan E. Bledsoe)

Procedure 15-1 Removal of Pinch-Point Injury Patient

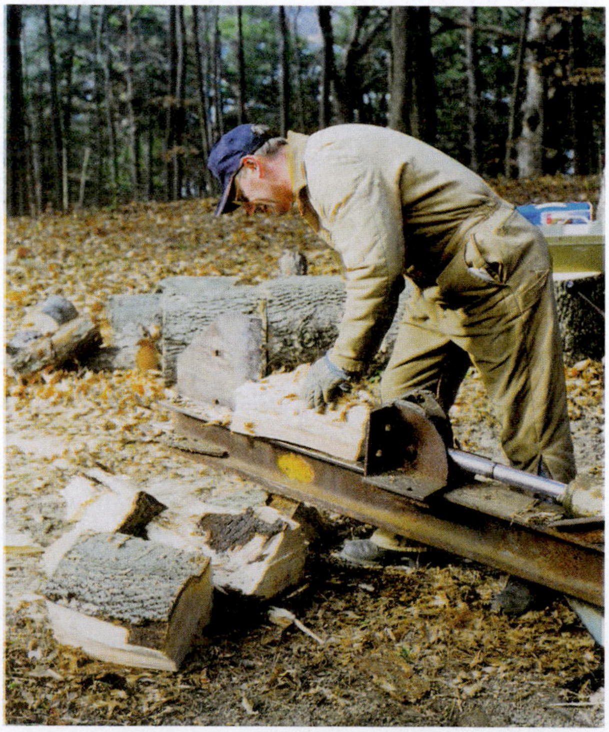

15-1a Log splitter—a typical mechanism for a pinch-point injury in a rural setting. Note the absence of protective gear on the farmer, except for lightweight work gloves.

(© Mark Foster)

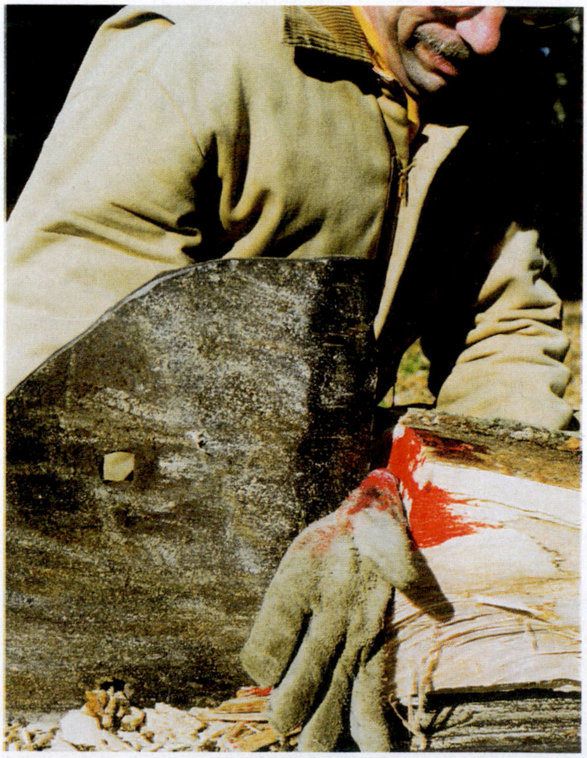

15-1b Hand caught in pinch-point mechanism of injury, with the possibility of compartment syndrome.

(© Mark Foster)

(Continued)

Procedure 15-1 *Continued*

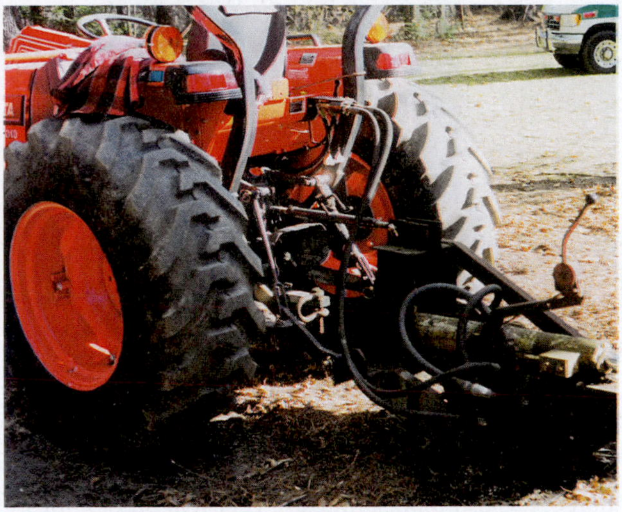

15-1c Determine whether machinery is operated by other equipment—in this case, a tractor. If so, use the machinery to extricate the patient. Then lock-out/tag-out the appropriate levers or switches.

(© Mark Foster)

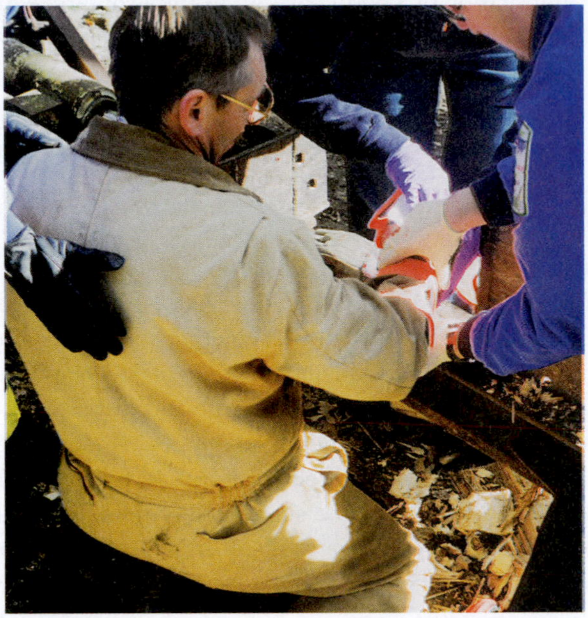

15-1d Stabilize both fractures and circulatory injuries during extrication.

(© Mark Foster)

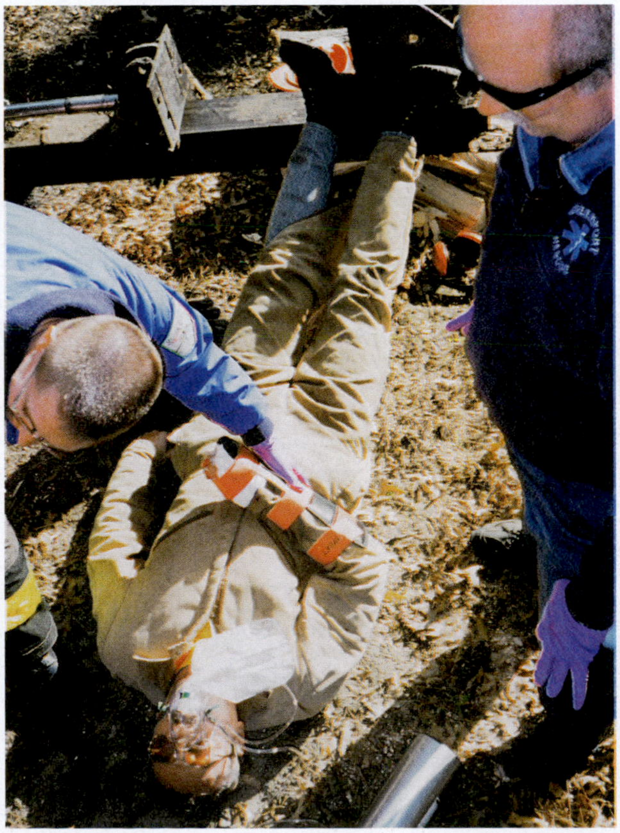

15-1e Provide rapid treatment for shock, especially if the call for help was delayed for a lengthy period.

(© Mark Foster)

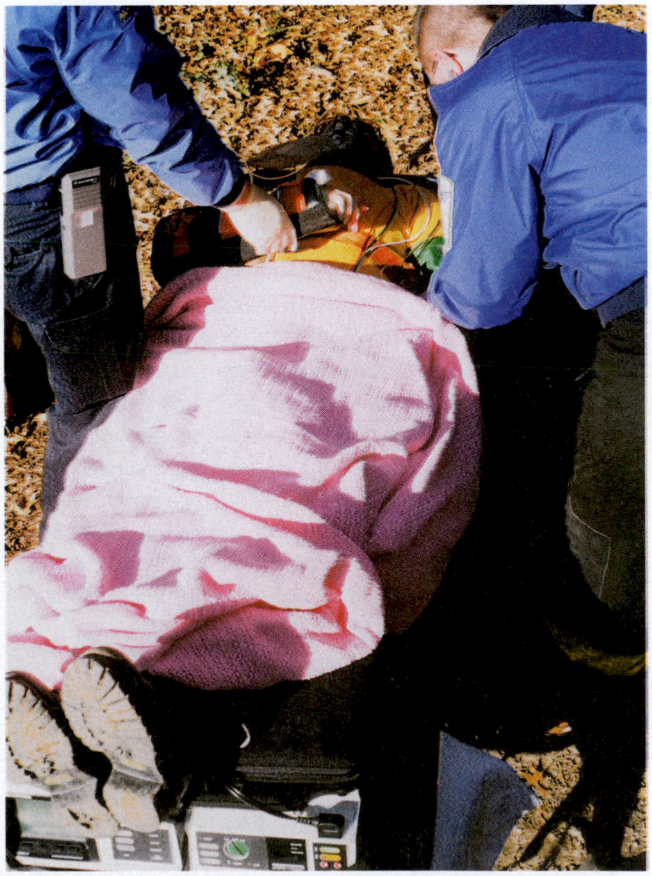

15-1f Package and transport to the nearest appropriate medical facility, using the most effective means of transport.

(© Mark Foster)

- ***Shear points:*** Like pinch points, **shear points** result when two objects come together. However, in this instance, the pinch points either meet or pass, causing amputation of a body part. An example of farm equipment able to cause a shear point is a sickle bar mower.
- *Crush **points:*** **Crush points** develop when two or more objects come together with enough weight or force to crush the affected appendage. A common crush point mechanism of injury is a tractor rollover.

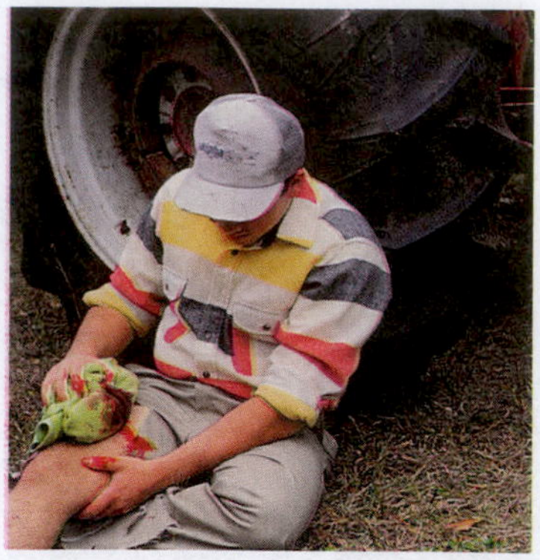

FIGURE 15-9 In rural settings, any serious bleeding injury can result in shock if distance delays treatment or transport.

Emergency Medical Care

In general, provide the same emergency medical care to patients involved in agricultural emergencies as you would to any other patient with similar injuries. However, at all times, keep in mind the effect of time and distance on the potential for shock. A farmer involved in a minor accident, for example, may lie injured for hours in harsh weather conditions before someone suspects any trouble. In cases involving long response and/or transport times, any serious bleeding injury can result in inadequate tissue perfusion if not treated promptly and effectively (Figure 15-9). In addition, because of unsanitary work conditions, sepsis and poisoning are very real possibilities.

To assess the decisions in an agricultural emergency, consider Rural Scenario 2.

Rural Scenario 2

It's late afternoon on a warm day in May. You are the on-duty paramedic at a rural rescue squad. The squad's staff consists of a 24-hour paid paramedic and a supplemental BLS ambulance crew. Having just completed a call, you are in the bay of the squad building restocking your ALS bag and checking your gear. Suddenly a car enters the squad's parking lot, and a very anxious man jumps out. The man rushes up to you. He declares, "My father is trapped under a tractor. He's hurt real bad, and I don't know what to do."

You load the four-wheel-drive quick response vehicle and tell the man that you will follow him to the scene of the accident. However, he speeds off before you can get precise directions to the farm.

En route to the emergency, you contact the county dispatcher and request that she tone out the BLS crew and the local fire rescue squad. Although you still cannot report an address, the dispatcher begins to assemble emergency personnel.

You follow the man into a field, using the four-wheel-drive vehicle to travel over the rough terrain. When you arrive at the site of the overturned tractor, you call county dispatch and provide your exact location before exiting the quick response vehicle. You also request that a helicopter be dispatched.

As you approach the scene, you see an elderly man trapped underneath a tractor from the waist down. Before beginning assessment, you ask the patient's son to make sure the tractor is shut down and the fuel shut-off switch is in place. You also look for fuel leaks, but find none.

On primary assessment, you observe that the patient has multiple contusions to his head and chest and an open humerus fracture on his right arm. Because of the position of the tractor, you are unable to access his lower extremities. The patient is unconscious, unresponsive, ashen, and diaphoretic. Vitals include pulse 132, respirations 32 and shallow, blood pressure 130/88 mmHg.

Ten minutes later, the fire and BLS crews arrive on the scene. The helicopter is still 30 minutes out.

1. What would have made this call go smoother in the response phase?

   (The best scenario would be to have the son ride in your vehicle. A car chase is never a good idea, especially when you do not have a clue about where you are going. You should also specify the need for extrication, giving the crew time to assemble the necessary equipment.)

2. During the 10 minutes you are alone, what care would you provide to the patient?

   (You would protect the airway and use all appropriate ALS procedures such as IV and monitor to treat for shock. Just because you are alone does not mean you cannot provide treatment.)

3. As the on-scene paramedic, what directions would you provide to BLS and fire crews?

   (Directions: Treat for shock and accomplish rapid extrication.)

4. What steps might you take to reduce compartment syndrome?

   (The best treatment is rapid extrication. If you suspect compartment syndrome may have set in, be prepared to treat for septic shock.)

5. What details of this scenario are common to other calls you might make in a rural setting?

   (Details might include use of volunteers, lengthy distances, patients located in isolated areas, the use of many organizations to facilitate the treatment of your patient, and consideration of air transport.)

Recreational Emergencies

Recreational activities have always drawn people to rural settings. Depending on the season and the activity, the population in a rural community can swell dramatically as vacationers, sports enthusiasts, music fans, or "adventure seekers" arrive in an area. Small hill towns, for example, can grow to two or three times their normal size when a ski slope opens. Such a situation presents unique challenges to EMS units in the area (Figure 15-10). A ski slope, for instance, may have its own first aid station and ski patrol, but cannot usually provide advanced care or transport to a patient involved in a skiing accident.

As a rural paramedic, you need to be familiar with the recreational or wilderness pursuits in your area. If you live near a lake, local lifeguards can perform basic first aid and CPR, but they cannot abandon their beach patrol. Further treatment and transport falls to local EMS units. In such cases, a paramedic would need to be well versed in the procedures and skills related to water emergencies.

If you live in a wilderness or mountainous area, you might need to be aware of the accidents commonly encountered by hunters, backpackers, mountaineers, rock climbers, or mountain bikers. You might decide to take courses to receive certification in wilderness rescue. You might also practice rescues in extreme weather conditions, such as those found on New Hampshire's Mt. Washington, where harsh and unpredictable weather patterns can trap or injure even the most experienced climber. (For more information on treating environmental emergencies, see the chapter "Environmental Trauma.")

In wilderness rescues, distance and extrication time play an important part in your decisions. For example, if a rock climber is injured in the Shawangunks in New Paltz, New York, several hospitals lie within a 30-minute range. However, if the patient is injured on the second pitch of a three-pitch climb, evacuation will delay transport, especially if the injury occurs on a class 5.10 or 5.11 route.

A helicopter might seem the obvious choice of transport for wilderness rescues. However, you must take into account weather conditions, availability of suitable landing zones, and the time it will take a helicopter to arrive. In some instances, ground transport may be more efficient, even if it means carrying a patient out in a basket stretcher. In other instances, a helicopter might be able to provide a higher level of care, depending on regional and state protocols. For example, if a rock climber has sustained a severe head injury and if ground transport lacks protocols for rapid sequence intubation, the patient's needs might be better served with helicopter transport.

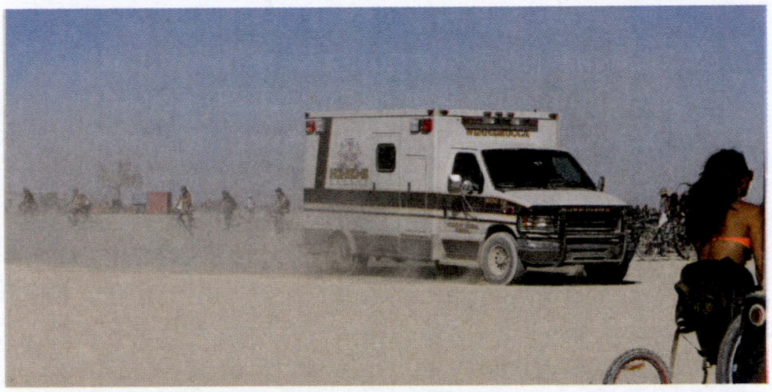

FIGURE 15-10 The recreational activities that draw people to rural settings for vacations, adventure, and sports activities also increase the chances for EMS involvement in environmental emergencies. The "Burning Man" event brings more than 50,000 people to the arid desert of northwestern Nevada.

(© Dr. Bryan E. Bledsoe)

Keep in mind that the helicopter is not a panacea. It has specific uses, tied to distance and level of care. Indiscriminate use of air transport can sometimes add dangerous minutes to patient treatment or even carry the risk of further patient injury. For example, high-altitude sickness can be worsened by an increase in altitude due to unpressurized flight. Decompression syndrome patients are definitely candidates for low-altitude transport. (For more on diving-related injuries, see the chapter "Environmental Trauma.")

To assess the decisions in a recreational emergency, consider Rural Scenario 3.

Rural Scenario 3

Shifting his weight from side to side, Jim compensates for the boat's wake as he glides across New York's Hudson River on water skis. His girlfriend, Renee, is piloting Jim's new boat, while two of Jim's friends enjoy the ride. As Jim shifts to tack in the opposite direction, he catches a wave and drops into the water. Renee sees Jim fall and turns the boat around to pick him up. She does her best to bring the boat gently to him, but piloting is new to her. She realizes too late that the boat is going to hit Jim and puts the motor in reverse.

When the boat strikes Jim, the motor sucks his legs into the propeller. Both of his legs become twisted in and around the shaft. Fearing the worst, Jim's friends jump into the water to hold up his head so that he does not drown. They then yell to the nearest boat for help. The owner of that boat uses his cell phone to call 911.

The 911 dispatcher receives the call. Using pre-arrival dispatch instructions, the dispatcher initiates bystander treatment and gathers the necessary information. Meanwhile, the dispatcher's partner tones out the local rescue squad and the fire department extrication team. Because of the seriousness of the situation, the dispatcher also tones out the nearest ALS unit, where you serve as a paid 24-hour paramedic. Listening to other dispatches on the scanner, you had already begun to move closer to the scene. You now respond rapidly.

On arrival, you find that members of the rescue squad and fire department have entered the water to relieve the patient's exhausted friends. By this time, the patient is unconscious and unresponsive. He has a patent airway and does not have any trauma to his upper body. Postextrication assessment reveals the following vitals: a weak, rapid pulse of 130; respirations 24 and shallow; blood pressure 90/PALP. On physical examination, you note that both legs have multiple fractures. Deep lacerations run from the patient's groin to his ankles. Included in the lacerations are two arterial bleeders.

1. What would be the appropriate BLS and ALS treatment for this patient?

   (BLS treatment includes high-concentration O_2, removal of wet clothing, passive warming for hypothermia, and direct pressure on the lesser bleeders. ALS treatment includes airway management, manual tamponading of arterial bleeders, IV therapy with moderate fluid challenges, monitoring, and rapid transport to a trauma center. Desired blood pressure should remain approximately 90/PALP.)

2. Would the PASG (pneumatic anti-shock garment) be appropriate in this situation? Explain.

   (PASG would not be advised due to the fact that application will not tamponade arterial bleeding and will hide large blood loss inside the pants.)

3. What could be done to ensure better long-term management of this patient in the rural emergency setting?

   (Because saline does not carry oxygen, better long-term management would include moderate fluid challenges instead of large fluid challenges. Also, tamponading of specific arterial bleeding, rather than tamponading of a large area, increases blood flow to the extremities. This makes the extremities more salvageable.)

4. Suppose air transport was unavailable. How would this change treatment provided by the paramedic?

   (The paramedic could transport the patient to the nearest local hospital for stabilization and possible blood transfusions. This action, of course, would depend on equipment and services rendered by the local hospital.)

5. How did the availability of universal access to a 911 number affect the outcome of this patient?

   (The 911 number provided rapid dispatch of all necessary equipment and personnel. It also allowed bystander actions to be guided by a highly trained dispatcher.)

Summary

Rural EMS presents the paramedic and other health care personnel with special challenges such as lengthy distances, radio dead spots, shortages of EMS providers and medical directors, lack of around-the-clock emergency departments, and fewer opportunities for skills practice. To meet these challenges, many rural EMS units have turned to creative problem solving. Counties have joined together to share in the cost of universal access to the 911 system. Squads have adopted flexible training sessions, making use of computerized instruction and networking through the Internet.

Paramedics play an important part in filling the "health care gap" between rural and urban areas. They take a leading role in training rural residents as CPR drivers and first responders. They intercept volunteer BLS units traveling over long distances and provide definitive care. They develop the specialized skills and training to handle the agricultural and/or recreational emergencies unique to their county or district. Because distance often increases the contact time between paramedics and their rural patients, decisions about treatment and use of air transport literally make the difference between life and death.

You Make the Call

The stone quarry in your district was abandoned after it flooded several years ago. Since then, the county has used it as a water source and placed it off limits to recreational users. However, the quarry's clear water and high cliffs serve as a magnet to teenagers who want to go swimming. To you, the quarry holds nothing but trouble for the teens. It is isolated and filled with old rusted equipment. Nothing—not even a well-traveled road—lies near the quarry.

One hot sunny afternoon in August, three teenagers—John, Todd, and Stacey—decide to hike into a remote part of the quarry for a swim. Once at the quarry, Todd rushes to the top of one of the 50-foot cliffs and jumps into the water. Misjudging the water's depth, he hits bottom. When Todd doesn't come up for air, Stacey realizes something is wrong. She and John dive into the water and pull Todd to shore.

The two teens now panic. Todd is breathing, but unconscious. Blood is pouring from a wound in his leg. Stacey tries to stop the bleeding by applying direct pressure. Meanwhile, John races to get help. It takes him nearly 30 minutes to reach a telephone. Lacking a universal access number, he calls the local fire department, which in turn places a call to your volunteer ALS unit. By the time you get into your ambulance, 45 minutes have passed since the accident took place. Although it will only take you about 10 minutes to reach the quarry, you will still need to gain access to the patient at the distant location where the teens chose to swim.

1. What apparatus or support are you going to need to perform this rescue?
2. Based on the mechanism of injury, what injuries should you suspect?
3. What will you do to stabilize this patient?
4. What factors made it impossible for you to meet response, treatment, and transport times in the rural setting when compared with the urban or suburban setting?

See Suggested Responses at the back of this book.

Review Questions

1. Every decision that a paramedic makes in a rural setting needs to be made with the primary thought of ____________ in mind.
   a. budget
   b. distance
   c. insurance
   d. rust out
2. A technological innovation that promises to improve communications in rural areas is the ____________
   a. CAD.
   b. computer.
   c. cell (or mobile) phone.
   d. base station.
3. Regardless of where a paramedic operates, positive relationships with a hospital depend on good ____________
   a. equipment.
   b. pay schedules.
   c. technology updates.
   d. communications.
4. Rural paramedics must be highly skilled and highly practiced to compensate for ____________.
   a. extended run times.
   b. more complicated logistics.
   c. patients with lower acuity.
   d. all of the above.
5. Because hazardous materials can be found in many places on a farm or ranch, which piece of equipment should be standard on every rural EMS unit?
   a. CAD
   b. SCBA
   c. QRU
   d. PTO
6. Common mechanisms of injury in accidents involving agricultural equipment include ____________
   a. wrap points.
   b. pinch points.
   c. shear points.
   d. all of the above.

See Answers to Review Questions at the end of this book.

References

1. Key, C. B. "Operational Issues in EMS." *Emerg Med Clin North Am* 20 (2002): 913–927.
2. Shah, M. N., T. V. Caprio, P. Swanson, et al. "A Novel Emergency Medical Services-Based Program to Identify and Assist Older Adults in a Rural Community." *J Am Geriatr Soc* 58 (2010): 2205–2211.
3. Whyte, B. S. and R. Ansley. "Pay for Performance Improves Rural EMS Quality: Investment in Prehospital Care." *Prehosp Emerg Care* 12 (2008): 495–497.
4. Studnel, J. R., A. R. Fernandez, and G. S. Margolis. "Assessing Continued Cognitive Competence among Rural Emergency Medical Technicians." *Prehosp Emerg Care* 13 (2000): 357–363.

5. Warren, L., R. Sapien, and L. Fullerton-Gleason. "Is On-Line Pediatric Continuing Education Effective in a Rural State?" *Prehosp Emerg Care* 12 (2008): 498–502.

6. Gilpen, J. L., Jr, H. Carabin, J. L. Regens, and R. W. Burden, Jr. "Agriculture Emergencies: A Primer for First Responders." *Biosecur Bioterror* 7 (2008): 187–198.

7. Shepherd, L. G. "Confined-Space Accidents on the Farm: The Manure Pit and Silo." *CJEM* 1 (1999): 108–111.

Further Readings

Farabee, C. R., Jr. *Death, Daring, and Disaster: Search and Rescue in the National Parks.* Boulder, CO: Roberts, Rinehart Publishers, 1999.

Tilton, Buck and Frank Hubbel, *Medicine for the Backcountry.* 3rd ed. Guilford, CT: Globe Pequot, 2000.

Wilkerson, James A. *Medicine for Mountaineering & Other Wilderness Activities.* 6th ed. Seattle, WA: The Mountaineers, 2010.

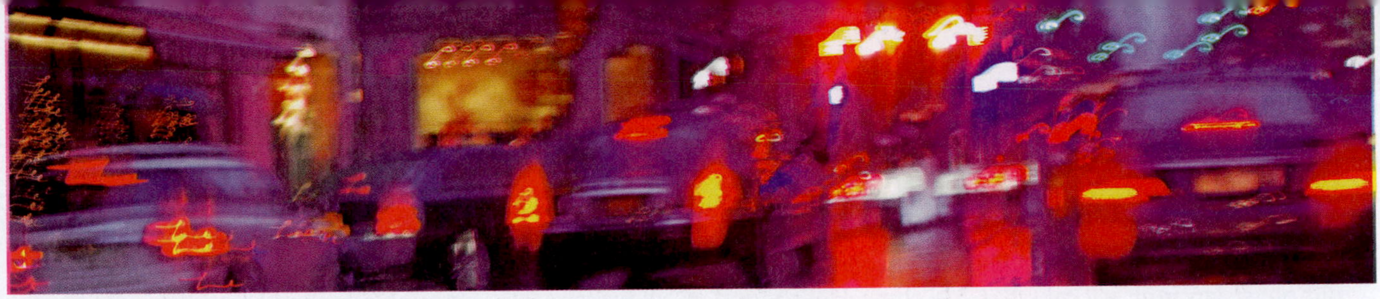

Chapter 16
Responding to Terrorist Acts

Bryan Bledsoe, DO, FACEP, FAAEM, EMT-P

STANDARD
EMS Operations (Terrorism and Disaster)

COMPETENCY
Applies knowledge of operational roles and responsibilities to ensure patient, public, and personnel safety.

Learning Objectives

Terminal Performance Objective: After reading this chapter, you should be able to effectively perform the expected functions of EMS personnel when responding to terrorist acts.

Enabling Objectives: To accomplish the terminal performance objective, you should be able to:

1. Define key terms introduced in this chapter.
2. Describe the characteristics of chemical, biological, radiologic, nuclear, and explosive (CBRNE) weapons used in terrorism, and injuries consistent with these mechanisms.
3. Describe the precautions EMS should take in responding to a known or suspected terrorist attack.
4. Given a variety of scenarios, identify assessment and treatment parameters for patients that have been harmed by various mechanisms used in a terrorist attack.

KEY TERMS

biological agents, p. 417
biotoxins, p. 415
CBRNE, p. 410
dirty bomb, p. 413
dosimeter, p. 413
erythema, p. 415
explosives, p. 411
fallout, p. 412
fasciculations, p. 414
Geiger counter, p. 413
incendiary agents, p. 411
Mark I kit, p. 414
miosis, p. 414
nerve agents, p. 414
nuclear detonation, p. 412
pulmonary agents, p. 415
rhinorrhea, p. 414
specific gravity, p. 414
terrorist act, p. 410
vesicants, p. 415
volatility, p. 414
weapons of mass destruction (WMDs), p. 410

Case Study

Late Monday morning, during the first real cold spell of winter, Adam and Sean are called to transport a 54-year-old physician from a local OB/GYN clinic. He is found to have some "chest tightness" but no ECG abnormalities, and the rest of his assessment is unremarkable. Shortly after delivering him to the emergency department, the pagers go off again, and Adam and Sean are requested to respond to the same address, where several people are now complaining of fatigue, shortness of breath, and headache. Adam remembers that the clinic was the subject of a news report a week earlier, when anti-abortion demonstrators became violent during a protest. As Adam and Sean call in service and en route, Adam requests that the fire department respond for a possible hazardous environment. Sean uses the cell phone (and a secure line) to contact the dispatch center to make his concerns known and suggests that dispatch call the clinic and request evacuation of the facility. Sean also requests that the center activate the community's weapons of mass destruction plan.

Adam and Sean are on the first unit to arrive, so they establish incident command. They size up the scene and notice a dozen or so people in the parking lot but no signs of any smoke or gas clouds coming from the clinic. Adam notes the flag blowing gently from a northwesterly breeze. Sean parks the ambulance north and west of the building and, using the ambulance's public address system, requests the clinic employees to approach his location. He also contacts dispatch with an approximate number of people at the scene and suggests that the fire department approach the building from the northwest. Both paramedics don high-efficiency particulate air (HEPA) respirators and gloves. Sean speaks with some of the employees to ensure that all personnel are accounted for and out of the building.

When the fire department arrives, Captain James approaches, receives a situation update from Adam, and assumes incident command. He reports that a team with self-contained breathing apparatus (SCBA) gear is entering the building to investigate the problem. Adam and Sean establish a treatment sector and begin to assess the victims and administer high-concentration oxygen to the patients with the worst complaints. Their initial evaluation reveals that most patients are complaining of general fatigue, headache, some ringing in the ears, and mild dyspnea. Two other ambulances arrive and, at the direction of Adam, begin oxygen administration to the remaining patients. A pulse CO-oximeter reveals the presence of elevated carboxyhemoglobin levels in virtually all clinic employees and patrons. Captain James answers a radio call from the entry team and reports that carbon monoxide readings are very high in the building.

Adam and Sean remain at the scene but direct the other ambulances to begin transporting patients to the two local hospitals. Sean contacts medical direction and provides the number of patients, their signs and symptoms, and the likely cause of their problems. As Sean and Adam prepare the last of the patients for transport, Captain James reports that the furnace flue was intentionally redirected into the furnace room, generating the carbon monoxide. It is presumed to be a terrorist act, as many believe the clinic to be an abortion clinic. The police are informed and the area becomes a crime scene.

Introduction

The events of September 11, 2001, have had a great impact on our society and our sensitivity to the threat of terrorist acts. The extensive planning and coordination needed to bring down the World Trade Center, damage the Pentagon, and achieve such a great loss of life show just how intent some people are on causing public harm. This new awareness forces the EMS community to prepare itself to respond to acts of terrorism. These acts can come in many forms.

The weapon of choice used by terrorist groups worldwide is the conventional explosive. Conventional explosives have been used frequently in the Middle East and in the British Isles and were used by the Unabomber in the United States. We have also experienced major explosive events, such as the destruction of the Physics Annex at the University of Wisconsin in the mid-1960s, the first attempt to destroy the World Trade Center in 1993, and the bombing of the Oklahoma City federal building in 1995. All of these incidents involved the use of vehicles filled with high-nitrogen-content fertilizer soaked with diesel fuel and parked under or adjacent to the facility.

It is clear that the 21st century will bring new terrorism threats using more unconventional means, such as commercial aircraft to bring down structures and **weapons of mass destruction (WMDs)** including chemical, biological, radiologic, nuclear, and explosive (**CBRNE**) weapons (Figure 16-1).[1,2] Harbingers of such acts include the attack on the Tokyo subway system with sarin gas in 1996 and letters laced with anthrax spores sent through the mail in North America in 2001. Both events underscore the real potential for massive and widespread injury and death caused by

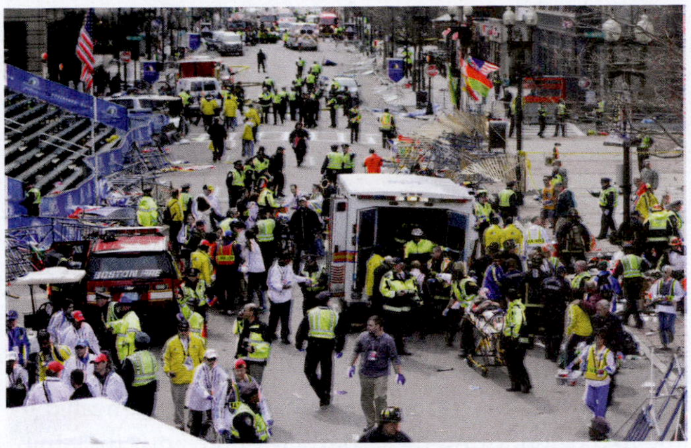

FIGURE 16-1 Providing treatment to a victim of the World Trade Center attack in New York City on September 11, 2001.

(© Charles Krupa/AP Images)

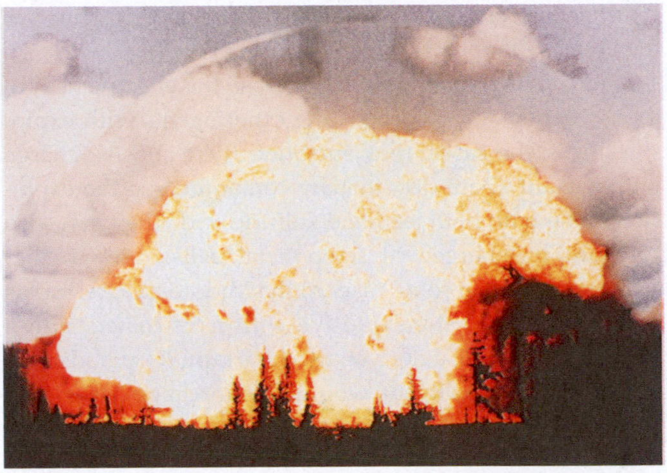

FIGURE 16-2 An explosion releases tremendous amounts of heat energy, generating a pressure wave, blast wind, and projection of debris.

(Reproduced from Bombing: Injury Patterns and Care. Office of Public Health Preparedness and Response, www.CDC.gov)

those intending to incite terror using WMDs. With the increasing likelihood of a **terrorist act**, EMS personnel become responsible for maintaining a higher index of suspicion for such an event. As a paramedic, you also must prepare to protect yourself and your crew, your patients, and the public from the effects of such an attack.

Terrorists may be of foreign or domestic origin. They are likely to target locations that are symbolic of the government (a federal building, such as the Pentagon) or that represent the influence of a country (such as an embassy). Domestic terrorists may further target corporations or their executives who represent a threat to their cause. They may also target their own employer or the public through their employer's products (as in tainted food or pharmaceuticals). The objective of both the domestic and the foreign terrorist is to incite terror in the public.

The likely mechanisms of mass destruction used by terrorists include explosive and incendiary agents, nuclear detonation or contamination, and the release of either chemical or biological agents.

Explosive Agents

Explosives are the most likely method by which terrorists will strike. The bomb may range from a suicide bomber carrying a few sticks of dynamite to a large vehicle filled with highly explosive material. More recently, terrorists have attempted to detonate explosives on commercial airliners (e.g., the "shoe bomber" on American Airlines Flight 63 on December 22, 2001, and the "underwear bomber" on Northwest Airlines Flight 253 on December 25, 2009). In an instant, the device detonates and causes damage to the human body through several mechanisms (Figure 16-2). The blast pressure wave causes compression/decompression injury as it passes through the lungs, the ears, and other hollow, air-filled organs. This damage may be enhanced when the explosion occurs in a confined space, such as the interior of a building or other structure. Debris thrown by the blast produces penetrating or blunt injuries, and similar additional injury occurs as the victim is thrown by the blast wind. Secondary combustion induces burn injury, and structural collapse causes blunt and crushing injuries. After the initial explosion, associated dangers include structural collapse, fire, electrical hazard, and combustible or toxic gas hazards. *Also be wary of secondary explosives set intentionally to disrupt rescue and to injure emergency responders.* After the blast, emergency responders are left to locate, extricate, and provide medical care for the victims. (See the chapter "Mechanism of Injury" for a detailed explanation of the blast process, the associated mechanisms of injury, and assessment and care of the blast victim.)

Incendiary agents are a special subset of explosives with less explosive power and greater heat and burn potential. Napalm, used extensively during the Vietnam War, is a military example, whereas the Molotov cocktail or gasoline bomb is more of a terrorist weapon. Some incendiary agents are of special concern. White phosphorus may spontaneously combust when exposed to air and may be a part of military munitions or a terrorist weapon. It can be very difficult to extinguish when it contacts the skin. Often, fire-resistant oil is used to exclude the air and extinguish any flame. Another example is magnesium, a metal that burns vigorously and at a high temperature (3,000°C). It also is difficult to extinguish. Incendiary agents are likely to cause severe and extensive burn injuries.

CONTENT REVIEW

➤ Examples of Incendiary Agents
- Napalm
- Gasoline
- White phosphorus
- Magnesium

(For more information on burn injuries and their care, see the "Burns" chapter.)

Terrorists may choose to increase the effectiveness of their weapons by incorporating other agents with explosives. In some cases, they surround the explosive charge with old auto batteries, thereby contaminating the explosion scene with both lead and sulfuric acid. They may also surround the charge with scrap metal, nails, or screws that act as shrapnel. In some cases in the Middle East, terrorists have surrounded the explosive with nails coated with a form of rat poison, a derivative of warfarin (Coumadin), to increase the severity of wound hemorrhage associated with shrapnel wounds.

Nuclear Detonation

Nuclear detonation is the release of energy that is generated when heavy nuclei split (fission) or light nuclei combine (fusion) to form new elements. The unleashed energy is tremendous and creates an explosion of immense proportion. In addition to the extremes of the injury-producing mechanisms associated with conventional explosions, radiant heat is likely to incinerate everything in the immediate vicinity of the blast and induce serious burn injury to exposed skin even at great distances from the blast epicenter. Burn injuries are likely to be the most lethal and debilitating injuries associated with a nuclear detonation.

The damage associated with a typical nuclear detonation is extreme and results in concentric circles of total destruction and mortality, severe destruction and very high mortality, heavy destruction and moderate mortality, and light destruction and limited mortality (Figure 16-3). The explosive energy disrupts communications, power, water and waste service, travel, and the medical, emergency medical, and public safety infrastructures. The destruction also disrupts access to the scene and limits the ability of the EMS system to identify, reach, and care for the seriously injured. It is an extreme disaster with great loss of life and injury and presents a great challenge to emergency responders.

The nuclear reaction also generates particles of debris and dust that give off nuclear radiation. Gases, heated by the explosion, draw these particles high into the atmosphere, where upper air currents carry the contamination until it returns to Earth as **fallout**. This uplifting of irradiated debris leaves the scene almost radiation free from moments after the blast until about 1 hour post-ignition. Thereafter, there is a serious danger from fallout at the scene and downwind for many, many miles.

Nuclear radiation cannot be felt, seen, or otherwise detected by any of our senses. However, it damages the cells of the human body as it passes through them. Radiation passage changes the structure of molecules and essential elements of the cells. Damaged cells then go on to repair themselves, to die, or to produce altered or damaged cells (cancer). As the intensity and duration of exposure increases, so do the degree and extent of cell damage and the risk to life. Nuclear radiation from the sun and other natural sources bombards us constantly. This exposure is very limited and the damage caused by it is minimal.

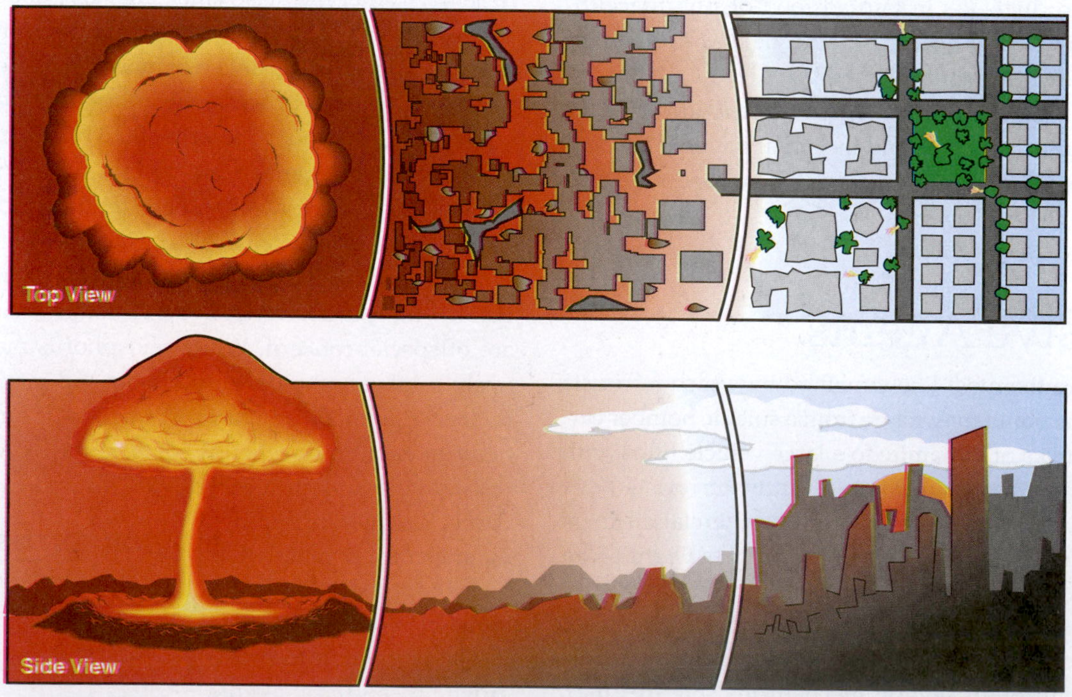

FIGURE 16-3 The concentric circles of destruction following detonation of a nuclear weapon.

However, the initial radiation produced by the nuclear chain reaction (the blast) and fallout can produce serious and life-threatening exposure. (See the chapter "Burns" for the types of radiation, mechanisms of injury, and the assessment and care of the irradiated patient.)

Nuclear Incident Response

The first hour post-ignition is generally spent moving the injured into structures that will protect them from fallout. Ideally, they are moved into the central areas of large, structurally sound buildings or at least to some cover from the falling contaminated dust. Simultaneously, emergency responders organize, determine the direction of fallout movement, and begin to extricate the walking wounded and seriously injured from the outer perimeter of the explosion. During this time, evacuation of those in the anticipated path of fallout occurs. (They should remain outside the fallout pathway for at least 48 hours and until radiologic monitoring determines it is safe to return.) Entry into the scene is made from upwind and laterally to upper air movement in order to limit radioactive fallout exposure to rescuers.

As the response is organized, egress and evacuation routes are cleared, the injured are located and evacuated, and the response moves closer and closer to the blast epicenter. In general, some limited medical care is provided where the victims are found, but most emergency medical care is provided at treatment sectors that are remote from the seriously damaged areas and away from where fallout is expected. Patients are brought to a decontamination area, monitored for contamination, and decontaminated as needed before care begins.

Care for victims of a nuclear detonation involves decontamination (as necessary), treatment as for a conventional explosion (compression/decompression, blunt and penetrating injury care), and treatment for thermal burns. Burns are the most common and most immediately life-threatening injuries associated with a nuclear detonation and will likely be the focus of most care.

Before victims of a nuclear detonation arrive at an emergency medical treatment sector, someone must monitor them for radioactive contamination. This monitoring is accomplished using a device called a **Geiger counter**. The Geiger counter measures the passage of radioactive particles or rays through a receiving chamber and requires some training to use properly. (Usually, someone specially trained—and other than EMS—provides radioactive monitoring and decontamination.) If any significant radioactivity is noted, the patient's clothing is removed and he is washed with soap, water, and gentle scrubbing and then rinsed. All contaminated clothing is bagged, and the wash water is collected for proper disposal. A properly decontaminated patient does not pose a radiation threat either to himself or to you. During a response to a suspected nuclear incident, you will likely wear a **dosimeter**, a pen-like device used to record your total radiation exposure. This device is then monitored to determine when your exposure level is such that you should leave the scene for your own safety. Specially trained scene responders or health physicists will monitor dosages and determine how long you, as a care provider, can safely work at the scene.

If the risk of fallout and continuing radiation exposure is serious, paramedics may be asked to help distribute potassium iodide (KI) tablets. These tablets reduce the uptake of radioactive iodine (a common component of radioactive fallout) by the thyroid, which reduces the risk of thyroid injury or cancer. You may also be involved in the effort to evacuate the public from the expected fallout path.

Generally, patients with serious radiation exposure present with nausea, fatigue, and malaise (a general ill feeling). Treatment for these patients is limited to support, such as keeping them warm and well hydrated. The sooner these symptoms appear after the incident, the more serious the exposure. Generally, if symptoms occur earlier than 6 hours after the detonation, the exposure was very high. However, the effects of radiation exposure differ widely among individuals, so early diagnosis of the exposure extent and survivability from symptoms is unreliable. Because of the severity and nature of a nuclear detonation, disaster triage is necessary and many serious-to-critical burn and radiation-exposure patients will not survive—in part because of the inability of a medical system to care for the sheer number of victims.

Radioactive Contamination

Radioactive contamination may also be spread using conventional explosives (the "**dirty bomb**"). This type of blast is of conventional origin and does not cause the great magnitude of destruction that a nuclear detonation would. However, the explosion distributes radioactive material over a large area and into the surrounding air. The result is an explosion site with radioactive material contaminating the immediate vicinity. The greatest danger of this terrorist weapon is that the nature of the risk (the radiation) may not be recognized until well after the incident. Consequently, many more individuals and rescuers may be exposed or contaminated. Emergency care for victims of a recognized dirty bomb ignition includes radioactive decontamination and treatment (at a remote sector) for injuries that would be expected from a conventional bomb blast.

Chemical Agents

Another terrorist WMD is the release of chemical agents. Potential chemical weapons range from simple hazardous materials common in our society, such as chlorine gas, to sophisticated chemicals, such as nerve agents specifically designed to harm humans. Because these chemical weapons are often gases or aerosols that will disperse in an open or windy area, the more common targets for their use are confined spaces such as subways or large buildings, which have central heating or air conditioning, or areas where many people congregate, such as arenas, shopping malls, and convention centers.

The concepts of volatility (vapor pressure) and specific gravity are important to understanding how chemical weapon agents are distributed. **Volatility** is the ease with which a chemical changes from a liquid to a gas. Most chemical weapons are liquids that are moderately volatile. They are often deployed by an explosion or sprayed into the atmosphere, creating an aerosol. A chemical that remains a liquid is said to be *persistent* and poses a contact or absorption threat, whereas vapors, gases, or aerosols present an inhalation danger. An example of a persistent chemical weapon is mustard agent. An example of a volatile, inhalable chemical weapon is lewisite.

Specific gravity refers to the density or weight of the vapor or gas as compared with air. A vapor or gas with a specific gravity less than air rises and quickly disperses into the atmosphere. This limits the effectiveness of the agent as a weapon. A gas with a specific gravity greater than air sinks beneath it, stays close to the ground, and accumulates in low places. Closed spaces, such as a basement, or low areas, such as a river valley, resist dispersal of the vapor and maintain the danger. Common chemicals with high specific gravity include chlorine and phosgene.

Environmental conditions affect the dispersal of chemical weapons. In strong winds, the gas or vapor mixes with large quantities of air and dilutes and disperses very quickly, limiting its concentration and effectiveness. Light wind moves the cloud downwind as a unit, increasing its effectiveness and the area involved. In windless conditions (which are infrequent), the cloud remains stationary, decreasing the area affected by it. Trees and buildings retard dispersion, whereas open spaces enhance dispersal. Precipitation, especially rain, may deactivate or absorb some agents, such as chlorine. Early morning and the time just before sunset are best for agent release because the winds are usually at their lowest velocity. The interior of a building with few open windows, especially when being heated or air conditioned, is an especially controlled environment. When confined within a building, a chemical agent remains concentrated and deadly for a prolonged period.

Chemical weapons are classified according to the way they cause damage to the human body. These chemicals include nerve agents, vesicants, pulmonary agents, biotoxins, incapacitating agents, and other hazardous chemicals.

Nerve Agents

CONTENT REVIEW

➤ Classifications for Chemical Weapons
- Nerve agents
- Vesicants
- Pulmonary agents
- Biotoxins
- Incapacitating agents
- Other hazardous chemicals

Nerve agents and some insecticides damage nervous impulse conduction. These agents generally inhibit the degradation of a neurotransmitter (acetylcholine) and quickly cause a nervous system overload. This results in muscle twitching and spasms, convulsions, unconsciousness, and respiratory failure. Some common examples of nerve agents include GB (sarin), VX, GF, GD (soman), and GA (tabun). Although not designed as weapons, organophosphate (malathion, parathion) and carbamate (sevin) insecticides share a similar mechanism of action to nerve agents. They are much less potent, but they are still dangerous.

Nerve agents present as either vapor or liquid and are capable of being absorbed through the skin or inhaled and absorbed through the respiratory system. Exposure quickly leads to a series of signs and symptoms remembered as SLUDGE, or Salivation, Lacrimation, Urination, Diarrhea, Gastrointestinal distress, and Emesis. In addition to these signs, the patient may experience dyspnea, **fasciculations** (these are prominent), **rhinorrhea**, blurry vision, **miosis**, nausea, and sweating. Ultimately, the patient may become unconscious, seize, stop breathing, and die.

The actions of nerve agents can generally be reversed if the antidote is administered shortly after exposure. However, many nerve agents permanently bind to the agents, reabsorbing the neurotransmitters, and their effects become more difficult to reverse. The prognosis for a patient exposed to a nerve agent is good with aggressive artificial ventilation and quick administration of the antidote.

Treatment for nerve agent exposure includes the administration of atropine and then pralidoxime chloride. The military currently has these medications available in a two-part autoinjector set called a **Mark I kit**. As the threat of nerve agent release to the civilian population becomes greater, these kits may become increasingly available to the EMS provider. The autoinjectors are designed for self-administration or buddy-administration (mainly for military personnel) or may be administered by rescue personnel. They are quick to use and may be necessary when confronted with numerous patients exposed to a nerve agent. The antidote combination is often followed by the administration of diazepam to reduce seizure activity. The autoinjector is a convenient way to administer this regimen of medications; however, the intravenous route is more rapid and preferred when available and as time permits.

The Mark I kit contains 2 mg of atropine and 600 mg of pralidoxime chloride. It is administered for the first and mild symptoms of exposure (blurry vision, mild dyspnea, and rhinorrhea) and repeated in 10 minutes if symptoms do not improve. If serious signs and symptoms are present, three doses of both atropine and pralidoxime chloride may be administered. Intravenous administration should provide 2 mg of atropine every 5 minutes (until drying of secretions or 20 mg is administered) and 1 g of pralidoxime chloride every hour (until spontaneous respirations return). A pediatric version of the Mark I kit is available.[3]

Vesicants (Blistering Agents)

Vesicants are agents that damage exposed tissue, frequently causing vesicles (blisters). They are capable of causing damage to the skin, eyes, respiratory tract, and lungs, and are able to induce generalized illness as well. The mustard gas of World War I is an example of a vesicant. Other examples include sulfur mustard (HD), nitrogen mustard (HN), lewisite (L), and phosgene oxime (CX). With the exception of phosgene oxime, the vesicants are thick oily liquids that create a toxic vapor threat in warm temperatures. The liquid form, however, is highly toxic to the touch. Lewisite and phosgene oxime induce immediate irritation on contact or inhalation, whereas the mustards produce only slight discomfort that becomes more severe with time. The slow progression of signs and symptoms may prolong contact and increase the severity of exposure.

Patients exposed to vesicants present with the signs and symptoms of injury to the skin, mucous membranes, and lungs. Exposed skin exhibits the signs of a chemical burn, including pain, **erythema**, and eventually blistering. The eyes and upper airway display a burning or stinging sensation, with tearing and rhinorrhea. Respiratory tract exposure results in dyspnea, cough, wheezing, and pulmonary edema. Systemic signs and symptoms include nausea, vomiting, and fatigue. Signs and symptoms occur slowly with the mustard agents, which may prolong exposure.

Emergency care for the patient exposed to a vesicant is immediate decontamination. Exposure of even a few minutes can result in permanent injury. The exposed areas should be irrigated immediately with water from a hose (using limited pressure, if possible). Also irrigate the eyes, with a preference for saline over water, but do not delay irrigation to await the proper fluid. If blistering has occurred, treat the lesions as you would any chemical burn. Apply loose sterile dressings, gently bandage affected eyes, and medicate the patient for any serious pain.

Pulmonary Agents

Pulmonary agents are those that cause chemical injury primarily to the lungs. They include phosgene, chlorine, hydrogen sulfide, and similar agents, and some of the by-products that are created when synthetics such as plastic combust. These agents attack the mucous membranes of the respiratory system from the oral pharynx and nasal pharynx to the smaller respiratory bronchioles and alveoli. They produce inflammation and pulmonary edema, resulting in dyspnea and hypoxia. Early signs and symptoms of pulmonary agent exposure are related to irritation of the upper airway. They include rhinorrhea; nasal, oral, and throat irritation; wheezing; and cough. The victim may also experience tearing and eye irritation. Pulmonary edema is generally a late sign of exposure.

Emergency care for the individual exposed to a pulmonary agent is removal from the environment; exposure to fresh air; high-concentration oxygen; and rest. Endotracheal intubation and ventilation may be required. In cases of moderate to severe respiratory distress, consider 0.5 mL of albuterol by nebulized inhalation.

Biotoxins

Another type of agent that is classified as a biological agent but behaves more like a chemical agent is the **biotoxin**.[4] These toxins are produced by living organisms but are themselves not alive. Such agents include ricin, staphylococcal enterotoxin B (SEB), botulinum toxin, and trichothecene mycotoxins (T2). Ricin, a by-product of castor oil production, inhibits the body's ability to synthesize proteins. It may be either aerosolized and inhaled or ingested. Ricin causes pulmonary edema when inhaled and gastric symptoms when ingested. Poisoning by both routes may cause shock and multiple organ failure.

Staphylococcal enterotoxin is produced by a bacterium, *Staphylococcus aureus*, and is the agent most commonly responsible for food poisoning. Contamination may occur either orally, causing nausea and vomiting, or by inhalation, causing dyspnea and fever. Although only a small amount of toxin may cause symptoms and 50 percent of those contaminated may be incapacitated, SEB is rarely fatal.

Botulinum, the most toxic agent known, is an infrequent result of improper canning technique. It is 15,000 times more potent than VX, the most lethal nerve agent. Fortunately, the botulism toxin is very unstable, which limits its usefulness as a weapon of mass destruction. Like the nerve agents, botulinum attacks the nervous system. It interferes with impulse transmission and interrupts the central nervous system's control of the organs. The result is weakness, paralysis, and death by respiratory failure. Botulinum can be ingested or inhaled.

Trichothecene mycotoxins are a group of biotoxins produced by fungus molds. They prohibit protein and nucleic acid formulation and affect body cells that divide rapidly first. T2 acts very quickly, causing skin irritation (pain, burning, redness, and blistering), respiratory irritation (nasal and oral pain, rhinorrhea, epistaxis, wheezing, dyspnea, and hemoptysis), eye irritation (pain, redness, tearing, and blurry vision), and gastrointestinal symptoms (nausea, vomiting, abdominal cramping, and bloody diarrhea). T2 is most effective when absorbed through the skin. Generalized signs and symptoms include central nervous system signs, hypotension, and death.

Management of a victim of a biotoxin is supportive; antitoxins are generally not available. A special concern is directed to careful decontamination because even a very small amount of biotoxin can endanger rescuers and others.

Incapacitating Agents

Incapacitating agents include the riot control agents used by police and for personal protection, as well as newer agents being investigated by the military. These agents are intentionally selected or designed to incapacitate, not injure or harm, the recipient.

Riot control agents include CS, CN (mace), capsaicin (pepper spray), and CR. You may come into contact with these agents when they are released by police to suppress a large public disturbance or to subdue an assaultive or violent individual or are released by an individual for personal protection or possibly in the commission of a crime. These agents may, in the future, be used by those who wish to disrupt the public and incite terror.

The exposed patient often complains of eye irritation and tearing as well as rhinorrhea. If the agent is inhaled, these symptoms are often accompanied by airway irritation and dyspnea. These signs and symptoms are relieved by removal from the source, exposure to fresh air, and the administration of oxygen, when needed. The signs and symptoms further diminish with time.

The anticholinergic agents (atropine-like drugs) BZ and QNB are the prototype incapacitating agents for the military. The primary method of distribution of these agents is through the detonation of a mixture of explosive and agent. This explosion produces an aerosolized cloud. Exposure to BZ and QNB produces inappropriate affect, dry mucous beds, dilated pupils, slurred speech, disorientation, blurred vision, inhibition of the sweating reflex, elevated body temperature, and facial flushing. These effects become apparent after about 30 minutes of inhalation and last for up to 8 hours. The most dangerous effects of exposure include dysrhythmias and hyperthermia from the loss of the sweating reflex. The actions of BZ and QNB may be reversed by the administration of physostigmine.

Other Hazardous Chemicals

Any toxic chemical has a potential for use as a weapon of mass destruction. Industry produces countless hazardous materials with the potential to cause great harm if released into the air or water supply or ignited to release toxic gases. The only difference between an accidental release and one that is intended to incite terror is that the intentional release will likely be optimized to affect the greatest number of people. It may also be more difficult to identify the agent used by a terrorist because the container will likely not identify the agent. The Department of Transportation's *Emergency Response Guidebook,* which should be carried on every ambulance and fire apparatus, is a good guide to most common hazardous materials that might be used as a weapon as well as information on other WMD agents. It can also be helpful in denoting isolation and evacuation distances and suggesting specific care management steps.

Recognition of a Chemical Agent Release

A chemical weapon release may be visible as a cloud of mist, vapor, dust, or as puddles, or it may be completely unrecognizable. There may be an associated smell such as that of newly mown grass (phosgene), rotten eggs (hydrogen sulfide), or other strange or unusual odors. Suspect a chemical release if there are chemical odors when and where chemicals are not used or expected. However, never search out such an odor or touch any suspect liquid or material. You may also notice clusters of patients with chemical exposure symptoms or injured, incapacitated, or dead insects, birds, or animals. (You might remember that parakeets have been used in mines to detect toxic gas levels.) Given that the terrorist may be intent on optimizing the effect of the release, be especially wary of large public gatherings or large but confined spaces such as public buildings and low spaces that limit dissipation such as subway terminals. Terrorists may also target food or water supplies with either chemical or biological agents. This may result in very widespread effects.

A cardinal sign of a chemical release is the manifestation of similar signs and symptoms occurring rapidly among a group of individuals. Common signs of a chemical release include inflamed mucosa (eye, nasal, oral, or throat irritation), exposed skin irritation, chest tightness, burning and/or dyspnea, gastrointestinal signs (nausea, abdominal cramping, vomiting, and diarrhea), and central nervous system disturbances (confusion, lethargy, nausea/vomiting, intoxication, headache, and unconsciousness).

Management of a Chemical Agent Release

Approach the scene from upwind and higher ground and remain a good distance away from the site. Generally, evacuate the immediate area if the release is small and contained. However, if the release involves a great quantity of material, such as that in a railway tank car or large commercial storage container, evacuate the general population for a radius of 700 to 2,000 feet and 1.5 miles downwind during the day.

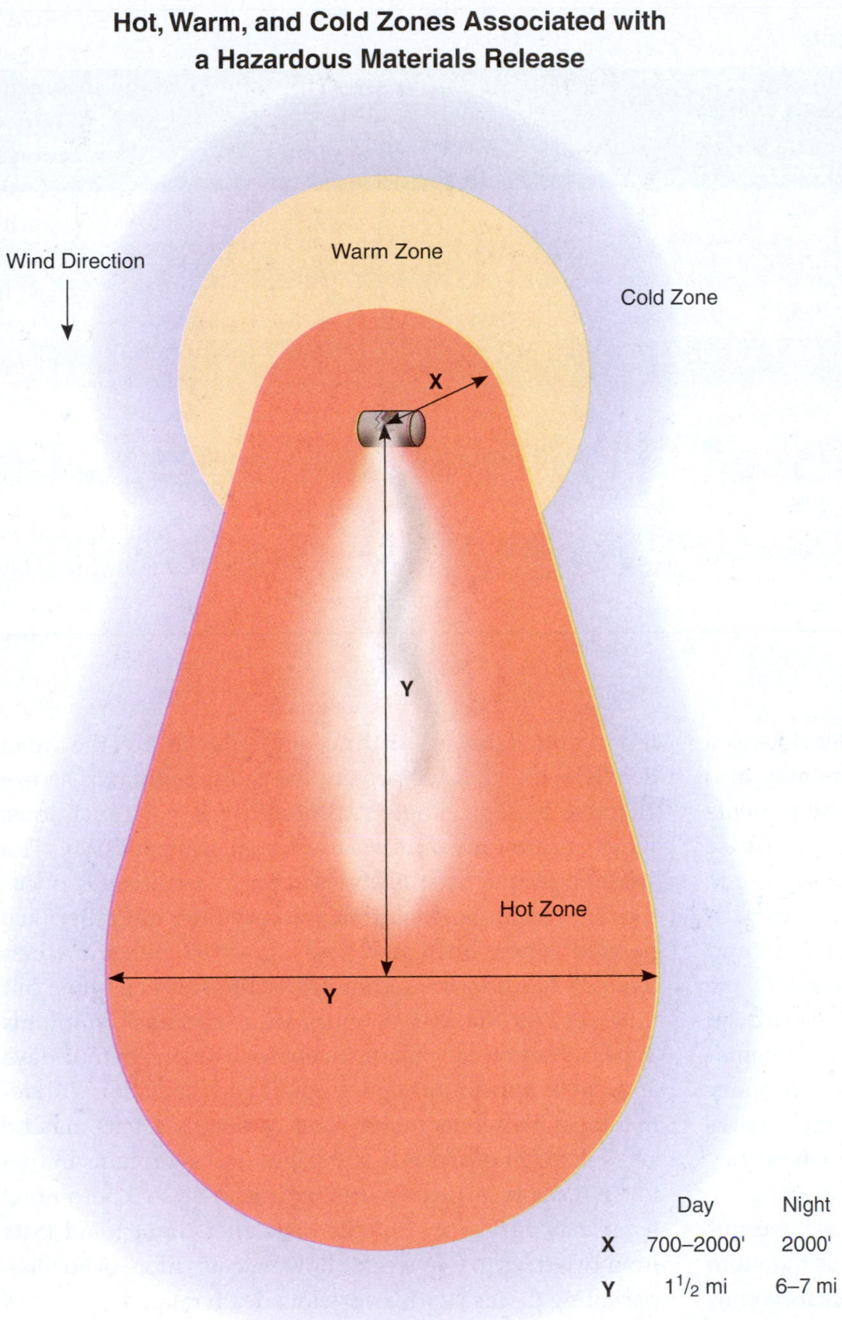

FIGURE 16-4 Hot, warm, and cold zones associated with a hazardous materials release.

If the release occurs at night, then evacuate a 2,000-foot radius and as much as 6 to 7 miles downwind (Figure 16-4).

Once the public danger is reduced by scene isolation, make sure that the injured are properly decontaminated before you begin care. Rescuers coming out of the danger zones must also be decontaminated. The agency that provides spill containment and decontamination at the hazardous materials incident generally provides decontamination for both nuclear and chemical weapons of mass destruction. This service is most commonly the fire department. (See the "Hazardous Materials" chapter.)

In addition to the specific emergency care steps noted earlier, most patients require decontamination, exposure to fresh air, oxygen administration, and possibly respiratory support. As a precautionary measure, use personal protective equipment (PPE), including a well-fitting HEPA filter mask, nitrile gloves (latex gloves do not offer much protection against chemical agents), and a Tyvek® disposable suit. Be careful of leather clothing items. Belts, watchbands, and shoes made of leather absorb many chemical agents and will present a continuing exposure danger once contaminated. These precautions provide very minimal protection against chemical agents and do not constitute the PPE necessary to work in a warm or hot zone.

Biological Agents

Biological agents are either living organisms or toxins produced by living organisms that are deliberately distributed to cause disease, incapacitation, and death. Generally, these agents are grouped as noncontagious (anthrax and biotoxins) or as contagious and capable of spreading from human to human (smallpox, Ebola, plague). Contagious agents are of greatest concern because the people originally infected can spread the disease, often before the medical community has recognized that a biological weapon attack has occurred. EMS and other medical systems are especially vulnerable because they are called to treat those who first display the disease's signs and symptoms, possibly before the nature and significance of the disease is known. Noncontagious agents affect only those who received the initial dose, thus limiting the scope of the disease and making it somewhat easier to identify when and where the contact took place.

Identification of a biological agent release is difficult because there is often no noticeable cloud of gas or any noticeable odor. This identification is especially challenging because any signs and symptoms of the disease occur at the end of the incubation period, often days or weeks after the initial contact. Rapid identification is further complicated because many potential biological weapons present with signs and symptoms typical of influenza or many other common and general illnesses (Table 16-1).

Most commonly, the existence of a biological attack is recognized when numerous patients report to the emergency department or medical clinic with similar signs

Table 16-1 Characteristics of Biological Agents

Disease	Incubation Period	Mortality	Signs and Symptoms				
			Fever	Chills	Cough	Malaise	Nausea/ Vomiting
Anthrax	1–6 days	90%	√		√	√	
Pneumonic plague*	1–6 days	57–100%	√	√	√	√	
Tularemia	3–5 days	35%	√		√	√	
Q fever	2–14 days	1%	√		√	√	
Smallpox*	12 days	30%	√			√	√
Venezuelan equine encephalitis	1–5 days	1%	√	√	√	√	√
Cholera	1–3 days	50%					√
Viral hemorrhagic fever	3–7 days	5–20%	√			√	
Ebola*	3–7 days	80–90%	√			√	

**Human-to-human contagious disease.*

and symptoms or when a health care provider notices a geographic cluster of patients. Care providers may also notice a disease occurring out of season (many patients with flu-like symptoms during the summer) or a disease outside its normal geographic regions (tropical disease in the northern latitudes). Only then can the health department begin to work to identify the disease's nature and when and where the exposure most likely happened. By the time the disease outbreak is recognized as a bioterrorism event, secondary exposures from those affected by contagious agents may already be occurring. These secondary exposures may include family members, friends, workmates, and the medical system, including EMS, emergency department personnel, and other health care providers.

Mother Nature may be the most sinister of all bioterrorists. Mutant strains of common diseases, such as the more serious variations of influenza, multiple-drug-resistant strains of tuberculosis, or the recent cold-like virus called *severe acute respiratory syndrome (SARS)*, may emerge and create epidemics of massive proportions. Outbreaks of naturally occurring disease may be more likely and more severe than a terrorist's use of a biological weapon. Tracking the origin and combating these naturally occurring diseases is exactly like tracking and combating a biological weapon used by terrorists.

Currently the list of potential WMD diseases is extensive and contains pneumonia-like agents, encephalitis-like agents, and others.

Pneumonia-Like Agents

Pneumonia-like bioterror agents include anthrax, plague, tularemia, and Q fever, and are the most likely agents for a terrorist attack.[5] They generally cause cough, dyspnea, fever, and malaise. Anthrax and plague are the most deadly, with 90 to 100 percent mortality. Anthrax is a very effective biological agent, although it is not contagious, which limits any human-to-human transmission. The strain of plague most likely used for bioterrorism is pneumonic, which carries not only a very high mortality (100 percent when untreated and about 57 percent when treated), but also has minimum victim survival when left untreated for the first 18 hours after signs and symptoms appear. Pneumonic plague incubates over one to four days and can be spread through droplets and inhalation. Tularemia (also known as rabbit fever or deerfly fever) may be aerosolized and presents with signs and symptoms in two to ten days. It carries a mortality rate of up to 5 percent. Q fever may appear in 10 to 20 days after contact and lasts from two days to two weeks; however, it is more of an incapacitating disease with a very low death rate.

Encephalitis-Like Agents

Smallpox and Venezuelan equine encephalitis (VEE) are influenza-like diseases with headache, fever, and malaise and a higher mortality, probably because these diseases attack the central nervous system. They are very effective as biological weapons because small amounts of aerosolized agent can cause the disease. Smallpox is very contagious through airborne droplets via the respiratory route. Signs and symptoms usually appear after about 12 days in about 30 percent of those exposed, with about a third of that number dying within five to seven days. Smallpox is considered eradicated as a naturally occurring disease, but it is thought that it may exist in the WMD programs of some countries. With VEE, human-to-human transmission does not occur, and mortality is generally less than 20 percent.

Other Biological Agents

Cholera is a common disease in underdeveloped countries and is frequently linked to poor sanitation. It is most commonly transmitted by the fecal-oral route and primarily causes severe dehydration and shock because of profuse diarrhea. It is one of the few agents that is not transmitted by the inhalation route and may be delivered as a weapon by way of contamination of food or untreated water.

Viral hemorrhagic fever (VHF) is a class of disease that includes the deadly Ebola virus. As the name suggests, hemorrhagic fever attacks the bloodstream and damages blood vessels, causing them to leak and the patient to bleed easily. The patient may bruise easily and display petechiae (tiny red patches of dermal hemorrhage). Most diseases of this class can be spread through the inhalation route or through direct contact with infectious material. VHFs may carry a high mortality rate (90 percent) and are aerosolized easily, although they are difficult to cultivate.

Protection against Biological Agent Transmission

Protection against the most common biological weapons includes the prudent care steps used to prevent ordinary communicable disease transmission. If there is a heightened alert status for a WMD release or terrorist event, employ a more aggressive use of standard precautions. Gloves are very effective in protecting against biological agent transmission from body fluids, as is rigorous and frequent hand washing. Almost all biological agents are transmitted by the respiratory route, so be sure to take droplet inhalation precautions. A properly fitted HEPA filter mask is very effective in preventing agent transmission (Figure 16-5). Consider applying a mask to your patient if he displays any signs or symptoms of respiratory disease. A sodium hypochlorite solution (0.5 percent) or other disinfectants are very effective in killing many biological agents. The ambulance interior and any equipment used or possibly contaminated should be cleaned vigorously with the solution.

Immunizations against many biological agents are not available. The immunizations that are available usually carry a small risk of associated reaction. Hence, the prophylactic administration to a very large number of health care workers may not be warranted unless or until a significant risk becomes apparent. Consult with your medical director for your system's recommendations and the method used to provide you with immunizations if the need arises.

Emergency care for most patients affected by biological weapons is limited to supportive care—maintain body temperature, administer oxygen, and provide hydration (and, in some cases, IV fluids). Because some of the biological agents may produce respiratory compromise, protocols may call for an albuterol or other nebulized treatment. If practical, consider the use of metered-dose inhalers (MDIs) rather than nebulization, because MDIs limit aerosolized-droplet formation and subsequent risk of contaminating inhalation. Once the exact organism is isolated (after prehospital care), then a regimen of antibiotic therapy may be prescribed.

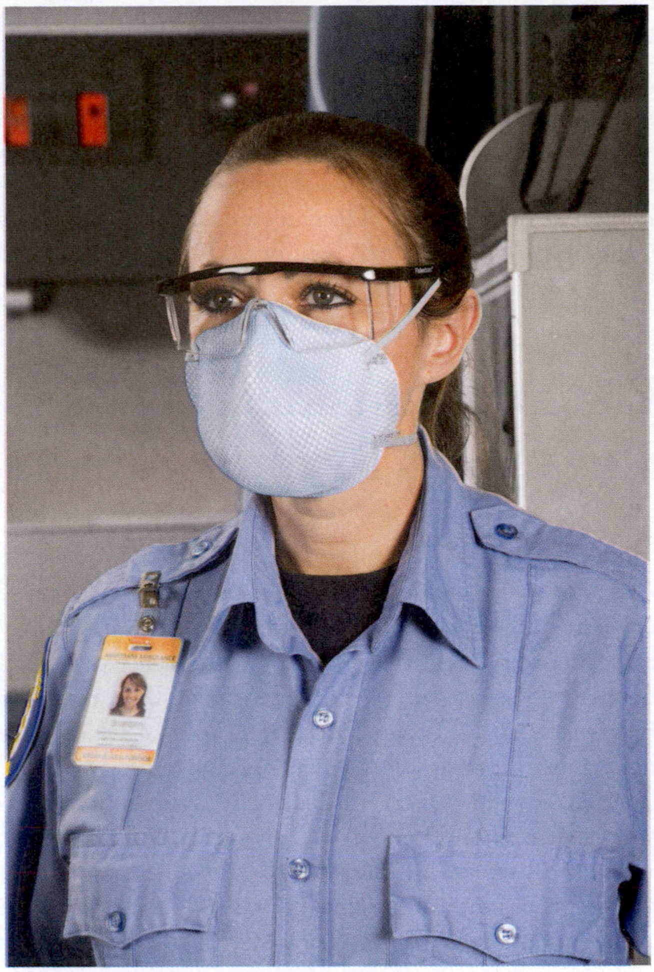

FIGURE 16-5 A HEPA filter mask.

If a biological attack is suspected, health officials will interview the victims carefully. They will try to determine when the patients first noticed symptoms and identify any close personal contacts since that time. These people may be infected if the agent is indeed contagious. The public health approach to biological terrorism may also involve isolation and quarantine. The patient or caregiver exposed to a highly contagious disease may be quarantined through a restriction to home or may be confined within a commandeered facility such as a motel. A person with the signs and symptoms of the disease may be isolated through a similar arrangement. There is a danger associated with placing affected patients or caregivers in a hospital or other medical facility because they can then endanger other patients or care providers who are receiving or providing care there.

Mass Shootings

Although guns are not usually considered weapons of mass destruction, some terrorist attacks may involve mass shootings. Paramedic response would be the same as for any multiple or mass shooting. Review the relevant information in the chapters "Mechanism of Injury," "Multiple Casualty Incidents and Incident Management," and "Crime Scene Awareness."

General Considerations Regarding Terrorist Attacks

Scene Safety

One of every five victims of the World Trade Center collapse on September 11, 2001, was a member of an emergency response team. This great number of emergency personnel deaths underscores the need to recognize the dangers to EMS providers and ensure that safety is an active concern during the response to any potential act of terrorism.

Terrorists in other countries often set secondary explosive devices with the intent to disrupt any rescue attempt. A chemical release or radioactivity can linger and affect those who attempt unprotected rescue of patients. Biological agents are likely to affect the EMS provider as well. It is imperative that you carefully analyze a scene to determine the risk to you and other rescuers. Then ensure that the scene is entered only by those properly equipped and trained to enter a hazardous or deadly environment.

Recognizing a Terrorist Attack

It is relatively easy to recognize a nuclear or conventional explosion. However, remember that radioactive fallout travels with the upper wind current (not just currents at ground level), so watch cloud movement. Stay upwind. Remember, too, that terrorists may use the conventional explosion to distribute radioactive or other hazardous material (the "dirty bomb"), and they may set secondary detonations through booby traps or timers that are designed to target rescuers. Also be aware of structural collapse, because the explosion may weaken a building's structure. Do not enter the scene until you are sure it is safe from all hazards.

A chemical release may not be as obvious. There may or may not be a cloud of gas or aerosolized material. There also may or may not be any unusual odors. However, groups of victims will be complaining of similar symptoms, although symptom development may take some time. Suspect a chemical incident when you notice incapacitated small animals, birds, and insects. You may also be alerted to a possible chemical incident when confronted with chemical-exposure-like symptoms where chemicals are not usually used. Stay upwind and uphill of the site and request that victims and potential victims evacuate (or be evacuated) to you. Only personnel who are specially trained and equipped to deal with hazardous materials should enter the scene. However, to protect yourself, don nitrile gloves, a well-fitting HEPA filter mask, and a Tyvek coverall when caring for a patient who has been decontaminated. These precautions provide only limited protection while working on decontaminated patients. They are not considered adequate for entry into the scene (warm or hot zone).[6,7]

Identifying a biological agent at the time of release is probably impossible. There might be a cloud of dust or aerosolized material but there are no immediate signs and symptoms from those exposed. Such contamination also may be distributed by the mail (anthrax-laced letters, for instance) or other mechanisms. The incident is likely to be recognized after the incubation period and only after several patients report to the emergency departments or clinics with the disease. Then the local health department will investigate what all victims have in common to identify where the biological agent release took place. If you happen to notice many patients presenting with signs and symptoms of illness at or around the same time, consider a possible biological attack. As with any potential disease, don gloves and a well-fitted HEPA filter mask. (See the chapter "Infectious Disease and Sepsis.") It is important to remember that you may be inadvertently exposed to a contagious agent, contract the disease, and then become a carrier. If you become aware of possible exposure or notice the signs and symptoms of a contagious disease, contact the proper health resource (your medical director, service infection control agent, or other person, according to protocols or your service policies) and ensure that you do not transmit the disease to others.

Legal Considerations

Training for Nontraditional Roles in a WMD Attack. The role of EMS personnel in a WMD attack is primarily patient care. However, such attacks can quickly overwhelm responding agencies, forcing personnel on scene to assume nontraditional roles. Assuming a role for which you have not been trained (e.g., decontaminating persons exposed to radiation in a "dirty bomb" attack), though, will put both you and the victim at risk. Because of this, regional response systems must establish response plans. Personnel who *may* be called on to provide a role in a WMD response outside their traditional area of responsibility must receive the necessary training. A significant amount of cross-training and crossover of on-scene roles may be essential for an adequate response to a WMD incident that does not put the victims or responders at increased risk.

Responding to a Terrorist Attack

Your first role in responding to a possible act of terrorism is to ensure your own safety and that of your patient, other rescuers, and the public. Once safety is ensured, make certain that all patients are properly decontaminated (if need be) and then begin to provide the appropriate emergency medical care.

Your role as an emergency care provider for a terrorist attack is very similar to the other emergency responses you are more likely to encounter during your career. A nuclear incident is handled as a conventional explosion with a hazardous material (radiation) involved. The release of a chemical agent is a hazardous material incident. A biological weapon release is handled like an infectious disease outbreak. Although the location of the attack may maximize the number of people it affects, it is still a hazardous material incident (chemical or radiation agent), an infectious disease incident (biological event), a conventional explosion, or a combination of these. Use the training you already have for these situations and follow your system's protocols and disaster plans for each.

Once a WMD incident is identified, begin preparing for the casualties. Often this will entail instituting the incident command system and establishing extrication, decontamination, triage, treatment, and transport sectors. Carefully match the available resources against the nature, number, and severity of injuries. Review the chapter "Multiple-Casualty Incidents and Incident Management."

Summary

Many of the mechanisms of injury used by terrorists (toxic gases, radiation contamination, or biological agents) induce their damage subtly so that there is little scene evidence. Your responsibility is to maintain an enhanced lookout for any signs of CBRNE release or exposure and limit the contact that you, the general population, and your patients have to such an agent. In general, it is not the role of EMS to deal with CBRNE agents. Your role as a paramedic is likely to be providing supportive care after patient decontamination.

You Make the Call

You are dispatched to "an explosion with possible injuries." Your emergency vehicle is the first to arrive at a synagogue with smoke pouring from broken windows and obviously injured people on the lawn.

1. What special safety considerations would you observe for this scene?
2. What are the likely injuries to expect from this mechanism of injury?
3. Should you enter the synagogue?

See Suggested Responses at the back of this book.

Review Questions

1. What is the most common method by which terrorists strike at their targets?
   a. Explosives
   b. Chemical weapons
   c. Anthrax exposures
   d. Poisonings of public water supplies
2. After an initial explosion, associated dangers include ____________
   a. fire.
   b. electrical hazard.
   c. structural collapse.
   d. all of the above.
3. Which type of injuries are likely to be the most lethal and debilitating injuries in conjunction with a nuclear detonation?
   a. Burn injuries
   b. Inhalation injuries
   c. Blunt trauma injuries
   d. Penetrating trauma injuries

4. If there is serious risk of fallout and continuing radiation exposure, paramedics may be asked to help distribute ______________
   a. iron tablets.
   b. magnesium capsules.
   c. potassium iodide tablets.
   d. sodium chloride solution.
5. Which of the following is an insecticide that is occasionally used by terrorists because its effects are similar to those of a nerve agent?
   a. GB (sarin)
   b. GD (soman)
   c. GA (tabun)
   d. Carbamate (sevin)
6. Emergency care for the patient exposed to a vesicant is immediate ______________
   a. transport.
   b. fluid therapy.
   c. oxygenation.
   d. decontamination.
7. Which of the following agents is not considered contagious?
   a. Ebola
   b. Anthrax
   c. Plague
   d. Smallpox
8. What is a common disease in underdeveloped countries that is frequently linked to poor sanitation?
   a. Cholera
   b. SARS
   c. Tularemia
   d. VEE
9. As a result of terrorist attacks and their reliance on nerve agents, EMS systems are starting to carry which antidote kit, developed by the military?
   a. Mark I kit
   b. AT kit
   c. Atro-Prad kit
   d. SNAP kit
10. Almost all biological agents are transmitted by which route?
   a. Ingestion
   b. Absorption
   c. Injection
   d. Inhalation

See Answers to Review Questions at the end of this book.

References

1. Stevens, G., A. Jones, G. Smith, et al. "Determinants of Paramedic Response Readiness for CBRNE Threats." *Biosecur Bioterror* 8 (2010): 193–202.
2. Grace, M. B., K. D. Cliffer, B. R. Moyer, et al. "The U.S. Government's Medical Countermeasure Portfolio Management for Nuclear and Radiological Emergencies: Synergy from Interagency Cooperation." *Health Phys* 10 (2011): 238–247.
3. Sandilands, E. A., A. M. Good, and D. N. Batemen. "The Use of Atropine as a Nerve Agent Response with Specific Reference to Children: Are Current Guidelines Too Cautious?" *Emerg Med J* 26 (2009): 690–694.
4. Aas, P. "The Threat of Mid-Spectrum Chemical Warfare Agents." *Prehosp Disaster Med* 18 (2003): 306–312.
5. Daya, M. and Y. Nakamura. "Pulmonary Disease from Biological Agents: Anthrax, Plague, Q Fever, and Tularemia." *Crit Care Clin* 21 (2005): 747–763.
6. Castle, N., R. Owen, S. Clark, et al. "Comparison of Techniques for Securing the Endotracheal Tube while Wearing Chemical, Biological, Radiological, or Nuclear Protection: A Manikin Study." *Prehosp Disaster Med* 25 (2010): 589–594.
7. Castle, N., Y. Pillay, and N. Spencer. "Comparison of Six Different Intubation Aids for Use while Wearing CBRN-PPE: A Manikin Study." *Resuscitation* 82(12) (2011): 1548–1552.

Further Readings

Bevelacqua, A., and R. Stilp. *Terrorism Handbook for Operational Responders.* 3rd ed. Clifton Park, NY: Cengage Learning, 2009.

Buck, G. *Preparing for Biological Terrorism: An Emergency Services Guide.* Albany, NY: Delmar Publishing, 2002.

Byrnes, M. E., D. A. King, and P. M. Tierno. *Nuclear, Chemical, and Biological Terrorism: Emergency Response and Public Protection.* Chelsea, MI: Lewis Publishers, 2003.

De Lorenzo, R. A., and R. S. Porter. *Tactical Emergency Care: Military and Operational Out-of-Hospital Medicine.* Upper Saddle River, NJ: Pearson/Prentice Hall, 1999.

Emergency Response Guidebook (ERG2012). Washington, DC: U.S. Department of Transportation, 2012.

Marks, M. E. *Emergency Responder's Guide to Terrorism.* Chester, MD: Red Hat Publishers, 2003.

Sachs, G. *Terrorism Emergency Response: A Workbook for Responders.* Upper Saddle River, NJ: Pearson/Prentice Hall, 2003.

Sidell, F. R., W. C. Patrick III, and T. R. Dashiell. *Jane's Chem-Bio Handbook.* 3rd ed. Alexandria, VA: Jane's Information Group, 2005.

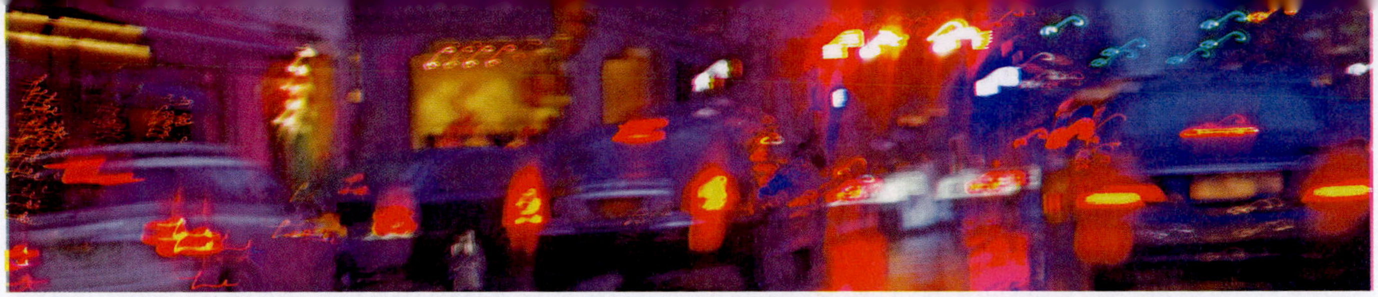

Precautions on Bloodborne Pathogens and Infectious Diseases

Prehospital emergency personnel, like all health care workers, are at risk for exposure to bloodborne pathogens and infectious diseases. In emergency situations it is often difficult to take or enforce proper infection control measures. However, as a paramedic, you must recognize your high-risk status. Study the following information on infection control carefully.

Infection control is designed to protect emergency personnel, their families, and their patients from unnecessary exposure to communicable diseases. Laws, regulations, and standards regarding infection control include:

- ***Centers for Disease Control and Prevention (CDC) Guidelines.*** The CDC has published extensive guidelines on infection control. Proper equipment and techniques that should be used by emergency response personnel to prevent or minimize risk of exposure are defined.
- ***The Ryan White Act.*** The Ryan White Act of 1990 allows emergency personnel to find out if they were exposed to an infectious disease while rendering patient care. Employers are required to name a "designated officer" to coordinate communications with the treating hospital.
- ***Americans with Disabilities Act.*** This act prohibits discrimination against individuals with disabilities, including those with contagious diseases. It guarantees equal employment opportunities and job protection if the infected individual can perform essential job functions and does not pose a threat to the safety and health of patients and coworkers.
- ***Occupational Safety and Health Administration (OSHA) Regulations.*** OSHA has enacted a regulation entitled Occupational Exposure to Bloodborne Pathogens that classifies emergency response personnel as being at the greatest risk of occupational exposure to communicable diseases. This regulation requires employers to provide hepatitis B (HBV) vaccinations free of charge, maintain a written exposure control plan, and provide personal protective equipment. These requirements primarily apply to private employers. Applicability to local and state governmental employees varies by locality. Many states have developed their own OSHA plans.
- ***National Fire Protection Association (NFPA) Guidelines.*** This is a national organization that has established specific guidelines and requirements regarding infection control for emergency response agencies, particularly fire departments and EMS services.

Standard Precautions and Personal Protective Equipment

Emergency response personnel should practice Standard Precautions by which ALL body substances are considered to be potentially infectious. To practice Standard Precautions, all emergency personnel should utilize personal protective equipment (PPE). Appropriate PPE should be available on every emergency vehicle. The minimum recommended PPE includes the following:

- ***Gloves.*** Disposable gloves should be donned by all emergency response personnel BEFORE initiating any emergency care. When an emergency incident involves more than one patient, you should attempt to change gloves between patients. When gloves have been contaminated, they should be removed as soon as possible. To properly remove contaminated gloves, grasp one glove approximately 1 inch from the wrist. Without touching the inside of the glove, pull the glove halfway off and stop. With that half-gloved hand, pull the glove on the opposite hand completely off. Place the removed glove in the palm of the other glove, with the inside of the removed glove exposed. Pull the second glove completely off with the ungloved hand, only touching the inside of the glove. Always wash hands after gloves are removed, even when the gloves appear intact.

- ***Masks and Protective Eyewear.*** Masks and protective eyewear should be present on all emergency vehicles and used in accordance with the level of exposure encountered. Masks and protective eyewear should be worn together whenever blood spatter is likely to occur, such as during arterial bleeding, childbirth, endotracheal intubation, invasive procedures, oral suctioning, and cleanup of equipment that requires heavy scrubbing or brushing. Both you and the patient should wear masks whenever the potential for airborne transmission of disease exists.
- ***HEPA and N-95 Respirators.*** Due to the resurgence of tuberculosis (TB), prehospital personnel should protect themselves from TB infection through use of an N-95 or a high-efficiency particulate air (HEPA) respirator, as approved by the National Institute of Occupational Safety and Health (NIOSH). It should fit snugly and be capable of filtering out the tuberculosis bacillus. An N-95 or HEPA respirator should be worn when caring for patients with confirmed or suspected TB. This is especially true when performing "high-hazard" procedures such as administration of nebulized medications, endotracheal intubation, or suctioning on such a patient.
- ***Gowns.*** Gowns protect clothing from blood splashes. If large splashes of blood are expected, such as with childbirth, wear impervious gowns.
- ***Resuscitation Equipment.*** Disposable resuscitation equipment should be the primary means of artificial ventilation in emergency care. Such items should be used once, then disposed of.

Remember, the proper use of personal protective equipment ensures effective infection control and minimizes risk. Use ALL protective equipment recommended for any particular situation to ensure maximum protection.

Consider ALL body substances potentially infectious and ALWAYS practice Standard Precautions.

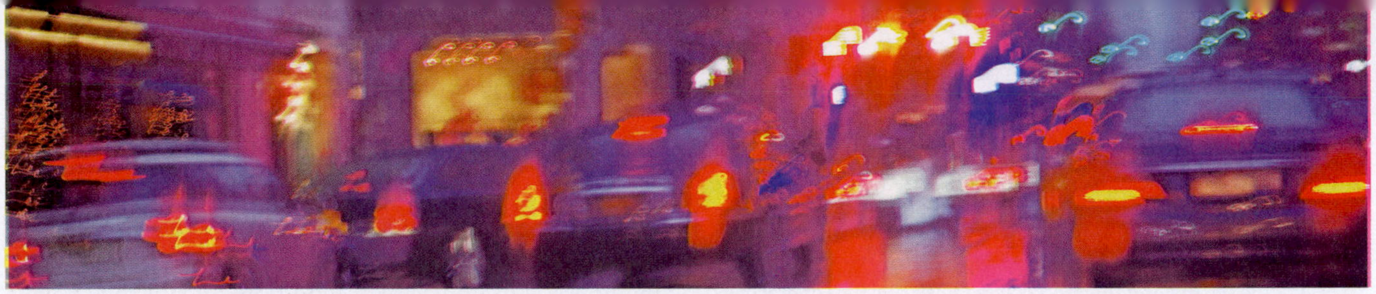

Suggested Responses to "You Make the Call"

The following are suggested responses to the "You Make the Call" scenarios presented in each chapter of Volume 5, Special Considerations/Operations. Each represents an acceptable response to the scenario but should not be interpreted as the only correct response.

Chapter 1—Gynecology

1. *What is your first priority?*

Your first priority is to assess the patient, obtain intravenous access, and prepare the patient for transport to the local emergency department by placing her on your stretcher in the position of comfort.

2. *What else should you do?*

You should try to obtain information regarding who performed the abortion so you can relay the information to the receiving facility. The receiving facility will most likely want to consult with the person who performed the abortion and even have him or her come in to see the patient right away.

3. *What do you suspect is the likely cause of her signs and symptoms?*

The fever is most likely secondary to an infection that is related to the recent abortion. The foul-smelling discharge, as well, is most likely necrotic tissue left over from the abortion.

In your assessment, you should determine whether the patient's "abortion" was an actual procedure or the result of her ingesting an "abortion pill." With an abortion pill, at some point the patient will be expected to bleed and slough off the results of pregnancy. Most procedure-based abortions will include removing the tissue and fetus. In any event, it is imperative to treat and transport the patient.

4. *Because your patient is a minor, do you have any legal requirements to notify her parents or obtain their consent before treating her?*

No. In this case, the patient is a minor who is in need of medical attention and treatment. It is implied that the parents would give consent (implied consent) for you to treat and transport the patient.

Chapter 2—Obstetrics

1. *What is your first priority?*

Your first priority is to apply oxygen and package the patient, being prepared for aggressive airway maneuvers if necessary.

2. *What do you suspect is the likely cause of the patient's signs and symptoms?*

This patient is clearly suffering from preeclampsia (hypertensive disorders of pregnancy) and could be subject to eclampsia and seizures if not treated quickly.

3. *Your patient's husband is very concerned about the well-being of his wife and baby. What should you tell him?*

Tell him the truth. Explain what you have found and that it is serious, but it is also a common situation that typically has normal births and outcomes if treated appropriately.

4. *How should this patient be transported to the hospital?*

She should be placed on the stretcher in a left lateral recumbent position with padding under her abdomen. The lights in the back of the unit should be kept down to a minimum, if not turned off completely. Consider magnesium sulfate administration if indicated. The transport should be made routine, without sirens or anything else that could aggravate or agitate the patient any more than she already is.

Chapter 3—Neonatology

1. *Should you stimulate this baby to breathe as soon as it is delivered? Why or why not?*

No. When thick meconium is present, and the infant is nonvigorous, consider positive-pressure ventilation if the infant is not breathing or the heart rate is less than 100 beats per minute.

2. *What is the major danger associated with this type of problem?*

Meconium can cause airway obstruction. In addition, the infant could inhale the meconium, potentially setting up an infection that could be life threatening.

3. *Once you have stabilized this infant, where should he be transported?*

This infant should be transported to a facility with a NICU.

Chapter 4—Pediatrics

1. *What are your assessment priorities for this patient?*

Initial assessment priorities are to determine the patient's level of consciousness, apply pressure to the bleeding scalp wound, and stabilize the cervical spine before doing a more thorough assessment.

2. *What interventions would you perform on scene and en route to the receiving hospital?*

On-scene interventions would be kept to a minimum, only handling the bleeding scalp wound, spinal precautions, and any other significant findings; otherwise, the majority of the treatment would be performed en route to the hospital.

3. *Describe possible transport considerations, including a potential refusal of transport by the angry parents.*

Clearly, in this case the patient should be transported for further evaluation and to give the proper authorities time to assess the situation for possible abuse. There is a possibility that the parents will refuse treatment and transport for the patient. In this case, the only option you will have is to contact the proper authorities and notify them of what you have found, making sure to thoroughly document your objective findings.

4. *What are the important factors in reporting this incident and documenting the call?*

It is very important that you do not accuse or confront the parents while on scene. Make sure you pay attention to the surroundings and scene. Document only the things you see, hear, touch, or smell. Do not document any feelings or assumptions.

Chapter 5—Geriatrics

1. *What general impression do you have of this patient?*

Your first impression should be of a possible stroke. It would be prudent, if possible, to determine when the symptoms began in order to determine whether the patient is within an interventional treatment window.

2. *Do you suspect that this is an acute or chronic problem? Explain.*

This is probably an acute problem because the patient's wife says that he normally takes care of her. Additionally, the house is in immaculate condition. Even if they have a housekeeper or housecleaner, there would be a few things out of place if he was normally like this, considering that the wife is very arthritic and can barely ambulate around the home.

3. *Aside from the patient's presentation and response to your interventions, what other information should be included in your hospital report?*

It would be important to record the inability of Mrs. Jones to navigate the home, the location of the patient, and, most important, to record the last known time the patient was "normal."

4. *What support do you provide for Mrs. Jones?*

If there is no one immediately available to come help take care of Mrs. Jones, you should allow her to ride with you to the hospital, where she would be able to receive assistance. Additionally, check with your local resources to see if an elder assistance program may exist that you or the hospital could contact to help. It would not be out of line to ask her whether she has someone she would like for you to contact, such as family members or a religious group.

Chapter 6—Abuse, Neglect, and Assault

1. *What do you suspect is taking place?*

This situation is highly indicative of child abuse.

2. *What physical evidence do you have to support this suspicion?*

Bruises on the child's arms and back in various stages of healing.

3. *What emotional evidence do you have to support this suspicion?*

The fact that the boy has a flat affect and does not look toward his parents.

4. *What other clues lead you to believe that abuse might be taking place?*

Additional clues that may not individually be representative of abuse but can be confirming evidence would include law officers being on scene for "domestic disturbance," and the fact that the boy is dressed only in underwear in the winter.

5. *What are your priorities in this case?*

In this case, the priorities are the child's welfare and making sure that he is not suffering from any medical emergency. Carefully document your findings in the patient care report.

Chapter 7—The Challenged Patient

1. *Why did the patient's doctor tell her that she has an increased risk of infection from communicable diseases?*

The medical treatments she is receiving (e.g., chemotherapy)—including the recent mastectomy, which includes a removal of lymph nodes responsible for helping with infections—all put her at high risk for obtaining an infection.

2. *What signs indicate that this patient has cancer?*

You would notice that she has a recent mastectomy and is wearing a scarf around her head with a wig at her bedside, indicating that she most likely has lost her hair from the cancer treatment.

3. *Is it necessary for all three of you to wear a mask? Explain.*

It is safer for the patient if all three of you wear masks. This will provide additional filtration for the patient and protection from communicable disease. Once in the ambulance, the patient compartment can be secluded by closing doors separating it from the cab and turning on the ventilation system. Once this has been accomplished, it would then be acceptable for the driver to remove his or her mask.

4. *Will you start a peripheral IV on this patient? Explain.*

Most likely, this patient will not require a peripheral IV. If she does, it would be important to avoid the side from which she has had her mastectomy. Mastectomies involve the removal of lymph nodes, which, in turn, makes the patient very susceptible to lymphedema secondary to any trauma or pressure on the arm.

5. *What information will you include in your patient report so the emergency department is prepared for this patient?*

You should include information about the additional respiratory precautions that you are taking.

Chapter 8—Acute Interventions for the Chronic Care Patient

1. *What does the condition of the apartment tell you?*

A messy, dirty apartment may indicate that the patient is on her own and has little support from family or friends. It may also show that she is receiving inadequate home care. These social factors may help you understand the patient's state of mind and interact with greater compassion.

2. *Why is it important to immediately interview the home care worker?*

The home care worker usually knows the patient well and can tell you exactly what is different, if anything, about the patient. If you don't fully understand the patient's baseline mental status and disability, you cannot adequately assess and compare your own findings.

3. *What are some of the causes of urinary incontinence?*

Causes include seizures, spinal injury, abdominal trauma, and overdose, among others.

4. *How can you rule out spinal injury to this patient?*

You can't. The possibility of spinal injury in a patient with a preexisting neurologic deficit cannot be ruled out without knowing the exact nature of his or her baseline deficit. That decision is best left to the patient's own physician or the ED staff.

5. *Why do you think the patient denies a history of diabetes and seizures if she takes Tegretol and Glucophage?*

Imagine how you would feel if confined to a wheelchair at age 18 for the rest of your life. Such patients can become unhappy, lonely, resentful, and bitter. They may also deny certain aspects of their disability in an attempt to feel better or to gain acceptance. In this case, because the patient exhibited no complicating factors related to diabetes or seizures, the crew decided not to argue with her. However, they had a responsibility to report all medications—and suspicions—as a part of their transfer of care.

6. *Why is it acceptable to defer the glucose test when patient medications indicate a possible blood sugar problem?*

The patient seems to be sensitive to her condition. Because she shows no signs of hypoglycemia, it is probably better to keep the patient calm than to argue with her about the test. If the crew had any doubts about their actions, they should, of course, consult with medical direction.

7. *Was there any need for an IV?*

No. The patient was showing no signs of shock, nor did she need to have any medications given.

8. *Should the patient have been placed on oxygen?*

Oxygen would not have hurt the patient in any way, but there was no indication for its use. The patient exhibited no shortness of breath, was in no distress, and had good skin color. (She was getting enough oxygen from room air.)

Chapter 9—Ground Ambulance Operations

1. *Should you drive down the open eastbound right lane with your lights and siren on? Explain.*

No—you should always use the left to pass vehicles. Motorists are taught to "move to the right when you see the lights" and by attempting to pass on the right, there is a potential that motorists may move to the right, into your path, as they try to make room.

2. *Should you enter the oncoming traffic by going around the left side of the vehicle that is currently stopped in the left-hand, eastbound lane? Explain.*

Yes—passing to the left is the safest place to pass. By cautiously moving into the oncoming traffic lane, you will be able to capture the westbound traffic's attention and move around other vehicles in the eastbound lane safely. Remember, this should be done cautiously and at a rate of speed slow enough to allow you to stop and maneuver as necessary to avoid obstacles.

3. *How can you best deal with this very dangerous intersection?*

The best method for dealing with this intersection is to make sure all your warning devices are operating (lights, siren, air horn). If your unit is equipped with an emergency horn, such as an air horn or horn on the siren, you should sound it as you approach the intersection. Changing the siren function from wail to high/low, yelp, or even phaser (depending on the type of siren) will also help to capture attention.

Begin to move to the left lane slowly so that all vehicles (that are aware of you) see where you are moving to. Slow down to a contained, slow, safe speed as you approach the intersection. Watch in all directions for traffic movement and be prepared to stop. When you get to the intersection, you should stop, make sure traffic has stopped in all directions, and then proceed through the intersection slowly.

Chapter 10—Air Medical Operations

1. *Would you go ahead and allow the patient to be transported by helicopter when her condition clearly does not warrant helicopter transport?*

Not based on the current findings. If the patient was showing signs of shock or decomposition, then it might be an option, but currently she is not showing those signs and does not require the use of an emergency helicopter service.

2. *What would you tell her husband and the first responders to explain your decision to not transport by helicopter?*

You must be very diplomatic in these situations to avoid upsetting the squad/fire department and/or the family. Explain to the family and squad the indications for helicopter transport and the importance of keeping the helicopter available for other emergencies. You can also explain to them your ability and commitment to keep the patient comfortable for the duration of the ride.

3. *What options are available to you to assist in dealing with the situation?*

If necessary, you can contact medical control to help you in making these decisions. Your medical director may very well talk with the family member if necessary to help mitigate the situation.

Additionally, based on your protocols, you can provide this patient with pain relief medications that will help with her comfort for the ride.

Chapter 11—Multiple-Casualty Incidents and Incident Management

1. *What two roles in the Incident Management System will you and your partner fill, as you are first on scene?*

One of you will be incident command while the other will begin size-up and triage as necessary.

2. *How would you size up the incident?*

You need to determine a safe location to stage the EMS units, as well as how many confirmed patients and how many suspected patients/victims you have. Determine the number of resources that are on the way and how many additional resources you are going to need. Make a radio call to give a brief report of what you have determined and what you have found.

3. *What additional resources would you anticipate, and what instructions would you provide for them?*

You can anticipate the need for more ambulances, medical first responders, and fire units. Let the ambulances and medical first responders know where the staging area will be and who the contact will be for that area so they can receive orders when they arrive.

4. *How would you use the Incident Management System to organize this incident?*

At this point you know that you will need an incident commander, medical operations chief, and fire operations chief. Under the medical operations you will need triage, treatment, and transport divisions. Depending on the number of resources, you can assign those to different people or overlap roles. Additionally, you will need a safety officer and potentially a public information officer.

5. *What would your initial radio report sound like in this incident?*

Medic One is on scene assuming command. We have a multiple-story motel with heavy smoke showing from the back. We have reports of twenty-plus victims. Requesting an additional eight transport units. Have all EMS stage at [give the staging location].

Chapter 12—Rescue Awareness and Operations

1. *What are your immediate considerations as you size up the scene?*

Immediate considerations include safety, hazards, number of patients, control of traffic and bystanders, and need for additional resources (implementation of the IMS).

2. *Why would you consider this a rescue operation?*

Because the patient is unconscious and entrapped in a potentially unstable vehicle/environment.

3. *What additional resources would you request?*

Additional resources might include police, fire department, another EMS unit, and possibly a low-angle rescue team to help move the patient up the embankment.

Chapter 13—Hazardous Materials

1. *What do you suspect has happened based on your quick scene size-up?*

You suspect hazardous materials are involved in the incident. The tractor-trailer is carrying a placard, it is leaking some kind of liquid, and occupants are drooling, tearing, sweating, and experiencing respiratory distress.

2. *What are your initial priorities?*

Your initial priorities are life safety, incident stabilization, and property conservation.

3. *How will you identify the substance involved in the accident?*

Identification of the substance can be performed by interpreting the placard that indicates some kind of poison. An NAERG will identify the specific chemical. Based on the poison placard and the SLUDGE symptoms exhibited by the occupants of the truck, you suspect an organophosphate insecticide. Positive identification can be made using the shipping papers found with the driver of the truck or in the cab. You might also consult one or more of the computerized data banks or telephone hotlines mentioned in this chapter.

4. *What additional resources would you request?*

You will ask for a hazmat team and special fire apparatus. These units will be needed for entry, removal of the patient from the car, hazard control, and decontamination. You will also request three additional ambulances. Counting your unit, there will be one ambulance for each patient and one for the hazardous materials team.

5. *Is this a fast-break or a long-term incident? Explain.*

This is a fast-break incident. Two patients exhibiting critical symptoms have self-rescued and brought themselves to your ambulance.

6. *What are your first actions?*

Your first actions are to secure the scene, set up a perimeter to prevent further decontamination, and request assistance. On arrival of fire apparatus, available PPE can be donned, and two-step decontamination performed on the two occupants of the truck who are near your ambulance.

Chapter 14—Crime Scene Awareness

1. *What is your evaluation of this situation from a safety perspective?*

There is a significant potential for danger. The son's apparent intoxication, combined with the patient's warning that he "isn't quite right when he's drinking," clearly indicates the need for immediate action.

2. *What are your options?*

The two immediate options both involve retreat. You either retreat with the patient or without the patient. In this case, both you and the son want the same thing—for you to leave. However, unless you can calm down the son, you may have to leave the patient behind, at least temporarily. Even though this action may be tactically and legally correct, thoughts of abandonment charges can be haunting. You may try to buy some time until the police arrive, but your main priority is personal safety. You also know that further agitation may only worsen the patient's condition. No matter how unsatisfactory, you may have to leave the scene until the police arrive to take charge of the situation.

Chapter 15—Rural EMS

1. *What apparatus or support are you going to need to perform this rescue?*

As soon as the mechanism of injury and scene environment are known, additional personnel should be summoned. Because the water is surrounded by high cliffs and is remote, you should request a water rescue team. Following the request for adequate support and specialized rescue teams, you determine whether to transport the patient by helicopter or a ground unit. The transport time to the trauma center, the weather, the difficulty accessing the patient, and the overall time from the onset of the injury should be considered. It is better to ask for help that you may not need than to need help and realize it has not been requested.

2. *Based on the mechanism of injury, what injuries should you suspect?*

The victim jumped into the water from a 50-foot cliff and landed in water of unknown depth, but apparently shallow. The history that he "jumped" rather than "dove" into the water indicates that the patient may have lower extremity injuries in addition to head and chest injuries. Because the patient is unresponsive, it is likely that he has sustained a head injury. A chest injury is possible, as is the possibility of barotrauma if he held his breath when he jumped. If the patient landed on his feet, you should expect lower extremity injuries, including possible calcaneal fractures, lumbar spine fractures, and a cervical spinal injury. Always assume the worst and hope for the best.

3. *What will you do to stabilize this patient?*

Stabilization of this patient is primarily surgical. However, you can attempt "field stabilization" while rescue resources prepare for egress from the quarry. The airway should be controlled if the GCS is less than or equal to 8. Full spinal immobilization should occur. Special attention should be paid to the chest because the patient is at risk for direct trauma and barotrauma. The on-scene time could be prolonged. Therefore, initiate fluid therapy per protocols and splint any fractures. If the patient has a neurologic deficit consistent with a spinal cord injury, consider beginning high-dose methylprednisolone therapy. Be sure to protect body temperature.

4. *What factors made it impossible for you to meet response, treatment, and transport times in the rural setting when compared with the urban or suburban setting?*

The location, mechanism of injury, required rescue resources, distance to the trauma center, and many other factors indicate that this patient will not be in a trauma center within an hour, much less an operating room. You may have to provide extended care while extrication is carried out. You have to do the best you can with what you have available. This victim undertook a high-risk exposure with some knowledge that transport to a hospital might be quite prolonged. He has to accept those risks.

Chapter 16—Responding to Terrorist Acts

1. *What special safety considerations would you observe for this scene?*

In addition to concerns about broken glass, structural collapse, smoke inhalation, electricity, and fire dangers, you should have concerns about secondary explosives that may have been set to injure rescuers and about possible chemical or radioactive contamination associated with the blast.

2. *What are the likely injuries to expect from this mechanism of injury?*

Suspect pressure injuries to the hollow organs—ears, bowel, sinuses, and lungs—with a special concern for injury to the lungs. Anticipate penetrating trauma from debris thrown by the blast or injury secondary to the patient being thrown by the blast. Smoke inhalation may also affect patients as may the emotional stress of the incident.

3. *Should you enter the synagogue?*

No, await the fire service because of the smoke and advise them to use caution in case there are secondary explosive devices. Treat patients upwind and at a safe distance from the incident.

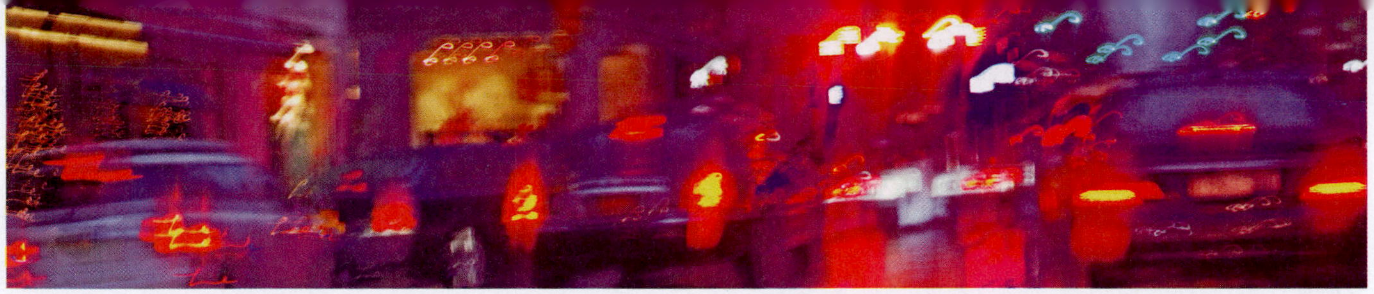

Answers to Review Questions

Below are the answers to the Review Questions presented in each chapter of Volume 5.

Chapter 1—Gynecology

1. b
2. c
3. c
4. b
5. c
6. c
7. c
8. d

Chapter 2—Obstetrics

1. b
2. d
3. b
4. c
5. d
6. c
7. a
8. a
9. b
10. b
11. d
12. c
13. d
14. a
15. a

Chapter 3—Neonatology

1. a
2. b
3. a
4. d
5. d
6. d
7. b
8. c
9. c
10. d
11. d
12. c

Chapter 4—Pediatrics

1. b
2. c
3. b
4. d
5. b
6. b
7. a
8. b
9. a
10. d
11. b
12. d
13. b
14. d
15. c
16. c
17. c
18. b
19. b
20. c
21. a
22. d

Chapter 5—Geriatrics

1. a
2. a
3. b
4. b
5. d
6. d
7. c
8. c
9. b
10. b

Chapter 6—Abuse, Neglect, and Assault

1. c
2. b
3. a
4. a
5. a
6. b
7. d
8. b
9. d
10. b

Chapter 7—The Challenged Patient

1. c
2. b
3. d
4. b
5. d
6. a
7. d
8. d

Chapter 8—Acute Interventions for the Chronic Care Patient

1. d
2. c

3. b
4. d
5. b
6. c
7. a
8. b
9. b
10. a

Chapter 9—Ground Ambulance Operations

1. c
2. b
3. c
4. d
5. c
6. a
7. a
8. b
9. c

Chapter 10—Air Medical Operations

1. a
2. d
3. a
4. c
5. d
6. b
7. a
8. b
9. b
10. c
11. b
12. d
13. d
14. a
15. a

Chapter 11—Multiple-Casualty Incidents and Incident Management

1. b
2. b
3. d
4. c
5. b
6. b
7. a
8. a
9. c
10. a

Chapter 12—Rescue Awareness and Operations

1. d
2. c
3. a
4. c
5. b
6. a
7. d
8. a
9. c
10. c

Chapter 13—Hazardous Materials

1. c
2. b
3. d
4. b
5. c
6. d
7. a
8. a
9. b
10. c

Chapter 14—Crime Scene Awareness

1. c
2. b
3. d
4. b
5. c
6. c
7. c
8. b

Chapter 15—Rural EMS

1. b
2. c
3. d
4. d
5. b
6. d

Chapter 16—Responding to Terrorist Acts

1. a
2. d
3. a
4. c
5. d
6. d
7. b
8. a
9. a
10. d

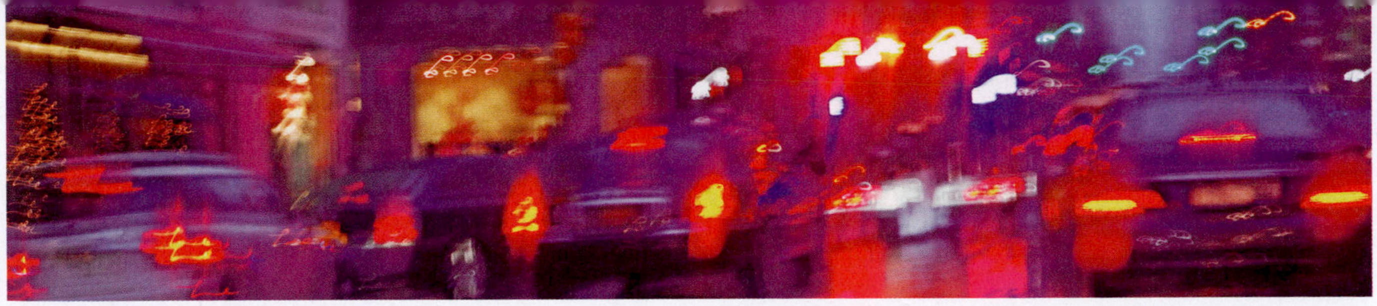

Glossary

abortion termination of pregnancy before the 20th week of gestation. The term refers to both miscarriage and induced abortion. Commonly, "abortion" is used for elective termination of pregnancy and "miscarriage" for the loss of a fetus by natural means. A miscarriage is sometimes called a "spontaneous abortion."

acetylcholinesterase (AChE) enzyme that stops the action of acetylcholine, a neurotransmitter.

acrocyanosis cyanosis of the extremities.

active rescue zone area in which special rescue teams operate; also known as the "hot zone" or "inner circle."

acute effects signs and/or symptoms rapidly displayed on exposure to a toxic substance.

acute respiratory distress syndrome (ARDS) respiratory insufficiency marked by progressive hypoxemia due to severe inflammatory damage.

ADAMS Atlas and Database of Air Medical Services, created by the Center for Transportation Injury Research and the Association of Air Medical Services, that includes information on air medical service providers, their communication centers, base helipads, rotor and fixed wing aircraft, and receiving hospitals.

advance directive legal document prepared when a person is alive, competent, and able to make informed decisions about health care. The document provides guidelines on treatment if the person is no longer capable of making decisions.

afterbirth the placenta and accompanying membranes that are expelled from the uterus after the birth of a child.

ageism discrimination against aged or elderly people.

air bags inflatable high-pressure pillows that, when inflated, can lift up to 20 tons, depending on the make.

air-purifying respirator (APR) system of filtering a normal environment for a specific chemical substance using filter cartridges.

Alzheimer's disease a progressive, degenerative disease that attacks the brain and results in impaired memory, thinking, and behavior. It affects 4 million American adults.

amniotic fluid clear, watery fluid that surrounds and protects the developing fetus.

amniotic sac the membranes that surround and protect the developing fetus throughout the period of intrauterine development.

aneurysm abnormal dilation of a blood vessel, usually an artery, due to a congenital defect or a weakness in the wall of the vessel.

ankylosing spondylitis a form of inflammatory arthritis that primarily affects the spine.

anorexia nervosa eating disorder marked by excessive fasting.

anoxic hypoxemia an oxygen deficiency due to disordered pulmonary mechanisms of oxygenation.

antepartum before the onset of labor.

aortic dissection a degeneration of the wall of the aorta.

aortocaval compression compression of the aorta and vena cava by the gravid uterus in the supine pregnant patient.

APGAR score a numerical system of rating the condition of a newborn. It evaluates the newborn's heart rate, respiratory rate, muscle tone, reflex irritability, and color.

aphasia absence or impairment of the ability to communicate through speaking, writing, or signing as a result of brain dysfunction; occurs when the individual suffers a brain injury due to stroke or head injury and no longer has the ability to speak or read. In *sensory aphasia*, the patient cannot understand the spoken word. In *motor aphasia*, the patient can understand what is said but cannot speak. A patient with *global aphasia* has both sensory and motor aphasia.

ARDS acute respiratory distress syndrome.

assisted living housing for the elderly or disabled that provides nursing care, housekeeping, and prepared meals as needed.

asthma a condition marked by recurrent attacks of dyspnea with wheezing due to spasmodic constriction of the bronchi, often as a response to allergens or to mucus plugs in the arterial walls.

autonomic dysfunction an abnormality of the involuntary aspect of the nervous system.

bacterial tracheitis bacterial infection of the airway, subglottic region; in children, most likely to appear after episodes of croup.

bend fractures fractures characterized by angulation and deformity in the bone without an obvious break.

bias-motivated crime a hate crime based on bias.

biological agents either living organisms or toxins produced by living organisms that are deliberately distributed to cause disease and death.

biotoxins poisons that are produced by a living organism but are themselves not alive.

biotransformation changing a substance in the body from one chemical to another; in the case of hazardous materials, the body tries to create less toxic materials.

BiPAP bilevel positive airway pressure.

birth injury avoidable and unavoidable mechanical and anoxic trauma incurred by the newborn during labor and delivery.

blood spatter evidence the pattern that blood forms when it is splattered or dropped at the scene of a crime.

body armor vest made of tightly woven, strong fibers that offer protection against handgun bullets, most knives, and blunt trauma; also known as "bulletproof vests."

brain ischemia injury to brain tissues caused by an inadequate supply of oxygen and nutrients.

branches functional levels within the IMS based on primary roles and geographic locations.

bronchiectasis chronic dilation of a bronchus or bronchi, with a secondary infection typically involving the lower portion of the lung.

bronchiolitis viral infection of the medium-sized airways, occurring most frequently during the first year of life.

buckle fractures fractures characterized by a raised or bulging projection at the fracture site.

CAMEO® Computer-Aided Management of Emergency Operations; website developed by the EPA and NOAA as a source of information, skills, and links related to hazardous substances.

cardiogenic shock the inability of the heart to meet the metabolic needs of the body, resulting in inadequate tissue perfusion.

cataract medical condition in which the lens of the eye loses its clearness.

CBRNE acronym for *chemical, biological, radiologic, nuclear, and explosive*, developed following the increase in terrorism; refers to situations in which any of these five hazards is or may be present.

cellulitis inflammation of cellular or connective tissue.

central IV line intravenous line placed into the superior vena cava for the administration of long-term fluid therapy.

C-FLOP mnemonic for the main functional areas within the IMS command: finance/administration, logistics, operations, and planning.

chain of evidence legally retaining items of evidence and accounting for their whereabouts at all times to prevent loss or tampering.

CHEMTEL Chemical Telephone, Inc.; maintains a 24-hour, toll-free hotline at 800-255-3924; for collect calls and calls from other points of origin, dial 813-248-0585.

CHEMTREC Chemical Transportation Emergency Center; maintains a 24-hour, toll-free hotline at 800-424-9300; for collect calls and calls from other points of origin, dial 703-527-3887.

child abuse physical or emotional violence or neglect toward a person from infancy to 18 years of age.

choanal atresia congenital closure of the passage between the nose and pharynx by a bony or membranous structure.

cleft lip congenital vertical fissure in the upper lip.

cleft palate congenital fissure in the roof of the mouth, forming a passageway between oral and nasal cavities.

closed incident an incident that is not likely to generate any further patients; also known as a contained incident.

cold zone location at a hazmat incident outside the warm zone; area where incident operations take place; also called the green zone or the safe zone.

colostomy a surgical diversion of the large intestine through an opening in the skin where the fecal matter is collected in a pouch; may be temporary or permanent.

command the individual or group responsible for coordinating all activities and who makes final decisions on the emergency scene; often referred to as the incident commander (IC) or officer in charge (OIC).

command staff officers who report directly to the incident commander; officers who handle public information, safety, and outside liaisons, also known as management staff.

comorbidity having more than one disease at a time.

compartment syndrome condition that occurs when circulation to a portion of the body is cut off; after a period of time toxins can develop in the blood, leading to shock when circulation is restored.

concealment hiding the body behind objects that shield a person from view but offer little or no protection against bullets or other ballistics.

conductive deafness deafness caused when transmission of the sound waves through the external ear canal to the middle or inner ear is blocked.

congenital present at birth.

congregate care living arrangement in which the elderly live in, but do not own, individual apartments or rooms and receive select services.

consensus standards widely agreed-on guidelines, such as those developed by the National Fire Protection Association and others.

CONTOMS Counter-Narcotics Tactical Operations; program that manages the training and certification of EMT-Ts and SWAT-Medics.

cor pulmonale congestive heart failure secondary to pulmonary hypertension.

cover hiding the body behind solid and impenetrable objects that protect a person from bullets.

CPAP continuous positive airway pressure.

cribbing wooden slats used to shore up heavy equipment.

croup laryngotracheobronchitis; a common viral infection of young children, resulting in edema of the subglottic tissues; characterized by barking cough and inspiratory stridor.

crowning the bulging of the fetal head past the opening of the vagina during a contraction; it is an indication of impending delivery.

crush points mechanisms of injury in which two or more objects come together with enough weight or force to crush the affected appendage.

cystitis infection of the urinary bladder.

cytochrome oxidase enzyme complex, found in cellular mitochondria, that enables oxygen to create the adenosine triphosphate (ATP) required for all muscle energy.

deafness the inability to hear.

delayed effects signs, symptoms, and/or conditions developed hours, days, weeks, months, or even years after the exposure.

delayed cord clamping (DCC) recommended delay in clamping the umbilical cord in a newly born infant who does not require immediate resuscitation to minimize the likelihood of intraventricular hemorrhage.

delirium an acute alteration in mental functioning that is often reversible.

dementia a deterioration of mental status that is usually associated with structural neurologic disease. It is often progressive and irreversible.

demobilized released for use outside the incident, as occurs when resources including personnel, vehicles, and equipment are no longer needed at the scene.

demographic pertaining to population makeup or changes.

demyelination destruction or removal of the myelin sheath of nerve tissue; found in Guillain-Barré syndrome.

Department of Homeland Security (DHS) a cabinet-level department of the U.S. government, created in response to the terrorist attacks of September 11, 2001. It is charged with protecting the United States and its territories from terrorist attacks and overseeing the response to terrorist attacks, man-made accidents, and natural disasters.

deployment strategy used by an EMS agency to maneuver its ambulances and crews in an effort to reduce response times.

diabetic ketoacidosis complication of diabetes due to decreased insulin secretion or intake; characterized by high levels of blood glucose, metabolic acidosis, and, in advanced stages, coma; often referred to as diabetic coma.

diabetic retinopathy slow loss of vision as a result of damage done by diabetes.

diaphragmatic hernia protrusion of abdominal contents into the thoracic cavity through an opening in the diaphragm.

dirty bomb a conventional explosive device that distributes radioactive material over a large area.

disaster management management of incidents that generate large numbers of patients, often overwhelming resources and damaging parts of the infrastructure.

disentanglement process of freeing a patient from wreckage, to allow for proper care, removal, and transfer.

distributive shock marked decrease in peripheral vascular resistance with resultant hypotension; examples include septic shock, neurogenic shock, and anaphylactic shock.

domestic elder abuse physical or emotional violence or neglect when an elder is being cared for in a home-based setting.

domestic incidents multiple-casualty incidents or disasters within the United States.

dosimeter an instrument that measures the cumulative amount of radiation absorbed.

DOT KKK 1822F specs the manufacturing and design specifications produced by the Federal General Services Administrative Automotive Commodity Center.

ductus arteriosus channel between the main pulmonary artery and the aorta of the fetus.

due regard legal terminology found in the motor vehicle laws of most states that sets up a higher standard for the operators of emergency vehicles.

dysmenorrhea painful menstruation.

dyspareunia painful sexual intercourse.

dysphagia inability to swallow or difficulty swallowing.

dysphoria an exaggerated feeling of depression or unrest, characterized by a mood of general dissatisfaction, restlessness, discomfort, and unhappiness.

dysuria painful urination often associated with cystitis.

ectopic pregnancy the implantation of a developing fetus outside the uterus, often in a fallopian tube.

eddies water that flows around especially large objects and, for a time, flows upstream around the downside of an obstruction; provides an opportunity to escape dangerous currents.

effacement the thinning and shortening of the cervix during labor.

elderly aged 65 or older.

Emergency Medical Services for Children (EMSC) federally funded program aimed at improving the health of pediatric patients who suffer from life-threatening illnesses and injuries.

emergency operations center (EOC) a site from which civil government officials (municipal, county, state, and/or federal) exercise direction and control in an emergency or disaster.

emesis vomitus.

EMS communications officer person who notifies hospitals of incoming patients from a multiple-casualty incident; reports to the transportation officer; may also be called the EMS COM or MED COM.

EMT-Tacticals (EMT-Ts) EMS personnel trained to serve with a technical emergency medical service or a law enforcement agency.

endometriosis condition in which endometrial tissue grows outside the uterus.

endometritis infection of the endometrium.

endometrium the inner layer of the uterine wall where the fertilized egg implants.

enucleation removal of the eyeball after trauma or illness.

epiglottitis bacterial infection of the epiglottis, usually occurring in children older than age four; a serious medical emergency.

epistaxis nosebleed.

erythema general reddening of the skin due to dilation of the superficial capillaries.

essential equipment equipment/supplies required on every ambulance.

estimated date of confinement (EDC) the approximate day the infant will be born. This date is usually set at 40 weeks after the date of the mother's last menstrual period (LMP).

exocrine disorder involving external secretions.

explosives chemical(s) that, when ignited, instantly generate a great amount of heat, resulting in a destructive shock wave and blast wind.

extrauterine outside the uterus.

extrication use of force to free a patient from entrapment; also a group or branch responsible for removing patients from entanglements and transferring them to the treatment area, also known as a rescue group.

facilities unit unit that selects and maintains areas used for rehabilitation and command.

fallout radioactive dust and particles that may be life threatening to people far from the epicenter of a nuclear detonation.

fasciculations involuntary contractions or twitchings of muscle fibers.

febrile seizures seizures that occur as a result of a sudden increase in body temperature; occur most commonly between the ages of six months and six years.

fibrosis the formation of fiber-like connective tissue, also called scar tissue, in an organ.

finance/administration section section responsible for maintaining records for personnel, time, and costs of resources/procurement; reports directly to the IC.

fixed-wing aircraft vehicles capable of flight that use fixed wings to generate lift; airplanes.

foreign body airway obstruction (FBAO) blockage or obstruction of the airway by an object that impairs respiration; in the case of pediatric patients, tongues, abundant secretions, and deciduous (baby) teeth are likely to block airways.

functional impairment decreased ability to meet daily needs on an independent basis.

gangrene death of tissue or bone, usually from an insufficient blood supply.

Geiger counter an instrument used to detect and measure the radiation given off by an object or area.

geriatric abuse a syndrome in which an elderly person is physically or psychologically injured by another person.

geriatrics the study and treatment of diseases of the aged.

gerontology scientific study of the effects of aging and of age-related diseases on humans.

glaucoma group of eye diseases that results in increased intraocular pressure on the optic nerve; if left untreated, it can lead to blindness.

glomerulonephritis a form of nephritis, or inflammation of the kidneys; primarily involves the glomeruli, one of the capillary networks that are part of the renal corpuscles in the nephrons.

glottic function opening and closing of the glottic space.

gold standard ultimate standard of excellence.

greenstick fractures fractures characterized by an incomplete break in the bone.

growth plate the area just below the head of a long bone in which growth in bone length occurs; the epiphyseal plate.

Guillain-Barré syndrome acute viral infection that triggers the production of autoantibodies, which damage the myelin sheath covering the peripheral nerves; causes rapid, progressive loss of motor function, ranging from muscle weakness to full-body paralysis.

gynecology the branch of medicine that deals with the health maintenance and the diseases of women, primarily of the reproductive organs.

hate crimes crimes committed against a person solely on the basis of the individual's actual or perceived race, color, national origin, ethnicity, gender, disability, or sexual orientation.

hazardous materials (hazmat) any substance that causes adverse health effects on human exposure.

heat escape lessening position (HELP) developed by Dr. John Hayward, it is an in-water, head-up tuck or fetal position designed to reduce heat loss by as much as 60 percent.

heatstroke life-threatening condition caused by a disturbance in temperature regulation; in the elderly, characterized by extreme fever and, in extreme cases, delirium or coma.

hemoptysis expectoration of blood arising from the oral cavity, larynx, trachea, bronchi, or lungs; characterized by sudden coughing with production of salty sputum with frothy bright-red blood.

hepatomegaly enlarged liver.

herniation protrusion or projection of an organ or part of an organ through the wall of the cavity that normally contains it.

herpes zoster an acute eruption caused by a reactivation of latent varicella virus (chickenpox) in the dorsal root ganglia; also known as *shingles*.

hiatal hernia protrusion of the stomach upward into the mediastinal cavity through the esophageal hiatus of the diaphragm.

hospice program of palliative care and support services that addresses the physical, social, economic, and spiritual needs of terminally ill patients and their families.

hot zone location at a hazmat incident where the actual hazardous material and highest levels of contamination exist; also called the red zone or the exclusionary zone.

human trafficking the trade of humans; the illegal movement of people, usually for forced labor or commercial sexual exploitation.

hyperbilirubinemia an excessive amount of bilirubin—the orange-colored pigment associated with bile—in the blood. In newborns, the condition appears as jaundice. Precipitating factors include maternal Rh or ABO incompatibility, neonatal sepsis, anoxia, hypoglycemia, and congenital liver or gastrointestinal defects.

hyperglycemia abnormally high concentration of glucose in the blood.

hypertrophy an increase in the size or bulk of an organ or structure; caused by growth rather than by a tumor.

hypochondriasis an abnormal concern with one's health, with the false belief of suffering from some disease, despite medical assurances to the contrary; commonly known as *hypochondria*.

hypoglycemia abnormally low concentration of glucose in the blood.

hypovolemic shock decreased amount of intravascular fluid in the body; often due to trauma that causes blood loss into a body cavity or frank external hemorrhage; in children, can be the result of vomiting and diarrhea.

immune senescence diminished vigor of the immune response to the challenge and rechallenge by pathogens.

incendiary agents a subset of explosives with less explosive power but greater heat and burn potential.

incident command post (ICP) place where command officers from various agencies can meet with each other and select a management staff.

Incident Command System (ICS) a management program designed for controlling, directing, and coordinating emergency response resources; sometimes used as a synonym for ***Incident Management System (IMS)***.

incident commander (IC) the person responsible for coordinating all activities at a multiple-casualty scene.

Incident Management System (IMS) See *Incident Command System.*

incontinence inability to retain urine or feces because of loss of sphincter control or cerebral or spinal lesions.

information officer (IO) person who collects data about the incident and releases it to the press or media.

institutional elder abuse physical or emotional violence or neglect when an elder is being cared for by a person paid to provide care.

instrument flight rules (IFR) regulations that permit an aircraft to operate in instrument meteorological conditions.

intermittent mandatory ventilation (IMV) respirator setting in which a patient-triggered breath does not result in assistance by the machine.

intracerebral hemorrhage bleeding directly into the brain.

intractable resistant to cure, relief, or control.

intrapartum occurring during childbirth.

isolette also known as an incubator; a clear plastic enclosed bassinet used to keep prematurely born infants warm. The temperature of an isolette can be adjusted regardless of the room temperature. Some isolettes also provide humidity control.

kyphosis exaggeration of the normal posterior curvature of the spine.

labor the time and processes that occur during childbirth; the physiologic and mechanical process in which the baby, placenta, and amniotic sac are expelled through the birth canal.

labyrinthitis inner ear infection that causes vertigo, nausea, and an unsteady gait.

liaison officer (LO) person who coordinates all incident operations that involve outside agencies.

life-care community communities that provide apartments/homes for independent living and a range of services, including nursing care. Usually the elderly own their own homes.

local effects effects involving areas around the immediate site; should be evaluated based on the burn model.

lochia vaginal discharge following birth that contains blood, mucus, and placental tissue.

lock-out/tag-out locking off of a machinery switch, then placing a tag on the switch stating why it is shut off; method of preventing equipment from being accidentally restarted.

logistics section section that supports incident operations, coordinating procurement and distribution of all medical resources.

maceration process of softening a solid by soaking it in a liquid.

manual lateral uterine displacement (LUD) the technique of cupping the uterus to lift it upward and leftward off the maternal blood vessels.

Marfan syndrome hereditary condition of connective tissue, bones, muscles, ligaments, and skeletal structures characterized by irregular and unsteady gait, tall lean body type with long extremities, flat feet, and stooped shoulders. The aorta is usually dilated and may become weakened enough to allow an aneurysm to develop.

Mark I kit a two-part auto-injector set that the military uses as treatment for nerve agent exposure; involves the administration of atropine followed by pralidoxime chloride.

meconium dark green material found in the intestine of the full-term newborn. It can be expelled from the intestine into the amniotic fluid during periods of fetal distress.

medical supply unit unit that coordinates procurement and distribution of equipment and supplies at a multiple-casualty incident.

melena a dark, tarry stool caused by the presence of "digested" free blood.

menarche the onset of menses, usually occurring between ages 10 and 14.

Ménière's disease a disease of the inner ear characterized by vertigo, nerve deafness, and a roar or buzzing in the ear.

meningomyelocele herniation of the spinal cord and membranes through a defect in the spinal column.

menopause the cessation of menses and ovarian function due to decreased secretion of estrogen.

menorrhagia excessive menstrual flow.

menstruation sloughing of the uterine lining (endometrium) if a fertilized egg is not implanted. It is controlled by the cyclical release of hormones. Menstruation is also called a *period*.

mesenteric ischemia or infarct death of tissue in the peritoneal fold (mesentery) that encircles the small intestine; a life-threatening condition.

minimum standards lowest or least allowable standards.

miosis abnormal contraction of the pupils; pinpoint pupils.

miscarriage commonly used term to describe a pregnancy that ends before 20 weeks' gestation; may also be called *spontaneous abortion*.

mittelschmerz abdominal pain associated with ovulation.

morgue area where deceased victims of an incident are collected.

morgue officer person who supervises the morgue; may report to the triage officer or the treatment officer.

mucoviscidosis cystic fibrosis, so called because of the abnormally viscous mucoid secretions associated with the disease.

multiple-casualty incident (MCI) incident that generates large numbers of patients and that often makes traditional EMS response ineffective because of special circumstances surrounding the event; also known as a mass-casualty incident.

mutual aid agreements agreements or plans for sharing departmental resources.

mutual aid coordination center (MACC) an aspect of the NIMS system that oversees the coordination and utilization of resources from outside the local public safety entity.

myasthenia gravis disease characterized by episodic muscle weakness triggered by an autoimmune attack of the acetylcholine receptors.

myometrium the thick middle layer of the uterine wall, made up of smooth muscle fibers.

nasogastric tube/orogastric tube a tube that runs through the nose or mouth and esophagus into the stomach; used for administering liquid nutrients or medications or for removing air or liquids from the stomach.

National Incident Management System (NIMS) national system used for the management of multiple-casualty incidents, involving assumption of responsibility for command and designation and coordination of such elements as triage, treatment, transport, and staging.

neonatal abstinence syndrome (NAS) a generalized disorder presenting a clinical picture of central nervous system (CNS) hyperirritability, gastrointestinal dysfunction, respiratory distress, and vague autonomic symptoms. It may be due to intrauterine exposure to heroin, methadone, or other less potent opiates. Nonopiate CNS depressants may also cause NAS.

neonate an infant from the time of birth to one month of age.

nephrons the functional units of the kidneys.

nerve agents chemicals that inhibit the degradation of a neurotransmitter (acetylcholine) and quickly facilitate a nervous system overload.

neutropenia a condition that results from an abnormally low neutrophil count in the blood (less than 2,000/mm^3).

newborn a baby in the first few hours of its life; also called a newly born infant.

night vision goggles (NVG) electro-optical goggles used to detect visible and infrared energy to provide a visible image in the dark.

nocturia excessive urination during the night.

noncardiogenic shock types of shock that result from causes other than inadequate cardiac output.

nuclear detonation the release of energy that is generated when heavy nuclei split (fission) or light nuclei combine (fusion) to form new elements. The unleashed energy is tremendous and creates an explosion of immense proportion.

obstetrics the branch of medicine that deals with the care of women throughout pregnancy.

old-old an elderly person aged 80 or older.

omphalocele congenital hernia of the umbilicus.

open incident an incident that has the potential to generate additional patients; also known as an uncontained incident.

operations section fulfills directions from command and does the actual work at an incident.

osteoarthritis a degenerative joint disease, characterized by a loss of articular cartilage and hypertrophy of bone.

osteoporosis softening of bone tissue due to the loss of essential minerals, principally calcium.

otitis media middle ear infection.

ovulation the release of an egg from the ovary.

Parkinson's disease chronic, degenerative nervous disease characterized by tremors, muscular weakness and rigidity, and a loss of postural reflexes.

particulate evidence evidence such as hairs or fibers that cannot be readily seen with the human eye; also known as microscopic or trace evidence.

partner abuse physical or emotional violence from a man or woman toward a domestic partner.

peak load the highest volume of calls at a given time.

PEEP positive end-expiratory pressure.

pelvic inflammatory disease (PID) an acute infection of the reproductive organs that can be caused by a bacterium, virus, or fungus.

perimetrium the serous peritoneal membrane that forms the outermost layer of the uterine wall.

persistent fetal circulation condition in which blood continues to bypass the fetal respiratory system, resulting in ongoing hypoxia.

personal-care home living arrangement that includes room, board, and some supervision.

phototherapy exposure to sunlight or artificial light for therapeutic purposes. In newborns, light is used to treat hyperbilirubinemia or jaundice.

Pierre Robin syndrome unusually small jaw, combined with a cleft palate, downward displacement of the tongue, and an absent gag reflex.

pill-rolling motion an involuntary tremor, usually in one hand or sometimes in both, in which fingers move as if they were rolling a pill back and forth.

pinch points mechanisms of injury in which two objects come together and catch a portion of the patient's body in between them.

placenta the organ that serves as a lifeline for the developing fetus. The placenta is attached to the wall of the uterus and the umbilical cord.

planning/intelligence section provides past, present, and future information about an incident.

polycythemia an excess of red blood cells. In a newborn, the condition may reflect hypovolemia or prolonged intrauterine hypoxia.

polypharmacy multiple drug therapy in which there is a concurrent use of a number of drugs.

postpartum depression the "let down" feeling experienced during the period following birth, occurring in 70 to 80 percent of mothers.

premenstrual dysphoric disorder (PMDD) condition in which a woman has severe depression symptoms, irritability, and tension before menstruation.

premenstrual syndrome (PMS) a variety of signs and symptoms, such as weight gain, irritability, or specific food cravings, associated with the changing hormonal levels that precede menstruation.

presbycusis progressive hearing loss that occurs with aging.

pressure ulcer ischemic damage and subsequent necrosis affecting the skin, subcutaneous tissue, and often the muscle; result of intense pressure over a short time or low pressure over a long time; also known as *pressure sore* or *bedsore*.

primary area of responsibility (PAR) stationing of ambulances at specific high-volume locations.

primary contamination direct exposure of a person or item to a hazardous substance.

primary triage triage that takes place early in the incident, usually on first arrival.

prompt care facilities hospital agencies that provide limited care and nonemergent medical treatment.

pruritus itching; often occurs as a symptom of some systemic change or illness.

puerperium the time period surrounding the birth of the fetus.

pulmonary agents chemicals that primarily cause injury to the lungs; commonly referred to as choking agents.

rape penile penetration of the genitalia or rectum without the consent of the victim.

rapid intervention team ambulance and crew dedicated to stand by in case a rescuer becomes ill or injured.

recirculating currents movement of currents over a uniform obstruction; also known as a "drowning machine."

reportable collisions collisions that involve more than $1,000 in damage or a personal injury.

reserve capacity the ability of an EMS agency to respond to calls beyond those handled by the on-duty crews.

retinopathy any disorder of the retina.

rhinorrhea watery discharge from the nose.

rotor-wing aircraft vehicles that use rotating blades (rotors) to provide lift and propulsion; helicopters.

rust out an inability to keep abreast of new technologies and standards.

safety data sheet (SDS) easily accessible sheet of detailed information about chemicals found at fixed facilities; formerly called *material safety data sheet (MSDS)*.

safety officer (SO) person who monitors all on-scene actions and ensures that they do not create any potentially harmful conditions.

SALT acronym for a mass triage system that reflects the components of the assessment: **S**ort, **A**ssess, **L**ifesaving Interventions, and **T**reatment/Transport.

scene-authority law state or local statute specifying who has ultimate authority at a multiple-casualty incident.

scrambling climbing over rocks and/or downed trees on a steep trail without the aid of ropes. This can be especially dangerous when the surface is wet or icy.

scree loose pebbles or rock debris that can form on the slopes or bases of mountains; sometimes used to describe debris in sloping dry stream beds.

secondary contamination transfer of a hazardous substance to a noncontaminated person or item via contact with someone or something already contaminated by the substance.

secondary triage triage that takes place after patients are moved to a treatment area to determine any change in status.

section chief officer who supervises major functional areas or sections; reports to the incident commander.

sector interchangeable name for a branch, group, or division; does not, however, designate a functional or geographic area.

semi-decontaminated patient another name for field-decontaminated patient.

senile dementia general term used to describe an abnormal decline in mental functioning seen in the elderly; also called *organic brain syndrome* or *multi-infarct dementia*.

sensorineural deafness deafness caused by the inability of nerve impulses to reach the auditory center of the brain because of nerve damage either to the inner ear or to the brain.

sensorium sensory apparatus of the body as a whole; also the portion of the brain that functions as a center of sensations.

sexual assault unwanted oral, genital, rectal, or manual sexual contact.

shear points mechanisms of injury in which pinch points meet or pass, causing amputation of a body part.

shipping papers documents routinely carried aboard vehicles transporting hazardous materials; ideally should identify specific substances and quantities carried; also known as bills of lading.

short haul a helicopter extrication technique in which a person is attached to a rope that is, in turn, attached to a helicopter. The aircraft lifts off with the person attached to it. Obviously this means of evacuation requires highly specialized skills.

shunt surgical connection that runs from the brain to the abdomen for the purpose of draining excess cerebrospinal fluid, thus preventing increased intracranial pressure.

Shy-Drager syndrome chronic orthostatic hypotension caused by a primary autonomic nervous system deficiency.

sick sinus syndrome a group of disorders characterized by dysfunction of the sinoatrial node in the heart.

silent myocardial infarction a myocardial infarction that occurs without exhibiting obvious signs and symptoms.

silo gas toxic fumes (oxides of nitrogen, or NO_2) produced by the fermentation of grains in a silo.

singular command process in which a single individual is responsible for coordinating an incident; most useful in single-jurisdictional incidents.

situational awareness using scene size-ups to enable awareness of everything that is happening in a multiple-casualty incident.

span of control number of people or tasks that a single individual can monitor.

special weapons and tactics (SWAT) team a trained police unit equipped to handle hostage holders and other difficult law enforcement situations.

specific gravity refers to the density or weight of a vapor or gas as compared with air.

spondylosis a degeneration of the vertebral body.

spotter the person behind the left rear side of the ambulance who assists the operator in backing up the vehicle.

staff functions supervisory roles in the Incident Management System.

staging area location where ambulances, personnel, and equipment are kept in reserve for use at an incident.

staging officer person who supervises the staging area and guards against premature commitment of resources and freelancing by personnel; reports to the branch director.

START acronym for the most widely used disaster triage system; stands for **S**imple **T**riage **a**nd **R**apid **T**ransport.

status epilepticus prolonged seizure or multiple seizures with no regaining of consciousness between them.

Stokes-Adams syndrome a series of symptoms resulting from heart block, most commonly syncope. The symptoms result from decreased blood flow to the brain caused by the sudden decrease in cardiac output.

stoma a permanent surgical opening in the neck through which the patient breathes.

strainer a partial obstruction that filters, or strains, the water, such as downed trees or wire mesh; causes an unequal force on the two sides.

stroke injury to or death of brain tissue resulting from interruption of cerebral blood flow and oxygenation.

subarachnoid hemorrhage bleeding that occurs between the arachnoid and dura mater of the brain.

substance abuse misuse of chemically active agents such as alcohol, psychoactive chemicals, and therapeutic agents; typically results in clinically significant impairment or distress.

sudden infant death syndrome (SIDS) illness of unknown etiology that occurs during the first year of life, with the peak at ages two to four months.

synergism a standard pharmacological principle in which two substances or drugs work together to produce an effect that neither of them can produce on their own.

system status management (SSM) a computerized personnel and ambulance deployment system.

systemic effects effects that occur throughout the body after exposure to a toxic substance.

tactical emergency medical service (TEMS) a specially trained unit that provides on-site medical support to law enforcement.

terrorist act the use of violence to provoke fear and influence behavior for political, social, religious, or ethnic goals.

thyrotoxicosis toxic condition characterized by tachycardia, nervous symptoms, and rapid metabolism due to hyperactivity of the thyroid gland.

tiered response system system that allows multiple vehicles to arrive at an EMS call at different times, often providing different levels of care or transport.

tinnitus ringing or tingling in the ear.

tocolysis the process of stopping labor.

tracheostomy small surgical opening that a surgeon makes from the anterior neck into the trachea, held open by a metal or plastic tube.

transient ischemic attack (TIA) reversible interruption of blood flow to the brain; often seen as a precursor to a stroke.

transportation unit supervisor person who coordinates operations with the staging officer and the transportation supervisor; gets patients into the ambulance and routed to hospitals.

treatment group supervisor person who controls all actions in the treatment group/sector.

treatment unit leader EMS member who manages the various treatment units and reports to the treatment group supervisor.

triage act of sorting patients based on the severity of their injuries.

triage group supervisor person who supervises a triage group or triage sector at a multiple-casualty incident.

triage officer person responsible for triage, or sorting patients into categories based on the severity of their injuries.

turgor ability of the skin to return to normal appearance after being subjected to pressure.

two-pillow orthopnea the number of pillows—in this case, two—needed to ease the difficulty of breathing while lying down; a significant factor in assessing the level of respiratory distress.

umbilical cord structure containing two arteries and one vein that connects the placenta and the fetus.

UN number a four-digit identification number specific to a given chemical; some UN numbers are assigned to a group of related chemicals, but with different characteristics, such as the UN 1203 designation for diesel fuel, gasohol, gasoline, motor fuels, motor spirits, and petrol. (The letters UN stand for "United Nations." Sometimes the letters NA for "North American" appear with or instead of the UN designation.)

unified command process in which managers from different jurisdictions—law enforcement, fire, EMS—coordinate their activities and share responsibility for command.

urosepsis septicemia originating from the urinary tract.

urostomy surgical diversion of the urinary tract to a stoma, or hole, in the abdominal wall.

vagal stimulation stimulation of the vagus nerve, causing a parasympathetic response.

Valsalva maneuver forced exhalation against a closed glottis, such as with coughing. This maneuver stimulates the parasympathetic nervous system via the vagus nerve, which, in turn, slows the heart rate.

varicosities an abnormal dilation of a vein or group of veins.

vertigo the sensation of faintness or dizziness; may cause a loss of balance.

vesicants agents that damage exposed skin, frequently causing vesicles (blisters).

visual flight rules (VFR) regulations under which a pilot operates an aircraft in weather conditions clear enough for the pilot to see where the aircraft is going.

volatility the ease with which a chemical changes from a liquid to a gas; the tendency of a chemical agent to evaporate.

warm zone location at a hazmat incident adjacent to the hot zone; area where a decontamination corridor is established; also called the yellow zone or contamination reduction zone.

warning placard diamond-shaped graphic placed on vehicles to indicate hazard classification.

weapons of mass destruction (WMDs) variety of chemical, biological, nuclear, or other devices used by terrorists to strike at government or high-profile targets; designed to create a maximum number of casualties.

windshield survey a survey of the emergency scene conducted by the incident commander through the windshield of his vehicle as it arrives at the scene.

wrap points mechanisms of injury in which an appendage gets caught and significantly twisted.

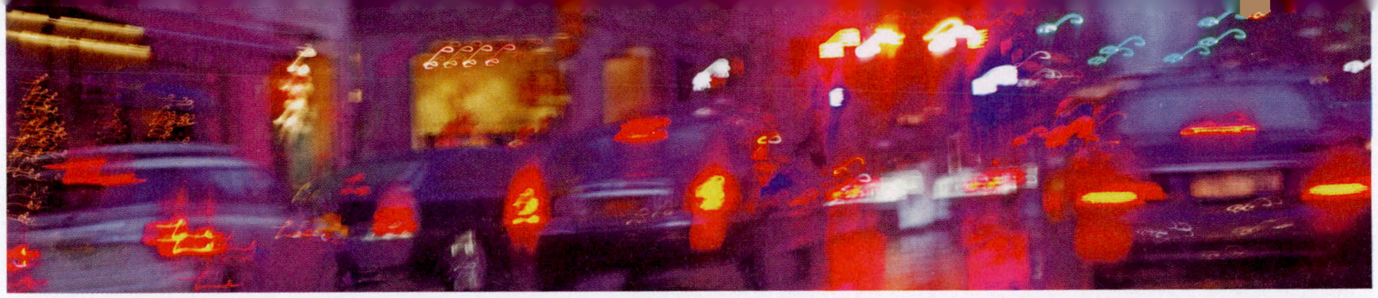

Index

A

Abdomen, pediatric patients, 89
Abdominal injuries, child abuse and, 206
Abortion, 29–30
Abruptio placentae, 31–32
Absorption, 370
Abuse
- child, 141–143, 204–207
- elder, 203–204
- geriatric, 194
- partner, 201–202

Acetylcholinesterase (AChE), 368
Acrocyanosis, 74
Active rescue zone, 332
Acute effects, 367
Acute infections, 254–255
ADAMS, 285
Adolescents, 86
Advance directives, 156
Advanced life support (ALS), 82
Afterbirth, 20
Ageism, 154
Agricultural emergencies. *See also* Rural EMS
- emergency medical care, 404
- farm machinery, 400
- hazardous materials, 400
- mechanisms of injury, 402–404
- safety, 399–400
- trauma potential, 400–402

Air bags, 401
Air medical transport. *See also* Helicopters
- aircraft, 278–281
- aircraft departure, 289
- aircraft loading, 289
- approach, 287–288
- controversies, 285–286
- for disaster assistance, 276
- guidelines for dispatch, 282–284
- history, 277–278
- initial information, 286
- for interfacility transport, 275–276
- introduction to, 275–277
- landing zone, 286–287
- limitations of, 284–285
- for organ procurement, 276
- patient handoff, 288–289
- role in EMS, 281–286
- scene operations, 286–289
- for search and rescue, 276
- for specialty care, 276
- staffing, 285
- uses for, 275–277, 281

Aircraft. *See also* Air medical transport
- departure, 289
- in EMS system, 281
- fixed-wing, 278–279
- loading, 289
- rotor-wing, 278, 279–281

Air-purifying respirator (APR), 373
Airway
- control, pediatric emergencies, 136
- pediatric assessment, 91
- pediatric patients, 86–87

Airway management
- pediatric, 99–109
- in pregnancy, 48–49

Alcohol abuse, 191–192
Alpha radiation, 365
Alzheimer's disease, 180
Ambulances
- checking, 263–264
- collisions, reducing, 266–267
- deployment, 261, 264–265
- design, 261–262
- due regard standard, 267–268
- escorts, 269
- essential equipment, 261
- guidelines, 263
- intersections and, 269–271
- lights and siren, 268–269
- loading, 269
- medical equipment standards, 262–263
- at multiple-casualty incident, 314–315
- multiple-vehicle responses, 269
- operation, 261–271
- parking, 269, 270
- peak load, 264
- primary areas of responsibility (PARs), 264–265
- provider eduction, 266
- safe operation, 265–271
- spotters, 266
- staffing, 265
- standard operating procedures (SOPs), 267
- standards, 261
- system status management (SSM), 265
- tired response system, 265
- traffic congestion and, 265
- types of, 262
- vehicle/equipment checklist, 263

Amniotic fluid, 21
Amniotic sac, 21
Analgesia and sedation, pediatric, 137–138
Analgesics, 190–191
Anaphylactic shock, 125
Anatomy and physiology
- gynecology, 3–8
- obstetrics, 19–21
- pediatrics, 86–90

Aneurysms, 176–177
Angina pectoris, 175
Angiotensin-converting enzyme (ACE) inhibitors, 188
Ankylosing spondylitis (AS), 185–186
Anorexia nervosa, 163

Anoxic hypoxemia, 169
Antepartum, 55
Anticoagulant therapy, 251
Anticoagulants, 189
Antidepressants, 189
Antihypertensives, 188
Anti-inflammatory agents, 190–191
Antipsychotics, 189–190
Antiseizure medications, 190
Aortic dissection, 176–177
Aortic stenosis, 58, 59
Aortocaval compression, 47–48
APGAR score, 40–41, 61, 65
Aphasia, 180, 218
Apnea, 57, 71, 245
Apnea monitors, 144
Apparent life-threatening event (ALTE), 141
Arrhythmias
  bradyarrhythmias, 127
  geriatrics, 176
  pulseless arrest, 127–129
  tachyarrhythmias, 126–127
Arthritis, 223
Articulation disorders, 219
Assessment
  abortion, 29
  abruptio placentae, 32
  asthma, 121
  bacterial tracheitis, 119
  bronchiolitis, 122
  congenital abnormalities, 59–61
  croup, 118
  ectopic pregnancy, 30–31
  elderly patients, 163–166
  epiglottitis, 119
  foreign body airway obstruction (FBAO), 123
  foreign body aspiration, 120–121
  gestational diabetes, 34
  gynecologic, 8–10
  home care, 239–242
  hypertensive disorders of pregnancy, 33
  hypoglycemia, 131
  meningitis, 130
  newborns, 59–63
  obstetric patient, 25–28
  pediatric, 90–99
  placenta previa, 31
  pneumonia, 122
  poisoning and toxic exposure, 133
  preterm labor, 35
  rescue, 330–331
  respiratory disorders (home care), 249–250
  seizures, 129
  sexual assault, 14
  special needs infants/children, 145–146
  sudden infant death syndrome (SIDS), 141
  supine hypotensive syndrome, 33–34
  trauma (elderly), 193–194
Assisted living, 155
Asthma
  defined, 121
  home respiratory support, 243–244
  pediatric, 121–122
Asystole, 127
Atrial septal defect, 57, 58
Automobile anatomy, 344–345
Autonomic dysfunction, 177

B

Bacterial tracheitis, 120
Bag-valve mask (BVM) ventilation, 82
Baptism request, 76
Behavioral/psychological disorders, elderly patients, 192–193
Bend fractures, 139
Beta radiation, 365
Beta-blockers, 188
Biotransformation, 367
BiPAP, 243, 249
Birth injuries
  common, 75–76
  risk factors, 75–76
  statistics, 75
Bleeding, in pregnancy, 29
Blood spatter evidence, 390
Body armor, 387
Body surface area (BSA), 89
Boiling point, 364
Bowel obstruction, 183
Bradyarrhythmias, 127
Bradycardia, 71–72
Brain ischemia, 178
Branches
  defined, 305
  EMS, 305–316
  example, 306
  groups and divisions, 305
  sectors, 305
  units, 305
Braxton-Hicks contractions, 35
Breathing, pediatric assessment, 91–93
Breech presentation, 42
Bronchiectasis, 245
Bronchiolitis, 122
Bronchitis, 243
Bronchopulmonary dysplasia (BPD), 244
Broviac catheter, 250
Buckle fractures, 139
Bullying, 378
Burns
  child abuse and, 206
  elderly patients, 195
  pediatric patients, 136, 139–140
  rule of nines, 140

C

CAMEO®, 362
Cancer
  lung, 175
  neutropenia and, 224
  as pathological challenge, 223–224
Capnography, 99
Caput succedaneum, 76
Cardiac arrest
  neonate, 76
  in pregnancy, 47–49
Cardiac conditions (home care), 251
Cardiac syncope, 177
Cardiogenic shock, 124, 125–126
Cardiomyopathy, 126
Cardiovascular system
  elderly patients, 169
  pediatrics, 89
  pregnancy and, 21–22
Caregivers, responding to, 83
Car-versus-pedestrian injuries, 135
Cataracts, 164, 165
Cave-ins, 342
Cellulitis, 237
Central IV lines, 144–145
Cephalopelvic disproportion, 44
Cerebral palsy, 224–225
Cerebravascular disease, 178–179
Cervix, 5
C-FLOP, 299
Chain of evidence, 210
Challenged patients
  developmental disabilities, 221–223
  hearing impairments, 216–217
  introduction to, 215
  mentally and emotionally, 221
  obesity, 219–221
  paralysis, 221
  pathological challenges, 223–227

physical challenges, 216–221
speech impairments, 218–219
visual impairments, 217–218
Chemical asphyxiants, 368–369
CHEMTEL, 362–364
CHEMTREC, 362–364
Chest, pediatrics, 87–89, 139
Chest compressions
neonatal resuscitation, 67
in pregnancy, 47
Child abuse and neglect. *See also* Pediatrics
abused characteristics, 204–205
abuser characteristics, 204
assessment, 142–143
defined, 204
emotional abuse and, 207
identification of, 205–206
management of, 143
maternal drug abuse and, 206
perpetrators of, 141
physical exam, 205–206
recording and reporting, 207
resources for, 143
sexual, 142
signs of neglect, 206–207
types of, 141–142
Children. *See also* Pediatrics
adolescents, 86
anatomic and physiologic characteristics, 87, 88
BLS maneuvers, 100
endotracheal intubation, 106–107
foreign body airway obstruction (FBAO), 99
home care, 255–256
legal considerations, 90
multiple-casualty incidents, 146–147
nasogastric intubation, 110
nonambulatory, modifications for, 147
normal vital signs, 95
pre-school, 85
school-age, 85
with special needs, 143–146
toddler, 84
Choanal atresia, 59
Chronic hypertension, 33
Chronic obstructive pulmonary disease (COPD), 173–174, 243–244
Circulation
pediatric assessment, 93–94
pediatric patients, 109–111
Cleft lip, 59
Cleft palate, 59
Clitoris, 4
Closed incidents, 300
Coarctation of the aorta, 58
Cold zone, 364
Cold-protective response, 337–338
Colostomy, 221, 253
Comfort care, 256–257
Command. *See also* Incident Management System (IMS)
defined, 299
establishing, 299
incident command post (ICP), 301
incident commander, 299
incident communications, 301
incident size-up, 299–300
incident stabilization, 300
information officer (IO), 304
liaison officer (LO), 304
life safety, 300
mental health support, 304
procedures, 302–303
property conservation, 300
resource utilization, 301–302
safety officer (SO), 303–304
section chief, 303
singular, 300
span of control, 299
staff, 303–304
staff functions, 303
staging area identification, 301
support of, 303–305
termination of, 303
unified, 300–301
vest, 302
Communicable diseases, patients with, 228
Communications
difficulties in elderly, 162, 164–165
incident, 301
multiple-casualty incidents (MCIs), 316
rural EMS, 396, 397
situational awareness, 387
Comorbidity, 160
Compartment syndrome, 401
Compensated shock, 123
Concealment, 385–386
Conductive deafness, 216
Confined-space hazards. *See also* Hazardous atmosphere rescues
protections in the workplace, 341–342
risks, 340–341
Congenital abnormalities
airway establishment and, 62
APGAR score and, 61
assessment, 59–61
heat loss prevention and, 62–63
treatment, 62–63
types of, 57–59
Congenital heart disease, 125–126
Congestive heart failure (CHF), 244
Congregate care, 155
Consensus standards, 297
Contact and cover, 386
Contamination, 365–366
CONTOMS, 388
Contraceptives, 9
COPD (chronic obstructive pulmonary disease), 173–174, 243–244
Cor pulmonale, 244
Corpus luteum, 6
Corrosives, 368
Corticosteroids, 191
CPAP, 243, 249
Cribbing, 401
Crime scene awareness
advised of danger en route, 379
approach to, 379–381
cover and concealment, 385–386
danger observation on arrival, 380–381
dangerous crowds and bystanders, 382
distraction and evasion, 386
domestic violence, 384
drug laboratories, 383–384
drug-related crimes, 383
EMS and, 388–390
eruption of danger during care/transport, 381
evidence preserving, 389–390
highway encounters, 381
introduction to, 378–379
murder, assault, robbery, 382
police operations and, 388–389
retreat, 385
safety tactics, 385–386
scenarios, 379–381
situational awareness, 386–387
specific scenes, 381–384
street gangs, 382–383
tactical considerations, 384–388
tactical patient care, 387–388
violent street incidents, 382–383

Critical incident stress management (CISM), 318
Croup, 118
Crowning, 28
Crush points, 404
C-spine stabilization, pediatric, 113
Culturally diverse patients, 227
Cystic fibrosis (CF), 225, 244
Cystitis, 12
Cysts
 defined, 11
 ovarian, ruptured, 11–12
Cytochrome oxidase, 368

D

Dams/hydroelectric intakes, 336–337
Dangerous crowds and bystanders, 382
Dead/nonsalvageable (BLACK) victims, 147
Deafness, 216–217
Decision making, decontamination, 370–371
Decompensated shock, 124
Decontamination. *See also* Hazmat incidents
 absorption, 370
 approaches to, 369–372
 decision making, 370–371
 dilution, 369
 field, 371–372
 isolation/disposal, 370
 methods of, 369–370
 neutralization, 370
 semi-decontaminated patients, 371
Defibrillation, in pregnancy, 48
Delayed cord clamping (DCC), 63
Delayed effects, 367
Delirium, 179–180
Delivery
 abnormal situations, 42–44
 breech presentation, 42
 cephalopelvic disproportion, 44
 complications of, 44–45
 field, 38–40
 limb presentation, 43
 maternal complications, 45–47
 meconium staining, 45
 multiple births, 44
 normal, 38–39
 normal blood loss, 40
 postpartum hemorrhage, 45–46
 precipitous, 44
 prolapsed cord, 42–43
 pulmonary embolism, 47
 at scene decision, 37
 shoulder dystocia, 44–45, 46
 uterine inversion, 47
 uterine rupture, 46–47
Dementia, 180
Demobilized resources, 303
Demographic changes, 264
Demyelination, 245
Department of Homeland Security (DHS), 297, 298
Depression
 elderly patients, 192
 postpartum, 255
Developmental disabilities. *See also* Challenged patients
 accommodations for, 222
 Down syndrome, 222
 fetal alcohol syndrome (FAS), 223
 overview, 221–222
Diabetes
 elderly patients and, 181–182
 gestational, 34–35
 obstetrics and, 26–27
Diabetic ketoacidosis, 132
Diabetic retinopathy, 217
Dialysis shunts, 251
Diaphragmatic hernia, 59, 71
Diarrhea, 75, 131
Digitalis (digoxin), 188–189
Dilution, 369
Disaster management
 defined, 316
 mental health services, 318
 mitigation, 317
 planning, 317
 recovery, 317
 response, 317
Disasters, 296
Disentanglement
 defined, 328, 331
 EMS responsibilities, 332
Distraction and evasion, 386
Distressed newborns
 apnea, 57, 71
 assessment parameters, 64–65
 bradycardia, 71–72
 cardiac resuscitation, postresuscitation, and stabilization, 76
 common birth injuries, 75–76
 diaphragmatic hernia, 71
 diarrhea, 75
 fever, 73–74
 hypoglycemia, 74–75
 hypothermia, 74
 hypovolemia, 73
 maternal narcotic use and, 69
 meconium-stained amniotic fluid, 70–71
 neonatal transport and, 70
 overview, 63–64
 prematurity, 72
 respiratory distress/cyanosis, 72–73
 resuscitation, 64–69
 resuscitation illustration, 65
 seizures, 73
 specific situations, 70–76
 vomiting, 75
Distributive shock, 125
Diuretics, 188
Dizziness/vertigo, 179
Do Not Resuscitate (DNR) orders, 156, 157, 242
Documentation
 evidence, 390
 sexual assault, 15
Domestic elder abuse, 203
Domestic incidents, 298
Domestic violence, 384
DOT KKK 1822F specs, 261
Down syndrome, 222
Drug abuse, 191
Drug laboratories, 383–384
Drug-related crimes, 383
Ductus arteriosus, 55
Due regard standard, 267–268
Dysfunctional uterine bleeding, 13
Dysmenorrhea, 8
Dyspareunia, 8
Dysphagia, 160
Dysphoria, 192
Dysuria, 12

E

Eclampsia, 32–33
Ectopic pregnancy, 12–13, 30–31
Eddies, 337
Effacement, 35
Eight-step field decontamination, 371–372
Elder abuse
 abused characteristics, 203
 abuser characteristics, 204
 causes of, 203
 domestic, 203
 identification of, 203

institutional, 203
theories about, 203
Elderly patients
alcohol abuse, 191–192
altered mental status and confusion, 165–166
Alzheimer's disease, 180
angina pectoris, 175
ankylosing spondylitis (AS), 185–186
aortic dissection/aneurysms, 176–177
arrhythmias, 176
assessment of, 163–166
behavioral/psychological disorders, 192–193
body system changes illustration, 167
bowel obstruction, 183
burns, 195
cardiovascular disorders, 175–178
cardiovascular system, 169
cerebrovascular disease, 178–179
chronic obstructive pulmonary disease (COPD), 173–174
common medical conditions, 172–193
communication difficulties, 162
continence and elimination problems, 162–163
defined, 153
delirium, 179–180
dementia, 180
depression, 192
diabetes mellitus, 181–182
dizziness/vertigo, 179
drug abuse, 191
endocrine system, 170
environmental emergencies, 186–187
ethics, 156–157
financing/resources for health care, 157–159
gastrointestinal disorders, 182–183
gastrointestinal system, 170
general health assessment, 163
genitourinary system, 171
GI hemorrhage, 182–183
head and spinal injuries, 195–196
heart failure, 176
hematologic system, 172
history, 164–166
home safety for, 161
hospital alternatives, 158
hypertension, 177
hyperthermia (heatstroke), 187
hypothermia, 187
immune system, 171
integumentary system, 170–171
living environments, 154–156
lung cancer, 175
management of, 166–167
mesenteric ischemia/infarct, 183
metabolic and endocrine disorders, 181–182
mobility and falls, 161–162
multiple-system failure, 160
musculoskeletal disorders, 184–186
musculoskeletal system, 171
myocardial infarction (MI), 175
nervous system, 169–170
neurologic disorders, 178–181
orthopedic injuries, 195
osteoarthritis, 184
osteoporosis, 184–185
Parkinson's disease, 180–181
pathophysiology of, 160–163
pharmacology in, 160–161
physical exam, 166
pneumonia, 172–173
population characteristics, 154
poverty and loneliness, 154–155
pressure ulcers (decubitus ulcers), 183–184
prevention and self-help, 158–159
pulmonary edema, 174
pulmonary embolism, 174
pulmonary/respiratory disorders, 172–175
renal system, 171
respiratory system, 168–169
seizures, 179
skin diseases, 183
skin disorders, 183–184
social support, 155–156
societal issues, 154–157
stroke, 178–179
substance abuse, 191–192
suicide, 192–193
syncope, 177–178
system pathophysiology in, 167–172
thermoregulatory system, 170
thyroid disorders, 182
toxicologic emergencies, 187–191
transient ischemic attack (TIA), 178–179
trauma in, 193–196
urinary disorders, 186
Electrical therapy, pediatrics, 113
Elimination, 162
Emergency Medical Services for Children (EMSC), 81
Emergency operations center (EOC), 298
Emergency response guidebook, 361–362
Emesis, 240
Emphysema, 243
EMS communications officer, 316
EMS groups. *See also* Incident Management System (IMS)
communications, 316
extrication/rescue unit, 315
morgue, 313
overview, 305–306
rehabilitation (rehab) unit, 315–316
on-scene physicians, 314
staging, 314–315
transport unit, 315
treatment, 313–314
triage, 306–313
EMT-Tacticals (EMT-Ts), 388
Endocrine system, elderly patients, 170
Endometriosis, 12
Endometritis, 12
Endometrium, 5
Endotracheal intubation
anatomic and physiologic concerns, 105
indications, 105
pediatric patients, 105–108
pediatric techniques, 107–108
tube placement verification, 108
Enucleation, 217
Environmental emergencies, elderly patients, 186–187
Environmental Protection Agency (EPA), 357
Epiglottitis, 119–120
Epistaxis, 177
Essential equipment, ambulance, 261
Estimated data of confinement (EDC), 23
Ethics, geriatrics, 156–157
Evidence
blood spatter, 390
documenting, 390
particulate, 390
preserving, 389–390
prints, 389
on-scene observations, 390
types of, 389–390
Exocrine, 244

Exposure treatment. *See also* Hazmat incidents
chemical asphyxiants, 368–369
corrosives, 368
hydrocarbon solvents, 369
overview, 367–368
pesticides, 368
pulmonary irritants, 368
Extraglottic airways, 109
Extrauterine, 55
Extremities, pediatrics, 89, 139
Extrication, 315, 331

F

Facilities unit, 304–305
Fallopian tubes, 5, 6
Falls
elderly, 161–162
pediatric patients, 134–135
Farm machinery, 400
Febrile seizures, 129
Female reproductive organs
clitoris, 4
cross-sectional anatomy, 4
external genitalia, 3–4
fallopian tubes, 6
internal genitalia, 4–6
labia, 4
mons pubis, 3
ovaries, 6
perineum, 3
uterus, 5–6
vagina, 4–5
Fetal alcohol syndrome (FAS), 223
Fetal circulation, 24–25
Fetal development, 22–23
Fetal heart tones (FHTs), 24
Fever, 73–74
Fibrosis, 169
Field decontamination. *See also* Decontamination
eight-step process, 371
transportation considerations, 371–372
two-step process, 371
Field delivery, 38–40
Finance/administration section, 304
Financial challenges, patients with, 228
Fixed-wing aircraft, 278–279
Flammable/explosive limits, 364–365
Flash point, 365
Flat water
cold-protective response, 337–338
location of submerged victims, 338
overview, 337
personal flotation devices, 337
rescue versus body recovery, 338
survival factors, 337
in-water patient immobilization, 338
Fluency disorders, 219
Fluid management, pediatric emergencies, 137
Fluid therapy, 111–112
Focal clonic seizures, 73
Foot/extremity pins, 335
Foreign body airway obstruction (FBAO)
infant risk, 84
pediatric airway management, 99–100, 104
respiratory emergency (pediatric), 122–123
Foreign body aspiration, 120–121
Fractures, child abuse and, 206
Fundus, 5

G

Gamma radiation, 365
Gangrene, 235
Gastric feeding tubes, 145
Gastroenteritis, 130
Gastrointestinal disorders, 182–183
Gastrointestinal system
elderly patients, 170
pediatric patient emergencies, 130–131
pregnancy and, 22
Gastrointestinal tract devices. *See also* GI/GU crises
colostomy stoma locations, 254
complications, 253–254
Gastrostomy tubes, 145
Genitourinary system, elderly patients, 171
Geriatrics. *See also* Elderly patients
abuse/neglect, observing, 193–194
analgesics and anti-inflammatory agents and, 190–191
angiotensin-converting enzyme (ACE) inhibitors and, 188
anticoagulants and, 189
antihypertensives/diuretics and, 188
antipsychotics/antidepressants and, 189–190
antiseizure medications and, 190
assessment considerations, 163–166
behavioral/psychological disorders, 192–193
beta-blockers and, 188
burns, 195
cardiovascular considerations, 194
cardiovascular disorders, 175–178
cardiovascular system, 169
common medical conditions, 172–193
corticosteroids and, 191
defined, 154
digitalis (digoxin) and, 188–189
endocrine system, 170
environmental emergencies, 186–187
ethics, 156–157
financing and resources, 157–159
gastrointestinal disorders, 182–183
gastrointestinal system, 170
genitourinary system, 171
head and spinal injuries, 195–196
hematologic system, 172
immune system, 171
integumentary system, 170–171
introduction to, 153
management considerations, 166–167
medications for Parkinson's disease and, 190
metabolic and endocrine disorders, 181–182
musculoskeletal disorders, 184–186
musculoskeletal system, 171
nervous system, 169–170
neurologic disorders, 178–181
orthopedic injuries, 195
pathophysiology, 160–163
pulmonary/respiratory disorders, 172–175
renal considerations, 194
renal system, 171
respiratory considerations, 194
respiratory system, 168–169
skin disorders, 183–184
substance abuse, 191–192
thermoregulatory system, 170
toxicologic emergencies, 187–191
transport considerations, 194
trauma and, 193–196
urinary disorders, 186
Gerontology, 154
Gestational age, estimation of, 47
Gestational diabetes, 34–35
GI hemorrhage, 182–183

GI/GU crises
gastrointestinal tract devices, 253–254
psychosocial implications, 254
response to, 236
urinary tract devices, 252–253
Glasgow Coma Scale (GCS), 96, 97
Glaucoma, 164, 217
Glottic function, 66
Gold standard, ambulance, 261
Governmental agencies, 159
Graafian follicles, 6
Green treatment unit, 314
Greenstick fractures, 139
Groshong catheter, 250
Ground ambulance. *See* Ambulances
Growth plate, 89
Guillain-Barré syndrome, 235, 245
Gynecologic emergencies
abdominal pain management, 13
cystitis, 12
ectopic pregnancy, 12–13
endometriosis, 12
endometritis, 12
management of, 10–11
medical, 11–13
mittelschmerz, 12
nontraumatic vaginal bleeding, 13
pelvic inflammatory disease (PID), 11
ruptured ovarian cyst, 11–12
sexual assault, 13–15
traumatic, 13–15
Gynecology
anatomy and physiology, 3–8
assessment, 8–10
defined, 3
female reproductive organs and, 3–6
history, 8–10
menstrual cycle and, 6–8
physical exam, 10

H

Hate crimes, 211, 382
Hazard control, 329
Hazardous atmosphere rescues. *See also* Rescue
cave-ins and structural collapses, 342
confined-space hazards, 340–342
overview, 340
Hazardous materials (hazmat)
agricultural, 400
alpha radiation, 365
beta radiation, 365
boiling point, 364
defined, 356
emergency response guidebook and, 361–362
flammable/explosive limits, 364–365
flash point, 365
gamma radiation, 365
ignition temperatures, 365
monitors and testing, 362
NFPA 704 System, 360–361
placard classifications, 359–360
recognition of, 359–361
safety data sheets (SDSs), 362, 363
shipping papers, 362
specific gravity, 365
substances, identification of, 361–364
terminology, 364–365
terrorism and, 356
vapor density, 365
vapor pressure, 365
water solubility, 365
zones, 364
Hazardous terrain rescues. *See also* Rescue
environmental issues, 351
extended care assessment, 350
flat, rough terrain evacuation, 349
helicopter use, 350
high-angle, 347–348
low-angle, 348
low-angle/high-angle evacuation, 349–350
overview, 346–347
packaging and evacuation practice, 350
patient access, 347–348
patient packaging, 348
patient removal, 349–350
types of terrain, 347
warning placard, 358
Hazmat incidents. *See also* Hazardous materials (hazmat)
awareness, 358–359
cold zone, 364
contamination, 365–366
cycles and actions of poisons, 367
decontamination, 369–372
entry readiness, 373
heat stress factors, 373
hot zone, 364
ICS and, 357–358
introduction to, 356
levels of training, 357
post-exit rehab, 373
practice importance, 374
protection equipment, 372–373
requirements and standards, 357
role of the paramedic in, 356–357
routes of exposure, 367
size-up, 357–364
terrorism and, 359
transportation, 358–359
treatment of exposures, 367–369
warm zone, 364
Head, pediatric patients, 86, 138
Head and spinal injuries
child abuse and, 206
elderly patients, 195–196
Head-tilt/chin-lift method, 93
Hearing impairments. *See also* Physical challenges
accommodations for, 217
recognition of deafness, 216–217
types of, 216
Heart disease, obstetrics and, 27
Heart failure, 176
Heat escape lessening position (HELP), 334
Heat stress factors, 373
Heatstroke, 186
Helicopters. *See also* Air medical transport; Aircraft
approach, 287–288
departure, 289
in EMS system, 281
HOTSAW mnemonic, 287
instrument flight rules (IFR), 280
landing zone, 286–287
limitations of use, 284–285
loading, 289
patient handoff, 288–289
safe utilization of services, 282
scene operations, 286–289
types of, 279–280
visual flight rules (VFR), 280
weather and, 279–280
Hematologic system, elderly patients, 172
Hemoptysis, 244
Hepatomegaly, 176
Herpes zoster, 183
Hiatal hernias, 170
Hickman catheter, 250
High-angle rescues, 347

High-impact incidents, 296
Highway encounters, 381
History
gynecologic, 8–10
obstetric patient, 25–27
pediatric assessment, 96–97
Hmong, medicinal practices of, 205
Home artificial ventilators, 144
Home care
acute infections, 254–255
acute situations, 242–257
airway complications, 235
ALS response to patients, 234–237
alterations in peripheral circulation, 235
altered mental status, 235
artificial airways/tracheostomies, 246–248
assessment, 239–242
BiPAP, 243, 249
cardiac conditions, 251
cardiac decompression, 235
commonly found devices, 237–238
CPAP, 243, 249
epidemiology of, 233–239
equipment malfunction, 236–237
GI/GU crises, 236, 252–254
home oxygen therapy, 246
hospice and comfort care, 256–257
infections and septic complications, 236–237
injury control and prevention, 238–239
interventions by home health care practitioner or physician, 238
introduction to, 233
legal considerations, 234
maternal and newborn care, 255–256
medical therapy in, 245–250
mental status, 241
other medical disorders and, 237
patient milieu, 240
patients receiving, 233–234
PEEP, 243, 249
preparing home for, 238
respiratory disorders, 242–250
respiratory failure, 235
scene safety, 239–240
scene size-up, 239–240
transport and management treatment plan, 242
vascular access devices (VADs), 250–251
ventilation, 248–249
Home oxygen therapy, 246
Hospice
ALS intervention, 256–257
care, 256–257
defined, 238
Hospital alternatives, 158
Hot zone, 364
Human trafficking, 209–211
Hybrid vehicles, 345
Hydrocarbon solvents, 369
Hymen, 4
Hyperbilirubinemia, 63
Hyperglycemia, 132
Hypertension, 27, 177
Hyperthermia (heatstroke), 187
Hypertrophy, 169, 235
Hypochondriasis, 192
Hypoglycemia, 74–75, 131–132
Hypoperfusion. *See* Shock
Hypothermia, 74, 187
Hypovolemia, 73
Hypovolemic shock, 124

I

Ignition temperatures, 365
Immediately dangerous to life and health (IDLH), 365
Immune senescence, 171
Immune system, elderly patients, 171
Incident command post (ICP), 301
Incident Command System (ICS)
C-FLOP, 299
defined, 297
hazmat emergencies and, 357–358
Incident Management System (IMS)
command, 299–303
consensus standards, 297
defined, 297
disaster management, 316–317
division of operations, 305
EMS branch, 305–316
finance/administration section, 304
illustrated, 303
logistics section, 304–305
operations section, 305
origins of, 297–299
planning/intelligence section, 305
regulations and standards, 297–298
scene-authority law, 297
as uniform, flexible system, 298–299
Incident tactical worksheet, 302
Incidents. *See also* Hazmat incidents
closed, 300
communications, 301
open, 300
stabilization of, 300
Incontinence, 162
Infants. *See also* Pediatrics
airway, clearing, 101
anatomic and physiologic characteristics, 87, 88
BLS maneuvers, 100
common complications, 255–256
defined, 84
foreign body airway obstruction (FBAO), 100
normal vital signs, 95
with special needs, 143–146
treatment of, 84
Infections, pediatric, 116
Information officer (IO), 304
Institutional elder abuse, 203
Instrument flight rules (IFR), 280
Integumentary system, elderly patients, 170–171
Intermittent mandatory ventilation (IMV), 244
Intracerebral hemorrhage, 178
Intraosseous infusion, pediatric patients, 111
Intrapartum, 55
Intrauterine devices (IUDs), 9
In-water patient immobilization, 338
Irreversible shock, 124
Isolation/disposal, 370
Isolette, 70

J

Jaw-thrust method, 93
JumpSTART system
algorithm, 146
defined, 309–311
illustrated, 311
objectives, 311
using, 146–147

K

Kyphosis, 168

L

Labia, 4
Labor
active, 27
defined, 36
effacement and, 35
management of, 37–38
maternal complications, 45–47

preterm, 35–36
stages of, 36–37
Labyrinthitis, 216
Landing zone, 286–287
Language disorders, 218
Laryngeal mask airway (LMA), 109
Lethal concentration/lethal doses (LCt/LD), 365
Level of consciousness, in pediatric assessment, 91
Liaison officer (LO), 304
Life-care communities, 155
Limb presentation, 43
Living environments, elderly, 154–156
Local effects, 367
Lochia, 37
Lock-out/tag-out, 400
Logistics section, 304–305
Low-angle rescues, 348
Lower GI bleed, 182–183
Low-impact incidents, 296
Lung cancer, 175
Lung transplants, patients awaiting, 245

M

Maceration, 184
Manual lateral uterine displacement (LUD), 48
Marfan syndrome, 170
Mass-casualty incidents. *See* Multiple-casualty incidents (MCIs)
Maternal narcotic use, 69
Maternal/newborn care, 255–256
Meconium, 62
Meconium staining, 45, 70–71
Medicaid, 157–158
Medical supply, 304
Medical treatment, rescue, 330–331
Medicare, 157
Medications
ACE inhibitors, 188
analgesics, 190–191
anticoagulants, 189
antipsychotics/antidepressants, 189–190
antiseizure, 179, 190
beta-blockers, 188
corticosteroids, 190–191
digitalis (digoxin), 188–189
for Parkinson's disease, 190
in pediatric advanced life support, 112
pediatrics, 112
Medi-Port, 251
Melena, 182
Menarche, 6
Ménière's disease, 165
Meningitis, 130
Meningomyelocele, 59
Menopause, 8
Menorrhagia, 13
Menstrual cycle
ischemic phase, 7
menstrual phase, 7–8
overview, 6
phases illustration, 7
proliferative phase, 6
secretory phase, 7
Menstruation, 7
Mesenteric ischemia/infarct, 182, 183
Metabolic and endocrine disorders, elderly patients, 181–183
Metabolic emergencies, pediatric patients, 131–132
METTAG, 311, 313
Minimum standards, ambulance, 261
Miscarriage, 12
Mitral (pulmonary) stenosis, 58, 59
Mittelschmerz, 12
Mobility problems, elderly, 161–162
Mons pubis, 3
Morbid obesity, 220–221
Morgue, 313
Morgue officer, 313
Motor vehicle collisions, 135
Moving water. *See also* Water rescues
dams/hydroelectric intakes, 336–337
eddies, 337
foot/extremity pins, 335
overview, 334–335
recirculating currents, 335
strainers, 335, 336
Mucoviscidosis, 225
Multifocal seizures, 73
Multiple births, 44
Multiple sclerosis (MS), 225
Multiple-casualty incidents (MCIs). *See also* Incident Management System (IMS)
ambulances at, 314–315
with children, 146–147
classification of, 296
common problems, 317
communications, 316
defined, 295
disaster, 296
disaster management, 316–317
extrication/rescue unit, 315
high-impact incident, 296
introduction to, 295–297
low-impact incident, 296
meeting challenge of, 317–318
mental health services, 318
morgue, 313
preplanning, drills, and critiques, 318
rehabilitation (rehab) unit, 315–316
on-scene physicians, 314
transport unit, 315
treatment, 313–314
triage, 305–313
Multiple-system failure, 160
Murder, assault, robbery, 382
Muscular dystrophy (MD), 225–226, 245
Musculoskeletal system
elderly patients, 171, 184–186
pregnancy and, 22
Mutual aid agreements, 305
Mutual aid coordination center (MACC), 298–299
Myasthenia gravis, 227, 235, 245
Myocardial infarction (MI), 175
Myoclonic seizures, 73
Myometrium, 6

N

Nasogastric intubation, 109
Nasogastric tube, 66
Nasopharyngeal airways, 103
National Fire Protection Association (NFPA), 357
National Incident Management System (NIMS)
defined, 297
function of, 298
mutual aid coordination center (MACC), 298–299
subsystems, 298
Nausea and vomiting, pediatric patients, 130
Needle cricothyrotomy, 104–105
Negative-pressure ventilators, 248
Neonatal abstinence syndrome (NAS), 75
Neonatal resuscitation
algorithm, 60
chest compressions, 67
drying, warming, position, suctioning, and tactile stimulation, 64–66

Neonatal resuscitation (*continued*)
- illustrated, 65
- inverted pyramid for, 64–69
- medications and fluids, 67
- supplemental oxygen, 67
- ventilation, 66–67

Neonates. *See also* Distressed newborns; Newborns; Pediatrics
- APGAR scoring, 40–41
- defined, 54, 83
- routine care of, 40
- stimulating, 41
- transport, 70

Neonatology, 54
Nephrons, 171
Nervous system
- elderly patients, 169–170
- pediatrics, 89

Neurogenic shock, 125
Neurologic emergencies, pediatric patients, 129–130
Neuromuscular degenerative diseases, 244–245
Neuromuscular disorders, obstetrics and, 27
Neutralization, 370
Neutropenia, 224
Newborns. *See also* Distressed newborns; Pediatrics
- assessment, 59–63
- congenital abnormalities, 57–59
- defined, 54, 83
- epidemiology, 55
- hemodynamic changes, 56
- home care, 255–256
- intubation and tracheal suctioning, 68–69
- pathophysiology, 55–59
- risk factors indicating possible complications, 55

NFPA 704 System, 360–361
Night vision goggles (NVG), 276, 286
Nocturia, 176
Noncardiogenic shock, 124–125
Nonsteroidal anti-inflammatory drugs (NSAIDs), 190, 223
Nontraumatic vaginal bleeding, 13

O

Obesity. *See also* Physical challenges
- accommodations for patients, 220
- etiologies, 219–220
- morbid, 220–221
- overview, 219

Obstetrics
- anatomy and physiology, 19–21
- assessment, 25–28
- defined, 3
- introduction to, 19
- labor, 36–38
- patient management, 28
- preexisting and aggravated medical conditions, 26–27
- prenatal care, 26
- prenatal period and, 19–25
- puerperium, 36–49
- terminology, 26

Occiput posterior position, 43
Occupational Safety and Health Administration (OSHA), 357
Old-old, 154, 155
Omphalocele, 59
On-scene observations, as evidence, 390
On-scene physicians, 314
Open incidents, 300
Operations section, 305
Orogastric tube, 66
Oropharyngeal airways, 102
Orthopedic injuries, elderly patients, 195
Orthostatic syncope, 177
Osteoarthritis, 184
Osteoporosis, 171, 184–185
Otitis media, 216
Ovarian cysts, 11–12
Ovaries, 5, 6
Ovulation, 6, 20
Oxygen saturation (SpO_2), 61
Oxygen therapy, home, 246
Oxygenation, 100–102

P

Pain, obstetric patient, 27
Paralysis, 221
Parents, responding to, 83
Parkinson's disease, 180–181
Particulate evidence, 390
Partner abuse
- abused characteristics, 202
- abuser characteristics, 201–202
- approaching patients, 202–203
- defined, 201
- identification of, 201
- reasons for not reporting, 201

Parts per million/parts per billion (ppm/ppb), 365
Patent ductus arteriosus, 57
Pathological challenges. *See also* Challenged patients
- arthritis, 223
- cancer, 223–224
- cerebral palsy, 224–225
- cystic fibrosis (mucoviscidosis), 225
- multiple sclerosis (MS), 225
- muscular dystrophy (MD), 225–226
- myasthenia gravis, 227
- poliomyelitis, 226
- previous head injuries, 226
- spina bifida, 227

Patient access
- hazardous terrain rescues, 347–348
- in rescue operations, 329–330

Patient handoff, air medical transport, 288–289
Patient packaging
- defined, 332
- hazardous terrain rescues, 348, 350
- vehicle rescues, 346

Pediatric airway management
- advanced, 104–109
- airway adjuncts, 102–103
- basic, 99–104
- endotracheal intubation, 105–108
- equipment guidelines, 102
- extraglottic airways, 109
- foreign body airway obstruction (FBAO), 99–100, 104
- manual positioning, 99
- nasogastric intubation, 109, 110
- nasopharyngeal airways, 103
- needle cricothyrotomy, 104–105
- oropharyngeal airways, 102
- oxygenation, 100–102
- rapid sequence intubation, 108–109
- suctioning, 100
- ventilation, 103–104

Pediatric assessment
- airway, 91
- basic considerations, 90
- basic steps in, 92
- breathing, 91–93
- cardiopulmonary arrest anticipation, 94–95
- circulation, 93–94
- general approach to, 90–99
- general impression, 91
- Glasgow Coma Scale (GCS), 96, 97
- history, 96–97
- level of consciousness, 91
- noninvasive monitoring, 98–99
- physical exam, 97–99

primary, 91–95
reassessment, 99
scene size-up, 90–91
secondary, 95–99
transitional phase, 95
transport priority, 95
vital functions, 91–94
vital signs, 97
Pediatric cardiac arrest algorithm, 128
Pediatric emergencies
airway control, 136
analgesia and sedation, 137–138
apparent life-threatening event (ALTE), 141
approach to, 82–83
arrhythmias, 126–129
burns, 136, 139–140
cardiomyopathy, 126
car-versus-pedestrian injuries, 135
chest and abdomen, 139
communication and psychological support, 82–83
congenital heart disease, 125–126
diarrhea, 131
extremities, 139
falls, 134–135
fluid management, 137
gastrointestinal, 130–131
head, face, and neck, 138
hyperglycemia, 132
hypoglycemia, 131–132
infections, 116
mechanisms of injury, 134–136
meningitis, 130
metabolic, 131–132
motor vehicle collisions, 135
nausea and vomiting, 130
neurologic, 129–130
penetrating injuries, 136
physical abuse, 136
poisoning and toxic exposure, 133–134
respiratory, 116–123
responding to parents and caregivers, 83
responding to patient needs, 82–83
seizures, 129–130
shock, 123–126
stabilization, 136–137
submersion/immersion injuries, 135–136
sudden infant death syndrome (SIDS), 140–141
trauma, 134–141
traumatic brain injury, 138
Pediatrics
abdomen, 89
abuse and neglect, 141–143
advanced life support skills, 82
airway, 86–87
anatomy and physiology, 86–90
cardiovascular system, 89
chest and lungs, 87–89
circulation, 109–111
continuing education and training, 81
C-spine stabilization, 113
electrical therapy, 131
extremities, 89
fluid therapy, 111–112
general management, 99–116
growth and development, 83–86
head, 86
health care and injury prevention, 81–82
intraosseous infusion, 111
medications, 112
metabolic differences, 89–90
multiple-casualty incidents, 146–147
nervous system, 89
paramedics role in, 81–82
respiratory system, 89
skin and body surface area, 89
special needs, 143–146
transport guidelines, 113–116
vascular access, 111
PEEP, 66, 243, 249
Pelvic inflammatory disease (PID), 11
Penetrating injuries, pediatric patient, 136
Perimetrium, 6
Perimortem Caesarean delivery (PMCD), 49
Perineum, 3
Peripherally inserted central catheters (PICC), 250
Persistent fetal circulation, 55
Personal flotation devices, 337
Personal-care homes, 155
Pesticides, 368
Pharmacology, in elderly patients, 160–161
Phototherapy, 75
Physical abuse, pediatric patients, 136
Physical challenges. *See also* Challenged patients
hearing impairments, 216–217
obesity, 219–221
overview, 216
paralysis, 221
speech impairments, 218–219
visual impairments, 217–218
Physical exam
child abuse and neglect, 205–206
elderly patient, 166
gynecologic, 10
obstetric patient, 27–28
pediatric assessment, 97–99
PID (pelvic inflammatory disease), 11
Pierre Robin syndrome, 59
Pill-rolling motion, 181
Pinch points, 402
Pinch-point injury patient removal, 402–403
Placards, warning
classifications, 359–360
colors, 360
defined, 358
illustrated, 360
NFPA 704 System, 360–361
UN number, 360
vehicle display, 359
Placenta, 20
Placenta previa, 31
Planning/intelligence section, 305
Pneumonia, 122, 172–173
Poisoning and toxic exposure
assessment, 133
management of, 133–134
pediatric, 133–134
Poisons, cycles and actions of, 367
Police operations, 388–389
Poliomyelitis, 226, 245
Polycythemia, 63
Polypharmacy, 160
Port-A-Cath, 251
Positive-pressure ventilators, 248
Post-exit rehab, 373
Postpartum depression, 255
Postpartum hemorrhage, 45–46
Precipitous delivery, 44
Preeclampsia, 32, 33
Pregnancy. *See also* Obstetrics
abortion, 29–30
abruptio placentae, 31–32
airway management in, 48–49
bleeding in, 29
Braxton-Hicks contractions, 35
cardiac arrest in pregnancy, 47–49
cardiovascular system during, 21–22
chest compressions in, 47

Pregnancy (*continued*)
complications of, 28–36
defibrillation in, 48
ectopic, 30–31
emergency drugs and, 49
fetal development, 22–23
gastrointestinal system during, 22
gestational diabetes, 34–35
hemodynamic changes, 23
hypertensive disorders of, 32–33
maternal-fetal circulation, 24–25
medical complications of, 32–36
medical conditions, 29–36
musculoskeletal system during, 22
physiologic changes of, 21–22
placenta previa, 31
preterm labor, 35–36
reproductive system during, 21
respiratory system during, 21
supine hypotensive syndrome, 33–34
trauma, 28–29
urinary system during, 22
uterine changes associated with, 22
Prematurity, 72
Premenstrual dysphoric disorder (PMDD), 8
Premenstrual syndrome (PMS), 8
Prenatal period, 19–25
Prepuce, 4
Presbycusis, 216
Preschoolers, 85
Pressure sores, 236
Pressure ulcers (decubitus ulcers), 183–184
Preterm labor, 35–36
Prevention and self-help, elderly patients, 158–159
Previous head injuries, 226
Primary apnea, 57
Primary assessment. *See also* Assessment
home care patient, 240–242
obstetric patient, 25
pediatric, 91–95
Primary contamination, 365
Primary triage, 306–307
Prolapsed cord, 42–43
Prompt care facilities, 398
Pruritus, 183
Pubic symphysis, 3
Pudendum, 3
Puerperium
abnormal delivery situations, 42–44
cardiac arrest, 47–49
defined, 36
delivery complications, 44–45
field delivery, 38–40
labor, 36–38
maternal complications, 45–47
neonatal care, 40–41
Pulmonary edema, 174
Pulmonary embolism, 47, 174
Pulmonary irritants, 368
Pulseless arrest, 127–129
Pulseless electrical activity, 129

R

Rape
characteristics of assailants, 208
characteristics of victims, 207–208
date rape drugs, 208–209
defined, 207
EMS responsibilities, 209
Rapid intervention team, 316
Rapid sequence intubation, 108–109
Recirculating currents, 335
Recreational emergencies, 405–406
Red treatment unit, 314
Rehabilitation (rehab) unit, 315–316
Religious organizations, 159
Renal system, elderly patients, 171
Reportable collisions, 266
Reproductive system, 21
Rescue
arrival, 328
crew assignments, 327
as dangerous activity, 324
disentanglement, 331–332
environments, 324
extrication, 331
hazard control, 329
hazardous atmosphere, 340–342
hazardous terrain, 346–351
highway operations and, 342–344
introduction to, 323–324
medical treatment, 330
operations, 328–333
paramedic role in, 324
patient access, 329–330
patient packaging, 332
preplanning, 327–328
protective equipment, 325–327
removal and transport, 332–333
safety procedures, 327
scene size-up, 328
standard operating procedures (SOPs), 327
surface water, 333–339
vehicle, 344–346
Rescue patients
access to, 329–330, 347–348
packaging, 332
protection, 326–378
quieting fears of, 331
removal and transport, 332–333
Rescuer protection, 325–326
Reserve capacity, ambulance staffing, 265
Respiratory arrest, 117
Respiratory disorders (home care)
assessment, 249–250
bronchopulmonary dysplasia (BPD), 244
chronic diseases, 243–245
chronic obstructive pulmonary disease (COPD), 243–244
congestive heart failure (CHF), 244
cystic fibrosis (CF), 244
management of, 250
neuromuscular degenerative diseases, 244–245
patients awaiting lung transplants, 245
sleep apnea, 245
Respiratory distress
newborns, 72–73
signs and symptoms, 94, 117
Respiratory emergencies (pediatric)
asthma, 121–122
bacterial tracheitis, 120
bronchiolitis, 122
croup, 118
epiglottitis, 119–120
foreign body airway obstruction (FBAO), 122–123
foreign body aspiration, 120–121
lower airway distress, 121–123
management of, 117–118
overview, 116
pneumonia, 122
respiratory arrest, 117
respiratory distress, 117
respiratory failure, 117
severity of, 116–117
upper airway obstruction, 118–121
Respiratory failure, signs and symptoms, 117
Respiratory system
elderly patients, 168–169

pediatrics, 89
pregnancy and, 21
Resuscitation
DNR orders and, 156–157, 242
neonatal, 41, 60, 64–69, 76
Retinopathy, 182
Rotor-wing aircraft, 278, 279–281
Rough terrain, patient packaging for, 348
Rule of nines, 140
Ruptured ovarian cyst, 11–12
Rural EMS
agricultural emergencies, 399–404
communication difficulties, 396
communications improvement, 397
distance and time, 395–396
distance factor, 398–399
enrollment shortages, 396
inadequate medical support, 396–397
ingenuity and increased responsibilities, 398
introduction to, 395
medical support improvement, 397–398
practicing, 395–398
problem solving, 397–398
recreational emergencies, 405–406
recruitment and certification, 397
situations and decisions, 398–406
special problems, 395–397
training and practice, 396
Rust out, 396

S

Safety data sheets (SDSs), 362, 363
Safety officer (SO), 303–304
Safety tactics, 385–386
SALT system. *See also* Triage
defined, 308
illustrated, 309
steps, 308
triage tags for, 310
Scene size-up
hazmat incidents, 357–364
home care, 239–240
pediatric assessment, 90–91
rescue, 328
vehicle rescues, 345
Scene-authority law, 297
School-age children, 85
Scrambling, 347
Scree, 347
Secondary apnea, 57
Secondary assessment. *See also* Assessment
home care patient, 240–242
pediatric, 95–99
Secondary contamination, 365–366
Secondary triage, 307
Section chief, 303
Sectors, 305
Seek cover, 386
Seizure disorders, obstetrics and, 27
Seizures
antiseizure medications, 179
causes, 179
febrile, 129
in neonatology, 73
pediatric, 129–130
syncope and, 178
Semi-decontaminated patients, 371
Senile dementia, 180
Senior centers, 159
Sensorineural deafness, 216
Sensorium, 236
Septic shock, 125
Sexual assault
characteristics of assailants, 208
characteristics of victims, 207–208
date rape drugs, 208–209
defined, 207
EMS responsibilities, 209
rape, 207
Shaken baby syndrome, 206
Shear points, 404
Shipping papers, 362
Shock (pediatric)
anaphylactic, 125
cardiogenic, 124, 125–126
categories of, 124
compensated, 123
decompensated, 124
distributive, 125
hypovolemic, 124
irreversible, 124
neurogenic, 125
noncardiogenic, 124–125
overview, 123
septic, 125
severity of, 123–124
Shoulder dystocia, 44–45, 46
Shunts, 145
Shy-Drager syndrome, 181
Sick sinus syndrome, 177
Silent myocardial infarction, 175
Silo gas, 400
Singular command, 300
Situational awareness. *See also* Crime scene awareness
contact and cover, 386
multiple-casualty incidents (MCIs), 299
warning signals and communication, 387
Skin, pediatric patients, 89
Skin disorders, elderly patients, 183–184
Sleep apnea, 245
Social support, elderly patients, 155–156
Span of control, 299
Special needs infants/children
apnea monitors, 144
assessment and management practices, 145–146
central IV lines, 144–145
gastric feeding tubes, 145
gastrostomy tubes, 145
home artificial ventilators, 144
home care devices, 143–145
overview, 143
shunts, 145
tracheostomy tubes, 143–144
Special weapons and tactics (SWAT) team, 387
Specific gravity, 365
Speech impairments. *See also* Physical challenges
accommodations for, 219
articulation disorders, 219
fluency disorders, 219
language disorders, 218
types of, 218–219
voice production disorders, 219
Spina bifida, 227
Spinal cord injury without radiographic abnormality (SCIWORA), 113
Spinal injuries, water rescues, 339
Spondylosis, 196
Spotters, 266
Stabilization
C-spine, 113
pediatric, in child safety seat, 114
pediatric emergencies, 136–137
pediatric system, applying, 115
Staging area
defined, 314
identifying, 301

Staging officer, 314
Standard operating procedures (SOPs)
ambulance, 267
rescue, 327
START system, 307–308. *See also* Triage
Status epilepticus, 129
Stokes-Adams syndrome, 177
Stoma, 144
Strainers, 335, 336
Street gangs, 382–383
Stroke, 178–179
Structural collapses, 342
Subarachnoid hemorrhage, 178
Submerged victims, water rescue, 338
Submersion/immersion injuries, pediatric patients, 135–136
Substance abuse
alcohol abuse, 191–192
defined, 191
drug abuse, 191
elderly patients, 191–192
Subtle seizures, 73
Suctioning, pediatric airway management, 100
Sudden infant death syndrome (SIDS), 140–141
Suicide, elderly patients, 192–193
Supine hypotensive syndrome, 33–34
Supraventricular tachycardia, 126–127
Surface water rescues. *See* Water rescues
Surgical menopause, 8
Syncope, 177–178
Syndromes, 57
Synergism, 367
System status management (SSM), 265
Systemic effects, 367

T

Tachyarrhythmias, 126–127
Tactical emergency medical service (TEMS), 379
Tactical EMS, 388
Tactical patient care, 387–388
Terminally ill patients, 228
Tetralogy of Fallot, 58
Thermoregulatory system, elderly patients, 170
Threshold limit value/ceiling level (TLV-CL), 365
Threshold limit value/short-term exposure limit (TLV/STEL), 365
Threshold limit value/time weighted average (TLV/TWA), 365
Thyroid disorders, 182
Thyrotoxicosis, 75
Tinnitus, 165
Tired response system, ambulance, 265
Tocolysis, 35
Toddlers, 84–85. *See also* Pediatrics
Tonic seizures, 73
Toxicologic emergencies, elderly patients, 187–191
Toxicologic terms, 365
Tracheostomy
common complications, 247
defined, 247
home care, 246–248
management of, 247–248
routine care, 247
tubes, 143–144
Transient hypertension, 33
Transient ischemic attack (TIA), 163, 178–179
Transport. *See also* Air medical transport; Ambulances
crime scenes and, 381
elderly patients, 194
field decontamination, 371–372
hazmat incidents, 358–359
home care and, 242
multiple-casualty incidents (MCIs), 315
neonates, 70
pediatric patients, 95, 113–116
rescue patients, 332–333
Transportation unit supervisor, 315
Transposition of the great vessels, 58
Trauma
agricultural emergencies, 400–402
gynecologic, 13–15
pregnancy, 28–29
Trauma (elderly)
assessment, 193–194
burns, 195
cardiovascular considerations, 194
contributing factors, 193
head and spinal injuries, 195–196
management of, 194
observing abuse/neglect, 193–194
orthopedic injuries, 195
renal considerations, 194
respiratory considerations, 194
specific injuries, 195–196
transport considerations, 194
Traumatic brain injury, 138
Treatment group supervisor, 313
Treatment unit leader, 314
Treatment units, 313–314
Triage
defined, 306
JumpSTART system, 309–311
METTAG, 311, 313
need for speed, 311–313
primary, 306–307
SALT system, 308–309, 310
secondary, 307
START system, 307–308
tags, 310, 311
Triage group supervisor, 306
Triage officer, 300
Turgor, 237
Two-pillow orthopnea, 176
Two-step field decontamination, 371–372

U

Umbilical cord
clamping and cutting, 40, 63
defined, 20
delayed cord clamping (DCC), 63
prolapsed, 42–43
UN number, 360
Unified command, 300–301
Upper GI bleed, 182
Urinary disorders, elderly patients, 186
Urinary system, pregnancy and, 22
Urinary tract devices, 252–253
Urosepsis, 186
Urostomy, 252
Uterine atony, 46
Uterine inversion, 47
Uterine rupture, 46–47
Uterine tubes. *See* Fallopian tubes
Uterus, 5–6

V

Vagal stimulation, 75
Vagina
defined, 4–5
dressings and, 10
Vaginal birth after Caesarean, 37–38
Vaginal bleeding, 27
Valsalva maneuver, 177
Vapor density, 365
Vapor pressure, 365
Varicosities, 177

Vascular access devices (VADs)
anticoagulant therapy, 251
complications, 251
defined, 250
types of, 250–251
Vascular access, pediatric patients, 111
Vasodepressor syncope, 177
Vasovagal syncope, 177
Vehicle rescues. *See also* Rescue
auto anatomy and, 344–345
circles of operation, 345
control hazards, 345
doors and, 345
downed lines and, 343
fire and fuel, 343
firewall and engine compartment and, 344
glass and, 345
highway operations and, 342–344
hybrid vehicles, 345
rolling and unstable vehicles, 344
scene size-up, 345
skills practice, 346
SRS airbags, 343
stabilization equipment, 347
strategies, 345–346
traffic hazards, 342–343
treatment, packaging, and removal, 346
Vehicle stabilization equipment, 347
Ventilation
BVM, 82
home care, 248–249
negative-pressure ventilators, 248
neonatal, 66–67
pediatric, 103–104
positive-pressure ventilators, 248
Ventricular fibrillation/pulseless ventricular tachycardia, 127–129
Ventricular septal defect, 57, 58
Ventricular tachycardia, 127
Vestibule, 4
Veterans Administration (VA), 158
Violent street incidents, 382–383
Visual flight rules (VFR), 280
Visual impairments. *See also* Physical challenges
etiologies, 217–218
recognizing and accommodating, 218
Vital functions, pediatric assessment, 91–94
Vital signs, pediatric patients, 97–99
Voice production disorders, 219
Vomiting, 75
Vulva, 3

W

Warm zone, 364
Warning placard, 358
Water rescues. *See also* Rescue
basic rescue techniques, 334
flat water, 337–339
general background, 333–334
heat escape lessening position (HELP), 334
moving water, 334–337
overview, 333
spinal injuries and, 339
water temperature, 333
Water solubility, 365
Weapons of mass destruction (WMD), 359
Weights and pound-kilogram conversion, 98
Wrap points, 402

Y

Yellow treatment unit, 314